*S Lakshmi Narayan's*

# Textbook of THERAPEUTIC EXERCISES

# *S Lakshmi Narayan's*
# Textbook of THERAPEUTIC EXERCISES

**Second Edition**

*Revised by*

**Basanta Kumar Nanda** BPT (Hons) MPT
Lecturer (Physiotherapy)
Swami Vivekanand National Institute of Rehabilitation Training and Research
Olatpur, Cuttack, Odisha, India

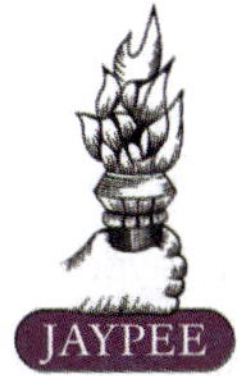


**JAYPEE BROTHERS MEDICAL PUBLISHERS**
*The Health Sciences Publisher*
New Delhi | London

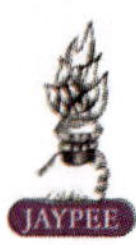

**Jaypee Brothers Medical Publishers (P) Ltd**

**Headquarters**
EMCA House, 23/23-B
Ansari Road, Daryaganj
New Delhi 110 002, India
Landline: +91-11-23272143,
+91-11-23272703+91-11-23282021,
+91-11-23245672
e-mail: jaypee@jaypeebrothers.com

**Corporate Office**
4838/24, Ansari Road, Daryaganj
New Delhi 110 002, India
Phone: +91-11-43574357
Fax: +91-11-43574314
e-mail: jaypee@jaypeebrothers.com

**Overseas Office**
JP Medical Ltd.
83, Victoria Street, London
SW1H 0HW (UK)
Phone: +44-20 3170 8910
e-mail: info@jpmedpub.com

**EU GPSR** Authorised Representative
Logos Europe, 9 rue Nicolas Poussin
17000, La Rochelle, France
Phone: +33 (0) 6 67 93 73 78
e-mail: contact@logoseurope.eu

Website: www.jaypeebrothers.com

Website: www.jaypeedigital.com



**Inquiries for bulk sales may be solicited at:** jaypee@jaypeebrothers.com

***S Lakshmi Narayan's Textbook of Therapeutic Exercises***

Second Edition: 2024

Reprint: **2026**

ISBN: 978-93-5696-661-1

Printed at Nutech Print Services Pvt. Ltd.

# Preface

The *Textbook of Therapeutic Exercises,* written by S Lakshmi Narayan, was a wonderful gift to the students of physiotherapy by the editor. To update the book with the latest information and to provide a few additional chapters with complete information on Exercise Therapy and Massage, the book has further been edited by me. By reading the book, a student will assimilate knowledge on basic principles and applications of Exercises, Massage, Joint Mobilization and Manipulation, Gait, Traction, Walking Aids, Hydrotherapy, etc. The chapter on Assessment of Patients has been updated with self-explanatory pictures. A total of 250 Multiple Choice Questions (MCQs) and Answers have been added as a separate chapter to fulfil the needs of the students.

I hope this current edition of the book will enhance the knowledge fund of the students of physiotherapy.

**Basanta Kumar Nanda**

# Acknowledgments

I sincerely acknowledge the students across the country and my colleagues for their inspiration to work on more and more books in the field of physiotherapy.

*Special acknowledgments to our publishers:*
My gratitude to Shri Jitendar P Vij (Group Chairman), Mr Ankit Vij (Managing Director), Mr MS Mani (Group President), Dr Madhu Choudhary (Director–Educational Publishing), Ms Pooja Bhandari [Director–Production (Books and Journals)], Ms Sunita Katla (EA to Group Chairman and Publishing Manager), Mr Ajay Kumar Sharma [DGM (Books and Journals)], Mr Sabyasachi Hazra [Associate Director (Publishing) and Team Lead (Diginerve, East)], and Ms Samina Khan (EA to Director–Educational Publishing).

I would also like to thank Dr Upma Tomar (Development Editor) and her entire team who brought the book to its present shape.

Thanks are due to Mr Rajesh Sharma (Production Coordinator), Ms Seema Dogra (Cover Visualizer), Mr Laxmidhar Padhiary (Quality Controller), Mr Kulwant Singh (Typesetter), Ms Neha Verma (Cover Designer), and Mr Sanjeev Kumar (Graphic Designer), for speedy completion of this mega task.

# Contents

# 1 CHAPTER Exercise Therapy

## INTRODUCTION

Exercise therapy is an important element of physical medicine. Physical medicine (physical medicine and rehabilitation) is a branch of medicine, that aims to enhance and restore functional ability and quality of life of people with impairments of various systems of the body or with disabilities. Physiotherapists, occupational therapists, speech therapists, use this as a method of treatment to remediate neuromuscular, musculoskeletal, cardiorespiratory and cognitive perceptual impairments. It can be defined as follows:

**Exercise therapy** is the systematic, planned performance of bodily movements, postures and activities, intended to provide a patient/client to optimize the overall health status, fitness or sense of well-being by preventing/remediating impairments, improving/restoring physical function, preventing/reducing health related risk factors, etc.

It is an essential tool used by therapists to treat patients/clients with neuromuscular, musculoskeletal, cardiopulmonary, disorders with the objectives of:

- Improvement/maintenance of joint range of motion.
- Improvement/maintenance of muscle bulk, strength and endurance.
- Decreasing pain of neuro-musculoskeletal origin.
- Improvement of respiratory function/lung capacities.
- Improvement of cardiovascular function.
- Improvement/maintenance of aerobic capacity/fitness.
- Improvement of overall function.

The exercise programs are designed by a qualified therapist to meet the unique need of the client. A patient/client who reports the therapist (physiotherapist/occupational therapist/speech therapist) with a functional impairment causing activity and participation limitation is evaluated by the therapist using the International Classification of Function (ICF) model **(Fig. 1.1)** and appropriate exercises are designed to remediate impairment, promote activity, restore participation in society and community.

However, a therapist/clinician should have adequate knowledge of muscles, joints, nervous system, to establish impairments and activity/participation limitations, and design/prescribe exercises to overcome such impairments and gain function.

### Muscles and its Types

There are three types of muscles found in the body, responsible for different functions. They are:

1. **Skeletal muscles:** These muscles, called as striated voluntary muscles are attached to bones, enabling production of voluntary movements.
2. **Cardiac muscles:** These muscles, called striated involuntary are found in heart, which help for pumping of blood.

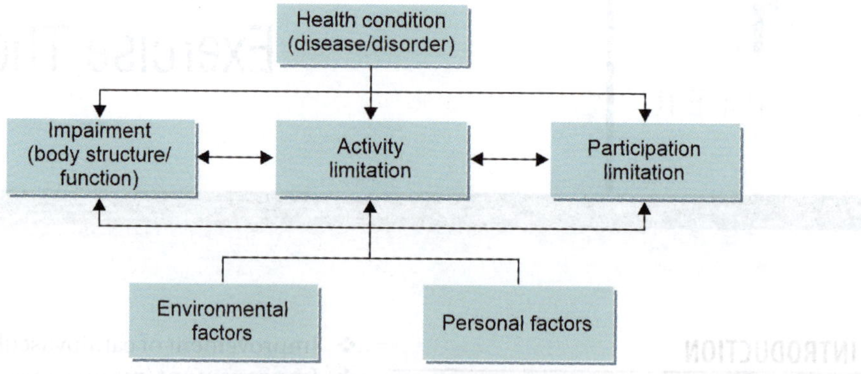


**Fig. 1.1:** The ICF model.

3. **Smooth muscles:** These muscles are found in the walls of hollow internal organs, such as blood vessels, gastrointestinal tract, bladder, uterus, etc., and are controlled by the autonomic nervous system.

The skeletal muscle fibers and their types are briefly discussed below:

### *Types of Skeletal Muscle Fibers*

These skeletal muscles in human body which are striated and voluntary are responsible for the activities or movements around a particular joint. They do not have the same structure and function and are made of three types of fibers, which are selectively recruited by the body depending on the types of activities the person performs.

The three main types of muscle fibers are:

1. Type I (slow-twitch)
2. Type IIa (fast-twitch oxidative)
3. Type IIb/Type IIx (fast-twitch glycolytic)

**Table 1.1** shows the muscle fiber types and their characteristics.

The different types of muscle fibers are briefly discussed below:

**Type I fibers (slow-twitch—fatigue resistant—red colored—oxidative muscle fibers)**

These slow oxidative (SO) fibers contract relatively slowly, and use aerobic respiration (oxygen and glucose) to produce ATP. These fibers can function for long periods without fatiguing, which makes them useful in maintaining posture, producing isometric contractions, stabilizing bones and joints, and activities requiring endurance/low intensity energy for longer period.

These fibers possess slower twitch speeds, produce less force and contain more number of the mitochondria, myoglobin and the blood capillaries. Because of the more number of myoglobin and blood vessels, the muscle fibers are red in color. These muscle fibers are of small diameter and are fatigue-resistant. They are recruited when performing activities for hours like long distance running and holding upright postures for longer duration. Triglycerides are the major storage fuel used, and they consume the produced lactic acid.

*Example:* Postural muscles like neck and trunk muscles.

**Type IIa fibers (fast-twitch oxidative—pink colored—fatigue resistant muscle fibers)**

Type-IIa fibers are sometimes called intermediate fibers because they possess characteristics that are intermediate between fast glycolytic fibers and slow oxidative fibers. They produce more force than type-I, and less force than type-IIb fibers. They possess high amount of mitochondria and do not possess significant myoglobin, and are lighter in color as compared to red slow oxidative fibers. They produce ATP relatively quickly through aerobic metabolism, more quickly than slow

**Table 1.1:** Types of muscle fibers.

| *Characteristic* | *Type I (slow twitch/slow oxidative)* | *Type IIa (fast twitch/fast oxidative)* | *Type IIb/Type-IIx (fast glycolytic)* |
|---|---|---|---|
| Activities | Maintenance of posture | Walking/running/ jogging | Weight lifting/gymnastic activities |
| Contraction speed | Slow | Fast | Very fast |
| Force produced | Low | High | Very high |
| Fiber size (diameter) | Smallest | Large | Largest |
| Color | Red | Pink | White |
| Fatigue resistance | High | Medium | Low |
| Motor neuron size | Small | Large | Very large |
| Oxidative capacity | High | Medium | Low |
| Mitochondrial density | High | Medium | Low |
| Capillary density | High | Medium | Low |
| Myoglobin | High | Medium | Low |
| ATPase level | Low | Medium | High |
| Metabolic type | Primarily aerobic/ oxidative | Primarily aerobic/ oxidative | Primarily anaerobic/ glycolytic |
| ATP production/ predominant energy system | Aerobic mechanism | Aerobic and anaerobic mechanism | Anaerobic mechanism |

fibers, and thus can produce relatively high amounts of tension through fast contractions without fatiguing quickly. These fibers are used primarily for movements, such as walking/ running, that require more energy than postural control but less energy than an explosive movement, such as sprinting.

*Example:* Leg muscles, which are responsible for walking and running.

### Type IIb/type IIx fibers (fast glycolytic—fast-twitch—early fatigable—white muscle fibers)

These muscle fibers are larger in diameter, possess high amount of glycogen and primarily use anaerobic glycolysis as their ATP source. These are the largest muscle fibers in human body. They do not possess substantial numbers of mitochondria, blood capillaries and significant amounts of myoglobin and/ therefore have a white color. These fibers are used to produce rapid, forceful contractions to make quick, powerful movements, and fatigue quickly. These muscle fibers are responsible for explosive movements like jumping/weight lifting.

*Example:* The muscles responsible for rapid movements such as shoulder flexors and abductors.

*Examples showing fiber recruitments:* The gymnastic people, who are performing the rapid movements and exercise will be having the more proportionate of the white fibers (type-IIx/type-IIb). The runners will be having more proportionate of the pink fibers (type IIa). The normal people like housewives, office clerks will be having more of red fibers (type I).

## *Shapes of Skeletal Muscles*

The different skeletal muscle shapes in the human body are parallel, oblique, circular, as per arrangement of fasciculi **(Figs. 1.2A to H)**, which are briefly discussed below:

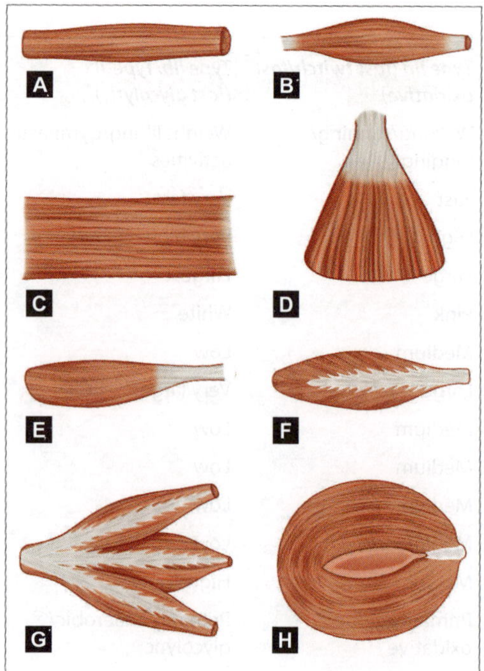


**Figs. 1.2A to H:** Shows shapes of different skeletal muscles: (A) Strap; (B) Fusiform; (C) Rhomboid; (D) Triangular; (E) Unipinnate; (F) Bipinnate; (G) Multipinnate; (H) Circular.

### Parallel Muscles

Parallel muscles have fibers that, as the name suggests, run parallel to each other. They are normally long muscles which cause large movements, and are not very strong but have good endurance. These muscles are again divided into four varieties. They are:

1. **Strap muscles:** In this muscle, fasciculi are parallel with each other and run the total length of the muscles and ends in flat tendon.
   *Example:* Sternocleidomastoid, sartorius.
2. **Fusiform muscles:** These are spindle-shaped muscles, with the muscle belly wider, than the origin and insertion.
   *Example:* Biceps brachii, brachioradialis.
3. **Rhomboidal muscles:** These muscles are of rhomboid shape or quadrangular in shape, having the broad attachments with the broad flat tendon.
   *Example:* Rhomboidus major, pronator quadratus.
4. **Triangular muscles:** The muscle fasciculi spread and ends with the flat and small tendon, giving the triangular or fan-shape.
   *Example:* Pectoralis major, temporalis.

### Oblique/Pennate Muscle Fibers

Oblique/pennate muscles have a large number of muscle fibers per unit and so are very strong, but tire easily. In this variety the fasciculi are short and the tendon runs maximum length of the muscle.

They are of three types such as:

1. **Unipinnate muscles:** These muscles have their fibers arranged to insert in a diagonal direction onto the tendon on one side, which allows great strength.
   *Example:* Tibialis anterior, lumbricals, extensor digitorum communis.
2. **Bipinnate muscles:** These muscles have two rows of muscle fibers, facing in opposite diagonal directions, with a central tendon, like a feather. This produces greater power/force, but through a lesser range of motion.
   *Example:* Intraosseous muscles of the hand, rectus femoris.
3. **Multipinnate muscles:** These muscles have multiple rows of diagonal fibers, with a central tendon that branches into two or more tendons.
   *Example:* Deltoid muscle.

### Circular Muscle Fibers

These muscles appear circular in shape, as the fasciculi are arranged in a circular manner, and help to close an orifice.

*Example:* Orbicularis oris, external anal sphincter.

## Anatomical Movements

### *Flexion (Fig. 1.3)*

The movement in the sagittal plane, where the angle between two segments of the body

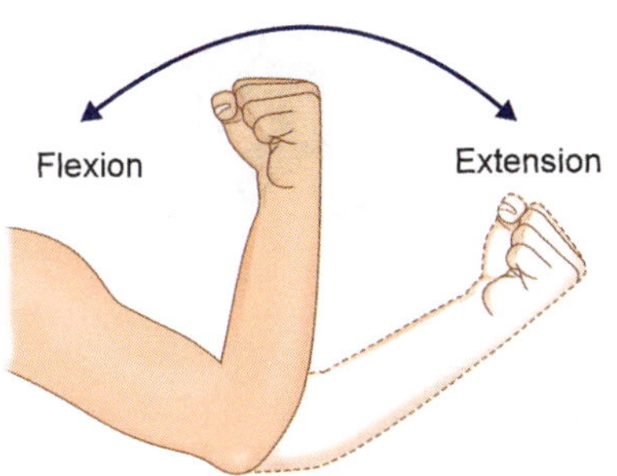


**Fig. 1.3:** Shows flexion/extension of elbow.

decreases. It is the act of bending forward. For example, in flexion of the elbow, the angle between the humerus and ulna decreases.

### *Extension (Fig. 1.3)*

This is the movement in the sagittal plane, where the angle between two body segments increases. It is the act of bending backwards. For example, in elbow extension from flexion, the angle between humerus and ulna increases.

### *Abduction (Fig. 1.4)*

This is the movement in coronal plane, where the segments of the body moves away from the midline of the body/body segment. For example, in shoulder abduction, the arm moves away to the sides, from the midlines of the body. In abduction of the index finger, by the 1st dorsal interosseous muscle, the index finger moves away from the midline of the hand, that passes through the middle finger. In great toe abduction by abductor hallucis, the great toe moves away from the 2nd toe (midline of foot).

### *Adduction (Fig. 1.4)*

This is the movement in coronal plane, where the segment of the body, moves towards the midline of the body/body segment. For example, in hip adduction, the thigh moves towards the opposite thigh/midline of the body.

### *Medial Rotation/Internal Rotation (Fig. 1.5)*

This is the movement in the transverse plane, where, the body segment moves inwards towards the midline of the body. For example, in shoulder medial rotation, the arm rotates inwards towards the midline of the body.

### *Lateral Rotation/External Rotation (Fig. 1.5)*

This is the movement in the transverse plane, where, the body segment moves outwards away from the midline of the body. For

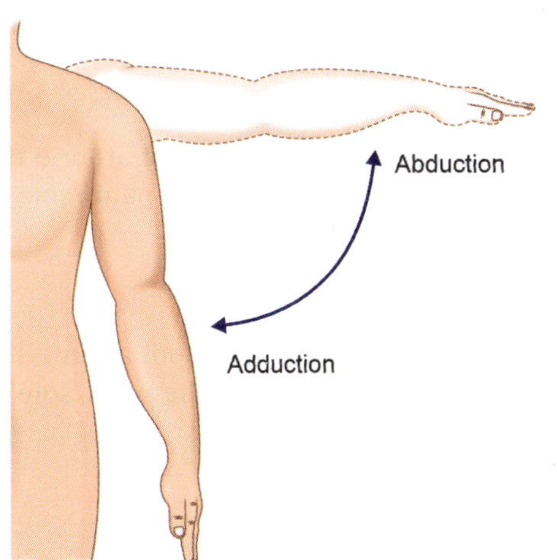


**Fig. 1.4:** Shows abduction and adduction of shoulder.

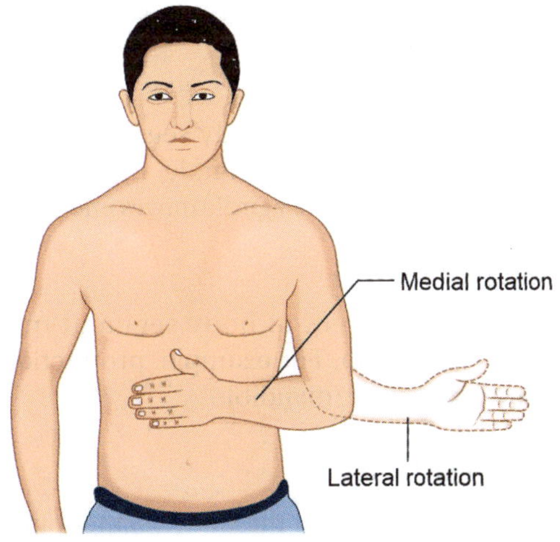


**Fig. 1.5:** Shows medial and lateral rotation of shoulder.

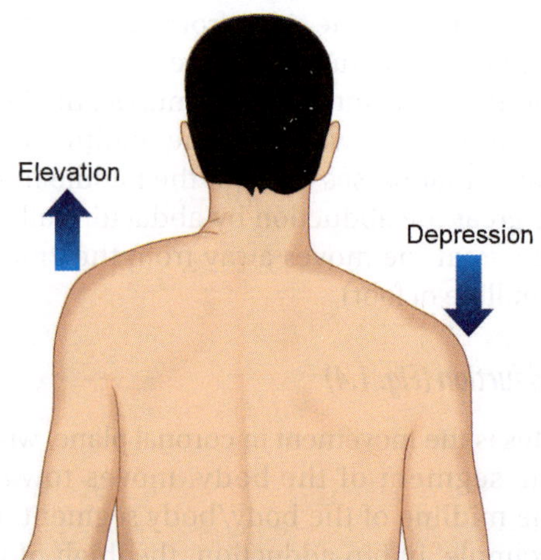


**Fig. 1.6:** Shows elevation/depression of shoulder girdle.

example, in shoulder lateral rotation, the arm rotates outwards away from the midline of the body.

### *Circumduction*

It is a circular/conical movement of a limb, which is the combination of flexion, extension, abduction, adduction, medial rotation, lateral rotation.

### *Elevation (Fig. 1.6)*

It is the movement of the body segment in a superior direction. For example, in shoulder shrug, the shoulder girdle moves superiorly.

### *Depression (Fig. 1.6)*

It is movement of the body segment in an inferior direction. For example, in shoulder depression, the shoulder girdle moves inferiorly.

### *Protraction (Fig. 1.7)*

It is the movement of body segment in a forward direction. For example, protraction of shoulder girdle/mandible.

### *Retraction (Fig. 1.7)*

It is the movement of the body segment in a backward direction. For example, retraction of shoulder girdle/mandible.

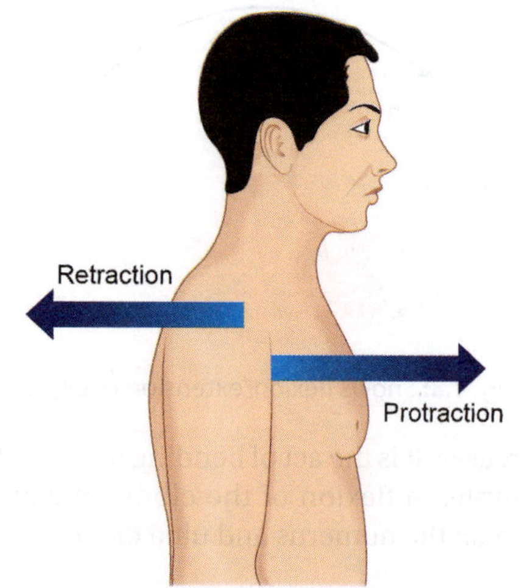


**Fig. 1.7:** Shows protraction/retraction of scapula.

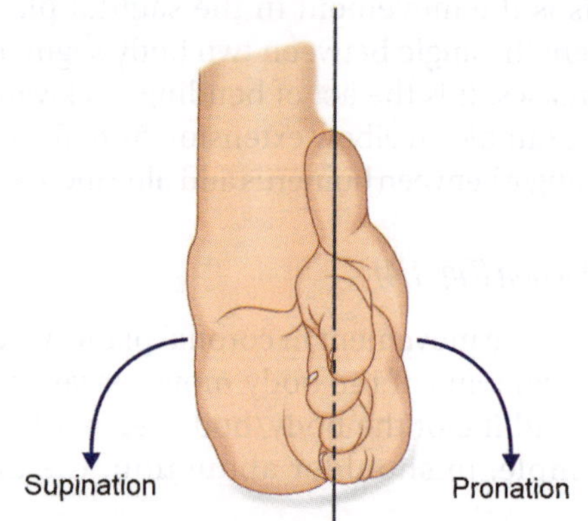


**Fig. 1.8:** Shows supination/pronation of forearm.

### *Supination (Fig. 1.8)*

It is the rotation of forearm/foot around the segment's long axis, where the palm/sole of foot faces upwards.

### *Pronation (Fig. 1.8)*

It is the rotation of forearm/foot around the segment's long axis, where the palm/sole of foot faces downwards.

### *Dorsiflexion (Fig. 1.9)*

It refers to flexion at the ankle, so that the foot moves superiorly, causing a reduction of leg-foot angle.

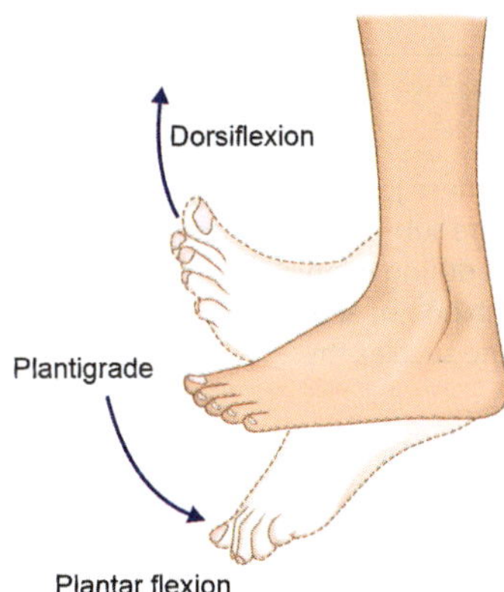


**Fig. 1.9:** Shows ankle dorsiflexion/plantar flexion.

### *Plantar Flexion (Fig. 1.9)*

It refers to extension at the ankle, so that, the foot moves inferiorly, causing an increase of leg-foot angle.

### *Inversion (Fig. 1.10)*

It is the rotation of foot, around its axis, causing movement of the sole towards the median plane, so that, the sole of the foot faces in a medial direction.

### *Eversion (Fig. 1.10)*

It is the rotation of foot, around its axis, causing movement of the sole away from the median plane, so that, the sole of the foot faces in a lateral direction.

- **Opposition of thumb (Fig. 1.11):** This is the movement, where, the thumb moves towards the little finger. This is the combination of CMC flexion, palmar abduction and medial rotation (pronation).
- Reposition is a movement that moves the thumb and the little finger away from each other, effectively reversing opposition.

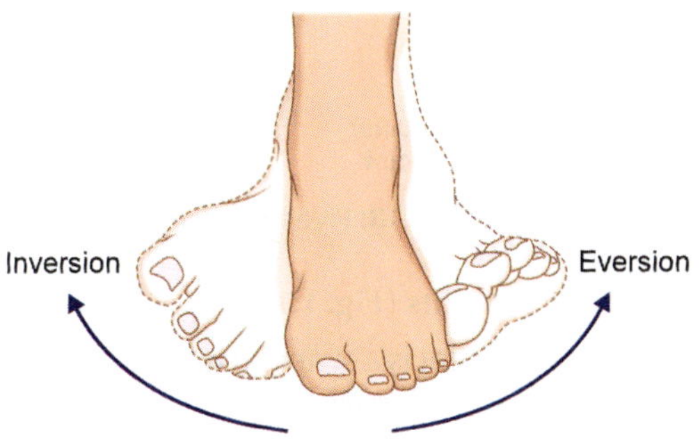


**Fig. 1.10:** Shows foot inversion/eversion.

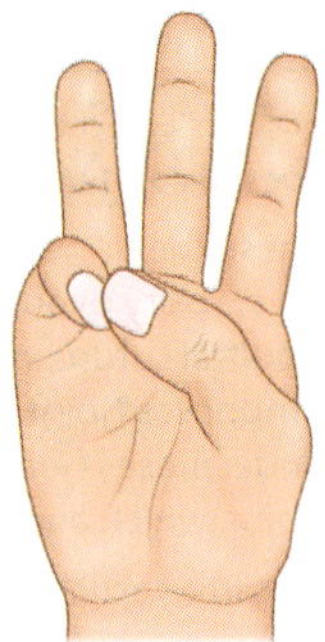

**Fig. 1.11:** Shows thumb opposition.

## Joints of Human Body

A joint is the structure, where two or more bones are connected by connective tissues to allow very little to significant movements for growth of the body and to perform function.

### *Classification of Joint*

Joints can be classified by the types of tissues present in the articulation (fibrous, cartilaginous, or synovial), or by the degrees of movements permitted (synarthrosis, amphiarthrosis or diarthrosis), which are briefly discussed in **Table 1.2**.

#### Hinged Joints (Fig. 1.12)

These joints produce movement in one plane, such as flexion/extension occurring in sagittal plane around the coronal axis, e.g., elbow joint, knee joint (called as modified hinged joint, as the axis of rotation changes during movement).

#### Pivot Joints (Fig. 1.13)

A pivot joint is a type of synovial joint that allows rotation around a single axis, e.g., atlantoaxial joint, proximal and distal radioulnar joint.

**Table 1.2:** Shows classification of joints in human body.

| *Classification by types of connecting tissues* | *Classification by degrees of movements* |
|---|---|
| **Fibrous joints**: In these the bones are connected by fibrous tissues. These joints exhibit strength and stability over range of movement. These joints are sub-classified into: Sutures (e.g., sagittal suture in skull, that allows little movement during infancy and childhood), gomphoses (joints between the teeth and jaw, which do not allow any movement), syndesmoses (joints held by interosseous membrane such as the middle radioulnar joint, which allows little movement). | Synarthrosis—immovable |
| **Cartilaginous joints:** In a cartilaginous joint**,** the bones are united by fibrocartilage or hyaline cartilage.<br>There are two main types: Synchondroses (primary cartilaginous) and symphyses (secondary cartilaginous). The joint between the diaphysis and epiphysis of a growing long bone, is the primary cartilaginous type, whereas the joints in the midline of the body, such as intervertebral joints, symphysis pubis, etc., are the examples of secondary cartilaginous joints. | Amphiarthrosis—slightly movable |
| **Synovial joints:** In these joints, the articulating surfaces are enclosed within a fluid-filled joint capsule lined by synovial membrane. These joints are freely movable and are the most common types of joints found in the human body. These joints are of different types which are briefly discussed separately below:<br>• Hinged joint<br>• Pivot joint<br>• Condyloid type joint<br>• Saddle type joint<br>• Plain type joint<br>• Ball and socket type joint | Diarthrosis—freely movable |

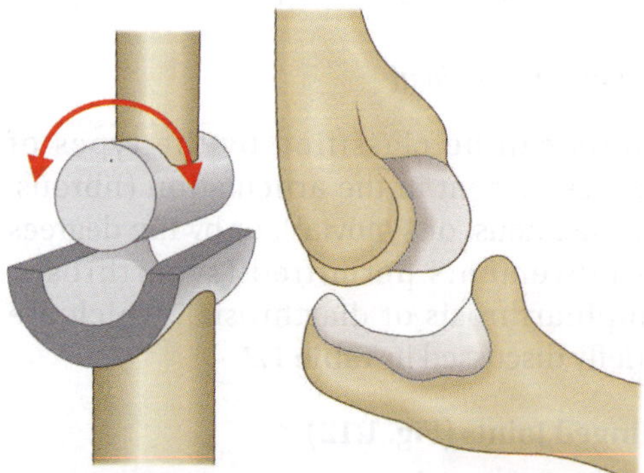
**Fig. 1.12:** Hinged joint (elbow).

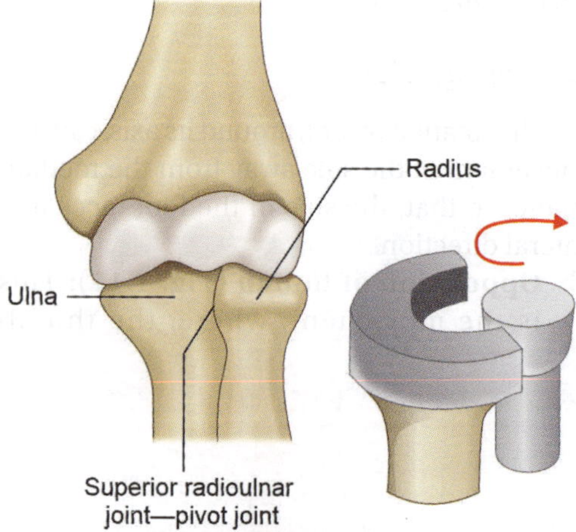

**Fig. 1.13:** Pivot joint.

## Condyloid Joints (Fig. 1.14)

A condyloid joint is a type of synovial joint, where an oval-shaped bone (convex surface) fits into an elliptical cavity (concave surface) of another bone, e.g., wrist joint, metacarpophalangeal joint, metatarsophalangeal joint.

## Saddle Type Joints (Fig. 1.15)

A saddle type joint is a synovial joint, in which, the opposing joint surfaces are reciprocally concave and convex. It is named saddle, as it

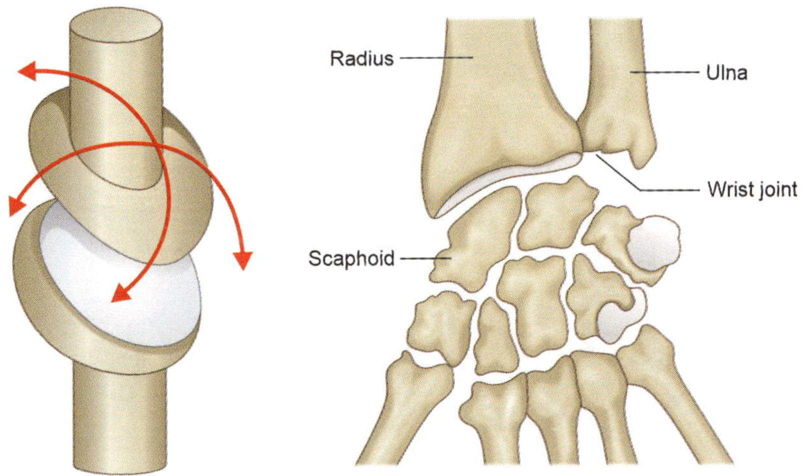


**Fig. 1.14:** Condyloid joint (wrist).

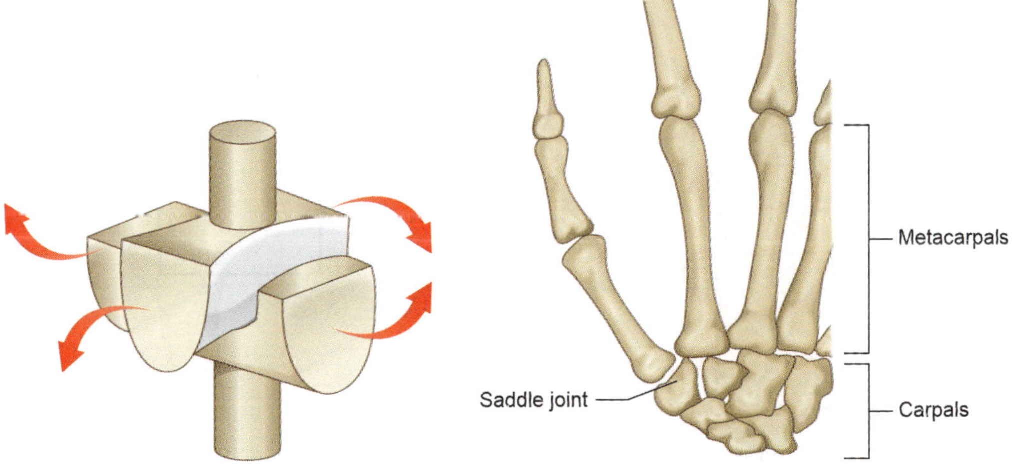


**Fig. 1.15:** Saddle joint (carpometacarpal joint of thumb).

resembles like the saddle on the horse's back, e.g., carpometacarpal joint of thumb.

### Plain Type Joints (Fig. 1.16)

The articular surfaces are relatively flat, allowing the bones to glide over one another, e.g., acromioclavicular joint, subtalar joint.

### Ball and Socket Type of Joint (Figs. 1.17A and B)

The ball-and-socket joint (or spheroid joint) is a type of synovial joint in which the ball-shaped surface of one rounded bone fits into the cup-like depression of another bone. The distal bone is capable of motion around a number of axes, which have one common center. This enables the joint to move in many directions, e.g., hip joint, shoulder joint.

## Range of Motion

Movement of the joints can be performed by the internal or external forces. The internal force can be produced by the muscles and

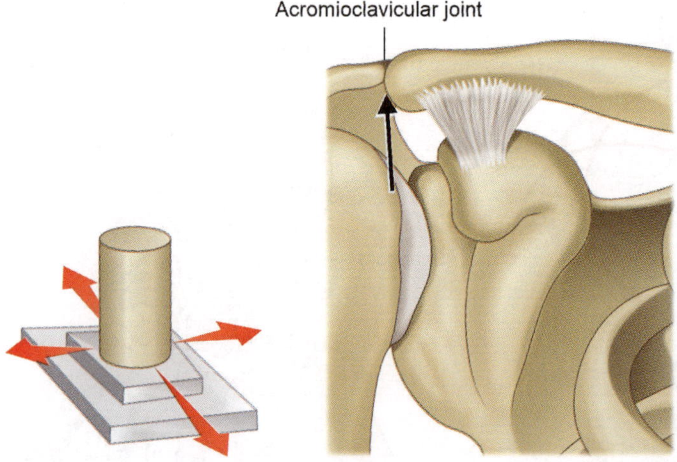


**Fig. 1.16:** Plane type of joint (acromioclavicular joint).

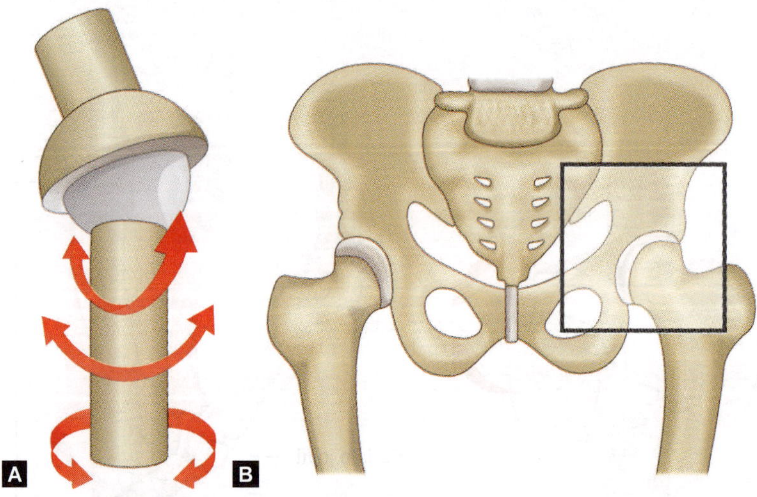


**Figs. 1.17A and B:** Ball and socket type joint (hip joint).

the external force may be produced manually or mechanically. The movement of a joint results in angulations of that particular joint. The angulation of the movements are referred as the range of motion. The range of muscle (ROM) will be perfect in a joint if the soft tissues and articulating surfaces are intact. In case of trauma/arthritis, if any change in length (shortening) occurs in soft tissues and if the joint space is reduced due to erosion/arthritis, it results in disturbance or alteration of the range of motion. Generally, in the hypomobile joint the ROM will be less than the normal prescribed ROM of that particular joint. In hypermobile joint it is *vise versa*. This ROM can be measured with the help of goniometer or inch tape (most commonly used for spine).

Ranges of motion measured in joint pathologies could be: (i) Active ROM, and (ii) Passive ROM.

### Active ROM

The ROM, which is achieved by the own effort of the individual, without any external force is called as active ROM. Generally, the active ROM, will be less in the hypomobile joint, as compared to the passive ROM.

### *Passive ROM*

The ROM which is achieved with the help of the external force is called as passive ROM. Normally, by the passive ROM we can achieve greater ROM than active ROM. In hypomobile joint, usually the passive ROM will be more than the active ROM because the tightened structures will be stretched by the passive force which cannot be achieved actively.

The ROM may be varying from each and every joint and each and every individual depending on the variety, size, and bony prominences. The same joint ROM may be differing from an individual to individual due to variation in muscle bulk and the bony prominence.

The prescribed ROM for joints of human body are shown in **Table 1.3**.

**Table 1.3:** ROM of joints of human body.

| | |
|---|---|
| • **Shoulder** | |
| Flexion | 0–180° (150–180°) |
| Extension | 0–45° (40–60°) |
| Abduction | 0–180° (150–180°) |
| Adduction | 0° |
| Internal rotation | 0–90° (70–90°) |
| External rotation | 0–90° (70–90°) |
| • **Elbow** | |
| Flexion | 0–135° (120–150°) |
| Extension | 0° |
| • **Forearm** | |
| Supination | 0–90° |
| Pronation | 0–90° |
| • **Wrist** | |
| Flexion | 0–90° (70–90°) |
| Extension | 0–70° (50–70°) |

*Contd...*

*Contd...*

| | |
|---|---|
| Ulnar deviation | 0–40° (25–40°) |
| Radial deviation | 0–20° (15–25°) |
| • **MCP (fingers)** | |
| Flexion | 0–90° |
| Extension | 0–10°–30° (nearly 10° in index finger and 30° in little finger) |
| Abduction | 0–20° |
| Adduction | 0° |
| • **PIP (fingers)** | |
| Flexion | 0–110° (90–120°) |
| Extension | 0° |
| • **DIP (fingers)** | |
| Flexion | 0–70° to 80° [digit 3 has highest range of flexion (80°), and digit 5 has lowest range of flexion (70°)] |
| Extension | 0° |
| • **Thumb** | |
| MCP flexion | 0–45° |
| IP flexion | 0–80° to 90° |
| IP extension | 0–10° (hyperextension in IP joint occurs in forceful movements of thumb) |
| • **HIP** | |
| Flexion | 0–120° (110–130°)—with knees flexed<br>0–90° to 100°—with knee extended |
| Extension | 0–30° (25–40°) |
| Abduction | 0–45° (45–55°) |
| Adduction | 0–20° |
| External rotation | 0–50° (45–50°) |
| Internal rotation | 0–40° (30–45°) |
| • **Knee** | |
| Flexion | 0–120° to 150° |
| Extension | 0° |
| • **Ankle** | |
| Plantar flexion | 0–45° to 50° |
| Dorsi flexion | 0–20° |
| Inversion | 0–40° to 45° |
| Eversion | 0–15° to 20° |

*Contd...*

*Contd...*

| | |
|---|---|
| • **MTP joint** | |
| Flexion | 0–30° to 45°—1st MTP<br>0–40°—2nd to 5th MTP |
| Extension | 0–35° to 40° (it may be as high as 70°)—1st MTP<br>0–40°—2nd to 5th MTP |
| Abduction | 0–15° |
| • **Interphalangeal joint—1st toe** | |
| Flexion | 0–90° |
| Extension | 0° |
| • **Proximal interphalangeal joint—2nd to 5th toes** | |
| Flexion | 0–35° |
| Extension | 0° |
| • **Distal interphalangeal joint—2nd to 5th toes** | |
| Flexion | 0–60° |
| Extension | 0–30° |

## *Ranges of Muscle Work (Figs. 1.18A and B)*

Range of muscle work means the degree of the movement done by the muscle contraction. As a muscle contracts, it undergoes shortening (concentric contractions) or lengthening (eccentric contractions). The amount of shortening or lengthening of muscle during contraction is about 50% of muscle's maximum length.

A muscle while produces movement, changes its position from full stretch to contracting to a position of maximal shortening. There are four types of ranges of muscle work.

### Full Range

Full range in which a muscle works, refers to the muscle changing from a position of full stretch, and contracting to a position of maximal shortening. The muscle moves the joint from the full stretched position to full contracted position (concentrically) or from full contracted position to full stretched position (eccentrically). The full range of movement rarely required in normal day-to-day activities. Full range exercises are required to be performed by the patients to maintain the full ROM of the joints.

### Outer Range

It refers to the muscle contracting from a position of full stretch, to a position half way through the full range of motion. The muscles move the joint from the fully stretched position to the minimal contracted position (concentrically) or from full contracted to the medium contracted position (eccentrically). Outer range movements are very much difficult to perform.

### Middle Range

It refers to the range, between the midpoint of the outer range (muscle partially shortened/lengthened) and the midpoint of the inner range (muscles partially shortened/lengthened). Muscle moves the joints between the minimal range to the medium range. This is the range which we use more in our day-to-day life. In this range the muscle has the maximum strength. Exercise in this range increases the muscle power, strength and tone.

### Inner Range

It refers to a position, halfway through the full range to a position, where a muscle is fully shortened (concentrically) or fully lengthened (eccentrically). The muscles move the joint from the medium contracted position to the full contracted position (concentrically) or from minimum contracted position to the full stretched position (eccentrically). Extreme inner range movements are difficult to perform and it requires the more numbers of motor unit contractions.

## Muscle Action

In normal muscle function, a single muscle cannot produce the effective movement. Depending on the function of the muscles they

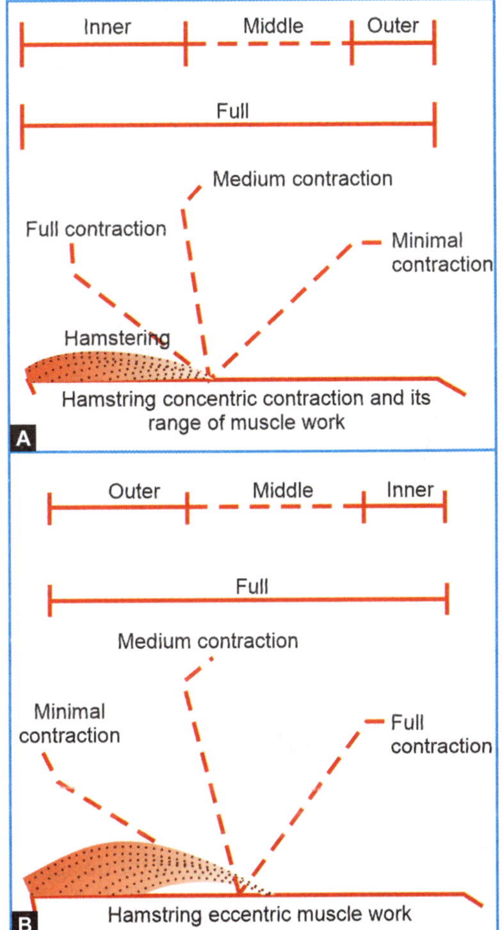


**Figs. 1.18A and B:** Hamstring concentric and eccentric muscle work at outer/middle/inner ranges.

are named as: (i) Agonists, (ii) Antagonists, (iii) Synergists, and (iv) Fixators.

### Agonists

These are chief muscles, which produce the effective movement. These groups of muscles are called as prime movers.

*Example:* For elbow flexion biceps brachii, brachioradialis and brachialis are helpful, but the brachialis has its major part in the contraction or movement. So, brachialis is called as the prime mover or agonists.

### Antagonists

These are the muscles, which act against the agonists. Their action is opposite to the action of the agonists.

*Example:* Triceps act as the antagonists to brachialis and biceps brachii while flexing the elbow. If the agonists contracts, the antagonist goes for relaxation as per Sherrington's principles of reciprocal inhibition. Same mechanism is used in the PNF techniques to reduce the spasm or the spasticity of the muscle group.

### Synergists (Syn-with)

These are the muscles, that help the agonists (prime mover) to perform function. The synergists act with the agonists, making stronger the action of agonists.

*Example:* Biceps brachii acts as synergists to brachialis for the elbow flexion.

### Fixators

Fixator muscles are those, that serve as stabilizer of one part of the body during movement of another part. It allows the agonist/synergists/antagonist muscle to work effectively by stabilizing the origin of the movement producing muscles to produce an effective contraction. A fixator muscle helps another muscle (the agonists) to move a different part of the body effectively.

*Example:* The muscles attached with the shoulder girdle to the trunk acts as the fixator for the deltoid action.

## Kinematic Chain

A kinematic chain is a series of interconnected bodies (links), that can move relative to each other. The human body, having so many segments joined together by different joints, is considered as a kinematic chain. The movement of one joint may require the motion over the proximal and distal joints, and sometimes it may not be required.

Two types of kinematic chains are present in human body.

- ❖ Closed kinematic chains
- ❖ Open kinematic chains.

### Closed Kinematic/Kinetic Chain Exercises

Closed kinematic/kinetic chain (CKC) exercises or closed chain exercises are exercises, or movements, where the distal aspect of the extremity is fixed to an object, that is stationary. With the distal part fixed, movement at any one joint in the kinetic chain requires motion as well at the other joints in the kinetic chain, therefore, both proximal and distal parts receive resistance training at the same time. Closed-chain exercises tend to offer more "functional" athletic benefits because of their ability to recruit more muscle groups.

These exercises are more functional than open kinematic/kinetic chain exercises, especially for rehabilitation of shoulder and knee. These exercises are often used to strengthen core muscles and stabilize posture. A benefit of closed kinetic chain exercises is that the movements they promote often relate better to activities of daily life, so they are considered more "functional.

*Example:* (1) Performing the sit-ups **(Fig. 1.19A)** and (2) performing the push-ups **(Fig. 1.19B)**.

In the first example the hip joint flexion and the ankle joint dorsiflexion occurs to produce the flexion over the knee to go for the sitting posture. The proximal joint (hip) is moving towards the distal (ankle) joint but the distal segment is fixed without any movement.

In the second example the shoulder extension and wrist extension produce the elbow flexion to perform the push-ups. The shoulder joint moves towards the fixed wrist.

### Open Kinematic/Kinetic Chain Exercises

A kinetic/kinematic chain is considered "open" when the part of the body moving (typically a limb) is free in space. In other words, the hand or foot are free to move and not pressing against a surface. This allows a muscle or muscle group to act in isolation. In an open kinematic chain, the segment furthest away from the body (e.g., hand/foot) is free and not fixed to any object. The movement occurs independently and not in predictable manner, with the distal joint moving and the proximal joint fixed without any motion.

*Example*

a. With the arm by the side, performing the elbow flexion and extension movement **(Fig. 1.19D).**
b. In standing posture, the leg is lifted from the ground and performing the knee flexion and extension movement **(Fig. 1.19C)**.

## Active and Passive Insufficiency

The terms active and passive insufficiencies are important concepts in exercise programs, the knowledge of which is essential for designing exercises which are less injurious and effective. Both active and passive insufficiencies are functional states that occur in multi-joint muscles only.

### Active Insufficiency

Active insufficiency occurs when a multi-joint muscle shortens over both the joints simultaneously. As the muscle shortens over the proximal joint, it becomes slack over the distal joint, so that, tension in the distal joint is lost. This usually occurs to agonist group of muscles.

*Example:* The long flexors of hand, such as flexor digitorum sublimis/profundus produce wrist flexion, MCP flexion PIP and

DIP flexion. If the above said movements are done in the same sequence, the person feels difficult in flexing the MCP of fingers after flexing the wrist, because the muscles are already shortened by wrist flexion. So, further shortening is difficult, resulting in inadequate grasp which is due to active insufficiency **(Fig. 1.20A)**. This is the reason, why, patients with wrist drop fail to make a grip, necessitating use of a short cock up splint to maintain the wrist in 20-30 degrees of extension.

A Achieving knee flexion by flexing the hip and dorsiflexing the ankle

C Isolated knee flexion

B Achieving elbow flexion by shoulder and wrist extension

D Isolated elbow flexion

**Figs. 1.19A to D:** (A and B) Closed kinematic chain; (C and D) Open kinematic chain exercises.

### *Passive Insufficiency*

Passive insufficiency occurs when a multi-joint muscle is lengthened simultaneously at both joints it crosses, resulting lack of full elongation of muscle in both the joints it crosses. If the muscle is fully elongated over the proximal joint, it will be shortened over the distal joint, thereby preventing the full range of motion at each joint it crosses. It occurs in the antagonists **(Fig. 1.20B)**.

*Example:* Extensor compartment muscles of the forearm. These muscles are responsible for wrist, MCP, PIP and DIP extension. While performing the opposite movement around these joints in a sequence, i.e., when wrist is flexed, the muscles cannot go for further more lengthening in the MCP, PIP and DIP. This phenomenon is called as passive insufficiency. Further, when the wrist is extended, the long flexors are stretched over the wrist, hence can not lengthen over the fingers, resulting in finger flexion (tenodesis effect). If the

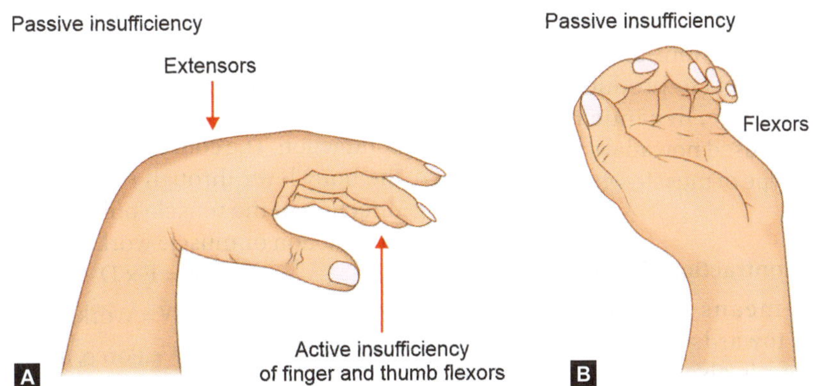


**Figs. 1.20A and B:** (A) Passive insufficiency of finger extensors, active insufficiency of finger flexors; (B) Passive insufficiency of finger flexors.

agonist muscle goes active insufficiency, the antagonist goes for the passive insufficiency.

## Types of Muscle Work

When muscles contract, force is produced and some works are done. Work is the product of force and the distance through which the force acts. The muscle works produced either help in holding a position (isometric/static muscle work), or lift a load (concentric muscle work) or lower a load (eccentric muscle work).

Muscle activity increases the intramuscular tension and changes in the muscle length. The muscle fibers are contracted and relaxed during the muscle work. We can categorize these muscle works by the change in the length and tone of the muscles into three varieties.

1. Isotonic (dynamic) contraction
2. Isometric contraction
3. Isokinetic contraction.

### *Isotonic Contraction (Muscle Work)/Dynamic Muscle Work*

Iso—equal, tonic—tone. By changing the length of the muscle, when same amount of tension is created throughout the contraction is said to be isotonic contraction.

In this type of muscle work, there is change in length of the contracting muscles producing movement. The term isotonic (maintenance of an even muscle tension/tone throughout the contraction period/movement) is not used nowadays, as muscle tone undergoes changes as muscle contracts to produce movement. In stead of isotonic, dynamic muscle work (contraction) is used nowadays to explain the event. These type of muscle works are divided into 2 types:

#### Concentric Contraction (Muscle Work)

Concentric means contraction causing movements towards the center. This type of contraction is also called as shortening contraction. The muscle isotonically shortens to produce the movement **(Fig. 1.21)**. The proximal and distal bones are drawn towards the center. Normally, one bony component is fixed and another will be moving to perform the movement. It can be movement of the distal component over the fixed proximal bony component, as in lifting the dumb-bell, or movement of the proximal component over the fixed distal component, as occurs in push-ups **(Figs. 1.22A to C)**. The concentric contractions are less tension producing contractions as compared to isometric and eccentric contractions/exercises.

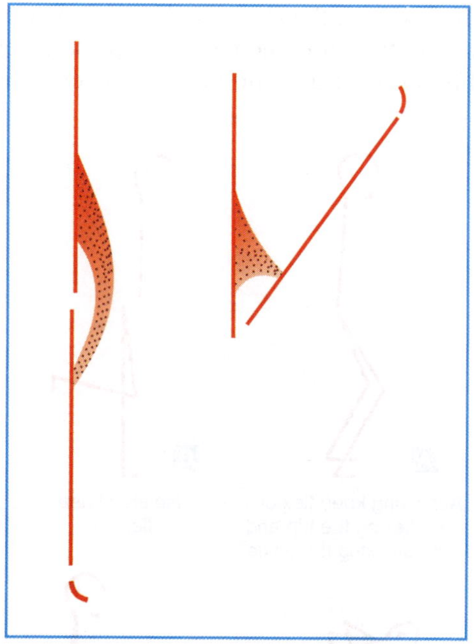

**Fig. 1.21:** Concentric contraction of elbow flexors.

Insertion of the muscle moves towards the origin or origin of the muscle moves towards the insertion during the concentric contraction. The concentric contraction moves the bony lever through some distance in the direction of the muscle pull. So that it results in an action or muscle work.

$$W = F \times D$$

| Where | W = Work, |
|---|---|
| | F = Force, and |
| | D = Distance |

Force, i.e., tension created inside the muscle, pulls the bony component to some

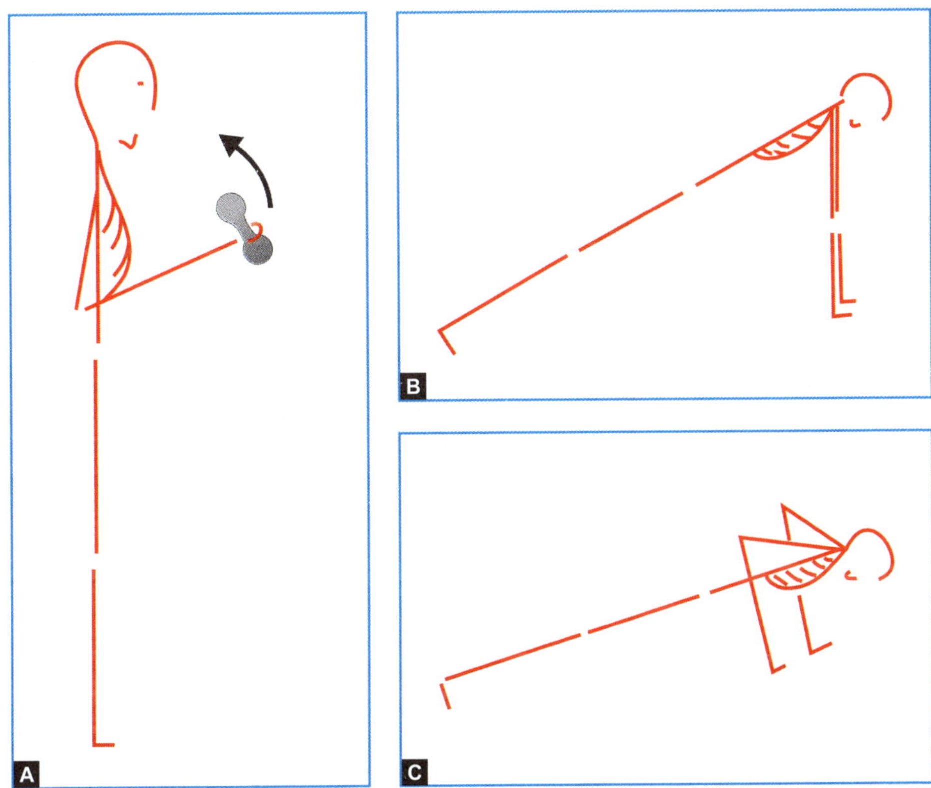

**Figs. 1.22A to C:** (A) Proximal component is fixed and the distal component is moving; (B and C) Distal component is fixed and the proximal component is moving.

distance, so that it results in movement. Concentric contractions are used to build up the muscle power and the muscle bulk and it requires more energy to perform exercises involving concentric muscle work. Normally, in the body-building exercise, the concentric exercises play a major role than the other varieties of contractions/exercises. Resisted concentric contractions are mostly useful to increase the muscle power and bulk.

### Eccentric Contraction/Exercise

Eccentric means contraction causing movements from the center **(Fig. 1.23)**. This is otherwise called as lengthening contraction. Here the proximal and distal bony components are pulled apart from the center. Eccentric contraction lengthens the muscle and the insertion of the muscle is pulled distally. The energy expenditure in this contraction is very less than the concentric contraction. However, the energy expenditure of eccentric exercises, depends on the duration of muscle contraction and the resistance applied, and in such cases the energy expenditure of eccentric exercises may exceed that of concentric exercises. The muscular tension moves the bony lever through a distance in the direction of the muscle pull.

The eccentric muscle work is said to be negative muscle work. Normally, these eccentric contractions are assisted by the gravitational force.

The contraction occurs inside the muscle even though it lengthens. For example, carrying a bucket by the hand and filling water from the tap. In this example the length of the muscle is increased and the bony components

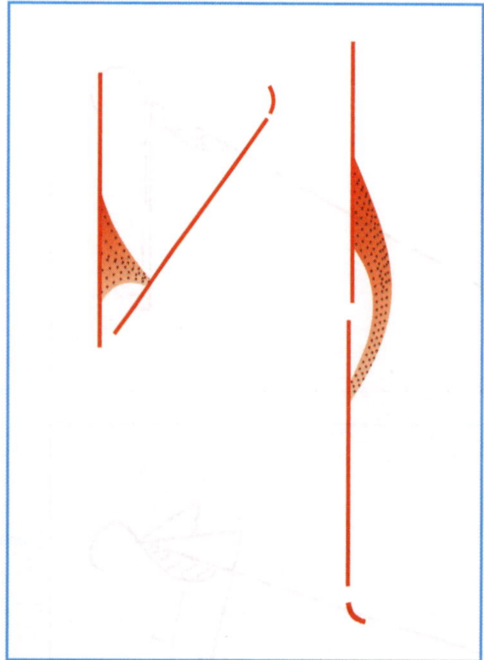

**Fig. 1.23:** Eccentric contraction of elbow flexors.

are drawn apart in the direction of the muscle pull and the tension generated inside the muscle slowly increases with the filling of the water in the bucket.

### *Isometric Contraction/Exercise*

An isometric exercise is a form of exercise involving the static contraction of a muscle without any visible movement in the angle of the joint. The term "isometric" combines the Greek words isos (equal) and -metria (measuring), meaning that in these exercises the length of the muscle and the angle of the joint do not change, though intramuscular tension is created, resulting in gain in strength.

There is no mechanical muscle work occurring in isometric contraction, because the force (F) generated, i.e., tension created is not moving the bony levers, as both the proximal and distal bones are fixed here. These types of contractions are also called as static or holding contraction. Isometric contractions produce muscle tension, which is higher than concentric and lower than eccentric. The energy expenditure by isometric contraction is usually higher than isotonic (concentric/eccentric), which depends on duration of muscle contraction and resistance applied (if any). Isometric contraction against resistance also can build up the muscle bulk and the power. This type of isometric exercise can help to improve the muscle strength. Less fatiguability is also seen in this type of contraction.

The three main types of isometric exercise are isometric presses, pulls, and holds. They may be included in a strength training regime in order to improve the body's ability to apply power from a static position or, in the case of isometric holds, improve the body's ability to maintain a position for a period of time. They can help maintain or build strength, especially in injured, arthritic, or immobilized areas of the body. They can also improve stabilization and core stability, which are important for posture, balance, and injury prevention.

However, isometric exercises have some limitations, such as not improving speed, power, or athletic performance, and not strengthening the muscles through their full range of motion. Isometric strength gain is specific to the joint angle. However, to increase the strength of muscles at different ranges of motion, multiangle isometrics are performed.

Resisted/weighted isometric exercises are performed to strengthen the muscles at specific angles using the principles of overload. The patient is asked to perform strong isometric contraction, not to move the part and the assessor/therapist will resist with almost equal amount of force to prevent any movement from occurring and also to ensure that patient exerts maximum effort.

*Example:* Isometric contraction of quadriceps/knee press **(Fig. 1.24)** is used to strengthen quadriceps femoris muscle, without producing knee movement. The plank is a type of isometric hold, which intensively activates the body's core musculature, resulting in postural stability **(Fig. 1.25)**.

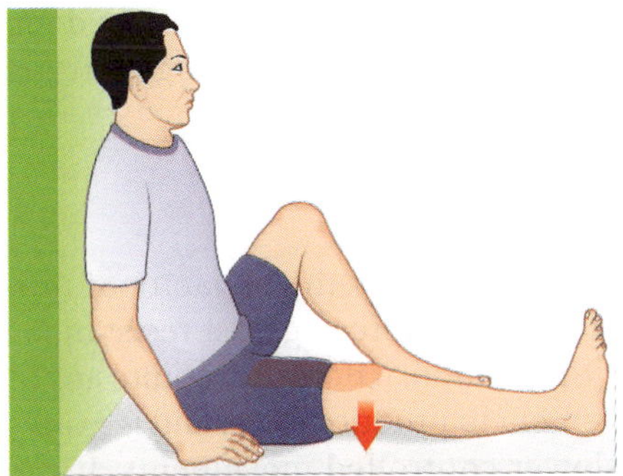

Fig. 1.24: Isometric quadriceps exercise.

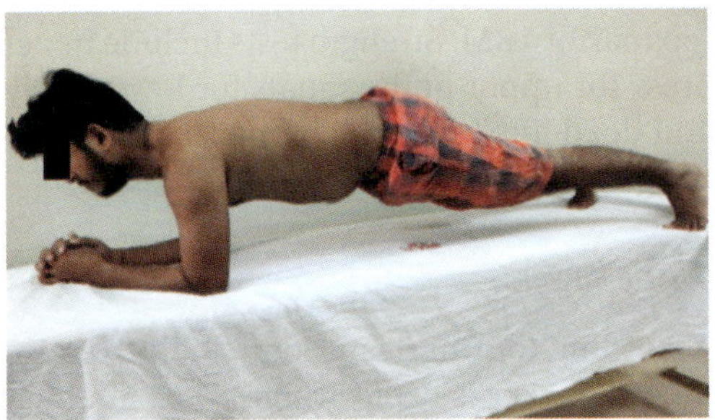

Fig. 1.25: The Plank exercise.

### *Isokinetic Contraction/Exercise*

Isokinetic exercise or accommodating variable-resistance exercise, is a type of therapeutic exercise which refers to force exertion against the isokinetic machine that leads to limb movement at a fixed velocity.

Iso—equal, kinetic—force. In isokinetic contractions/exercises the velocity/speed is same and the muscle force/resistance is variable. In isokinetic exercise whatever the torque produced in the muscle, the same amount of resistance is produced by the instrument. This type of contraction/exercise can be done with the help of the special equipment, called isokinetic dynamometer **(Fig. 1.26)**. The benefits of isokinetic movements vary by the speed (velocity) by which they are performed. Low-velocity exercises generally increase muscle strength, while high-velocity exercises are mainly used for the recovery of muscle endurance following an injury. Isokinetic exercises at a lower angular velocity (60°/sec) are more effective in increasing muscle strength, while exercises at a higher angular velocity (240°/sec) are more effective in enhancing the immune protection system.

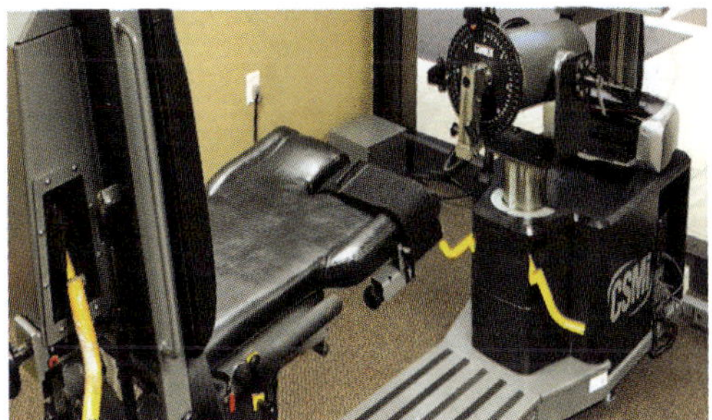

Fig. 1.26: Isokinetic dynamometer.

Slow to medium training velocities (60–80°/sec) are started initially, gradually progressing to higher training velocities.

**Benefits of Isokinetic Exercise**

- Resistance can be applied to the muscles throughout the entire range of motion.
- Muscle injuries are less likely to occur.
- Isokinetic exercise is considered safe and is associated with very few side effects.
- Isokinetic exercise may be safer than other types of training during rehabilitation because the resistance mechanism of the machine disengages the person, if one experiences any pain or discomfort. The controlled speed and resistance make it hard for the individual to push beyond limits.

**Uses of Isokinetic Exercise**

- Used in rehabilitation therapies and recovery of soft tissue injuries.
- It is used for testing of muscle function.
- It increases muscular control and development.
- It prevents injury.
- It increases muscle tone.

The tension created inside the muscle and strength gain, depends on the type of muscle contraction, i.e., eccentric/concentric/isometric **(Figs. 1.27A to C)**. The strength gain in the eccentric contraction is more than

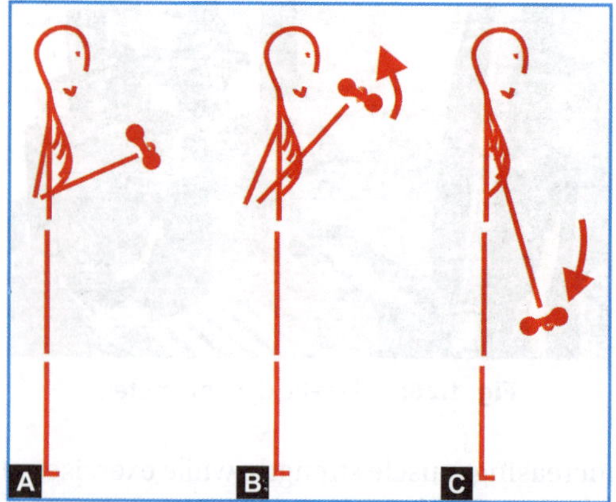


**Figs. 1.27A to C:** (A) Isometric; (B) Concentric; (C) Eccentric contraction.

the other contraction, i.e., strength gain and efficiency of eccentric contraction > isometric contraction > concentric contraction, which are briefly stated below.

**Difference Between Concentric, Eccentric and Isometric Contractions in Strength Training**

- **Concentric contraction:** A muscle shortens as it contracts and moves a load. It builds less strength/muscle tension and requires more energy than eccentric contraction.
- **Isometric contraction:** A muscle contracts isometrically and produces tension, but the length does not change. It builds intermediate tension between concentric and eccentric contractions, but the energy expenditure is higher than isotonic (concentric/eccentric) contractions, which depends on the resistance applied.
- **Eccentric contraction:** A muscle lengthens as it contracts and resists a load. It builds more strength and requires less energy than concentric contraction.

## Strength, Power and Endurance

Therapeutic exercises are designed for patients and athletes for gain of strength, power and endurance of muscles for improving performance. A knowledge of strength, power and endurance is essentially required for the therapist/clinician for designing exercises for the patients/athletes.

### *Muscle Strength*

Muscle strength is the capacity of muscle to exert strong force against resistance in a single repetition. It does not require any quick movement to produce force, and is expressed by slower controlled movements. It can be measured, based on the amount of weight lifted for a single repetition, referred to as one-rep max or 1RM. Strength tests include bench press for upper body, squats for lower body, and dead lifts (a loaded barbell/bar lifted off the ground) for lower back, etc.

### *Muscle Power*

According to American Council on Exercise, muscle power is explosiveness, i.e., ability to move weight with speed. It is the production of greatest amount of force in shortest possible time. Most power exercises include, vertical jumps, lateral hops, etc.

### *Endurance*

Endurance is the submaximal force produced by the muscle groups for sustained period of time. It refers to the body's physical capability to sustain an exercise for an extended period. Endurance exercise, also known as aerobic exercise is any physical activity, that increases heart rate and breathing for a sustained period of time. Endurance training through activities such as running, swimming, cycling builds the energy systems of the body, by increasing the mitochondrial content and respiratory capacity of the muscle fibers and enhancing the growth of the capillaries that uses oxygen as fuel to sustain long periods of exercise.

It is of two types namely:

- Muscular endurance.
- Cardiovascular endurance/general body endurance.

**Muscular Endurance**

Muscular endurance is the ability of a muscle or group of muscles to sustain repeated contractions against resistance for an extended period. The greater the muscular endurance, the more repetitions of a particular exercise one can perform. It is one of the components of muscular fitness, along with muscular strength, flexibility, and power. In endurance activities, a group of muscles contracts for a prolonged period of time without fatigue.

**Cardiorespiratory/General Body Endurance**

It is the capacity of heart, lungs and circulatory system to transport oxygen during prolonged exercise. Many groups of muscles of the body performing an activity for a prolonged period of time without fatigue, develop this endurance.

*Example:* Walking, jogging, running.

## Physiological Changes During Exercises (Exercise Physiology)

Exercise poses a substantial increase in demand for the body, as compared to the resting state. Exercise physiology involves the study of the acute responses and chronic adaptations (physiological changes) to exercise. It studies, specific changes in muscular, cardiorespiratory and neurohumeral systems, that lead to changes in functional capacity and strength due to strength and endurance training. The reactions to the exercises (adaptive responses), result from an elevation of metabolism produced by exercise. Controlled exercises, help to reduce or reverse disease progression due to the various adaptations.

The parasympathetic tone maintained by our nervous system at rest, that affects the respiratory rate, cardiac output, and various metabolic processes are altered by exercises. Exercises stimulate the sympathetic nervous system which work to maintain appropriate level of homeostasis for the increased demand in physical, metabolic, respiratory and cardiovascular efforts, to supply more oxygen and nutrients, remove $CO_2$ and metabolic waste products, maintain body temperature and acid balance and hormone levels.

### *Adaptations to Exercise*

**Acute Adaptations**

To accommodate the increased metabolic activity in skeletal muscles while exercising, the circulatory system, increases blood flow through increased cardiac output, and modulation of capillary blood flow, so that oxygen and $CO_2$ transport is properly controlled which helps to buffer the pH level of active tissues. Further, the nitric oxide (a local vasodilator) released from the endothelial cells helps to ensure adequate blood flow. As exercises progress, cardiac output increases in a linear fashion, in order to meet the increased demand of oxygen and food stuffs.

The consumption of oxygen, expressed as $VO_2$, is calculated by Fick equation [$VO_2$ = (Cardiac output) × (Difference in arterial and venous oxygen levels)]. $VO_2$ max (maximum energy consumption), a measure of aerobic capacity, is the highest rate of oxygen uptake, an individual can maintain during intense exercise, increases to 16 mL/100 mL of blood from the resting value of 4–5 mL/100 mL of blood. The various adaptation to exercise by different systems of body are briefly discussed below:

### *Effect of Exercise on Cardiovascular System*

**Effect on Heart**

A prolonged exercise causes the enlargement of heart. Generally, hypertrophy of the heart in athletes is caused by the strenuous exercises. This type of hypertrophic and enlarged heart is totally different from the diseased enlarged heart, i.e., cardiomegaly.

**Effect on Heart Rate**

There is significant increase of the heart rate observed at the beginning stage of the exercise, which comes down after some time. During the early stage of the exercise the rise of the heart rate is due to the cerebral activation of the medullary cardiac center. This heart rate rise differs from individual to individual. The athletes have the reduced heart rate than the normal man while performing exercise. As the stamina increases the heart rate decreases with the exercises.

**Effect on Cardiac Output**

Coronary blood flow is increased, supplying more nutrients to the myocardium, producing efficient cardiac output. The cardiac output tremendously increases with the strenuous exercise. In athletes the cardiac output may be more than 30 liters per minute, but the same is 5–6 liters per minute for the normal man. Cardiac output increases with the increased stroke volume mostly observed in the athletes.

**Effect on Venous Return**

During the muscular exercise the venous return increase. It may be due to: (1) continuous muscular contraction which squeezes and pumps blood towards the heart, (2) reflex venous constriction increases the venous return, and (3) respiratory movement increases the sucking effect on the right heart, as during the inspiration the intrathoracic and intra-abdominal pressure decreases which causes the rapid return of the blood to the heart.

**Effect on Blood Pressure (BP)**

There is linear increase in systolic blood pressure, however, the diastolic pressure value remains near resting value. Two to three hours post-exercise, blood pressure drops below pre-exercising values, known as post-exercise hypotension. A single bout of mild to moderate exercise can lead to a post-exercise decrease in blood pressure in hypertensive individuals (post-exercise hypotension). The raising of the BP is due to the: (1) Increased HR, (2) Increased cardiac output and (3) Increased vasoconstriction in the non-vital organ. The increasing of the HR and the cardiac and vasoconstrictor centers of the medulla stimulate the cerebral cortex to increase BP.

**Effect on Circulation**

During progressively increasing exercise intensity, the blood flow from the gastro-intestinal and renal systems is preferentially shunted towards the contracting muscles, through selective constriction and dilatation of capillary beds. During exercise blood supply to the active muscles and vital organ increases. It is found that the blood supply increases 30 times during exercise than the normal state. While performing exercise, the workload of the heart increases. In moderate exercise coronary flow increase depends on the $O_2$ requirement of the cardiac muscles. Sometimes due to strenuous exercise the cardiac muscle may not be getting the sufficient amount of $O_2$, and in that situation the person may feel the angina pain. The muscular exercise increases the pulmonary circulation but the blood supply to the brain remain normal. While performing exercise the blood flow to the active muscle, heart, and lung are increased but the same is decreased in the abdominal organs, kidney and other non-vital organ.

**Effect of Exercise on Respiratory System**

The respiratory system works along with the cardiovascular system, resulting in increased perfusion of the apex of the lungs, and increase in the surface area of the lungs for gas exchange, which in turn decreases the alveolar dead space. There is increase in respiratory rate. The following adaptations occur in respiratory system.

*Effect on Respiratory Rate*

The $O_2$ demand during the strenuous exercise increases the respiratory rate of an individual, it may be due to:

- Increased production of the $CO_2$ by the working muscles.
- Proprioceptive activation of the joint.

- Reflex effect by the respiratory centers.
- Increases temperature.
- Adrenaline hypersecretion.

*Effect on $O_2$ Exchange*

During the normal or moderate exercise the $O_2$ flow to the muscles, lung and the heart is increased. The $O_2$ tension rises in the alveoli and the arteries. Generally, the $O_2$ saturation goes up to 4 L/min. In the severe exercise the $O_2$ will be lacking due to production of lactic acid by the active muscles. So, the lactic acid quantity increases in the blood plasma and active muscles. To reduce the lactic acid accumulation and oxidize the lactic acid, excess amount of $O_2$ is needed; this lack is called $O_2$ debt (**Oxygen debt** is defined as the extra volume of oxygen, that is needed to restore all the energetic systems to their normal state after exercise. Where as **oxygen deficiency** is defined as the difference in oxygen volume between an ideal, hypothetical oxygen uptake, and the actual uptake in real life).

*Effect on Second Wind*

In early stage of the strenuous exercise the person feels the distress, headache, throbbing pain, breathlessness and irregular pulse, but if the exercise is continued, the distress comes down. This sense of relief is called as second wind. During the second wind distress disappears and the discomfort disappears. But the physiology of the second wind is not so clear.

**Effect of Exercise on Digestive System**

The mild exercise, like walking, increases the gastric juice secretion and the motility of stomach. But the strenuous exercise decreases the gastric juice secretion and the stomach motility, but increased secretion after cessation of the exercise will compensate the same.

**Effect of Exercise on Kidney Functions**

During the exercise the blood flow to the non-vital and the inactive muscles decreases. Due to the decreased blood flow to the kidney, there will be lacking of the urine formation and increased secretion of the ADH, which (ADH) increases the fluid reabsorption up to 1–2 hours from cessation of the exercise and there will be reduced urine flow. Normally, the exercises cause the increased amount of albumin in the urine. Sometimes physical exercise causes the red urine, which contain hemoglobin, it is due to the breakdown of the RBC during the strenuous exercises. It also breaks the myoglobin, which results in the black urine formation 24–48 hours after exercise.

**Effect of Exercise on Body Temperature**

Muscular activity produces the heat, if the heat loss is less the body temperature goes up. Normally, during exercise the body temperature goes up due to the temporary failure of the temperature regulation center activation.

**Effect of Exercise on Blood Fluid**

During the muscular exercise, there will be rapid loss of the water through sweating and expired air. In early stage of exercise the fluid enters into the tissue from the blood results in hemoconcentration and comes down by the fluid back to the blood. Sweating is observed during the early stage of exercises, however, if the exercise is prolonged the excessive sweating comes down.

**Effect of Exercise on Blood Cells**

During strenuous exercise the fluid enters into the tissue from the blood. So, the hemoconcentration occurs but the prolonged exercise may reduce the hemoconcentration by sending back the fluid into the blood. Sometimes during the strenuous exercise, the hemolysis may also occur. The WBC count increases in any sort of exercise. But the raising of the WBC may vary between the normal people to the athletes; it may be less for athletes as compared with the common men.

**Effect of Exercise on Endocrine Function**

Plasma levels of epinephrine, norepinephrine, cortisol and dopamine increase with maximal exercise, which returns to baseline after rest. There is release of growth hormone from the pituitary gland, with strenuous exercise, enhancing bone and tissue growth. There is increased insulin sensitivity after long-term exercises. Exercises increase levels of testosterone, resulting in enhanced growth, libido and mood. The antidiuretic hormone (ADH), that regulates water in the body also increases, but there is no change in the thyroid hormone.

**Effect of Exercise on Body Immunity**

Moderate intensity exercises, enhance the immune system of the body, whereas overstraining reduces the functionality of the immune cells.

**Muscle fiber recruitment in different types of exercise:**

Different muscle fibers are recruited for different type of exercises as under:

- The slow twitch type-I fibers, having abundant mitochondria, myoglobin and greater vascular supply, and having high oxidative and low glycolytic capacity, which are predominant in postural muscles, are recruited in exercises involving posture and balance.
- The fast-twitch oxidative, type-IIa fibers, having high oxidative and glycolytic capacity, are recruited for power activities, that require sustained effort, such as weight lifting for multiple repetitions, running, jumping, etc.
- The fast-twitch glycolytic, type-IIb fibers, having low oxidative and high glycolytic capacity, that undergo rapid fatigue, are recruited for high intensity, short duration exercises such as full effort sprints.

**Adaptations to Exercises in Strength Training**

With progressively overloading exercise training, the SAID principle, i.e., specific adaptations to increased demands, results in adaptation of the muscles to the increasing load, leading to hypertrophy of muscle fibers (an increase in diameter and volume) and increase of bone mineral density, to manage the overload. Isolated forces generated in the muscles contracting to overcome resistance, compresses the small arteries, thus increases the peripheral vascular resistance.

**Adaptations to Exercises in Endurance Training**

The slow twitch fibers are more recruited in endurance activities. There is increase in the number of mitochondria, and the gas exchange capacity of the myofibrils increases.

### *Chronic Changes (Adaptations) of Exercise*

**Endurance Training**

Aerobic exercises increase the cross sectional area of the slow twitch muscle fibers, and the fast-twitch fibers develop a higher oxygen capacity. The increased capillary bed density, resulting from endurance training, permits a greater blood flow to supply increased nutrients to the muscles.

The number of mitochondria, myoglobin content, glycogen storage capacity increase in the trained muscles. The ability to use fat as an energy source (gluconeogenesis) also increases.

Long-term aerobic exercises lead to positive cardiac adaptations, both morphologically and physiologically. The cardiac adaptations to aerobic exercise lead to increased cardiac output during exercise and higher $VO_2$ max after exercise. According to American College of Sports Medicine, dynamic aerobic training reduces blood pressure in individuals with hypertension.

Respiratory adaptations to prolonged endurance exercise, leads to increased blood flow in the upper regions of the lungs with increase of respiratory rate.

**Resistance/Strength Training**

It results in increase in size of muscle (muscle hypertrophy), due to increase of myofibril size and number of fast and slow twitch muscle fibers. It leads to greater force development by the trained muscles.

The cross-sectional area of ligaments and tendons increase (resulting in hypertrophy) in response to prolonged training, as the insertion sites of ligaments and tendons to bones become stronger.

# 2 CHAPTER

# Mechanics

## FORCE

Force is an external agent capable of changing a body's/system's state of rest or motion. It is the rate of change of momentum, which is used to accelerate/decelerate a moving system. It has a magnitude and a direction and is a vector quantity. In animals the contracting muscles produce the required force to move the body's levers to produce functional movements. In mechanical/motorized devices, forces are produced by the mechanical instruments such as weight and pulley systems/electric motors (as used in electrically operated traction devices) to make the systems function. In pathological states, where muscles are paralyzed, the forces required to move the body levers are not produced, resulting in impairment of function, activity and participation limitations and a decreased quality of life.

Force is applied on the object of particular weight to move it for particular distance. It is measured in Newton or Dyne. One newton is the force needed to accelerate one kilogram of mass at the rate of one meter per second square in the direction of the applied force. The relationship between newton and kilogram is: 10 Newton is equal to 1.019716 kg (approximately 1 kg). One dyne is defined as the force required to accelerate a mass of one gram at a rate of 1 centimeter per second square.

Clinicians, must understand, why the body/system is not able to produce the force to hold the static posture and/or produce momentum (mass X velocity of movement) for movement to maintain balance/equilibrium.

The force may act on object in states such as:
- **Static:** The force acting on the body at rest to hold a posture and to maintain static balance/equilibrium.
- **Dynamic:** The force acting on the body, in the states of motion.

Force acting on a system is found using the following formula.

Force = Mass × Acceleration,

where, force is measured in newton, mass in kilogram, acceleration in meter (m/s$^2$).

The forces acting on a system could be of the following types:

### Linear Force

The two or more forces acting along the same line and producing the straight-line motion is referred on the linear force.

*Example:*
- When two forces act on an object in same direction producing the linear motion, the forces are said to be the pushing linear force **(Fig. 2.1A)**.
- When the two forces pull an object in same direction it produces the linear motion, the force is said to be the pulling linear force **(Fig. 2.1B)**.
- When the two forces are acting opposite to each other with the equal magnitude it results in equilibrium **(Fig. 2.1C)**.
- When the two forces are acting opposite to each other with unequal magnitude the movement occurs towards the greater magnitude side.

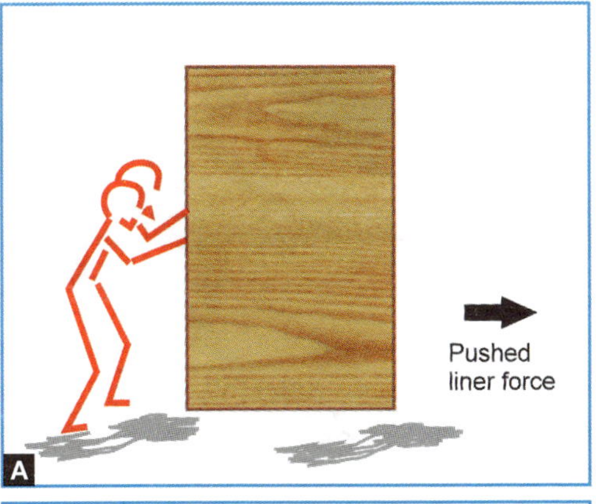


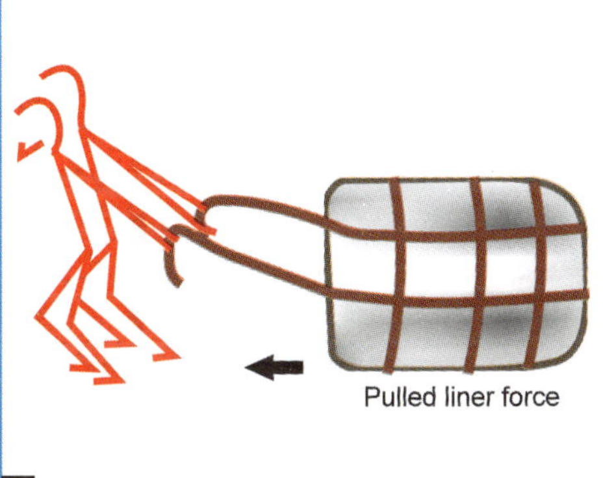


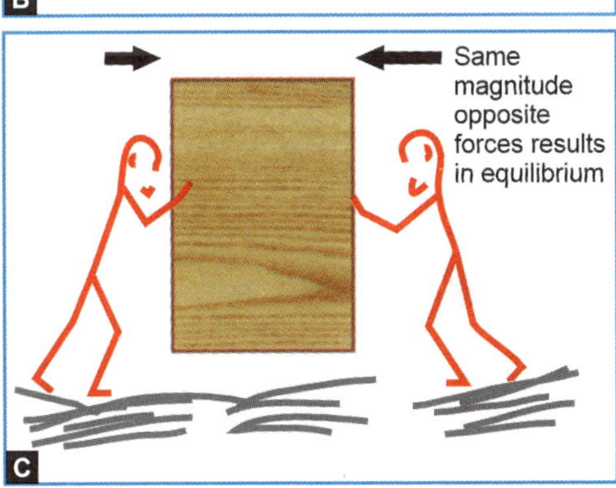


**Figs. 2.1A to C:** Linear forces.

## Parallel Force

Forces that act in the same or opposite direction at different points on objects, making the lines of action parallel to each other are called parallel forces. See-saw is an example of parallel forces **(Figs. 2.2A and B)**. The children on board when apply the two equal forces in the end, the fulcrum gives the counterforce to maintain the see-saw in neutral position. But, when the force exerted by one child exceeds other, a rotational movement is produced over the fulcrum.

The parallel forces could be:

- Like parallel forces, where all the forces act parallel to each other, and all of them act in the same direction.
- Unlike parallel forces, where all the forces act parallel to each other, and all of them do not act in the same direction, resulting in rotation.

## Rotational Force

In the parallel force system, when any one of the forces is greater than other, or the two parallel forces act in the opposite direction, it results in rotation of the system and that forces are said to be the rotational forces/force couple **(Figs. 2.3A and B)**.

### *Force Couple*

A force couple is a pair of parallel forces, oppositely directed, and displaced by a perpendicular distance or moment, resulting in rotational movement of the system. The simplest kind of force couple consists of two equal and opposite forces whose lines of action do not coincide. This is called a "simple force couple". The forces have a turning effect or moment called a torque about an axis which is perpendicular to the plane of the forces.

Torque is a measure of how much a force acting on an object causes that object to rotate. The magnitude of the torque = F (magnitude of force) × d (perpendicular distance between the line of action of force from the axis/fulcrum).

The force couples acting on various systems are of the following types:

**Clockwise Force Couple (Fig. 2.4A)**

Where the torque produced, tends to rotate the system in a clockwise direction.

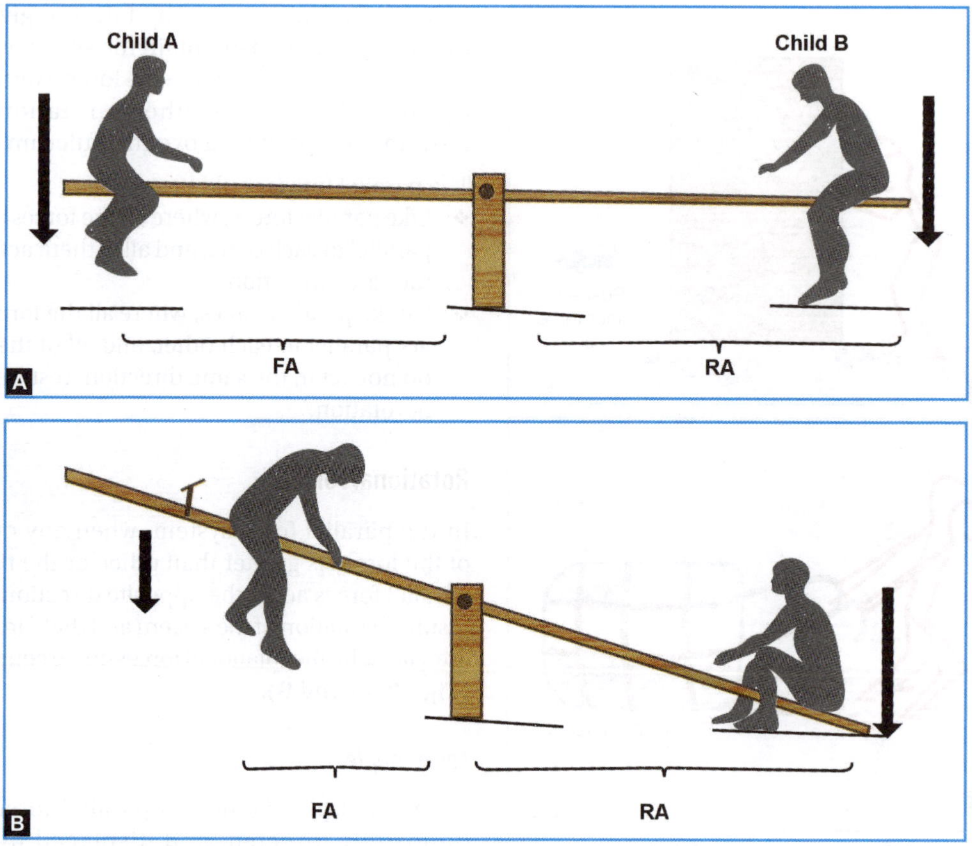

**Figs. 2.2A and B:** (A) Parallel forces with same magnitude; (B) Parallel forces with different magnitude.

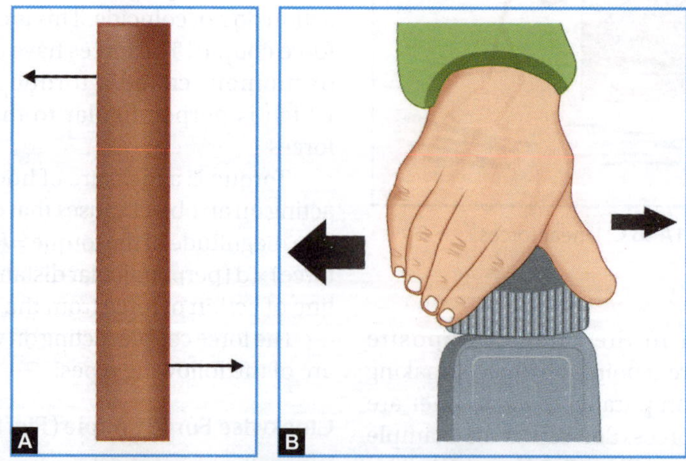


**Figs. 2.3A and B:** Rotational forces (force couple).

**Figs. 2.4A and B:** (A) Clockwise force couple; (B) Anticlockwise force couple.

### Anticlockwise Force Couple (Fig. 2.4B)

Where the torque produced, tends to rotate the system in the anticlockwise direction.

**Example of force couple in human body:** In the human body, upper trapezius—serratus anterior force couple, helps to rotate the scapula, in a upward direction, when the shoulder is abducted above 90 degrees in the frontal plane **(Fig. 2.5)**.

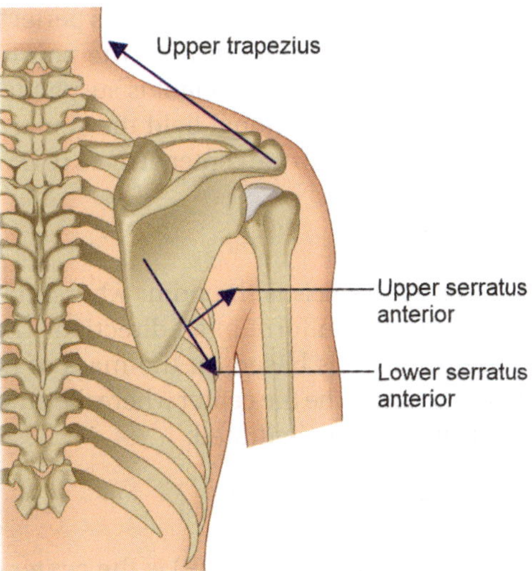


**Fig. 2.5:** Serratus anterior and upper trapezius force couple.

## Concurrent Force

If the two forces acting on the object in different directions are perpendicular to each other, the resultant force will be in between the two forces. It can be diagrammatically represented by the parallelogram method **(Fig. 2.6)**.

### *Center of Gravity*

The vertical projection of the COM is often defined as the center of gravity (COG). It is

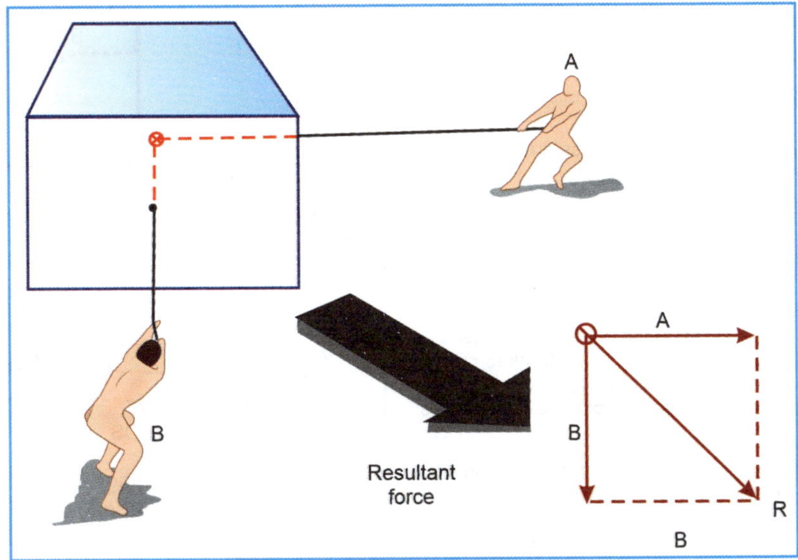


**Fig. 2.6:** Concurrent force system.

the point, at which the entire body is perfectly balanced in relation to gravity/the point at which the body's entire weight is suspended. In a uniform gravitational field the center of gravity is identical to the center of mass (COM).

### Center of Mass

The center of mass is the point where mass distribution is uniform in all directions. The center of mass is based on the mass of the body. It is said to be the center where the entire bodily mass is concentrated.

### Center of Pressure

The center of pressure (COP) is the center of the distribution of the total force applied to the supporting surface **(Fig. 2.7)**. The COP moves continuously around the COM to keep the COM within the support base (Benda et al., 1994; Winter et al., 1990).

The symmetrical objects will have the COG at the center of the object. It may depend on the size, shape, structure, weight, and portion of the particular object. In asymmetric object the COG is located in the heavier end where the mass is concentrated. In a rod the COG is located near to the upper end, if it is vertically placed and the same will be near to the ground if it is horizontally placed due to its height, weight difference, and the weight transmitted area. The center of gravity of human body in different postures are shown in **Figures 2.8A to C**.

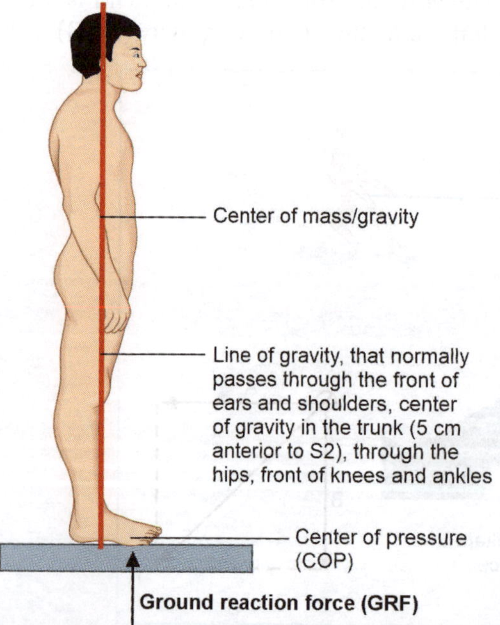


**Fig. 2.7:** Shows center of pressure (COP).

## Line of Gravity

The imaginary vertical line passing through the center of gravity is called as line of gravity **(Fig. 2.9)**. Normally, the center of gravity (COG) lies in front of the second sacral vertebra in the human body in the erect standing posture.

In the human body each and every segment of the body has its separate COG and the two or three segments together gives the different

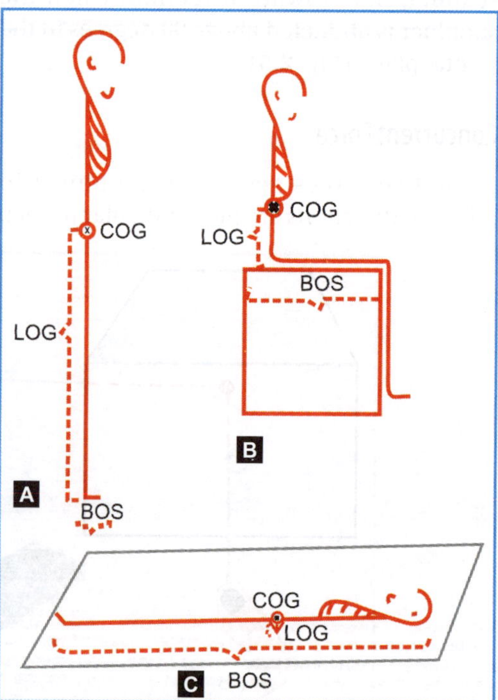


**Figs. 2.8A to C:** (A) Standing—COG in higher level, LOG is in highest height, less BOS; (B) Sitting—COG in lower level, LOG is in lesser height, BOS is more; (C) Lying—COG near to floor, LOG is in very much lesser height, BOS is very large.

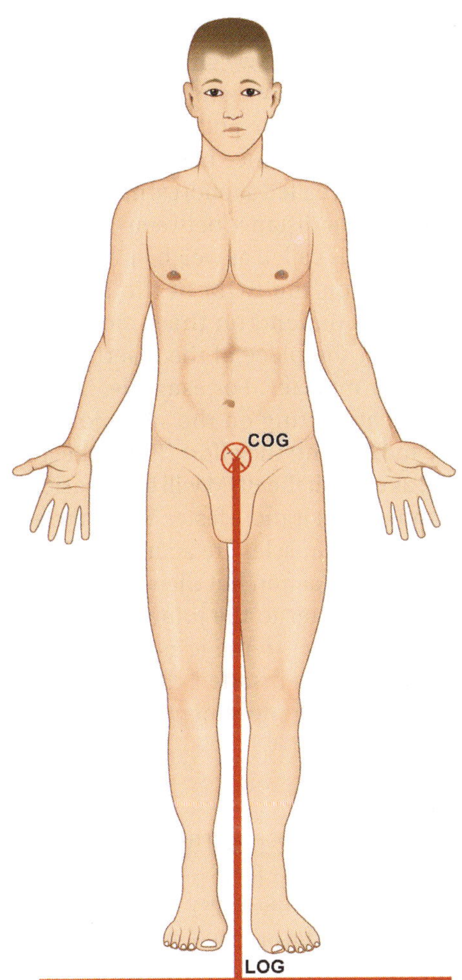

**Fig. 2.9:** The line of gravity.

COG. For example, the arm, forearm and hand will be having its own separate COG but the upper limb as a whole gives some other different COG.

## Base of Support

The base of support (BOS) means the area supported beneath the object. Whenever the base of support is more the stability will be more. Greater the BOS lower the COG of any object.

$$\text{BOS} \propto \frac{1}{\text{COG}}$$

For example, in the fundamental position of standing, the BOS is lesser than the lying, so COG in the standing position is in the higher level, whereas in the lying posture it will be just near to the ground. As a result lying posture is more stable than any other fundamental position and also it can be maintained for the longer period. The stability is directly proportional to BOS and inversely proportional to COG.

$$\text{Stability} \propto \text{BOS}$$

$$\text{Stability} \propto \frac{1}{\text{COG}}$$

### *Equilibrium*

it is the state of an object where all the forces acting on it are equal in magnitude and opposite in direction.

A state in which opposing forces or actions are balanced so that one is not stronger or greater than the other.

**Types of Equilibrium**

It is classified into the following three types:
- Stable equilibrium
- Unstable equilibrium
- Neutral equilibrium.

*Stable Equilibrium*

A body is in stable equilibrium if it comes back to its normal position on slight displacement. Generally, the equilibrium will be stable when the BOS is more and COG lies in the lower part of an object **(Fig. 2.10)**.

*Example:* Book placed on the table. When the force is applied on the book, the book regains its original state after the removal of the force.

*Unstable Equilibrium*

A state of equilibrium in which a small disturbance will produce a large change of the state of the object. A minimum force is enough to alter the equilibrium of an object in unstable equilibrium. The object with unstable equilibrium has less BOS and the COG is in

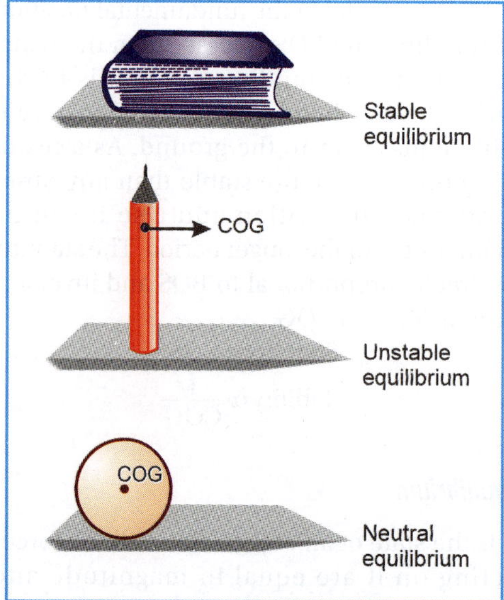


**Fig. 2.10:** Different types of equilibrium.

higher position. The object will be having the lesser equilibrium.

*Example:* A pencil balanced on the floor when applied with force, leads to alteration of its original state.

*Neutral Equilibrium*

It is the type of equilibrium in which the body comes to rest in its new position after being slightly displaced by some external force. The body does not move after attaining neutral equilibrium, that means it remains stationary.

Even though the movement or position changes in the object by the force exerted on it, there will not be any change in the COG of the object.

*Example:* Ball rolling on the floor.

## Lever

A lever is defined as the rigid bar, which moves about on some fixed point called fulcrum (F). To perform an activity or a movement, the bone acts as the lever arms and the joints acts as the fulcrum (F). The movement will be created by two types of forces, i.e., weight (W), and effort (E), in which the weight (W) is the opposing force and the effort (E) is action achieving force. The weight may be the weight of the body parts/weight held in hand and the effort may be the pull of the muscle. The perpendicular distance between the effort to the fulcrum is called as effort arm (EA) and the perpendicular distance between the weight to the fulcrum is called as weight arm (WA).

Achieving the ROM of the joints may sometimes depend on the strength of the muscles or the place of the insertion of the particular muscles. For example, if the two muscles are acting on the same joint for a same movement; the effort (E) will be added more, as a result the ROM will be so easier and also movement is more faster. When the equal powered two muscles are acting on the same joint for same action but their insertions are: (a) one is farther to the joint (fulcrum), (b) another is closer to the joint (fulcrum), the muscle, which is inserted closer to the joint produce stronger movement than the farther inserted muscles.

### Types of Levers

These are of three types. They are as under:

- First order lever (1°)
- Second order lever (2°)
- Third order lever (3°).

*First Order Lever*

The fulcrum (F) is between the effort (E) and the weight (W) **(Fig. 2.11)**. Sometimes the fulcrum is situated closer to the weight or effort. It is the lever of balance. Scissor **(Fig. 2.12A)**, see-saw, nail cutter, etc., are mechanical examples of 1st order lever. Nodding of head at the atlanto-occipital joint **(Fig. 2.12B)**, trunk bending at the lumbosacral joint with weight in hand are

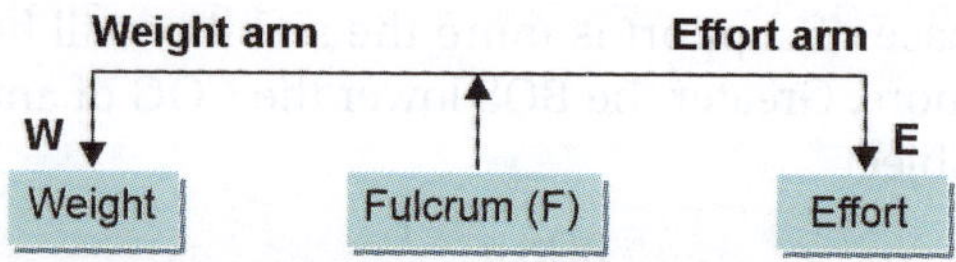


**Fig. 2.11:** The 1st order lever.

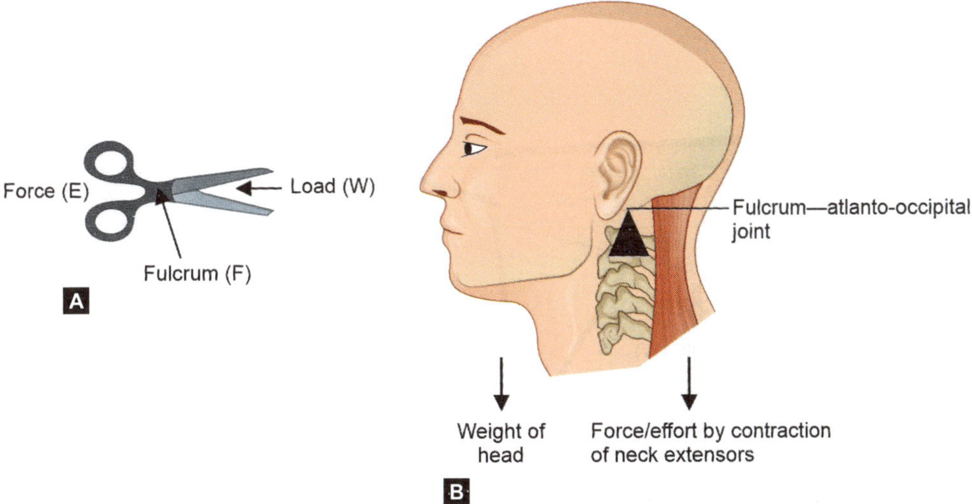


**Figs. 2.12A and B:** (A) Scissor—a 1st order lever; (B) Nodding of head at atlanto-occipital joint—a 1st order lever.

examples of 1st order lever in human body. During the nodding movement of the head, the neck extensors act as the effort (E), atlanto-occipital joint as fulcrum and the facial part is the weight (W). If the fulcrum is closer to the weight (W) it produces more speed or ROM but with less strength. If the fulcrum is close to the effort (E) it produces the less speed or ROM but with more strength. There are less number of first order levers seen in the human body.

*Second Order Lever*

The weight (W) lies between the fulcrum (F) and the effort (E) **(Fig. 2.13)**. These levers are the lever of the strength/power, but not the speed and ROM. These types of levers are less seen in the human body. A wheelbarrow **(Fig. 2.14A)**, a door operated by holding the handle, etc., are mechanical examples of 2nd order lever. Raising the body on the toes **(Fig. 2.14B)**, in which the metatarsophalangeal joints of the toes are the fulcrum (F), the tendo-Achilles tendon is the effort (E) and the body weight passing through the middle part of the foot is the resistance/weight (W). These types of lever always have the mechanical advantage, so these varieties of levers are called as the levers of the strength/power.

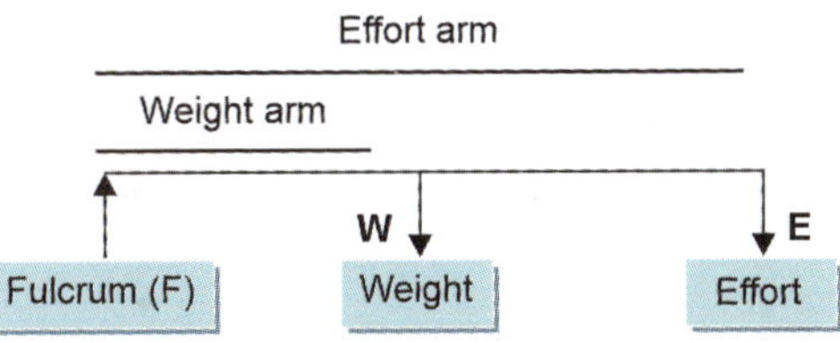


**Fig. 2.13:** The second order lever.

*Third Order Lever*

These are the levers in which the fulcrum is at one end and the force is applied in the middle and the weight is on the other end. The effort lies in between the fulcrum (F) and the weight (W) **(Fig. 2.15)**. These levers mostly have mechanical disadvantage, and are seen plentily in the human body. These are the levers of speed and also called as force multiplier lever. A forcep **(Fig. 2.16A)**, fishing stick, betel nut cutter, etc., are mechanical examples of 3rd order lever. In human body, flexing the elbow with weight in hand **(Fig. 2.16B)**, in which the elbow is the fulcrum

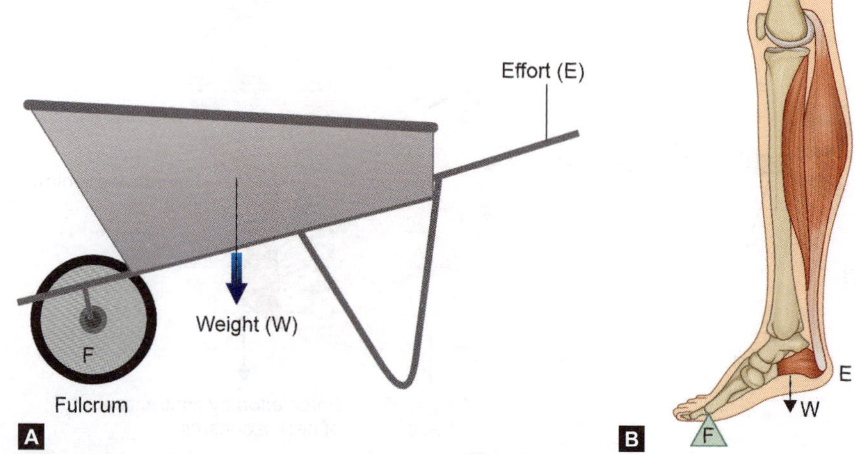


**Figs. 2.14A and B:** (A) Wheel barrow—2nd order lever; (B) Raising the body on toes—2nd order lever.

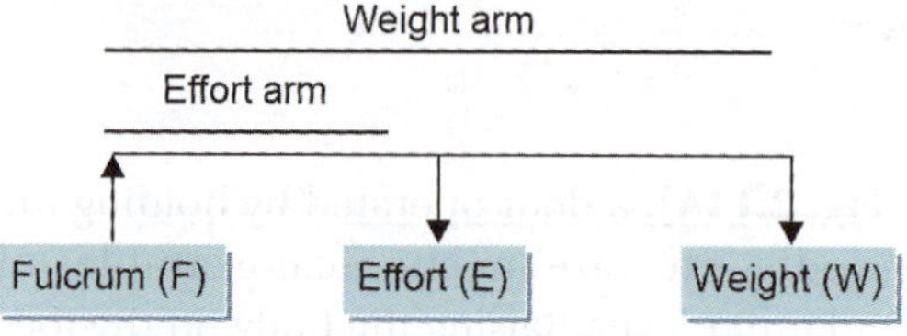


**Fig. 2.15:** The 3rd order lever.

(F) biceps insertion is the effort (E) and the weight on hand is load/weight (W), is the example of 3rd order lever.

### Mechanical Advantage

The mechanical advantage of a lever is a number that indicates how a lever performs as a simple machine by transforming the input force or effort into an output work. The ideal mechanical advantage of a lever is determined by dividing the distance from the fulcrum to the input force [effort (E)], by the distance from the fulcrum to weight (W)/ output force.

Mechanical advantage = Effort arm (EA)/ Weight (resistance) arm (WA)

If the weight arm (WA/RA) and effort arm (EA) are in same length, there may not be any mechanical advantage. The effort/force necessary to oppose the resistance/weight is same, and the mechanical advantage is: 1.

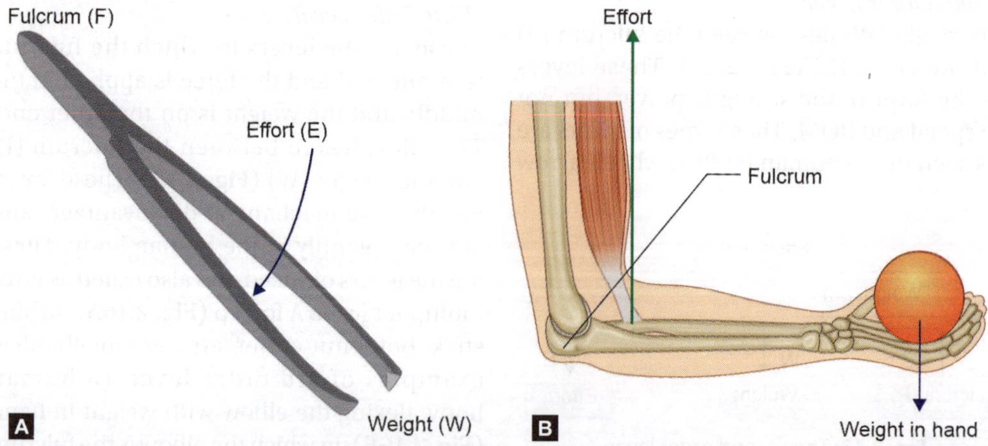


**Figs. 2.16A and B:** (A) Forcep—3rd order lever; (B) Flexing elbow with weight in hand—3rd order lever.

If the weight arm (WA/RA) is greater than the effort arm (EA), then the effort/force required is more to oppose the resistance, hence it is difficult to perform the movement. The mechanical advantage (MA) is <1.

If the effort arm (EA) exceeds the weight arm (WA/RA), less effort is required to oppose the resistance/weight. The mechanical advantage is >1, resulting in requirement of less force/effort to produce the movement. It can be achieved in all the second order levers and in some first order levers where the fulcrum is closer to the weight/resistance (W/R).

- In first order levers the effort arm (EA) may be greater, lesser or equal to weight arm (WA/RA). Among these, if the effort arm (EA) is greater than weight arm (WA/RA), it gives more mechanical advantage.
- In all second order levers the mechanical advantage is greater than one.
- In all third order levers the mechanical advantage is normally less than one. So, the effort should be more to produce the movement.

## Newton's Laws of Motion

Newton's laws of motion are three basic laws of classical mechanics that describe the relationship between the motion of an object and the forces acting on it. These laws can be stated as follows:

### *Law of Inertia*

A body remains at rest, or in motion at a constant speed in a straight line, unless acted upon by a force.

### *Law of Acceleration*

When a body is acted upon by a net force, the body's acceleration multiplied by its mass is equal to the net force, i.e., Force (F) = Mass (m) × Acceleration (a). Acceleration (a) = Force (F)/Mass (m).

### *Law of Action-Reaction*

If two bodies exert forces on each other to maintain equilibrium, these forces have the same magnitude but opposite directions. This says every action has equal and opposite reaction.

## Pulley

A pulley is a grooved wheel that rotates about a fixed axis by a rope that passes around it. The axis is supported by a framework or block and the whole structure may be used either as a fixed pulley or a movable pulley or a pulley combinations, called block and tackle. Pulleys are frequently used in exercise and traction equipment to increase or decreased the force magnitude and to change the direction of the force.

### *Mechanical Advantage of Pulleys*

There are two ways of determining the mechanical advantage of a pulley system. The simplest way to determine the mechanical advantage is counting the number of falls (or active lifting ropes) that are actually attached to the load. Alternatively, dividing the effort distance by the load distance also gives the mechanical advantage.

Two categories of pulleys are seen as under:

- Fixed pulley.
- Movable pulley.

#### Fixed Pulley

In a fixed pulley system, the pulley block is fixed to some suitable support and the rope which passes around the wheel is attached to the weight at one end and the effort is applied at the other. The fixed pulley may be a single fixed pulley **(Fig. 2.17)**, two fixed pullies, or more than 2 fixed pulley types.

A fixed pulley has an axle mounted in bearings attached to a supporting structure. A fixed pulley changes the direction of the force on a rope or belt that moves along its

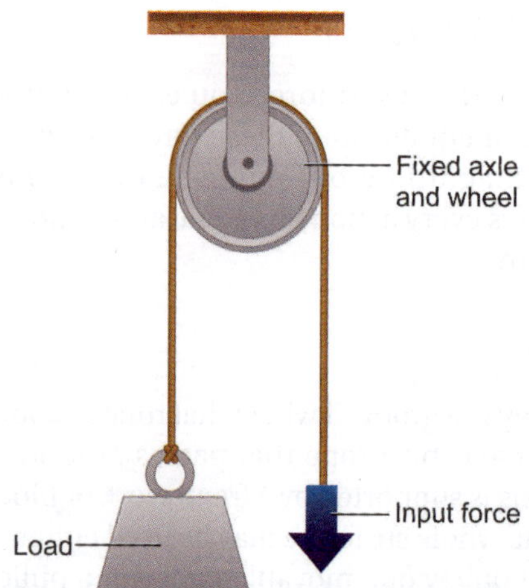


**Fig. 2.17:** Showing single fixed pulley.

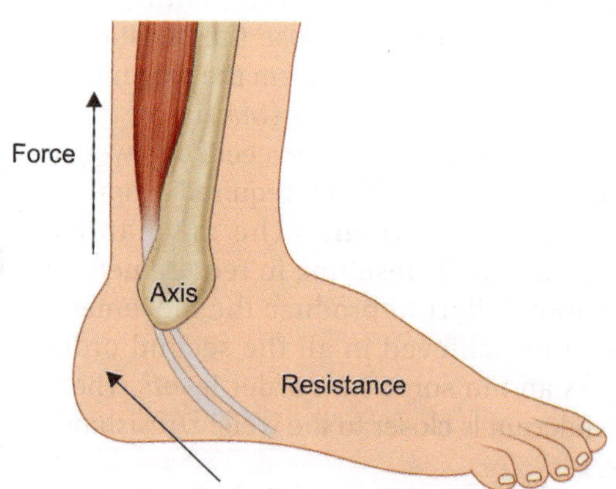


**Fig. 2.18:** Lateral malleolus acting as a fixed pulley.

circumference. Mechanical advantage is gained by combining a fixed pulley with a movable pulley or another fixed pulley of a different diameter. As the effort force is equal to the load force for the single fixed pulley, the mechanical advantage of a single fixed pulley is 1.

*Uses of Fixed Pulley System*

- This is used to alter the direction of force and enable traction or resistance to be applied at any angle. In physiotherapy such pulleys are used in shoulder pulley system to mobilize shoulder and to apply traction.
- The fixed pulley system is used in the body by some muscles to allow them to be inserted at a more advantageous angle. Example: Lateral malleolus acts as the fixed pulley for the peroneus longer tendon to reduce the resistance force of that muscle **(Fig. 2.18)**. The trochlea is a fixed pulley located in the elbow joint. It helps to change the direction of the force generated by the triceps muscles, allowing the individual to bend and straighten the elbow.

### Movable Pulley

A movable pulley is a pulley that is free to move up and down, and is attached to a ceiling or other object by two lengths of the same rope **(Fig. 2.19)**. A movable pulley has an axle in a movable block. A single movable pulley is supported by two parts of the same rope. This device is used to gain a mechanical advantage when lifting heavy weights. It acts as a second-class lever, which magnifies the force with a mechanical advantage of 2. Examples of movable pulleys in the human system include the patella which acts as a pulley for the quadriceps muscle, and the pulleys in the fingers and wrist that guide the flexor and extensor tendons. Movable pulleys are commonly found in the middle of a muscle or tendon's path, where they help to increase the mechanical advantage of the muscle.

Examples of movable pulleys in mechanics include construction cranes, modern elevators, and some types of weight lifting machines at the gymnasium. In physiotherapy, this type of pulley is used in the suspension therapy units which makes it easy to lift the body parts.

### *Compound Pulley*

These are combinations of pulleys, most commonly, combination of a fixed pulley with movable pulley, forming a block and tackle **(Fig. 2.20)**. A block and tackle is a pulley system, made up of fixed and movable pulleys, increasing the mechanical advantage. The simplest one is a combination of one fixed and

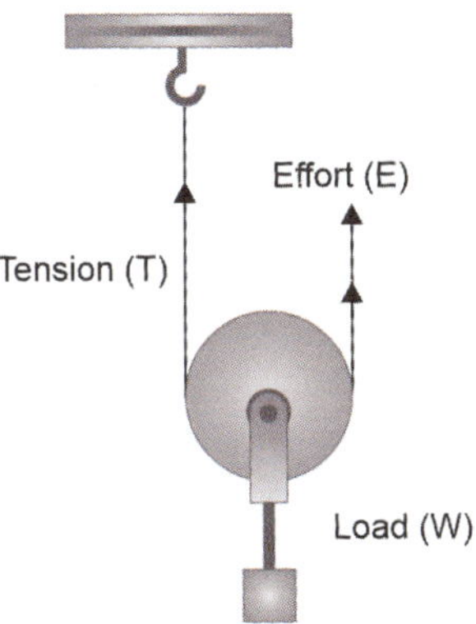


**Fig. 2.19:** The movable pulley.

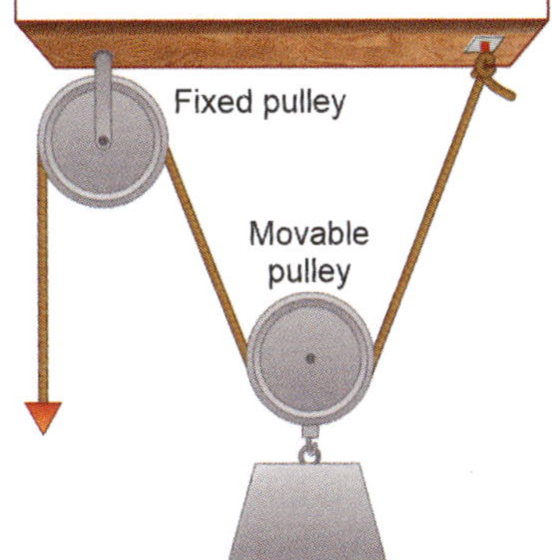


**Fig. 2.20:** Compound pulley—the block and tackle.

one movable pulley as used in the Guthrie-Smith suspension frame in suspension therapy.

The upper pulley is fixed to the overhead support to which one of the ropes is attached. The rope is then wound around the movable pulley to which the weight is attached and around the fixed pulley the effort being applied at the free end. It has a mechanical advantage of 2 or greater than 2. There are no examples of compound pulleys in the human body, as the musculoskeletal system does not use multiple pulleys mounted on a standard shaft or axle. However, the human body does use multiple anatomic pulleys, which can work together to create a mechanical advantage similar to a compound pulley system.

## Speed

Speed is measured as the ratio of distance to the time in which the distance was covered. Speed is a scalar quantity as it has only direction and no magnitude.

The formula for speed (s) = d/t.

Where,

- s is the speed in meter/second.
- d is the distance traveled in meter.
- t is the time taken in second.

## Work

Work is defined as the force, that moves an object for a particular distance. It is measured in joules or ergs.

$$\text{Work} = \text{Force} \times \text{Distance}$$

where, work measured in joules, force is measured in newtons, and distance is measured in meters.

## Power

Power is defined as the rate at which work is done upon an object. Power is a time-based quantity. Which is related to how fast a job is done. The formula for power is mentioned below.

$$P = W/t$$

It is the work done in unit time. The SI unit of power is Watt (W) which is joules per second (J/s).

## Elasticity

Elasticity is the ability of a body to resist a distorting influence and to return to its original size and shape when that influence or force is removed. The SI unit for elasticity is the pascal (Pa).

*Example:* Springs, elastic rubber, theraband, etc.

**Hook's law:** Hooke's law of elasticity was discovered by English scientist Robert Hooke in 1660. Hooke's law states that the strain of the material is proportional to the applied stress within the elastic limit of that material. That is for relatively small deformations of an object, the displacement or size of the deformation (strain), is directly proportional to the deforming force/load (stress), i.e., Stress α Strain.

Under these conditions, the object returns to its original shape and size upon removal of the load.

## Creep

Also called as cold flow, is the tendency of a solid material, to undergo slow deformation, while subjected to persistent mechanical stresses. It occurs as a result of long-term exposure to high levels of stress, that are still below the yield strength of the material. It is a rate dependent material nonlinearity, in which the material continues to deform under a constant load. It is highly time dependent and displays its effect over a long time. The materials subjected to heat for long periods have greater creep, which generally increases, as the melting point is approached.

In physiotherapy, when stretching exercises are given to elongate a tight soft tissue, creep (permanent deformation/change in length) is desired.

## Stress/Strain Curve

A stress-strain curve is the graphical representation, that demonstrates the reaction of a material, when subjected to load (stress) **(Fig. 2.21)**.

- **Proportional limit:** It is the region in the stress-strain curve which obeys Hooke's law, i.e., within the elastic limit the stress is directly proportional to the strain produced in the material. In this limit, the ratio of stress with strain gives a proportionality constant known as Young's modulus. The point OA in the graph is called the proportional limit.
- **Elastic limit:** It is the point in the graph up to which the material returns to its original position when the load acting on it is completely removed. Beyond this limit, the material does not return to its original position, and a plastic deformation starts to appear in it.

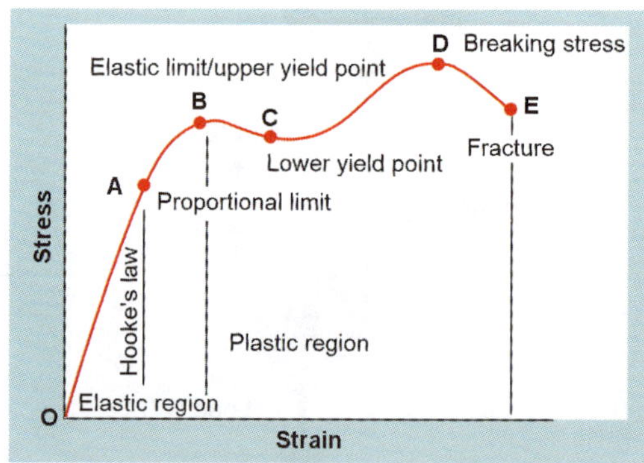


**Fig. 2.21:** Stress-strain curve.

- **Yield point:** The yield point is defined as the point at which the material starts to deform plastically. After the yield point is passed, permanent plastic deformation occurs. There are two yield points (i) upper yield point (ii) lower yield point.
- **Ultimate stress point:** It is a point that represents the maximum stress that a material can endure before failure. Beyond this point, failure occurs.
- **Fracture/breaking point:** It is the point in the stress-strain curve at which the failure of the material takes place.

### *Clinical Implication of Stress-Strain Curve*

While stretching a tight soft tissue, the therapist/clinician should apply a force of sufficient magnitude, for considerable time (minimum 30 seconds), to overcome elastic limit and achieve creep (plastic deformation). However, the force should not be too high to cause rupture.

## Springs

Springs are mechanical devices, used to assist or resist the movement in exercise therapy **(Fig. 2.22)**. Sometimes it is used for the passive mechanical stretching of the soft tissues. One end of the spring is attached to the body segment to move and the other end is

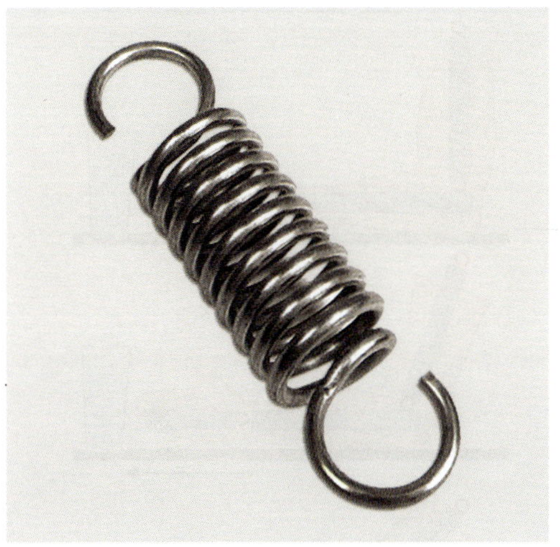

**Fig. 2.22:** The spring.

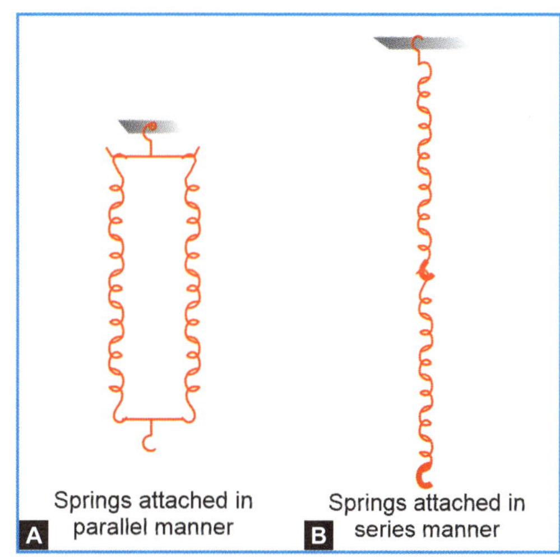


**Figs. 2.23A and B:** (A) Springs in parallel; (B) Springs in series.

attached to a rigid support. When the segment moves, the spring lengthens, thereby resisting movement, and when relaxed, the elastic recoil of the spring assists in moving the segment.

### *Weight of the Spring*

Sometimes the springs are graded in the weights.

*Example:* 20 lbs, 40 lbs, 50 lbs, 75 lbs. The 20 lbs springs needs the 20 lbs of force to elongate it. According to the pounds of the springs it requires the force to elongate it.

### *Springs in Parallel*

Two springs are said to be in parallel when they are connected side-by-side, so as to act as a single spring. The strain of the combinations is their common strain, and the stress of the combination is the sum of their stresses **(Fig. 2.23A)**.

### *Springs in Series*

Two or more springs are said to be in series when they are connected end-to-end or point to point. Any external stress applied to the combinations gets applied to each spring without change of magnitude and the amount strain (deformation) of the combination is the sum of the strains of the individual springs **(Fig. 2.23B)**.

## Energy

Energy is the capacity to perform the work. It is mainly of two types namely:

- Potential energy
- Kinetic energy

### *Potential Energy*

It is the capacity of doing the work with the help of the stored energy. For example, when the knee is flexed maximally in the standing position, the leg has the potential to fall down (extend) with the help of the gravity due to the position (stored potential energy).

### *Kinetic Energy*

This is the work done by an object as a result of motion. The potential and kinetic energy can be explained with the pendulum. The potential energy is stored in either side of the pendulum while moving. The potential energy is changed into kinetic energy while the pendulum falls with help of the gravitational force **(Fig. 2.24)**.

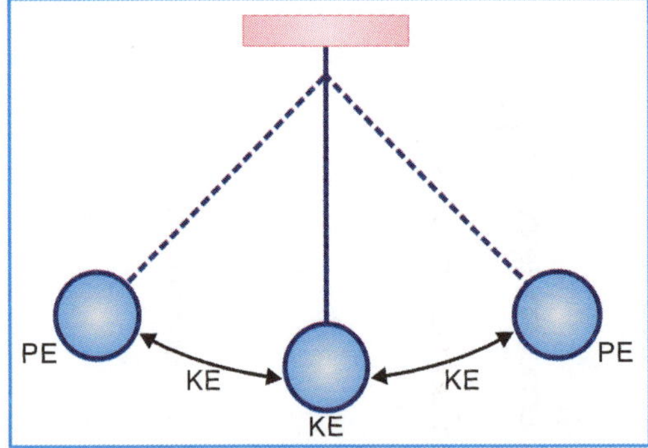


**Fig. 2.24:** Kinetic and potential energy.

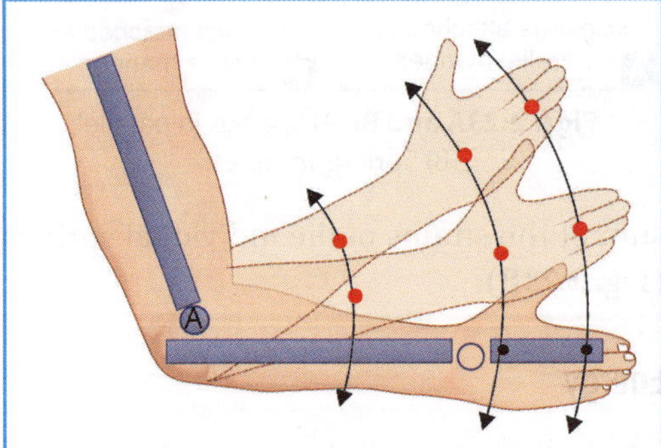


**Fig. 2.25:** Rotational motion.

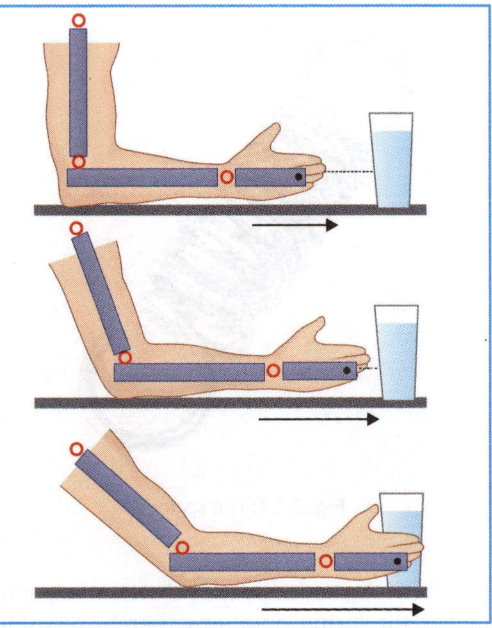

**Fig. 2.26:** Linear motion.

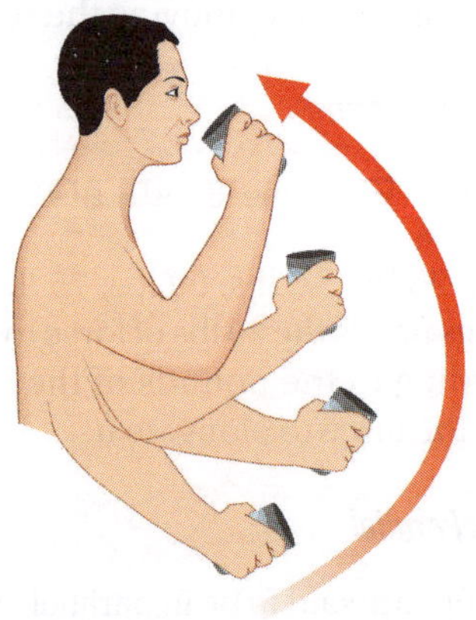

**Fig. 2.27:** Curvilinear motion.

## Types of Motion

### *Rotatory Motion (Fig. 2.25)*

- Rotation, or spin, is the circular movement of an object around a central axis. It is otherwisely called as angular motion. It is the motion of an object around a circular path, in a fixed orbit.
- Each segment moves through the same angle, same time at a constant distance from the axis. However, the rate of the angular motion/displacement may be constant (isokinetic) or variable,

### *Translatory Motion*

The motion in which all the particles of a body move through the same distance in the same time is called translatory motion. There are two types of translatory motions: linear motion; curvilinear motion.

In such a motion:

- Each segment or object moves in straight line.
- Each segment moves through same distance at the same time in parallel path. If the movement occurs in straight line is called as "linear motion" **(Fig. 2.26)**.
- If it occurs in curved pathway is called as "curvilinear motion" **(Fig. 2.27)**.

To perform osteokinematic movement there should be an axis and a plane.

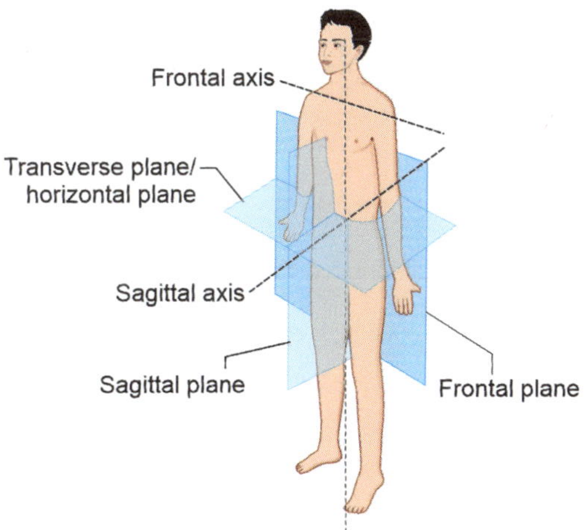


**Fig. 2.28:** The axes and planes of human body.

## Planes and Axes (Fig. 2.28)

Osteokinematic movements are produced in different planes around different axes.

### Plane

It is the surface which lies at right angles to axis and in which the movement take place. There are three types of planes.

#### Sagittal Plane

The sagittal plane lies vertically, passes through the sagittal suture and divides the body into right and left parts. Movement in this plane occurs around frontal axis **(Fig. 2.29)**. Flexion and extension movements of shoulder occur in sagittal plane, around the frontal axis.

#### Frontal/Coronal Plane

The frontal plane also lies vertically, passes through the coronal sutures and divides the body into anterior and posterior parts. Movement in this plane occurs around sagittal axis **(Fig. 2.30)**. Abduction and adduction movements of shoulder occur in the coronal/frontal plane around the sagittal axis.

#### Transverse Plane/Horizontal Plane

The transverse plane lies horizontally and divides the body into superior and inferior parts. Movement in this plane occurs around longitudinal/vertical axis **(Fig. 2.31)**. Medial

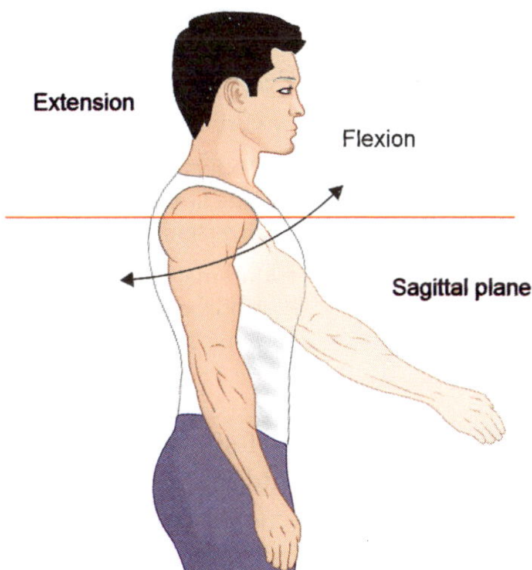


**Fig. 2.29:** Movement in sagittal plane.

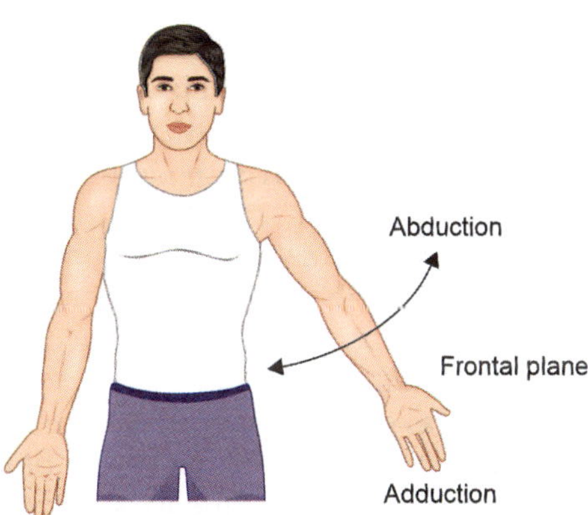


**Fig. 2.30:** Movement in frontal plane.

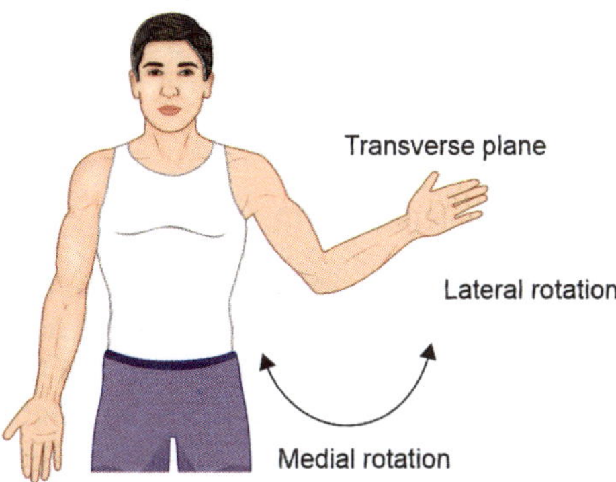


**Fig. 2.31:** Movement in transverse plane.

**TABLE 2.1:** Movements in different planes and axes.

| *Plane* | *Motion* | *Axis* |
|---|---|---|
| Sagittal | Flexion/extension | Frontal |
| Frontal | • Abduction/abduction<br>• Side flexion<br>• Inversion/eversion | Sagittal |
| Transverse | • Internal rotation/external rotation<br>• Horizontal adduction/abduction<br>• Supination/pronation | Vertical/longitudinal |

and lateral rotation of shoulder occurs in transverse plane around the vertical axis.

Examples of movements in different planes and axes are shown in **Table 2.1**.

### *Axes*

Axis is an imaginary line around which body rotates. Movements at a joint takes place in a plane about an axis. There are three axes of movement around which the body/body parts rotate. They are:

- **Sagittal axis:** This line runs from front to back through the center of the body. Movements around this axis occur in coronal/frontal plane.
- **Frontal axis:** This line runs from side to side through the center of the body. Movements around this axis occur in sagittal plane.
- **Vertical/longitudinal axis:** This line runs from top to bottom through the center of the body. Movements around this axis occur in transverse plane.

## Moment/Movement Arm

*Definition:* The moment arm, or the **distance from the axis of rotation**, is the perpendicular distance from the line of action of the force to the axis of rotation **(Fig. 2.32)**. By altering the moment arm, simple machines like a lever, pulley, gear, and most others produce mechanical advantage. In human body, the moment arm, i.e., distance between the line of action between the tendon of quadriceps, and knee axis, is the moment arm, which is maintained by the height of patella, produces mechanical advantage for the quadriceps to extend the knee. In surgeries, where the patella is removed (patellectomy), the moment arm significantly decreases, altering the mechanical advantage for quadriceps to cause knee extension (efficiency of quadriceps decreases), that results in quadriceps lag.

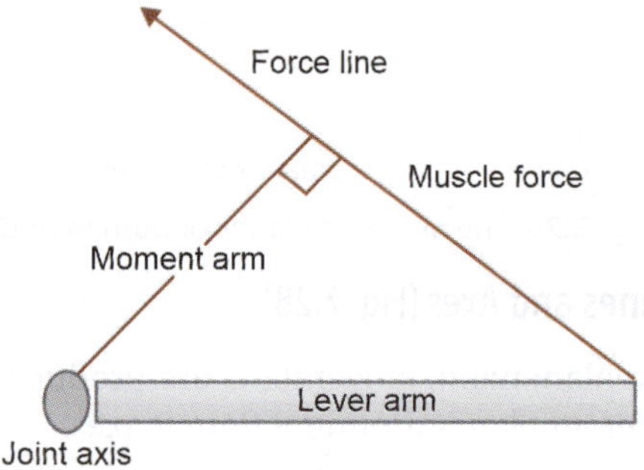


**Fig. 2.32:** The moment arm.

Rarely the movement arm comes in the line of the lever arm. Whenever the force is applied 90° to the lever arm, the perpendicular distance (the moment arm) is parallel to the lever arm (coinciding with the length of the lever arm, where the force acts) and is highest, than situations, where the force is not applied perpendicularly. In human joints most of the lines of forces are not perpendicular to the lever arm due to the muscular arrangement, so the movement (moment) arm will have the more short distance **(Figs. 2.33 and 2.34)**.

So, whenever the force is applied 90° to the lever arm, the movement arm coincides with the lever arm. If the line of force is applied 90° to

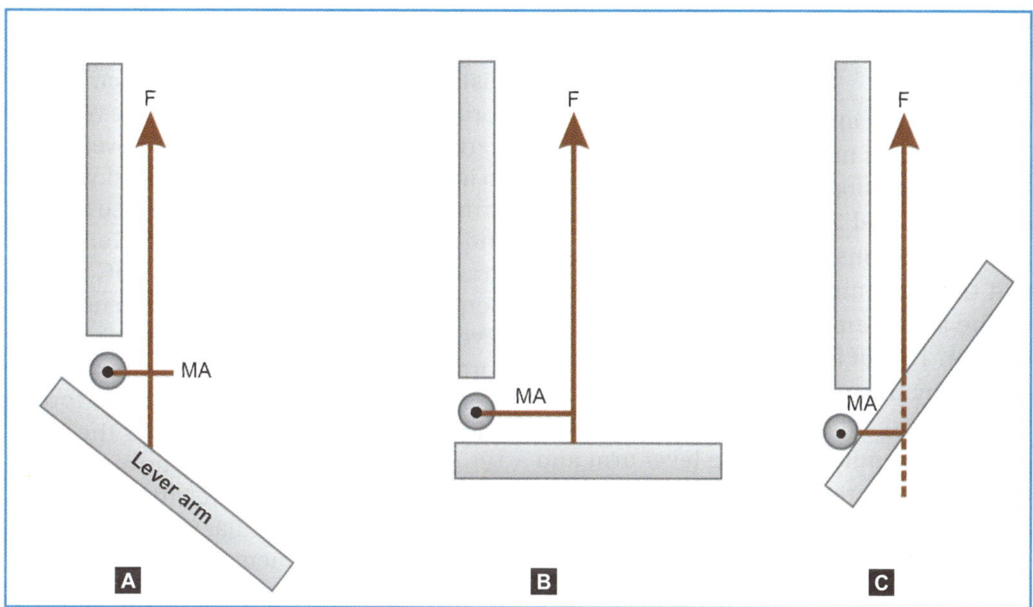


**Figs. 2.33A to C:** Hamstring exerting the force on the leg: (A) 45°; (B) 90°; (C) 125° flexion of knee.

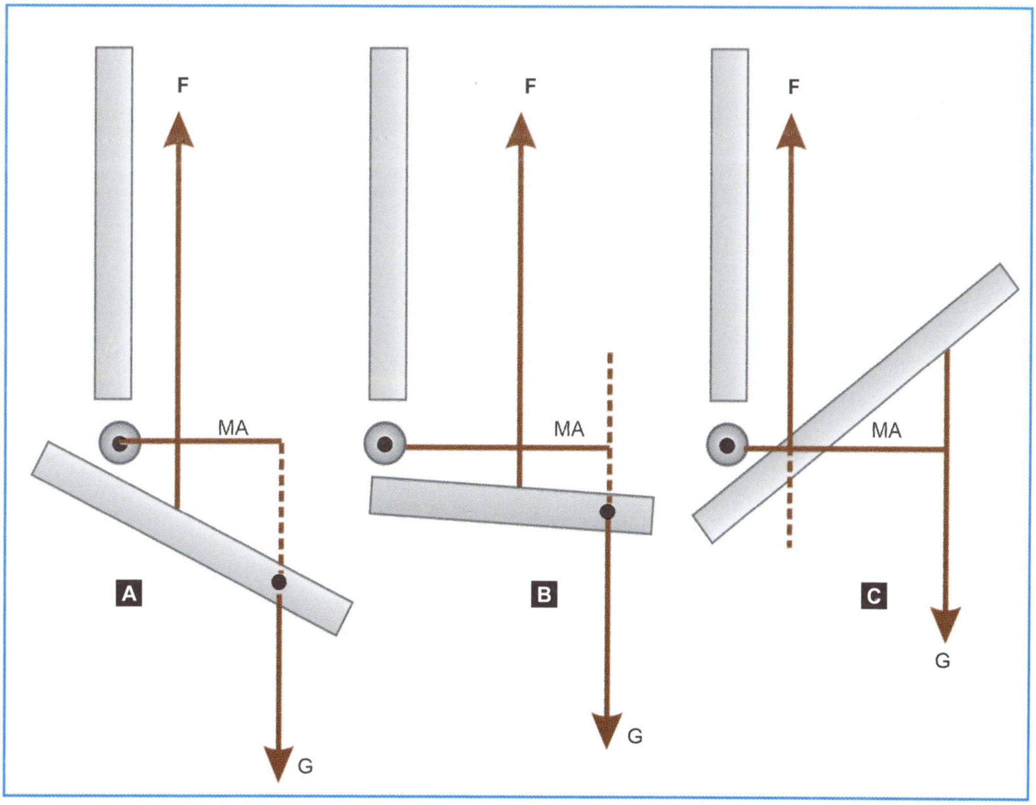

**Figs. 2.34A to C:** Movement arm in relation with gravitational force: (A) 45°; (B) 90°; (C) 125° flexion of knee.

the lever arm, the torque created in the muscle will be maximum.

$$T = f \times \perp d$$

$$\perp d = ma \text{ (moment arm)}$$

$$T = f \times ma \text{ (moment arm)}.$$

*For example:* During hamstring muscle action **(Figs. 2.33 and 2.34)**, generally, the lever arm will be constant and the line of force and the movement arm changes depend on the arrangement of the movement. In 45°, 90°, 125° of flexion of knee the torque created by the muscle will be more during 90°. Because whenever the line of force comes perpendicular to the lever arm and the movement arm distance will be more and also the movement arm coincides with the lever arm.

During 45° and 125°, i.e., below and above 90° of movement, the movement arm distance reduces and comes closer. So, the torque created in the muscle will be very less. Variation in the angulations of the lever results in increasing or decreasing of the movement arm. The application of the LOG also decides the moment arm of the lever. Generally, gravity acts vertically, so the LOG will be perpendicular to the lever arm. Whenever the lever is in 90° position the gravity exerts more torque on the lever. The muscular torque has to counteract the gravitational torque to generate the movement over the lever. Whenever the gravitational torque is less, i.e., during below or above 90° angulations, there will be less muscular torque needed to generate the movement on the lever.

# 3 CHAPTER

# Assessment, Examination and Evaluation of Neuro-musculoskeletal System

## INTRODUCTION

Management of patients with diseases and disorders involving various systems of the body and persons with disabilities, involves an interdisciplinary (involving many professionals in one campus) or multidisciplinary approach (involving professionals where services are not available in one campus, and patient is referred outside, if need arises). For effective management, the patient should be assessed by different professionals, and the problems of the patient/PWD need to be identified for deciding the treatment protocols after a thorough clinical reasoning. Besides, initial assessment, the client should be reassessed periodically to judge improvements of the condition.

### Assessment

Assessment is defined as a methodical way of acquiring, reviewing and using information about someone or something, so as to make improvement where necessary. It is a systematic process for measuring an individual's abilities based on collected data, received through examination.

### Examination

It involves both subjective examination (history of patient) to get qualitative data, and objective examination, where tests and measures are done for various systems to find quantitative data with a numerical value, showing the patient's impairments.

### Evaluation

It is an objective judgment of the skills and values of a person using well-defined criteria. It is one step away from standardized testing/examination helping to derive a working hypothesis. A good evaluation process should be valid, reliable, and practical.

### Documentation

It is the record of the patient's health status and medical condition, reflecting the patient's impairment data, care provided, the effect and continuity of care. Problem-oriented Medical Records (POMR), is a method of documentation, that records the healthcare status of the individual, the investigations performed and treatment planned.

### Problem-oriented Medical Record

Problem-oriented Medical Record (POMR), developed by Dr Lawrence Weed in late 1950s is a method of recording data, about the healthcare status of the patient in a problem-solving system, in an easily accessible way, that encourages ongoing assessment and revision of the healthcare plan. This approach provides the clinician a view of the patients' data as an orderly process to solve their problems, giving the opportunity to make explicit hypotheses and clinical decisions. The phases of POMR include:

### *Phase 1*

The formation of a database, including history, physical examination and laboratory and other test results.

### *Phase 2*

Identification of a specific problem list from the interpretation of the database, including specific impairment of function (physical, psychological, social and vocational) resulting from the disease process or from secondary impairments.

### *Phase 3*

Identification of a specific plan of care (POC) that includes interventions for each of the problems described; evaluative and progress notes are included for each problem.

### *Phase 4*

Determination of the effectiveness of the plan of care (POC) and subsequent changes as a result of patient progress.

SOAP, an acronym for subjective, objective, assessment plan, originates from POMR, for documenting the daily progress notes of the patient. SOAP notes are a highly structured format for documenting the progress of a patient during treatment and is only one of many possible formats that could be used by a health professional. They are entered in the patient's medical record by healthcare professionals to communicate information to other providers of care, to provide evidence of patient contact and to inform the clinical reasoning process. The four components of SOAP are:

1. **Subjective:** Where a client's subjective experiences, feelings, or perspectives are recorded. This might include subjective information from a patient's guardian or someone else involved in their care.
2. **Objective:** For a more complete overview of a client's health or mental status, objective information in the form of ROM, outcome measures of tests performed, etc., must also be recorded. This section records substantive data, such as facts and details from the therapy session.
3. **Assessment:** This involves, the clinician/therapist's analysis of various components of subjective and objective data.
4. **Plan:** This outlines the future actions for the patient. It talks about development of a best treatment strategy to reach the goals/objectives.

### *Procedure of Assessment of Neuromuscular System*

It consists of the followings:

**Demographic Data**

Name, age, gender, address.

**Subjective Examination**

- **History of present illness:** How and when the present problem started.
- **Past history:** History of past injury/illness, relevant to the current problems.
- **Family history:** Family structure (nuclear/joint family), family's support system, genetic inheritance (if any).
- **Personal history:** Educational qualification, occupation, marital status, number of children (if married), dietary habits, addictions of tobacco/alcohol, etc.
- **Socio-economic history:** Lives in urban/rural areas, family's monthly/annual income.
- **Functional history:** Information about patient's functional abilities/limitations.

**Objective Examination**

- Observation of posture and movements
- **Higher function examination:** Level of consciousness, speech, hearing, vision, memory, intelligence, orientation, concentration.
- Cranial nerve involvement (if any) **(Table 3.1)**.

**Table 3.1:** Clinical examination of cranial nerves.

| *Nerve number* | *Nerve name* | *Functional loss* | *Testing procedure* |
|---|---|---|---|
| 1st | Olfactory | Smell | A small amount of oil of peppermint and oil of cloves are taken in two small test tubes. The tubes are brought near each nostril separately, one after the other.<br>The patient is asked, if he can identify the smell or not. Inability to identify the smell, indicates injury to 1st cranial nerve, resulting in anosmia |
| 2nd | Optic | Visual acuity and visual field | Visual acuity is tested using a Snellen Eye Chart placed 20 feet away from the patient, making the patient read letters of various sizes. It must, of course, be remembered that loss of acuity of vision can be caused by errors of refraction, or by the presence of opacities in the cornea or the lens (cataract). Visual fields are tested by direct confrontation (the confrontation test). Each eye is tested individually, with the other eye covered **(Fig. 3.1)**. The examiner stands/sits 3 feet away from the patient, and the patient focuses on the examiner's eyes or nose. A pen or a finger is moved toward the center of the visual field in all four quadrants, and the patient will indicate when they can see the object. Alternatively, a select number of fingers are held up in a quadrant and have the patient identify how many fingers they see. This is repeated for all quadrants.<br>If an abnormality is detected, confirmation should be done through perimetry |
| 3rd | Oculomotor | Opening of eyelid affected, eyeball movement limitation causing double vision, as the affected eye turns slightly downward and outward and the unaffected eye looks straight. The affected eye may turn inward very slowly and may move only to the middle when looking inward. It cannot move up and down | The 3rd nerve has two major components, the outer parasympathetic fibers that supply the ciliary muscles and the sphincter pupillae, and the inner somatic fibers supply the levator palpebrae superioris in the eyelid (which retracts the upper eyelid) and the four extraocular muscles (superior, middle, inferior recti, and inferior oblique). In oculomotor nerve palsy, the involved eye would deviate downward and laterally at rest with ptosis. This nerve is tested by checking pupillary constriction and eyeball movement in upward/medial, upward/lateral, medial and downward/lateral direction. The pupillary light reflex is tested by shining a light into each eye and observing the pupil response. Ocular movements are tested by holding a pen or finger 30 to 40 cm in front of the patient and moving in an H-shaped pattern pausing during vertical and lateral gaze. The patient should follow the target with their eyes, carefully keeping their head still. The eyeball move normally 50° outwards, 50° inwards, 33° upwards, and 50° downwards. Limitations of movement of eyeball upwards (levator palpebrae superioris, superior rectus muscle), medial (medial rectus muscle), downwards (inferior rectus muscle) indicate 3rd nerve palsy |
| 4th | Trochlear | Intorsion (Internal rotation), depression, and abduction of the eyeball will be impaired | The trochlear nerve innervates the superior oblique muscle. Patients with trochlear nerve palsy often tilt their heads away from the affected eye and may have strabismus. It is tested in the same manner like oculomotor nerve, and any impairment of eyeball movement in the downward and outward direction suggests injury to this nerve. The dysfunction is usually incomplete as the oculomotor and abducens nerves also depress and abduct the eye |

*Contd...*

*Contd...*

| *Nerve number* | *Nerve name* | *Functional loss* | *Testing procedure* |
|---|---|---|---|
| 5th | Trigeminal | Sensation of face and posterior 1/3rd of tongue and chewing movements will be impaired | ***Motor Functions***<br>Motor function of the trigeminal nerve is tested by having the patient open their mouth against resistance. If weakness is present, the jaw will deviate to the side of weakness/paralysis, the healthy lateral pterygoid muscles pushing it to that side.<br>With the patient's teeth clenched, palpation of the masseter and temporal muscles, revealing reduced prominence on the affected side, showing asymmetry of face, indicate lesion to trigeminal nerve.<br>***Sensory Functions***<br>Testing for impairment of sensations for touch, pain and temperature over the entire face and over posterior one-third of the tongue reveals lesion to this nerve. Testing of the corneal reflexes on both sides and finding it is loss on one side, reveals injury to the 5th nerve. The sensation of the angle of the mandible should be tested if the facial sensation is diminished, as the C2 spinal root innervates this area. Sparing of the angle of the jaw is indicative of trigeminal pathology |
| 6th | Abducens | Impairment of movement of eyeball (laterally) | Abducens nerve innervates the lateral rectus muscle. It is tested in the same manner, such as oculomotor nerve, and any impairment of eyeball movement in the lateral direction suggests injury to this nerve |
| 7th | Facial | Facial muscle movements (except chewing) and closing of eyelids will be affected, causing ipsilateral facial palsy. Impairment of taste sensation over anterior 2/3rd of tongue | The facial nerve supplies the muscles of the face including the muscles that close the eyelids, and the mouth. The nerve is tested as follows:<br>The patient is asked to close his eyes firmly. In complete paralysis of the facial nerve, the patient will not be able to close the eye on the affected side. In partial paralysis, the closure is weak.<br>The person is asked to smile. In smiling, the normal mouth is more or less symmetrical, the two angles moving upwards and outwards. In facial paralysis, the angle fails to move on the paralyzed side.<br>The patient is asked to fill his/mouth with air. The clinician presses the cheek of the patient with the fingers and compare the resistance (offered by the buccinator muscle) on the two sides. The resistance is less on the paralyzed side. On pressing the cheek air may leak out of the mouth because the muscles closing the mouth are weak.<br>The sensation of taste should be tested on the anterior two-thirds of the tongue.<br>To evaluate taste, the patient is asked to stick out the tongue and close the eyes. A small amount of salt (for salty), quinine hydrochloride or caffeine strips (for bitter), tartaric acid (for sour), or sugar (for sweet) are applied to the lateral surface and side of the anterior tongue, then have the patient identify the substance |

*Contd...*

*Contd...*

| *Nerve number* | *Nerve name* | *Functional loss* | *Testing procedure* |
|---|---|---|---|
| 8th | Auditory (Vestibulocochlear) | Impairment of hearing and balance | This nerve is responsible for hearing (cochlear part) and for equilibrium (vestibular part).<br>Initial hearing testing is conducted by rubbing the fingers/ whispering close to one ear while occluding the other, then repeating for the other ear. Any asymmetry in response or hearing should be noted. Further evaluation using the Rinne and Weber tests is warranted if hearing loss is suspected, which helps to distinguish conductive from sensorineural hearing loss.<br>The Rinne test is performed by placing a vibrating 512-hertz tuning fork on the mastoid process, and once the sound is no longer heard, moving the fork to just outside the ear. In a normal (positive) Rinne test, air conduction is greater than bone conduction. In an abnormal (negative) Rinne test, bone conduction is greater than air conduction in the affected ear. A patient with profound sensorineural hearing loss may not hear anything from the tuning fork placed on the mastoid process or near the external auditory canal.<br>The Weber test is performed by placing a vibrating 512-hertz tuning fork on the center of the forehead. Sound is louder in, or "lateralizes to," the ear experiencing conductive hearing loss or opposite the ear with sensorineural hearing loss.<br>To assess vestibular function, testing for nystagmus is made and the direction, duration, and trigger of the nystagmus are noted. Note should be made for the patient experiencing vertigo during examination |
| 9th | Glossopharyngeal nerve | Taste sensation from posterior 1/3rd of tongue, may be affected. Unilateral damage to the glossopharyngeal nerve results in the absence of a gag response when that side of the pharynx is stimulated and poses difficulty in swallowing | Sensations of taste can be tested by applying substances that are salty (salt), sweet (sugar), sour (lemon), or bitter (quinine) to the posterior one-third of the tongue. The mouth should be rinsed and the tongue dried before the substance is applied.<br>The client is instructed to say "ah" and yawn to observe upward movement of the soft palate. The gag reflex should also be tested. Difficulty in swallowing and impaired gag reflex indicates damage to this nerve<br>The gag reflex, also known as the pharyngeal reflex, is an involuntary reflex involving bilateral pharyngeal muscle contraction and elevation of the soft palate on touching the palatal arches with cotton swab. If the glossopharyngeal nerve is damaged on one side, there will be no response when touched (unilateral absence of gag reflex) |
| 10th | Vagus | Sensation to larynx, motor function to soft palate, pharynx, larynx, and esophagus may be affected, causing difficulty in swallowing | The patient is asked to open the mouth wide and say 'aah'. The clinician observes the movement of the soft palate. In a normal person, the soft palate is elevated. When one vagus nerve is paralyzed the palate is pulled towards the normal side. When the nerve is paralyzed on both sides the soft palate does not move at all. The gag reflex may be absent. There is also hoarseness of voice, due to injury to superior laryngeal nerve (causing temporary hoarseness) and recurrent laryngeal nerve (causing permanent hoarseness) |

*Contd...*

*Contd...*

| *Nerve number* | *Nerve name* | *Functional loss* | *Testing procedure* |
|---|---|---|---|
| 11th | Accessory | Shrugging of shoulder, lateral flexion of neck to the tested side and rotation to the opposite side is weak/impaired | The clinician puts his/her hands on the right and left shoulders of the patient and ask him to elevate (shrug) the shoulders. In injury to this nerve, the movement will be weak/impaired. Testing the power of sternocleidomastoid also reveals impairment (if any) of functioning of this nerve |
| 12th | Hypoglossal | Impairment of movement of tongue | To test the nerve, the patient is asked to protrude the tongue. In a normal person, the protruded tongue lies in the midline. Atrophy, fasciculations, and deviation of the tongue in the direction of the lesion are associated with lower motor neuron pathology. The tongue deviates away from the lesion with upper motor neuron pathology, and there will not be atrophy or fasciculations |

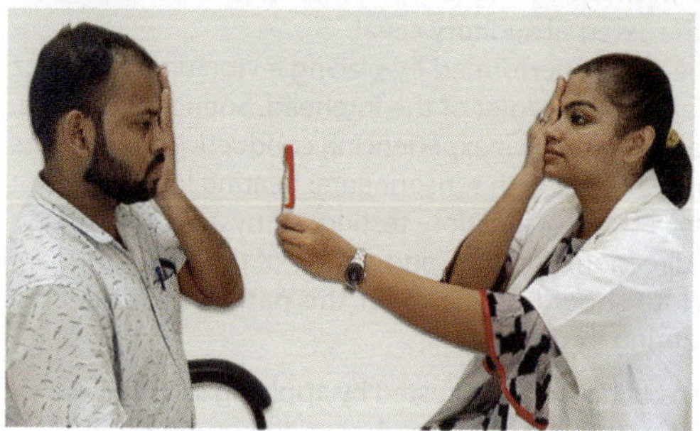

**Fig. 3.1:** The confrontation test.

### Sensory System Examination

Sensations may be classified into categories by various methods dependent on anatomic or functional criteria. An anatomic classification divides sensory function into:

1. Somatic sensation
2. Visceral sensation

However, clinically, only somatic sensation can be tested and documented.

One functional classification separates sensory modalities into simple affective sensations, termed protopathic, and sensations that provide discriminative analysis with regard to the environment, termed epicritic.

*The Epicritic Sensation/System*

It is concerned with touch discrimination and small changes in temperature. Epicritic neurons detect gentle touch, such as light vibrations; the ability to recognize the shape of an object being held (stereognosis), tactile localization, tactile discrimination, two-point discrimination, etc. Example: Fine touch, vibration, stereognosis.

*Protopathic Sensation/System*

It is primitive and concerned with diffuse pain, extremes of temperature, etc. It is the sensibility to strong stimulations of pain and temperature. It is low in degree and poorly localized, existing in the skin and in the viscera, and acting as a defensive agency against pathologic changes in the tissues. Example: Pain, pressure and temperature sensation.

A more practical classification that utilizes both anatomic criteria including the types and locations of end organs and functional criteria, classify sensory modalities into:

- **Exteroceptive sensation**
- **Proprioceptive sensation**
- **Cortical sensation**

*Exteroceptive Sensation (also Termed Superficial Sensation)*

Receptors are present in the skin and mucous membranes. These include:

- **Tactile or touch sensation (thigmesthesia):** Impairments could be:
  - *Anesthesia:* Absence of touch appreciation.

- *Hypoesthesia:* Decrease of touch appreciation.
- *Hyperesthesia:* Exaggeration of touch sensation.

❖ **Pain sensation (algesia): Impairments could be:**
- *Analgesia:* Absence of pain appreciation.
- *Hypoalgesia:* Decrease of pain appreciation.
- *Hyperalgesia:* Exaggeration of pain appreciation, which is often unpleasant.

❖ **Temperature sensation—both hot and cold (thermesthesia): Impairments could be:**
- *Thermanalgesia:* Absence of temperature appreciation
- *Thermhypesthesia:* Decrease of temperature appreciation
- *Thermhyperesthesia:* Exaggeration of temperature sensation.

**Sensory perversions:** In patients with sensory perversions, the sensory system is disordered; sensations may be diminished, increased, or distorted. These include:

❖ **Hyperpathia:** Indicates a lowered threshold for painful sensation.

❖ **Paresthesias:** Abnormal sensations perceived without specific stimulation. They may be tactile, thermal or painful and are either episodic or constant.

❖ **Dysesthesia:** Painful sensations, such as intense burning, elicited by a nonpainful cutaneous stimulus, such as a light touch or gentle stroking over affected areas of the body. Sometimes referred to as hyperpathia or hyperalgesia.

❖ **Allodynia:** Painful response to non-painful stimulus.

*Proprioceptive Sensation (also Termed Deep Sensation)*

Receptors are located in muscles, tendons, ligaments and joints. These include:

❖ **Joint position sense at rest/Proprioception (Arthresthesia)**

❖ Vibratory sense (Pallesthesia)

❖ **Kinesthesia:** Perception of motion

*Cortical Sensation*

Interpretative sensory functions that require analysis of individual sensory modalities by the parietal lobes to provide discrimination. The different sensory modalities are:

❖ **Stereognosis:** Ability to recognize and identify objects by feeling them. The absence of this ability is termed astereognosis.

❖ **Graphesthesia:** Ability to recognize symbols written on the skin. The absence of this ability is termed Agraphesthesia.

❖ **Two-point discrimination:** Ability to recognize simultaneous stimulation by two blunt points. Measured by the distance between the points required for recognition.

❖ **Touch localization (topognosis):** Ability to localize stimuli to parts of the body. Topagnosia is the absence of this ability.

❖ **Double simultaneous stimulation:** Ability to perceive a sensory stimulus when corresponding areas on the opposite side of the body are stimulated simultaneously. Loss of this ability is termed sensory extinction.

Before sensory examination, the clinician should be thorough about the dermatomes and sensory distribution of the peripheral nerves.

The dermatomes (areas of the skin whose sensory distribution is innervated by the afferent nerve fibers from the dorsal root of a specific single spinal nerve root,) of the upper limb, lower limb and trunk are shown in the following figures **(Figs. 3.2A to C)**.

For the sensory testing of a particular peripheral nerve, recording should be made on body chart **(Figs. 3.3A to C)**. The cutaneous distribution of nerves of upper limb and lower limb are shown in **Figures 3.4A to D**. Depending upon, the sensory impairment noted, body chart diagram showing the affected part should be drawn and sensory

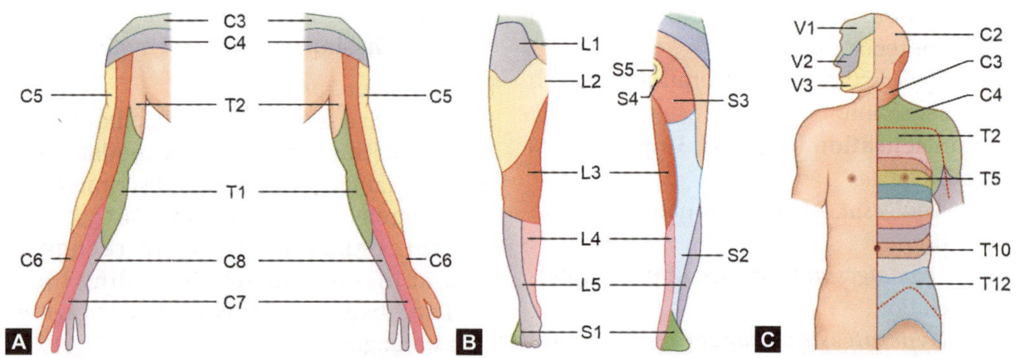


**Figs. 3.2A to C:** (A) Dermatomes of upper limb; (B) Dermatomes of lower limb; (C) Dermatomes of trunk.

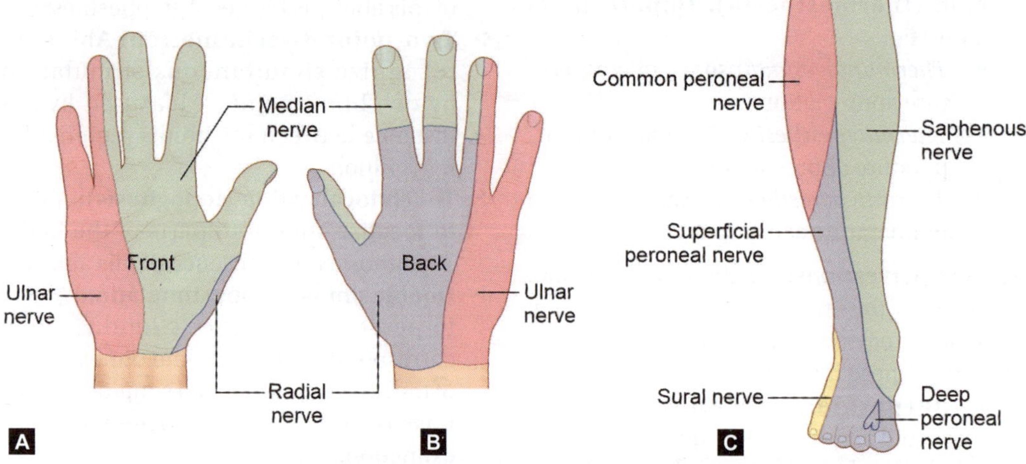


**Figs 3.3A to C:** (A and B) Body chart showing sensory supply of ulnar/median/radial nerve in hand; (C) Body chart showing the sensory distribution in the front of leg.

impairments in the form of "absent", "reduced", "normal" should be indicated symbolically.

### *Instruments Required for Sensory Testing*

The test requires instruments, such as cotton wisp, Neurotip pins, test tubes containing hot and cold water, 128 Hz tuning fork.

### *Grading of Sensory Impairments*

Sensation can be graded using 0–10 scale, such as VAS, where 0-Complete anesthesia, 10-Normal sensation. However, using ASIA, grading system, sensation can be graded using **Table 3.2.**

### *Methods of Testing of Different Sensations*

Before sensory testing, informed consent should be obtained from the patient/caregiver. The area to be tested, should be properly exposed, taking due precaution to maintain privacy of the individual. The methods of assessment are:

#### Light Touch

A wisp of cotton wool or fine brush is gently tapped over the manubrium or the vertex of skull or any other intact area as a reference point for normal feeling. The patient is asked to close the eyes, to eliminate the possibility

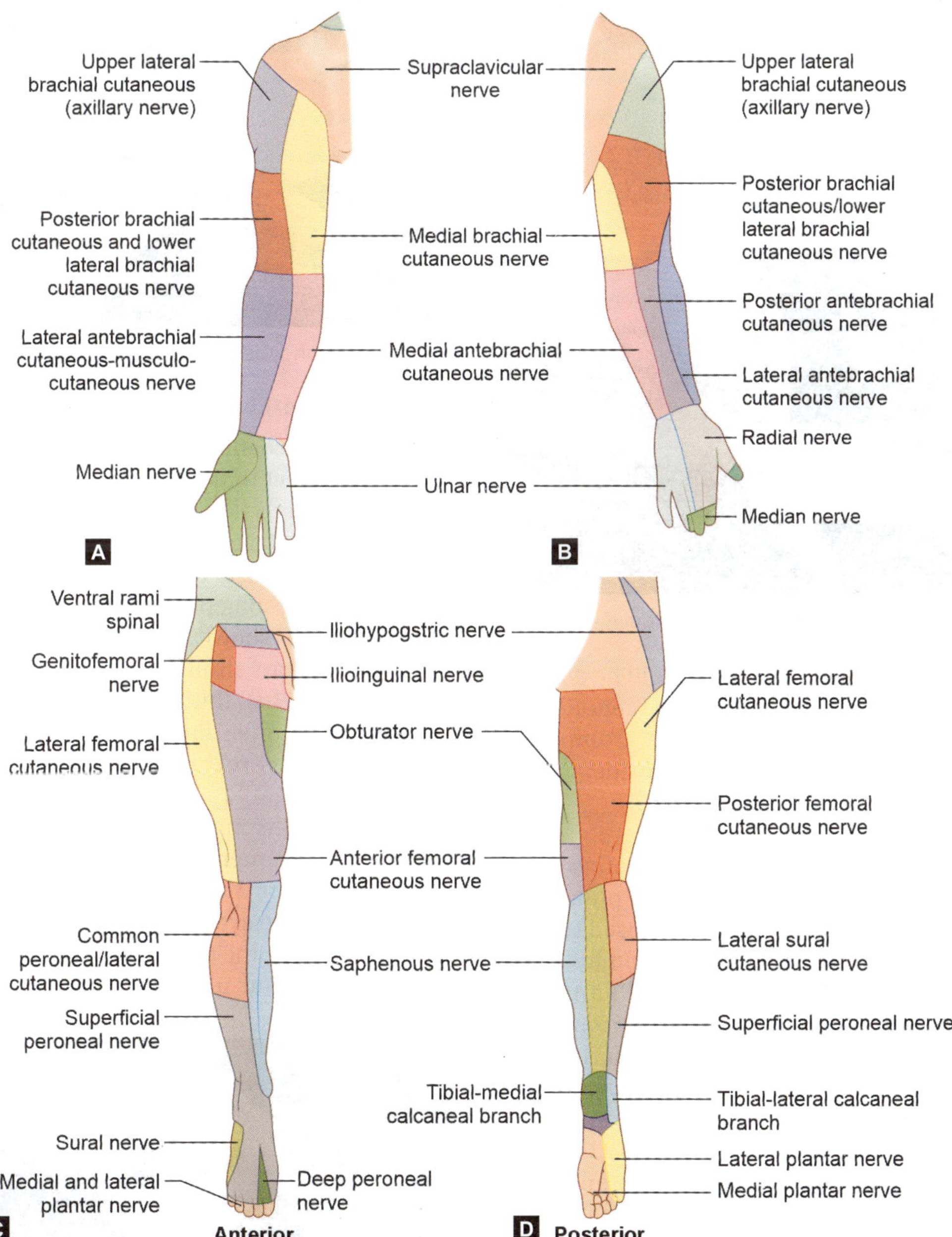


**Figs. 3.4A to D:** (A) Cutaneous/sensory distribution on front of upper limb; (B) Cutaneous/sensory distribution on back of upper limb; (C) Cutaneous/sensory distribution on front of lower limb; (D) Cutaneous/sensory distribution on back of lower limb.

of wrong information given due to visual substitution and respond when the stimulus is detected. The stimuli are then applied to dermatomal area/cutaneous supply zones of nerves **(Fig. 3.5)**, with random application and withholding, to get correct response

**Table 3.2:** Shows grading of sensation.

| *Grade* | *Criteria* |
|---|---|
| 0 | Absent |
| 1 | Altered |
| 2 | Normal |
| NT | Not testable |

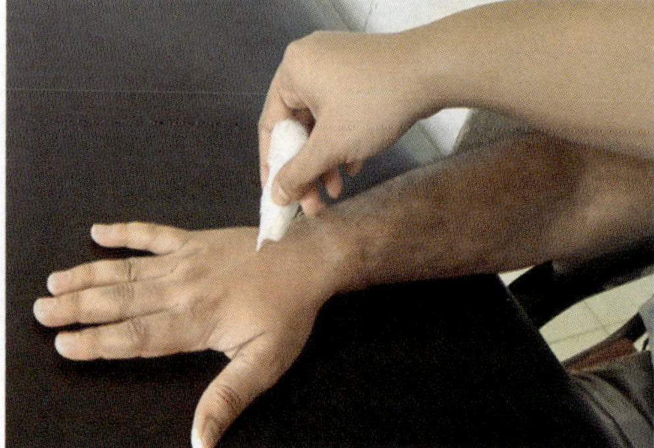

**Fig. 3.5:** Testing light touch.

from the patient. The test should be done in a caudocranial direction, and the cotton should not be dragged over the skin. Comparison should be done with the sound side.

### Pain

Neurological pins, such a Neurotips (single use neurological examination pins)/blunt end of percussion hammer are used to assess superficial pain. A reference stimulus should be established as was explained for the light touch stimulus using both the sharp and blunt end of the test instrument. The dermatomes should be assessed in an ascending manner, i.e., in distal to proximal direction and always a constant pressure is applied **(Fig. 3.6)**. Alternation between the sharp end of the neurological pin and the blunt end should be made randomly while testing. Patients with impaired superficial pain sensation will report the stimulus as being dull or not feeling it at all.

### Temperature

Both hot and cold test tubes are used randomly to find hot and cold sensitivity.

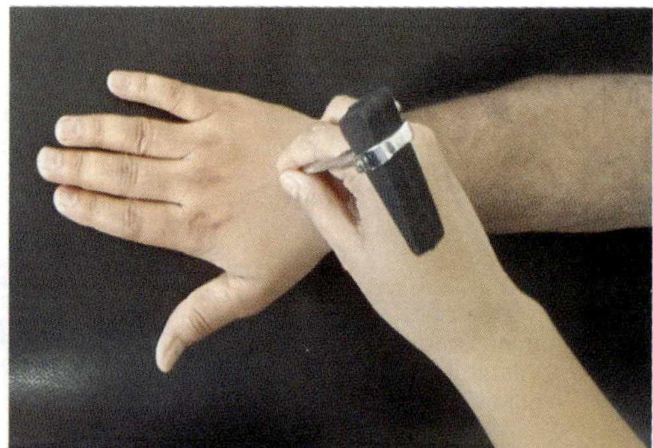

**Fig. 3.6:** Testing the superficial pain sensation.

### Proprioception/kinesthesia

The ability to recognize the location of a body part with respect to the environment (when the joint is at rest) is known as proprioception. This sensory modality is assessed by testing the joint position sense of the patient at rest. The procedure for testing proprioception for PIP joint of fingers is shown below.

The clinician should hold the DIP of patient's great toe/thumb/finger, between the thumb and index finger of left hand and gently holds the proximal phalanx with the right hand. Small amplitude movements using left hand is made to demonstrate up and down movements with the eyes open **(Fig. 3.7)**. Then the same procedure is repeated with the eyes closed. The patient is asked to indicate the position of the moving segment (whether placed up or down for

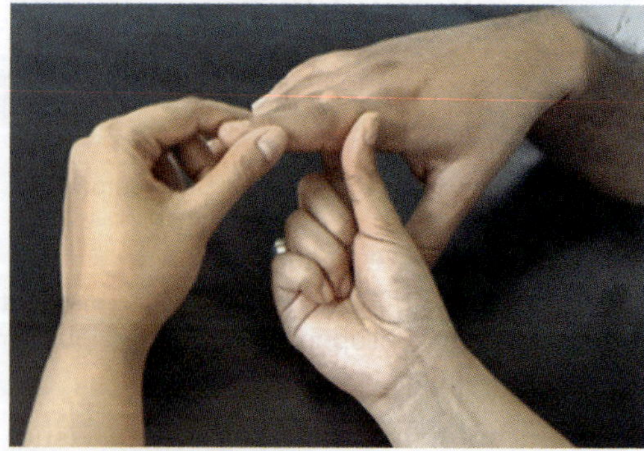

**Fig. 3.7:** Testing proprioception/kinesthesia of PIP joint of index finger.

proprioception and moving up and down for kinesthesia). If the patient fails to tell the joint position at rest/in motion, the amplitude of movement is increased to find the response. If no response is found in the distal joint testing of the proximal joints should be made in the following order.

The order of testing of proprioception/kinesthesia:

**Upper limb:** DIP → PIP → MCP → Wrist → Elbow → Shoulder

**Lower limb:** DIP → PIP → MTP → Ankle → Knee → Hip

### Vibration

Tested using a 128 Hz tuning fork. To initiate the test, the clinician strikes the prongs of the tuning fork against his/her thenar eminence of the hand to initiate vibration. By holding the tuning fork at the stem (not at the prongs), a reference stimulus is established by placing the foot piece of the vibrating tuning fork at the vertex of the head or the manubrium of the patient. Subsequently, the prongs are struck against the hand to restart the vibrations **(Fig. 3.8A)** and the foot piece of the vibrating tuning fork is placed on the most distal bony prominence (e.g., IP joint of great toe) with the patient's eyes closed **(Fig. 3.8B)**. The patient should be able to tell when he/she first noted the stimulus and when it stopped. If the patient is able to identify and characterize the stimulus at the most distal point, then there is no need to move to the next bony prominence. However, if he is unable to identify the stimulus, then the next bony prominence (i.e., the metatarsophalangeal joint of the great toe, medial malleolus, tibial tuberosity, anterior superior iliac spine) is tested in the ascending manner. The same procedure should be followed for the upper limbs.

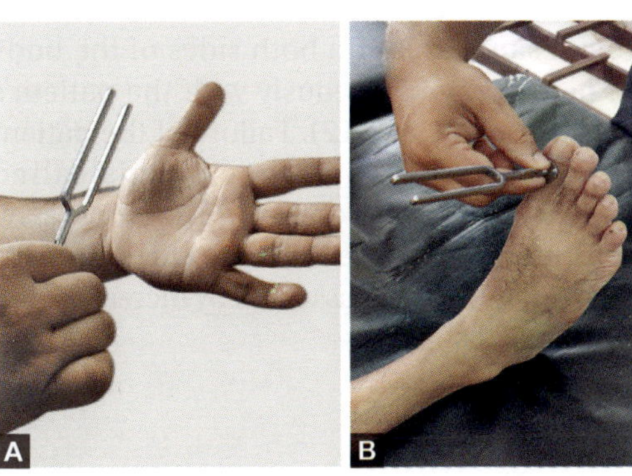

**Figs. 3.8A and B:** (A) Vibrating the tuning fork; (B) Testing vibration sensation on great toe.

## Cortical Sensation

Cortical sensation does not need to be assessed routinely. It is not necessary to test cortical sensation in patients with spinal cord or peripheral nerve lesions. If the patient's symptoms are due to lesion to right hemisphere, examination of cortical sensation may be helpful. The cortical sensory modalities, include tactile discrimination (graphesthesia, stereognosis, two point discrimination, extinction), tactile localization, barognosis.

## Graphesthesia

Graphesthesia refers to the ability to detect the tracing of letters or numbers on the skin just by feeling it (i.e., without visual input). It is assessed by using a blunt object to make tracings of letters or numbers on the palms of the patient while their eyes are closed **(Fig. 3.9)**. The patient should be able to tell the examiner what letter or number was outlined if this modality is intact.

### *Stereognosis*

Stereognosis (also known as haptic perception or tactile gnosis) is the ability to perceive and recognize the form of an object in the absence of visual and auditory information. It is tested by asking the patient to close the eyes, and placing a relatively common object like a pen, coin or a key **(Fig. 3.10)** in his palm. With stereognosis intact, the patient should be able to identify the object without trouble.

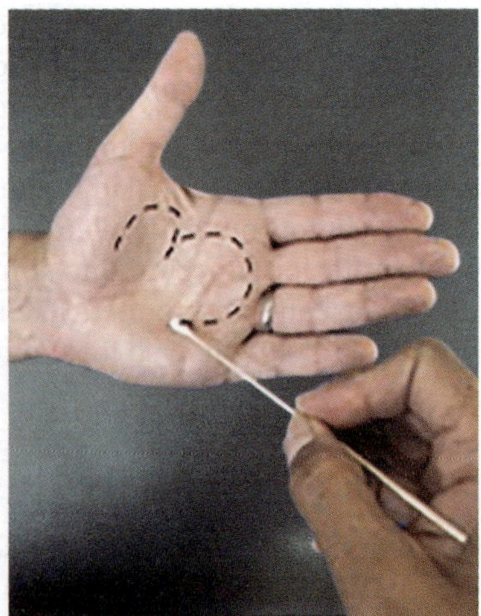

**Fig. 3.9:** Tests for graphesthesia.

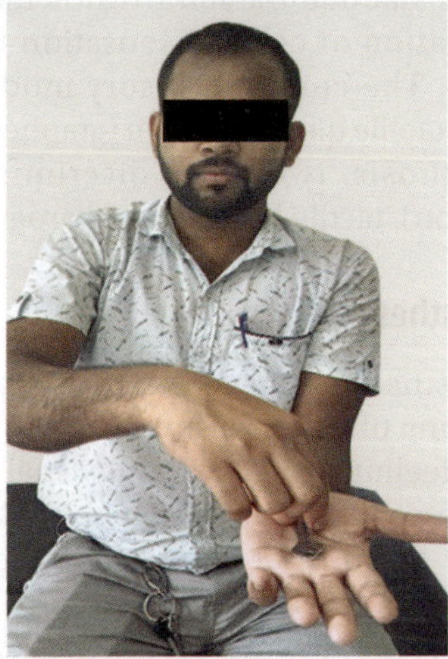

**Fig. 3.10:** Test for stereognosis.

### *Two Point Discrimination*

The two-point discrimination test is used to assess if the patient is able to identify two close points on a small area of skin. It is the most sensitivity test for cortical sensory impairment. It is a measure of tactile agnosia, or the inability to recognize these two points despite intact cutaneous sensation and proprioception. The examiner uses a paper clip, two-point discriminator, or calipers to apply pressure on two adjacent points in longitudinal direction and perpendicular to the long axis of the finger/body part **(Fig. 3.11)**. The distance between the two points are gradually reduced, till the patient begins to commit error. The minimal distance, between the two points, where two points are perceived separately, and beyond which the two points are perceived as 1, is noted and compared with the normal values.

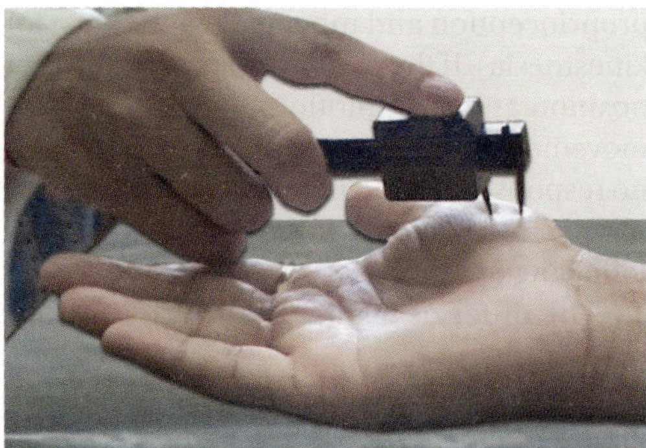

**Fig. 3.11:** 2-point discrimination test on palm of hand.

- Normal values of two point discrimination:
  - *Finger tips:* 2–8 mm
  - *Lips:* 2–4 mm
  - *Palm:* 8–12 mm
  - *Back of hand:* 20–30 mm
  - *Dorsum of foot:* 30–40 mm

### *Extinction*

To test for extinction, the examiner should touch same areas on both sides of the body of patient simultaneously with the patient's eyes closed **(Fig. 3.12)**. Failure of the patient to perceive touch on one side is called the extinction phenomenon. Normally, sensation is perceived on both sides. Severity of extinction can be assessed by increasing the intensity of stimulus.

### *Barognosis*

It is a test for tactile perception of weight. To test for intact barognosis, a set of small objects

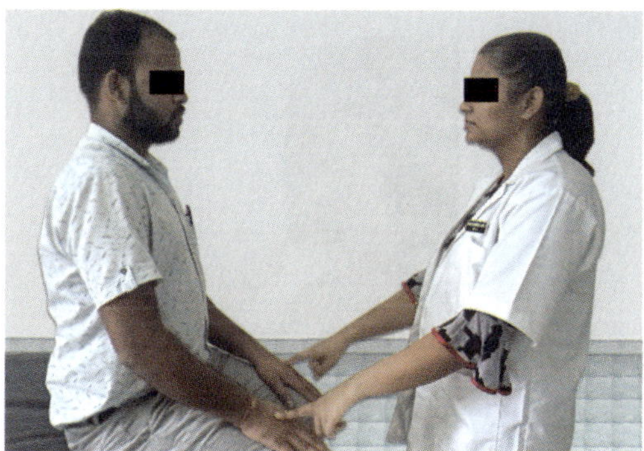

**Fig. 3.12:** Test for extinction.

with same size and shape, but differing in weight are placed one at a time in the same hand of the patient, sitting with the eyes closed. He/she is asked to identify the comparative weight of the objects, by saying, whether the object is heavy or light.

### *Tactile Localization (Topognosis)*

It is the ability to localize stimuli to parts of the body. Topagnosia is the absence of this ability. It is tested by asking the patient to point with his index finger to the point touched by the examiner.

#### Motor System Examination:

The clinical examination of the motor system consists of the following identities. It is as follows.

### *Bulk of Muscles*

The state of nutrition is examined by inspection and palpation of various muscles, and comparing these on the two sides. In muscular atrophy, the muscle mass decreases and the muscle gives a soft and flabby feeling. Atrophy may be general, following a prolonged illness. Physical exercise increases the bulk (hypertrophy) of the muscles. In some diseases of the muscles (dystrophies), the muscle mass increases (pseudohypertrophy), but these bulky muscles are weak despite their size. Calf and buttock muscles are especially involved.

#### Measurement of Muscle Bulk

The muscular weakness or the atrophy leads to the reduction of the muscle bulk. To measure the muscle bulk, the bulky area is selected. In general, muscle bulk measurements for lower limbs are done for the quadriceps and calf muscles, and for upper limbs, bulks of arm (biceps/triceps), and forearm (brachioradialis) are measured.

#### Quadriceps Muscle Bulk

From the base of the patella three points are marked in the bulky area with a difference of 2 or 3 inches. The circumference is measured from all the three marked areas by the inch tape. The difference is compared with the normal side limb **(Fig. 3.13)**.

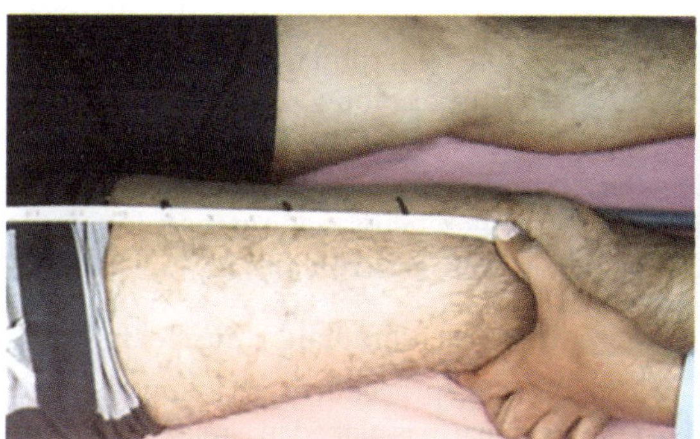

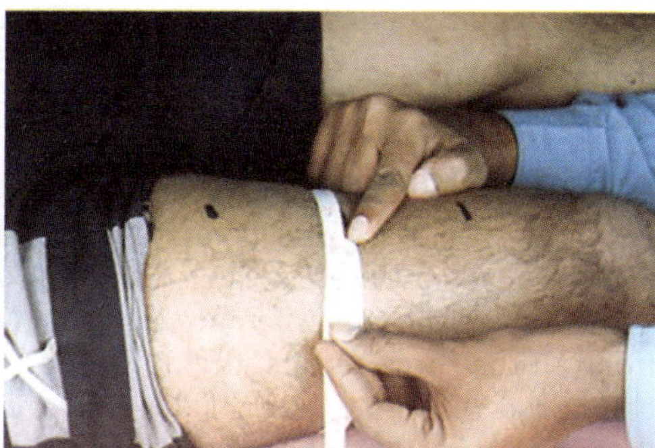

**Fig. 3.13:** Measurements of quadriceps muscle bulk with inch tape.

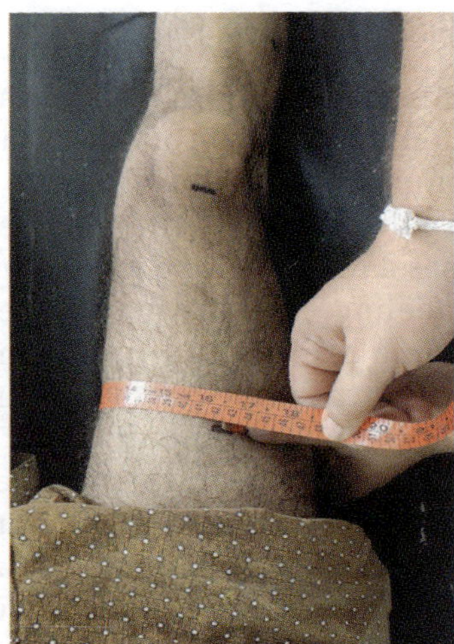

**Fig. 3.14:** Measurement of quadriceps bulk 15 cm from superior pole of patella.

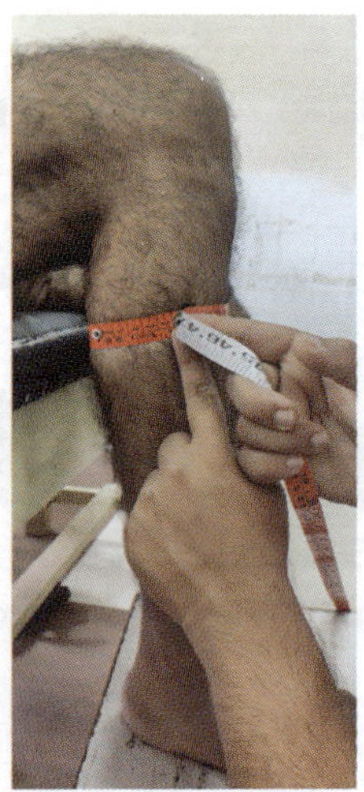

**Fig. 3.15:** Measurement of calf circumference.

However, the quickest method to measure the thigh circumference is followed as described under **(Fig. 3.14)**.

- The thigh area is maximally undressed.
- Markings are made on superior pole of patella and on the mid thigh region (at a distance of 15 cm from the superior pole of patella).
- Measurement of thigh circumference is made at the mark on mid thigh.

Alternatively, for people, who have standing stability, the thigh girth measurement is taken in standing as follows: The subject stands erect with his/her weight evenly distributed on both feet and legs slightly parted. The circumference measure is taken at the level of the mid-point of the thigh, midway between the greater trochanter of femur and medial knee joint line.

### Calf Muscle Bulk

From the apex of the patella three points are marked on the bulky area with a difference of 1 or 2 inches. The circumference is measured from all the three points, the difference is compared with the normal side. However, the simplest method of measurement of calf circumference include:

- Finding the widest part of the calf, usually around the middle of the upper leg **(Fig. 3.15)**.
- A flexible tape measure is wrapped around the calf, keeping it horizontal and not too tight and measurement is taken.
- The value is compared with the normal side, by measuring the circumference in the same way.

## *Arm Muscle Bulk Measurement*

The procedure involves:

### Finding the Mid Point of Arm

With the elbow flexed 90°, and arm by the side and palm facing up, mid point of arm is established by measuring the distance between the tip of shoulder (tip of acromion) and bony tip of elbow (most distal part of olecranon). After the mid point is established, the elbow is extended and measurement of the arm circumference is made at the midpoint as shown in **Figures 3.16A and B**.

### Forearm (Brachioradialis) Muscle Bulk

The following procedures are followed:

- The forearm is placed in a relaxed position by the side of the body, with the palms

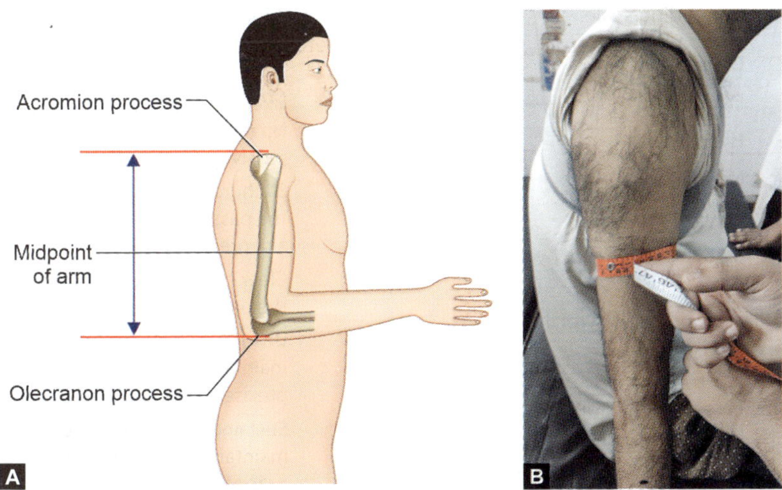


**Figs. 3.16A and B:** (A) Finding the midpoint of arm; (B) Measurement of arm circumference.

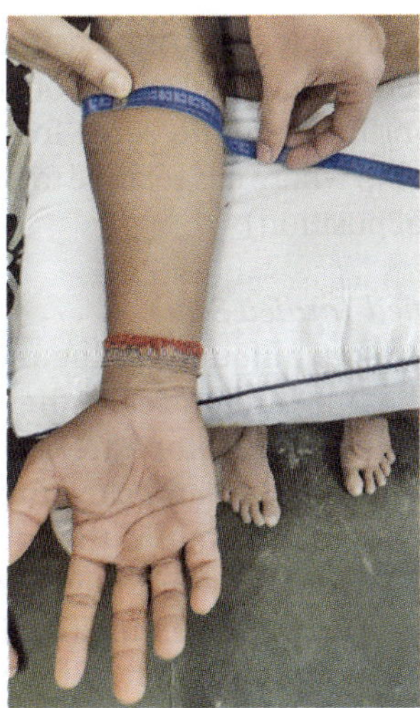

**Fig. 3.17:** Measurement of forearm circumference.

facing forwards in standing/elbow flexed to 90° and forearm resting on pillow and palm facing upwards in sitting.

- The measuring tape is wrapped around the upper 1/3rd, i.e., the most muscular part of the forearm and measurement is taken **(Fig. 3.17)**.

### *Muscle Tone Examination*

It is a state of sustained partial contraction of the muscles at rest, maintaining some tension. The muscle tension (tone) may increase or decrease during pathological conditions. Increased muscle tone (hypertonia is due to spasticity/rigidity), or decreased muscle tone (hypotonia), are tested by passively moving the parts of the limb and assessing the resistance offered by the muscles, as well as by palpating the muscle. The tone may increase (spastic/rigid states), fluctuate (dyskinetic disorders—chorea/athetosis/dystonia/ballismus), decrease (flaccid states). Muscle tone is graded by the tone grading scale:

#### Tone Grading

Muscle tone is graded using the tone grading scale **(Table 3.3)**.

#### Grading of Spasticity

Though different grading systems exist for grading of spasticity, presently, the Modified modified Asworth Scale **(Table 3.4)** is used to grade spasticity. The grade 1 plus, which was used in the Modified Asworth scale has been withdrawn in Modified modified Asworth scale.

#### The Tardieu Scale

**The Tardieu scale:** It assesses spasticity by passively moving the joint at three specified

**Table 3.3:** The tone grading scale.

| Grade | Criteria |
|---|---|
| 0 | Flaccid |
| 1+ | Hypotonia |
| 2+ | Normal |
| 3+ | Mild hypertonia |
| 4+ | Moderate-to-severe hypertonia |

**Table 3.4:** Modified modified Asworth Scale.

| Grade | Criteria |
|---|---|
| 0 | No increase in muscle tone |
| 1 | Slight increase in muscle tone, manifested by a catch and release or by minimal resistance at the end of the ROM when the affected part (s) is moved in flexion or extension, abduction or adduction, medial rotation or lateral rotation |
| 2 | Marked increase in muscle tone, manifested by a catch in the middle range and resistance throughout remainder of the range of motion, but affected part is easily moved |
| 3 | Considerable increase in muscle tone, passive movement is difficult |
| 4 | Affected part is rigid in flexion or extension, abduction or adduction, medial rotation or lateral rotation |

**Table 3.5:** Velocity of joint movement used in Tardieu scale.

| Velocity | Criteria |
|---|---|
| V1 | As slow as possible (slower than the natural drop of the limb segment under gravity) |
| V2 | Speed of the limb segment falling under gravity |
| V3 | As fast as possible (faster than the rate of the natural drop of the limb segment under gravity) |

velocities (slow, under gravity, fast) **(Table 3.5)**, while the intensity and muscle reaction to stretch is rated on a 6-point scale, with the joint angle recorded at where the muscle reaction is first felt **(Table 3.6)**.

**Table 3.6:** Tardieu scale (quality of muscle reaction to stretch).

| Grade | Criteria |
|---|---|
| 0 | No resistance throughout the course of the passive movement |
| 1 | Slight resistance throughout the course of the passive movement with no clear catch at a precise angle |
| 2 | Clear catch at precise angle, interrupting the passive movement followed by release |
| 3 | Unsustained clonus (<10 seconds when maintaining the pressure) occurring at a precise angle, followed by release |
| 4 | Sustained clonus (>10 seconds when maintaining the pressure) occurring at a precise angle |
| 5 | Joint is immobile |

Angle of muscle action is measured relative to the position of minimal stretch of the muscle (corresponding to angle zero) for all joints except the hip where it is relative to the resting anatomical position).

*The Modified Tardieu Scale*

Due to the large amount of time required to perform the full Tardieu scale, the Modified Tardieu scale was developed. It records the joint angle during fast and slow movements only. The angle of catch at the most rapid velocity (R1), and the joint angle, when the muscle length is at its maximum (R2) (assessed by moving the joint through full ROM, using slow passive movements) are determined **(Figs. 3.18A and B)**. The difference in degrees between the angles R2 and R1 is referred to as the dynamic components of spasticity.

*Pendulum Test*

(Wartenberg Pendulum Test)

This is most commonly done for knee joint, to find spasticity of quadriceps femoris. In this, the leg is made to move under the gravity, with the patient in high sitting/supine with leg hanging at the foot end of bed. The observer drops the leg from the extended position of knee and observes the number of

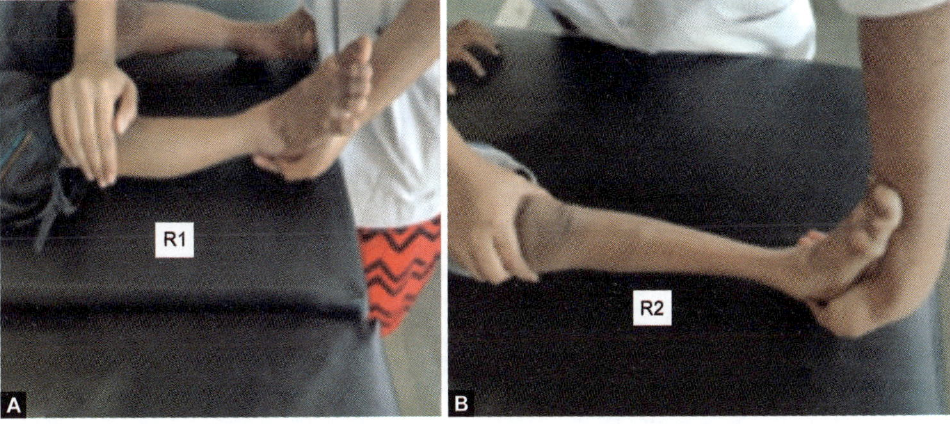


**Figs. 3.18A and B:** (A) Finding R1; (B) Finding R2.

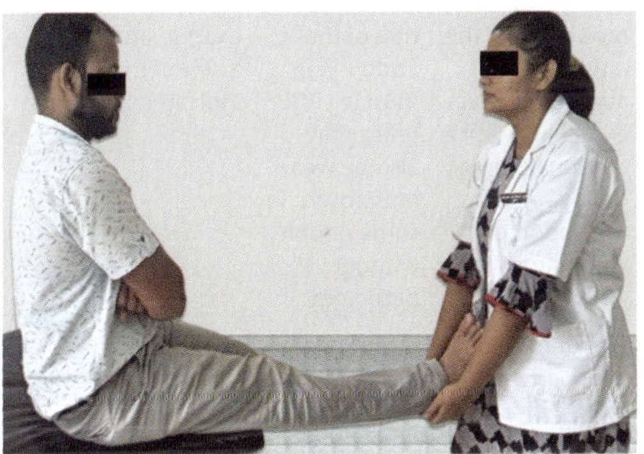

**Fig. 3.19:** The pendulum test.

oscillations made by leg, after the leg is dropped **(Fig. 3.19)**. The procedure is repeated after periodic intervals and increased oscillations of leg indicate reduction of spasticity.

*Examination of the Reflexes*

The reflexes which are of importance in clinical neurology can be divided mainly into the following groups:

- Superficial reflexes
- Deep or tendon reflexes
- Visceral reflexes of organic reflexes
- Pathologic reflexes

The following points must be remembered in all reflexes:

- Method of eliciting the reflexes
- Response or the result produced
- Afferent and efferent pathway
- Centers for the reflexes
- Clinical significance of each reflex

*Superficial Reflexes*

Superficial reflexes are usually elicited by stroking the skin or mucous membranes. Abnormal reflex response will show a combination of diminished or absent superficial reflexes. The various superficial reflexes and their clinical significance are shown in **Table 3.7**.

### Deep Tendon Reflexes

If the tendon of a slightly stretched muscle is sharply tapped with percussion hammer, the muscle contracts immediately. Deep reflexes are 'fractionated' stretch reflexes. The stimulus that initiates the reflex is the stretch of the muscle spindles and not the tendon receptors. Impulses originating in the muscle spindles are conducted to the CNS, and pass directly to the motor neurons, which supply the same muscle and cause muscle contraction. The deep tendon reflexes are graded on both sides, and compared for their speed, amplitude, and the duration of contraction and relaxation of the muscle in each case. The deep tendon reflexes serve as a guide to establish recovery from flaccid/shock stage. The reflex, which is usually absent in the shock/flaccid stage, when begins to appear indicates recovery. If the reflex presents as hyperreflexia, it indicates

**Table 3.7:** Superficial reflexes.

| *Type of reflex* | *Characteristics* | *Name of reflex* | *Segmental innervation* | *Stimulus* | *Normal Response* | *Clinical significance* |
|---|---|---|---|---|---|---|
| Skin reflex | Elicited by stroking/ tapping the skin | Abdominal reflex | Upper abdominal reflex: T8–T9, lower abdominal reflex: T10–T12 | Each quadrant of abdomen is stroked medially, above and below the umbilicus **(Fig. 3.20)** | Deviation of umbilicus towards the stimulus | Superficial abdominal reflexes disappear in both upper and lower motor neuron disease. In case of lower motor neuron disease, affecting the lower quadrants, the umbilicus is pulled towards the upper side, when the upper quadrant is stimulated |
| | | Deep abdominal reflex | Upper abdominal reflex: T8–T9, lower abdominal reflex: T10–T12 | This is elicited by tapping over the anterior rectus abdominal muscle sheath with a tendon hammer/ gently pressing the abdomen with fingers | Contraction of the abdominal muscles. This reflex may also be weak or is absent in some people without pathology | If the reflex is exaggerated/ asymmetrical it indicates CNS lesion |
| | | Anal reflex | S2–S4 | Stroking is done over perianal region, or a gloved finger is inserted into the rectum | Contraction of sphincter ani muscle | The absence of this reflex indicates that there is an interruption of the reflex arc, or damage to the spinal cord, which may be in the sensory afferent limb or the motor efferent limb. |
| | | Bulbocavernosus reflex | S2–S4 | With the gloved fingers, the clinician pulls glans penis in males or presses clitoris in females | Contraction of anal sphincter | Absence of the reflex is indicator of spinal shock |
| | | Cremasteric reflex | L1–L2 | Stroking done over inner thigh | Elevation of testicle | The absence of the reflex is considered to be diagnostic for testicular torsion. The cremasteric reflex has been |

*Contd...*

*Contd...*

| *Type of reflex* | *Character-istics* | *Name of reflex* | *Segmental innervation* | *Stimulus* | *Normal Response* | *Clinical significance* |
|---|---|---|---|---|---|---|
| | | | | | | reported to be absent in 100% of cases of testicular torsion, making it a potentially useful sign in this diagnosis |
| | | Plantar reflex (Babinski sign). | S1–S2 | Stroking is done over the lateral aspect of sole of foot from heel to base of 5th toe, and then, along the bases of the toes, medially up to the base of the 2nd toe **(Fig. 3.21)** | In healthy adults, there is a plantar flexion of the toes, especially the big toe, and the ankle is dorsiflexed and inverted<br>Stronger stimuli may produce withdrawal of the limb | The extensor plantar response or the Babinski's sign is a pathology occurring in UMN lesions. There occurs a extension of the big toe followed by extension and fanning of the other toes<br>Equivocal response: A partial flexion, followed by extension of great toe, indicating minimal damage to corticospinal system |
| | | Chaddock reflex:<br>Oppenheim reflex:<br>Gordon reflex: | | Chaddock reflex: Stroking over the lateral ankle and lateral aspect of foot..<br>Oppenheim reflex:<br>Stroking over anteromedial surface of tibia.<br>Gordon reflex: Squeezing of calf muscle firmly. | Same as Babiniski sign. | Same as Babiniski sign. This is an alternative test for individuals with hypersensitive skin. |
| Mucous membrane reflex | Elicited by stroking the mucous membrane | Corneal reflex | | The cornea is touched by wisp of cotton | Blinking | Absence of corneal reflex on one side indicates injury to 5th cranial nerve |
| | | Gag reflex | | The posterior part of pharynx-the uvula is stimulated by a wisp of cotton/tongue depressor | Bilateral pharyngeal muscle contraction and elevation of soft palate | Impaired in 9th and 10th cranial nerve lesions |

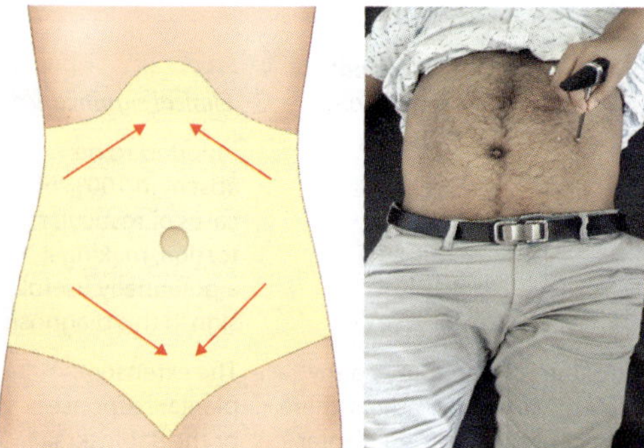

**Fig. 3.20:** Stroking pattern to elicit abdominal reflex.

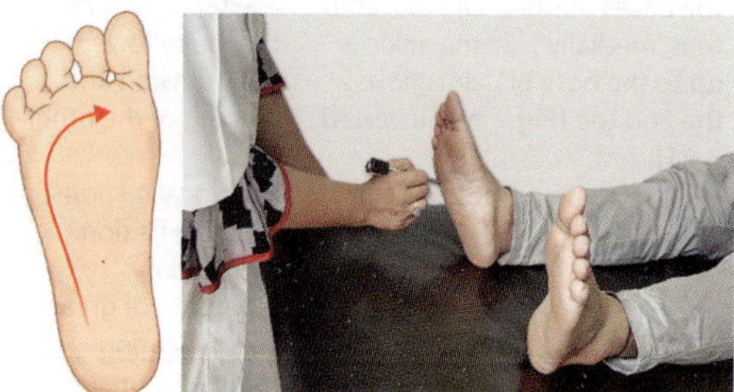

**Fig. 3.21:** Stroking pattern to elicit Babinski sign.

UMN lesion. However, in certain normal people, hyperreflexia (mostly knee jerk) may be found in the state of anxiety.

### Deep Tendon Reflex Grading

By convention the deep tendon reflexes are graded in a scale of 0 to 4 as shown in the table below **(Table 3.8)**.

*Jendrassik Maneuver*

This maneuver is followed during DTR testing, if the patient does not relax. The patient is asked to clench the teeth, flex both sets of fingers into a hook-like form and interlock the fingers of both hands **(Fig. 3.22)**. Then the patient's tendons are tapped using the percussion hammer.

**Table 3.9** shows the deep tendon reflexes tested in neuro-musculo-skeletal disorders.

### Visceral Reflexes

These are the pupillary reflexes, which are grouped into direct and indirect light reflexes.

**Table 3.8:** Deep tendon reflex grading.

| *Grade* | *Criteria* |
|---|---|
| 0 | No response |
| 1+ | Diminished |
| 2+ | Normal |
| 3+ | Brisk reflex, possibly but not necessarily abnormal |
| 4+ | Very brisk/exaggerated with clonus |

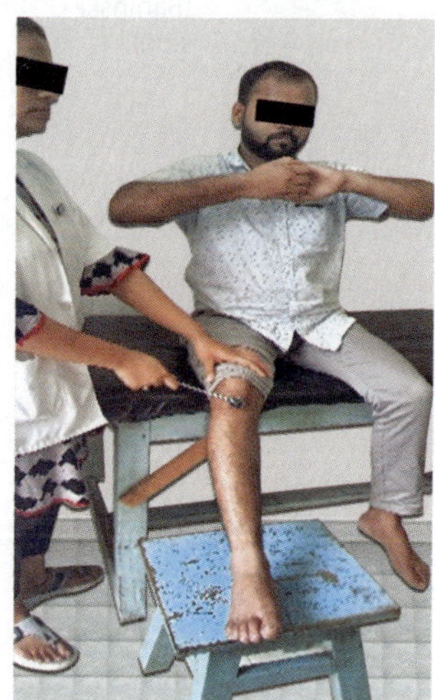

**Fig. 3.22:** Shows Jendrassik maneuver.

*Light Reflex (Direct Light Reflex)*

Each eye should be examined separately with the subject in a shady, indirectly illuminated place. A bright light is applied into the patient's eye being tested (the torch is brought from the side of the eye and never from directly in front of the eye as the subject will reflexly close his eyes). There is constriction of pupil almost immediately; then it dilates a little, and assumes a smaller size after undergoing a few oscillations. On switching off the light; the pupil quickly dilates to its previous size. The optic nerve is the afferent pathway; the center is in the midbrain (the concerned fibers leave the optic tract before the lateral geniculate body and end in the pretectal region of the midbrain on the Edinger-Westphal nuclei of both sides). The efferent pathway is the oculomotor nerve.

**Table 3.9:** Shows the deep tendon reflexes.

| *Name of reflex* | *Segmental innervation* | *Method of testing* | *Response* |
|---|---|---|---|
| Maxillary reflex | 5th cranial nerve (Both afferent and efferent) | Mandible of chin with the mouth open is struck with the percussion hammer over the thumb placed over mandible **(Fig. 3.23A)** | Sudden closure of jaw takes place |
| Biceps reflex/ jerk | C5,c6 (Musculocutaneous nerve) | The tendon of biceps brachii is tapped, using percussion hammer, with the elbow slightly flexed and forearm supported on clinician's forearm **(Fig. 3.23B)** | Contraction of biceps brachii. The response is decreased/ absent in LMN lesion and increased in UMN lesion |
| Triceps jerk | Radial nerve (C6, C7) | With the elbow slightly flexed, the tendon of triceps is tapped with the percussion hammer **(Fig. 3.23C)** | Contraction of the muscle with tendency for elbow extension. The response is decreased/ absent in LMN lesion and increased in UMN lesion |
| Supinator (Brachioradialis) reflex | Radial nerve (C6,C7,C8) | With the forearm in mid-prone position, tapping is done over the styloid process of radius **(Fig. 3.23D)** | Flexion and supination of forearm. The response is decreased/absent in LMN lesion and increased in UMN lesion |
| Knee jerk | Femoral nerve (L3,L4) | With the knee partially flexed in supine/high sitting, patellar tendon is tapped using percussion hammer **(Fig. 3.23E)** | Contraction of quadriceps with a tendency to cause knee extension. The response is decreased/absent in LMN lesion and increased in UMN lesion |
| Ankle jerk | Posterior tibial nerve (S1,S2) | With the ankle held in slight dorsiflexion, the Achilles tenon is tapped with the percussion hammer **(Fig. 3.23F)** | Contraction of ankle plantar flexors with slight plantar flexion of ankle. The response is decreased/absent in LMN lesion and increased in UMN lesion |

*Consensual Light Reflex (Indirect Light Reflex)*

The clinician place his/her hand between the patient's two eyes and focuses light into one eye, observing the effect on the pupil of the unstimulated side. There is constriction of the pupil in the other eye (i.e., both pupils constrict). The constriction of the pupil on the unstimulated side is called the consensual or indirect light reflex. This response is due to crossing of some of the fibers in the optic chiasma and their termination on the oculomotor nuclei of both sides. On switching off the light it is noted that, both pupils are dilated. The consensually mediated reaction is more active than the direct reaction of a pupil in some lesions of the optic nerve. Afferent pathway is by 2nd nerve, efferent pathway is by oculomotor nerve, and center is in midbrain.

*Accommodation Reflex*

When one looks at a near object the pupils constrict, the eyes converge, and the lenses become more convex. These three responses constitute accommodation reaction. The clinician, holds up his/her index finger close to the subject's nose and ask him to look at a distant object (or the far side of the room). Then the patient is asked to quickly focus his eyes at the clinician's finger. As the eyes converge the pupils constrict. If the patient is unable to see, he/she is asked to look at clinician's fingers held in front of his eyes. Afferent pathway is by

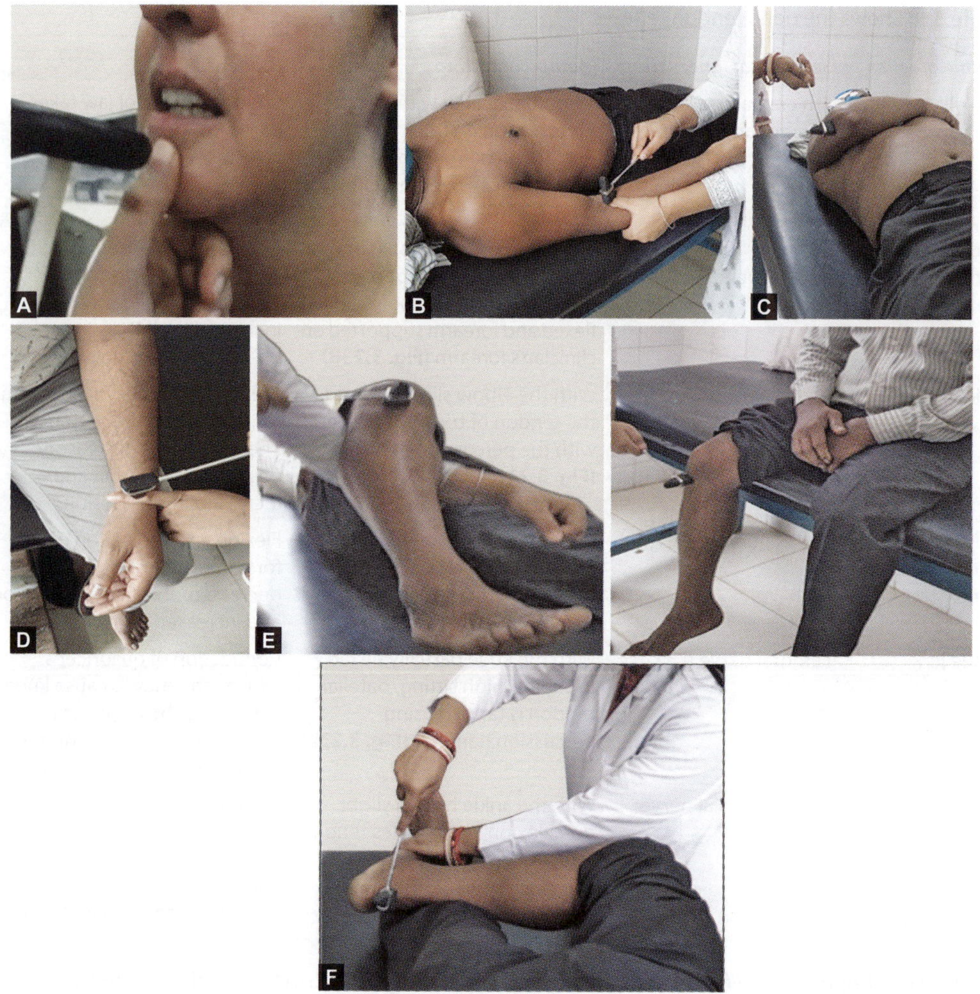

**Figs. 3.23A to F:** Shows testing of deep tendon reflexes.

2nd nerve, efferent pathway is by oculomotor nerve, and center is in visual cortex.

### *Pathological Reflexes*

This group includes some primitive responses, which appear only with lesions of UMN. Normally, they are suppressed by cerebral inhibition. The reflexogenic area is widened in upper motor neuron lesions, and the Babinski-like response is obtained from widespread areas. In children with cerebral palsy, these reflexes do not disappear as per schedule, making impairment of posture and movements (delayed motor milestones). For example, ATNR (Asymmetric tonic neck reflex), which normally should disappear in babies by 4–6 months, if fails to disappear due to brain insult, affects rolling of the child **(Fig. 3.24)**. These reflexes, also sometimes seen in adults with brain injury.

### *Tests for Joint Range of Motion*

The fourth chapter (Goniometry) explains in detail about the techniques of measuring the joint passive and active range of motion measurement.

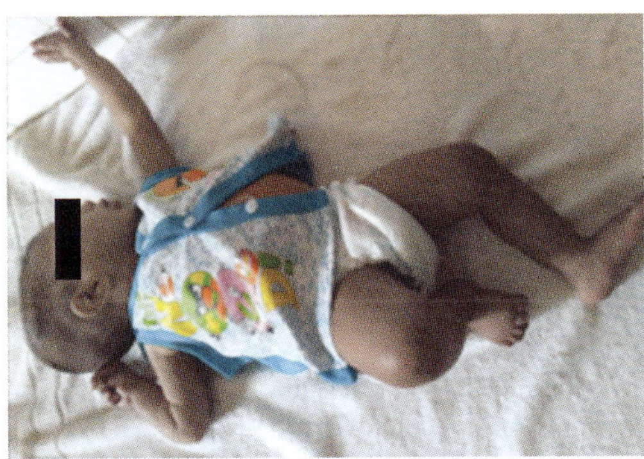

**Fig. 3.24:** ATNR (Asymmetric tonic neck reflex), preventing rolling.

### *Tests for Tightness/Contracture/Deformity*

Tightness (which can be stretched) of muscles/ joint capsules, contracture (which can not be stretched), deformity (abnormal alignment of joints, such as ankle equinus), should be found out for the spine and extremities, by doing specific tests, as for example, doing a Thomas test for hip flexion deformity/hip flexor tightness/contracture.

### *Strength of Muscles and Manual Muscle Testing*

Manual muscle testing (MMT) was developed by Wright and Lovett in 1912, as a means of testing and grading muscle strength, based on gravity and manually applied resistance.

The testing method was developed in response to the need to assess muscle strength losses during the polio outbreak in early part of the 20th century. Florence Kendall along with her husband Henry Otis Kendall, refined testing positions in the 1940s. The manual muscle testing taught today incorporates the anti-gravity testing methods of Wright and Lovett, with the refinement of Kendall. The commonly used methods of muscle testing are those as described by Daniels and Worthingham and Kendall et al., which are based on the work done by Wright and Lovett, that use arc of motion, gravity and manually applied resistance by the examiner to test and grade muscle power. The resistance is either applied throughout the range of motion, called make test/active resistance test or at one point in the arc of motion called break test.

Kendall et al., suggested a 0–10 scale, where as Daniel and Worthingham suggested a 0–5 scale. While grading muscle power, the scale used, is expressed by the score/grade divided by the maximum grade for that scale. For example, while assessing muscle power using numerical scales like Kendall's system with grades from 0–10, the power should be noted as 5/10, suggesting 5 is the score/grade obtained and the Kendall system of grading with maximum score of 10 was used. If the grade of muscle is represented as 3/5, it is understood that, the Daniel's system of grading was used and the score of muscle power is 3 out of a normal grade of 5.

Presently, the most commonly accepted way of assessing muscle power/strength is the Medical Research Council's scale (MRC scale) of muscle power. The MRC system has 6 grades like the Daniel's scale, where: 0-No contraction present, 1-Flickering contraction present, 2-Full range of movement present in the horizontal plane, where gravity is eliminated, 3-Full range of movement possible against gravity, 4-Full range of motion is possible against gravity with minimal resistance, 5-Full range of motion possible against maximum resistance.

While grading the muscle power using any system, first the clinician should assess the joint range of motion, so that, appropriate decision can be taken to grade the muscle considering the available range of motion. Most commonly, muscles should be graded within the available range of motion.

Plus (+) and Minus (-) Grades: Use of a plus (+) or minus (-) addition to a manual muscle test grades is discouraged except in three instances: Fair+/3+, Poor+/2+, and Poor-/2-.

Whatever, is the manual muscle testing scale, that is used to grade muscle power, the grades so derived are subjective and varies from clinician to clinician. To get more objective measure of muscle strength, hand held dynamometry/isokinetic dynamometry are the methods of choice.

**Tests for coordination**

It is the ability to execute smooth, accurate, controlled motor responses for accomplishment of function. Impairment of coordination (if any) are tested by the non-equilibrium and equilibrium coordination tests.

### *Non-equilibrium Coordination Tests*

(Finger to nose, finger to finger, tests for rapid alternating movements, finger to toe, heel to shin)

**For Upper Limb**

*Finger Nose Test (Fig. 3.25)*

The examiner sits in front of the patient and holds his/her index finger at arms length from the patient. Patient is asked to touch his/her nose and the clinician's index finger with own index finger first with eyes open, followed by with eyes closed. Difficulty in performing the movements/reaching the target, indicates incoordination. Cerebellar diseased patient may touch the nose by the wavering and oscillating fashion, or may miss the target. But the posterior column diseased person can touch accurately with opened eyes, but not with closed eyes.

*Finger-to-Finger Test (Fig. 3.26)*

Patient is asked to abduct both the shoulders 90° with elbow in extension and then to bring both the index fingers towards midline and touch each other. Cerebellar diseased patient may touch each other by the wavering and oscillating fashion. But the posterior column diseased person can touch accurately with opened eyes, but not with closed eyes.

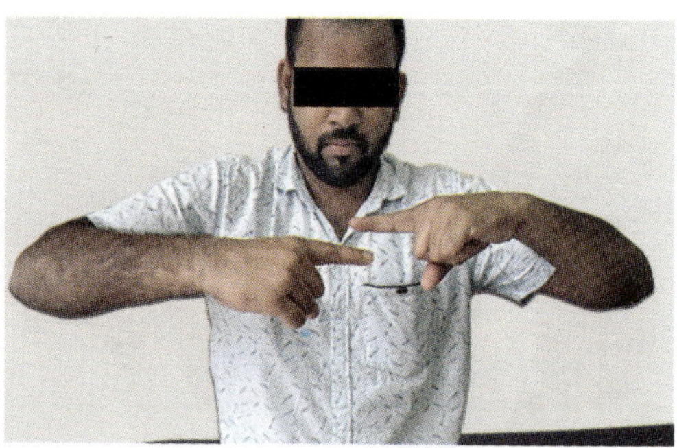

**Fig. 3.26:** Finger-to-finger test.

*Rapid Alternating Movement test*

The patient is asked to do the pronation and supination movement alternatively. In cerebellar lesion, the patient feels difficulty in performing this movement, this phenomena is called as dysdiadochokinesia.

**Lower Limb**

*Finger-Toe Test (Fig. 3.27)*

The therapist's/clinician's finger is pointed two feet above the patient's great toe and the patient is instructed to touch the clinician's finger with the great toe. The cerebellar disease patient can touch the finger with the oscillatory or light bouncing movements. But it can be done accurately with the opened eyes but not while closed, by the posterior column diseased patient.

*Heel-Shin Test*

Patient in supine lying. He/she is asked to move the heel up and down the opposite shin

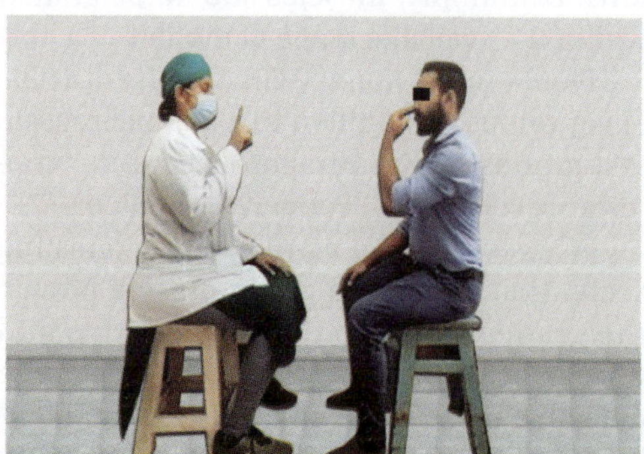

**Fig. 3.25:** Finger to nose test.

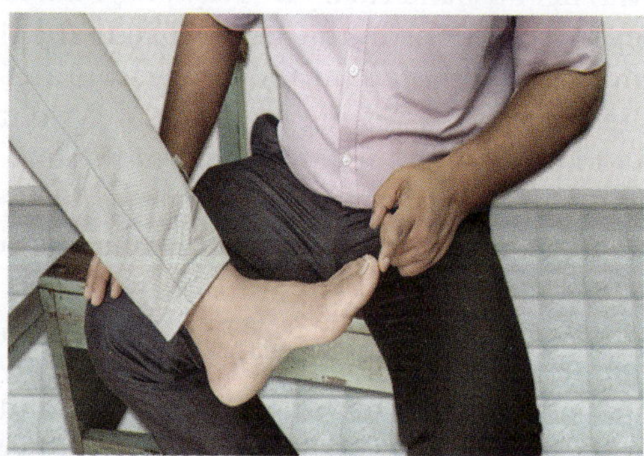

**Fig. 3.27:** Finger-toe test.

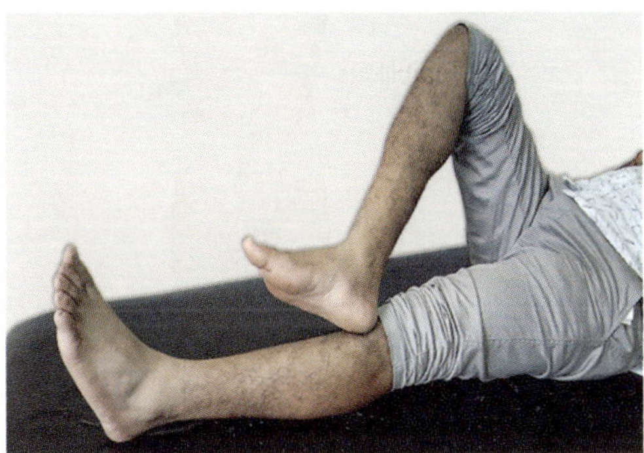

**Fig. 3.28:** Heel to shin test.

repeatedly for several times **(Fig. 3.28)**. The test is then performed in the similar manner for the opposite side. In cerebellar disease, the heel is carried up, to overshoot the knee. If the heel is carried down, it begins to execute an action tremor. In posterior column disease, the patient cannot perform it due to the inability to recognize the position of the joint.

### *Equilibrium Coordination tests*

(Rhomberg's test, Sharpened Rhomberg's test):

*Romberg's Test*

The Romberg's test is a test that measures sense of balance. It is typically used to diagnose problems with balance, which is composed of visual, vestibular (inner ear), and proprioceptive (positional sense) systems. Patient is made to stand straight, feet together with the eyes opened. Then the patient is instructed to shut the eyes **(Fig. 3.29)**

Patients with cerebellar ataxia, cannot stand with feet together, when the eyes are open, however, patients with sensory ataxia, can stand with feet together, with eyes open, but cannot stand when the eyes are closed, due to increased body sway and tendency to fall.

A Romberg's test is said to be positive, when there is imbalance in standing with the eyes closed.

Sharpened Romberg's test

This test is performed, if the Romberg's test is normal. The subject is asked to stand with

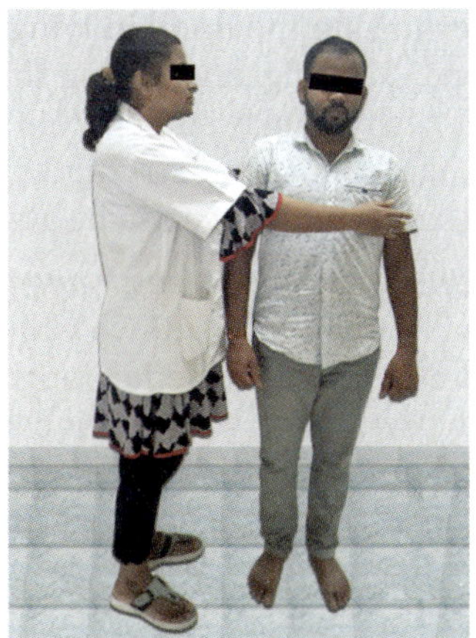

**Fig. 3.29:** Romberg's test.

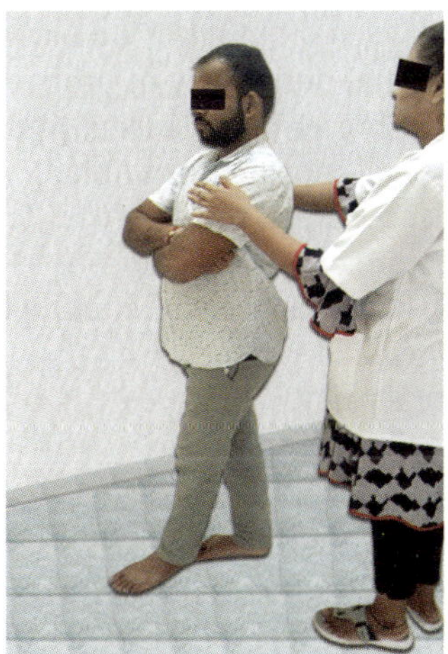

**Fig. 3.30:** Sharpened Romberg's test.

one heel of one foot, in front of the toes of the other, with the arms folded across the chest **(Fig. 3.30)**. The test is performed first with the eyes open, and then with the eyes closed. Inability to perform the test, indicates vestibular impairment.

### Assessment of Balance

Balance refers to **an individuals ability to maintain their line of gravity within their base of support (BOS)**. It can also be described as the ability to maintain equilibrium, where equilibrium can be defined as any condition in which all acting forces are cancelled by each other resulting in a stable balanced system.

By perturbing the body in lying, sitting, quadruped, standing, and testing supporting strategies such as ankle strategy/hip strategy, and change in support strategies such as stepping strategy, balance can be assessed.

*Leg Length Discrepancy Measurement*

In normal individual itself we can observe the mild difference in the leg length. If the leg length difference is ≤1 cm, it is considered as normal but the difference goes >1 cm is considered as abnormal. It needs the proper corrective treatment. First, the reason for the leg length discrepancy is analyzed before the treatment is carried out.

**Causes**

- Congenital deficiency of limb, e.g., congenital shortening of femur, phocomelia, congenital shortening of tibia.
- Trauma, e.g., malunited fracture, premature epiphyseal closure in fracture, loss of bony fragment after open fracture
- Poliomyelitis
- Cerebral palsy.
- Pelvic tilt or drop
- Scoliosis.
- Soft tissue shortening or contracture
- Bony abnormalities, e.g., coxa vara, coxa valga, genu varum and genu valgum.

*Limb Length Measurements (Lower Limbs)*

**Leg length discrepancy can be divided into 2 etiological groups:** True limb length discrepancy (LLD), defined as those which are associated with shortening of bony structures, and apparent limb length discrepancy (LLD), defined as those which are the result of altered mechanics of the lower extremities, or deformities of spine or pelvis.

A physiotherapist/clinician is very often asked to perform limb length measurements, mostly for the lower limbs (discussed below), though upper limb length measurement is also recommended, particularly, when limb lengthening procedures are warranted. The procedure for lower limbs involve:

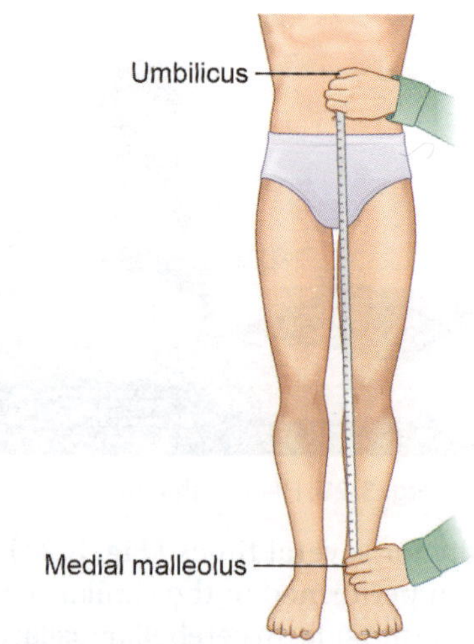


**Fig. 3.31:** Apparent limb length measurement.

*Apparent Limb Length Measurement*

Even though the true shortening measurement shows nil difference in the leg length but the examiner may feel the height difference by observation. That time the apparent limb length measurement has to be performed, and by this method we can know the leg length difference due to spinal or pelvic problem or due to deformities in hips and knees.

Patient in supine lying. Both the lower limbs are kept as straight and parallel as possible. Apparent limb length is measured from xiphisternum/umbilicus to the tip of medial malleolus **(Fig. 3.31)**. The length of both the lower limbs are to be measured, and difference in reading between the two (if any) is the apparent shortening/lengthening.

Pelvis Squaring

Squaring of the pelvis is done by making both the anterior superior iliac spine (ASIS) at the same level. This is done by further adducting the affected hip in presence of an adduction deformity (where the pelvis on the affected side is raised) **(Figs. 3.32A and B)**, or further abducting the affected hip in the presence of an abduction deformity (where the pelvis on the affected side is lowered) till both ASIS are at the same level (i.e., distance from umbilicus to

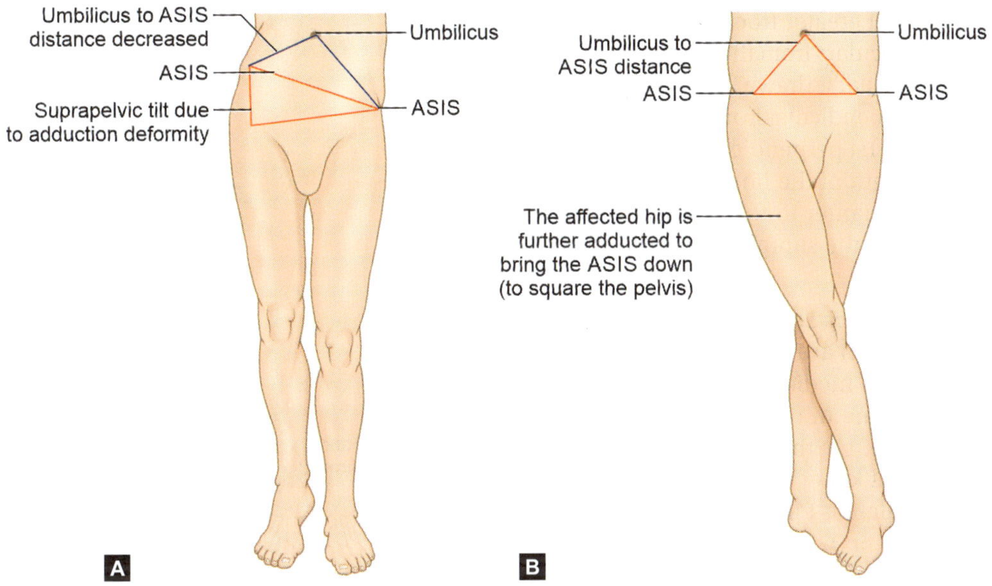


**Figs. 3.32A and B:** (A) Adduction deformity of hip, causing suprapelvic tilt; (B) Squaring of pelvis by further adducting the affected hip.
(ASIS: anterior superior iliac spine)

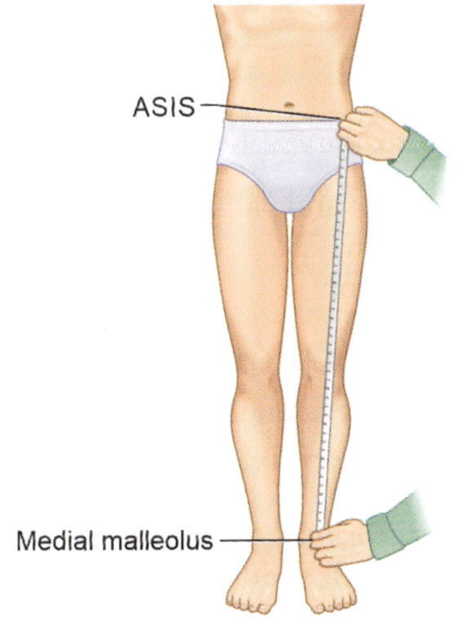


**Fig. 3.33:** Measurement of true limb length discrepancy.
(ASIS: anterior superior iliac spine)

ASISs on both sides are equal). If there is a fixed deformity in the hip, pelvis can not be squared.

True Limb Length Discrepancy

To measure the true shortening of the limb, the patient is positioned in supine lying. The legs are kept parallel to each other 15 to 20 cm apart. The measurement is taken from ASIS to the medial or lateral malleolus of the patient with the inch tape, if the pelvis is squared **(Fig. 3.33)**.

If the pelvis could not be squared, or fixed deformities are present in hip and knee joints, segmental limb length measure are done, which consists of:

### Supratrochanteric Length from Bryant's Triangle (Fig. 3.34)

The Bryant's triangle is a right angled triangle formed by: Anterior superior iliac spine

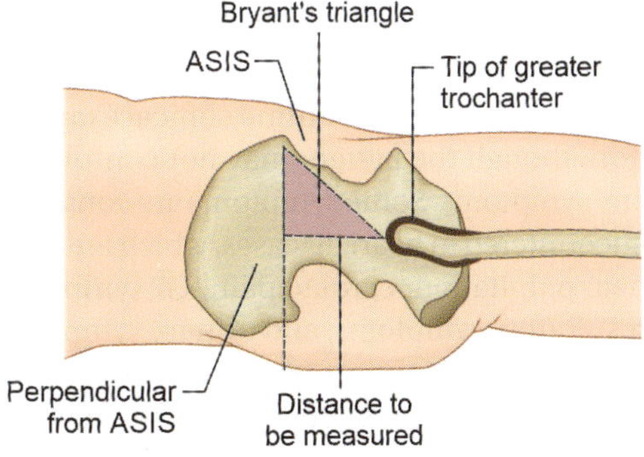


**Fig. 3.34:** Bryant's triangle.
(ASIS: anterior superior iliac spine)

(ASIS), tip of greater trochanter and junction of perpendiculars from the 2 points above (1st a perpendicular is drawn from ASIS to bed and another perpendicular from greater trochanter to meet the 1st perpendicular).

The length of the line from the tip of the greater trochanter to the perpendicular line from ASIS, is the supratrochanteric length to be measured.

*Infratrochanteric Length*

Measurements are done from tip of greater trochanter to medial knee joint line (lateral knee joint line in case of grossly atrophied quadriceps), for the thigh component and from medial knee joint line to the tip of the medial malleolus for the leg component.

For patients who can stand, an alternative method to find the lower limb length is to put slices of wooden blocks under the short limb **(Fig. 3.35)**, till both the ASIS are levelled. The thickness of the wooden block used under the short limb, gives the amount of shortening present.

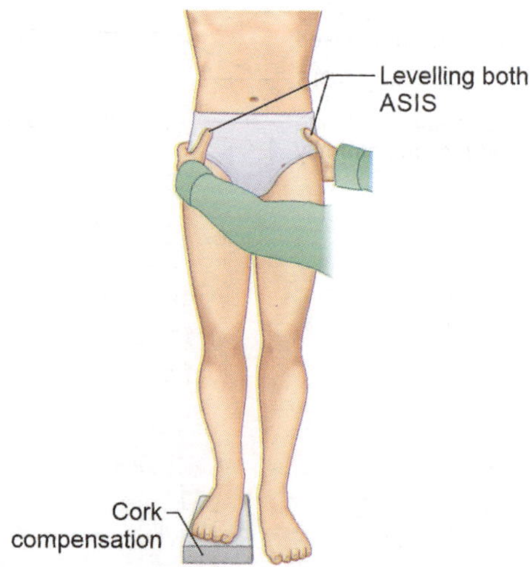


**Fig. 3.35:** Limb length measurement by wooden blocks/cork compensation.
(ASIS: anterior superior iliac spine)

### Pain Assessment

Pain scales are tools for clinicians to describe the level of pain patients experience. There are many pain scales, but the visual analogue scale (VAS) **(Fig. 3.36)**, is commonly used by clinicians.

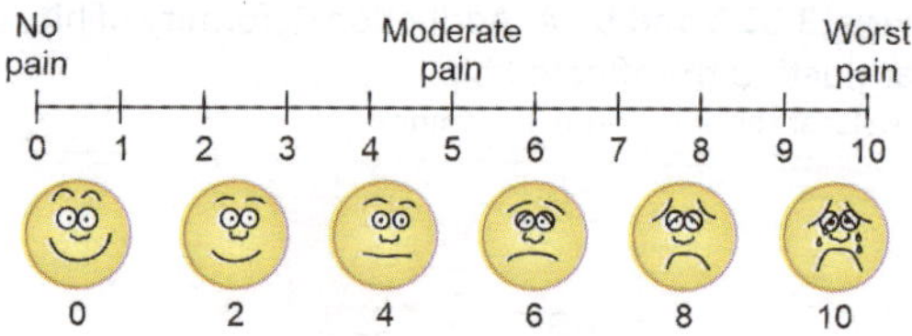


**Fig. 3.36:** The visual analogue scale (VAS).

## *Clinical Examination of the Cardiovascular System*

A person suffering from heart disease may present with many symptoms, some of which may not appear to be apparently connected with cardiovascular system. Heart disease may be detected during a routine clinical examination, though the patient may not complain of any symptoms. Some symptoms are constantly encountered in heart diseases, which are dyspnea, palpitation, cardiac pain, GI symptoms, respiratory symptoms, and urinary symptoms. Clinical examination of the cardiovascular system undergoes through different processes and it consists the following examinations:

- Examination of the arterial pulses
- Recording of the blood pressure
- Inspection and palpation of the system
- Percussion
- Auscultation

### Examination of Arterial Pulses

The pulse is the lateral pressure exerted by the walls of the blood vessels. It forms an elastic coiling and recoiling type. The pulse is usually felt by the tip of the three fingers (index, middle, and ring finger). Middle finger feels the pulse, index finger varies the pressure on the artery whereas ring finger is used to prevent the retrograde pulsation from the palmar arch. The examiner should notice for the rate, rhythm, volume, tension, and character of the pulse to find out the abnormal changes or pathology.

The normal pulse rate is 70–80 beats/min.

The pulses were felt all over the body, which are of, carotid artery pulse, superficial temporary artery pulse, brachial artery pulse, radial artery pulse, femoral artery pulse, posterior tibial artery pulse, popliteal artery pulse, dorsalis pedis, etc. Increase in pulse more than 100/min represents tachycardia and decrease in the rate less than 60/min represents bradycardia.

*Recording of the Blood Pressure*

This is done by auscultatory method, in which subject's blood pressure is measured by an apparatus called sphygmomanometer. Here subject's hand is tied by the cuff present in the apparatus around the arm above the elbow and pressure is raised by the hand pump. Then as the pressure is being released the pulse beats are auscultated with a stethoscope, noting down the appearance and disappearance of the sound. The readings at which sound of pulse beat appears and heard is the systole and the readings below it at which the pulse disappears is the diastole. Normal blood pressure is 120/80 mm of Hg. Increase in this pressure leads to hypertension and decrease in this pressure leads to hypotension.

*Inspection and Palpation*

The subject should be examined in good light, with chest bared, but without unnecessary exposure to chill, both in sitting and supine positions. Notice the shape of the chest and precordium and observe if there is any dyspnea and cyanosis. Subject should be examined for the pulsations of the veins, pulsations in the thoracic region, pulsations in the epigastrium, apex beat and the thrills and murmurs. Thrill is the palpable murmur.

**Percussion**

The clinician places the left middle finger firmly in contact with the skin and strikes its middle phalanx with the tip of the right middle finger 2–3 times. The percussing finger should be relaxed and should not be lifted up more than 3 inches or so and the movement of the hand should be loose and at the wrist and the finger joints and not at the elbow. Two things should be noticed while percussing—(a) the feeling imparted to the percussed finger and (b) the sound produced, which differs both quantitatively and qualitatively.

**Auscultation**

The auscultation takes a major role in the examination of the cardiovascular system. Here the heart sounds are being auscultated with the help of stethoscope. These sounds are heard due to the closure and opening of the valves present in the heart.

There are four heart sounds to be heard and these sounds can be heard in four places around the heart.

1. Aortic area—2nd right intercostal space close to sternum
2. Pulmonary area—2nd left intercostal space close to sternum
3. Tricuspid area—the 4th and 5th intercostal spaces near the lower sternal border.
4. Mitral area—5th left intercostal space in midclavicular line

The sounds which are heard is given below as follows:

- First sound (S1)—Louder and resembles LUBB sound heard during the closure of AV valves in ventricular systole.
- Second sound (S2)—Not louder resembles DUBB sound heard during the closure of semilunar valves in ventricular diastole.
- Third sound (S3)—Not heard loud, occurs in rapid ventricular filling.
- Fourth sound (S4)—Not heard loud, occurs in atrial contraction.

The first heart sound—lubb is created by the closure of atrioventricular valves at the beginning of ventricular systole and also it is more complex, louder and lasts longer than the second sound—dubb.

The third and fourth heart sound (S3 and S4) are two abnormal heart sound components which are proved to be indicators of heart failure during diastolic period.

A S3 can be a normal finding in children, pregnant females and well-trained athletes; however, a S4 heart sound is almost always abnormal.

Heart murmur is an abnormal sound that consists of a flow noise that is heard before, between, or after the normal heart sounds or that may mask the normal heart sounds.

**Exercise tolerance tests:** Before prescribing exercises to patients with cardiorespiratory illness, exercise tolerance tests are performed to decide the safe intensity of exercise. Exercise tolerance testing (also known as exercise testing or exercise stress testing) is used routinely in evaluating patients who present with chest pain, in patients who have chest pain on exertion, and in patients with known ischemic heart disease. The exercise tolerance tests could be simple tests like the 6 minute walk test, or symptom limited tests like treadmill tests.

- **Six-minute walk test:** The six-minute walk test is a submaximal exercise test used to assess aerobic capacity and endurance. It is a low-risk test that measures how far a person can walk in six minutes. The distance covered over a time of six minutes is used as the outcome by which to compare changes in performance capacity. It evaluates the functional capacity of the individual and provides valuable information regarding all the systems during physical activity, including pulmonary and cardiovascular systems, blood circulation, neuromuscular units, body metabolism, and peripheral circulation.
  - Before the test starts, the tester measures the participant's pulse, blood pressure, oxygen saturation level, and breathlessness.
  - The participant receives the instructions to walk back and forth at their own pace to a designated spot for six minutes.
  - The tester instructs the participant to say if they experience trouble breathing or chest pain.
- **Exercise stress tests (maximal exercise tolerance test):** These are symptom limited tests performed on a treadmill/bi-cycle ergometer, with a 12 lead ECG, to diagnose exercise induced myocardial ischemia, arrythmias, or abnormal blood pressure response. The test is performed, in the presence of a cardiologist, as the patient is made to exercise till symptoms develop. The patient is asked to report, when symptoms of chest pain/dyspnea develops and the clinician notes the heart rate at this point (maximum heart rate-MHR) and the intensity of exercise is gradually reduced and exercise is subsequently stopped. The Karvonen equation is used to find the training heart rate (THR)/exercise heart rate, from maximum heart rate (MHR).

There are four steps to using the Karvonen formula:

1. Estimation of max HR = 220 - Age for athletes/normal, from symptom limited exercise tests in patients.
2. Estimated max HR - resting HR = HR reserve (HRR)
3. HHR × percentage (e.g., 70% ) = percent of HRR
4. Percent of HRR + resting HR = target HR

Training heart rate/exercise heart rate = Resting heart rate (RHR) + (MHR-RHR) X% of intensity exercise.

The MHR, for athletes/healthy individuals should be found from 220-age, whereas for patients with cardiorespiratory diseases, it should be found from symptom limited exercise stress test.

For athletes and normal individuals, the intensity of exercise is measured by a percentage of max heart rate (measured in beats per minute, or BPM), which varies from person to person," The target heart rate for moderate intensity exercise is 50 to 70% of max heart rate. For vigorous exercise, it is 70 to 85%." There are different zones of intensity, such as lower intensity zone (50 to 60% of max. heart rate), temperate zone (60 to 70% of Max. heart rate), and aerobic zone (70 to 85% of max. heart rate).

For patients with cardiovascular disease:

- Exercise intensity appears to influence the number of cardioprotective benefits achieved from aerobic exercise. The current consensus recommends that exercise intensity prescribed for patients with CVD should be approximately 60% of the maximal heart rate (MHR), 50% of the heart rate reserve (HRR).
- Cardiopulmonary exercise test (CPET), is similar to exercise stress test, with the addition of ventilatory gas analysis to determine maximum oxygen consumption ($VO_2$ max). $VO_2$ max is typically measured in milliliters of oxygen consumed in a minute per kilogram of body weight. The $VO_2$ max is determined by performing a cardiorespiratory exercise, such walking on treadmill or running a static cycle. The patient is made to wear a face mask to record the oxygen consumption and $CO_2$ production while doing the exercise. The $VO_2$ max, should be compared with age specific normal values, to determine the cardiorespiratory function.

## Examination of Function

The ability to perform mobility on bed, mobility out of bed, activities of daily living (ADL), Instrumental activities of daily living should be examined and documented. Functional scales, such as functional independence measure scale, that measures the ability to perform daily tasks, are widely used by clinician's in clinical settings.

### *Examination of Gait*

For ambulatory patients with gait deviations, the walking pattern (gait) should be examined, by various methods described under the chapter on gait. The stance and swing phase abnormalities and the abnormalities of temporal and spatial parameters of gait should be found out and documented.

After a thorough assessment, the clinician makes a problem list, sets goal (short-term and long-term) and decides the plan of care (therapeutic strategies). Periodic re-evaluation should be done to know the beneficial changes with treatment.

# 4 CHAPTER Goniometry

## INTRODUCTION

The term goniometry is derived from two Greek words, gonia meaning angle, and metron, meaning measure. Goniometry refers to the measurement of angles created at human joints by the bones of the body. It is used to measure and document the amount of active and passive motion available in joints. To measure a range of motion of a particular joint the therapist/clinician should have the thorough knowledge on the range of motion of an individual joint, axis and plane of the joint for specific movements.

### Types of Goniometer

1. Universal goniometer:
   - Half circle goniometer
   - Full circle goniometer
2. Finger goniometer
3. Gravity dependent goniometer or fluid goniometer
4. Pendulum goniometer
5. Electrogoniometer
6. Digital goniometer

#### *Universal Goniometer*

A universal goniometer is an instrument that measures an angle of the joint . It may be made of either plastic or metal. It has four parts which are discussed below **(Fig. 4.1)**.

**Body**

Either a full circled protractor with scales from 0–360° **(Fig. 4.2A)** or a half circled protractor with scales from 0–180° **(Figs. 4.2B and C)**.

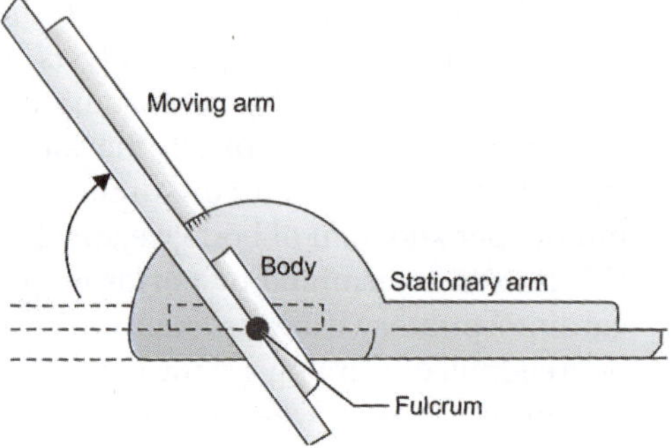


**Fig. 4.1:** The universal goniometer.

**Fulcrum**

It is a rivet or screw like device on the center of the body, that allows the moving arm to move freely on the body of the goniometer **(Fig. 4.1)**. The fulcrum of the goniometer is placed over the axis of the joint to be measured.

**Stationary Arm (Fig. 4.1)**

This arm is aligned over the inactive part (proximal segment) of the joint to be measured.

**Moving Arm (Fig. 4.1)**

The moving arm is placed on the part (segment)of the limb that moves with the joint motion.

#### *Finger Goniometer*

Though half circled universal finger goniometers can be used to measure the range of motion of small joints of fingers, thumb and toes (mostly for abduction/adduction), specially designed goniometers are used for

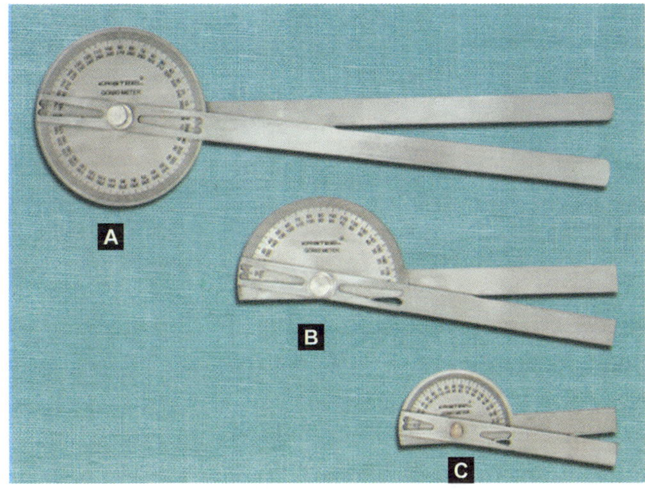


**Figs. 4.2A to C:** (A) Full circle bodied goniometer; (B and C) Half circle bodied goniometer.

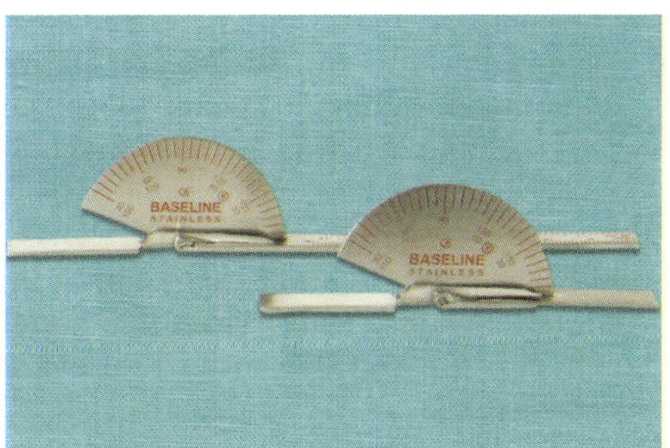


**Fig. 4.3:** The finger goniometer.

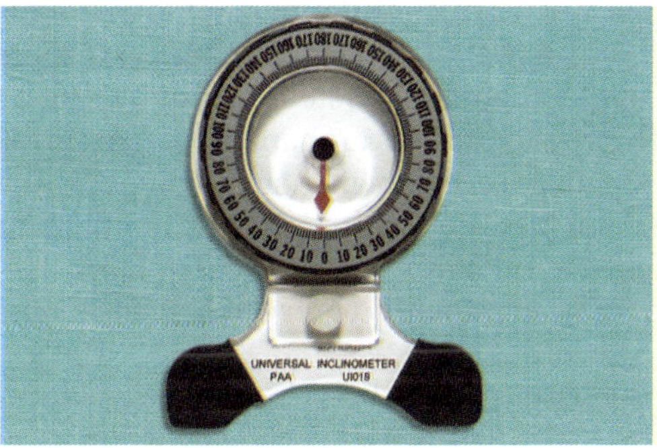


**Fig. 4.4:** The Inclinometer/gravity dependent goniometer.

measurement of flexion/extension of such small joints **(Fig. 4.3)**. It has a head with scales, that show the degrees of flexion, extension and hyperextension of the joints. It also has linear scales on the arm, that measure the proximal and distal segments of the joints.

### *Gravity Dependent Goniometer/Fluid Goniometer/Inclinometer*

It is also called **inclinometer**. It uses gravity's effect on pointers and fluid level to measure the joint range of motion **(Fig. 4.4)**. It was designed by Schenkar in 1956. It is having gravity effecting pointer and the fluid filled chamber with the air bubbles. It resembles like the carpenter's level meter. It is mostly used for measuring the pelvic tilt or drop, though, it can be used to measure range of motion of spine and certain peripheral joints.

### *Electrogoniometer*

These goniometers convert angular motion of the joint into an electric signal (voltage). It is designed by Karpovich and Karpovich in 1959. It has two arms. One arm is attached with the proximal segment and another is attached with the distal segment of the measuring joint. The potentiometer is connected with these two arms. Changes in the joint position show the angulations in the potentiometer **(Fig. 4.5)**.

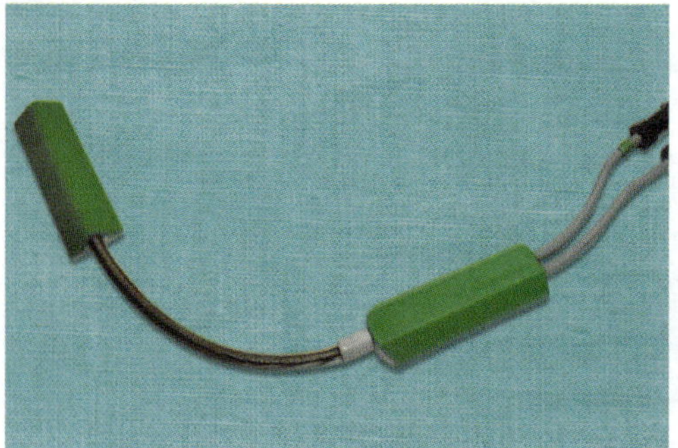

**Fig. 4.5:** The electrogoniometer.

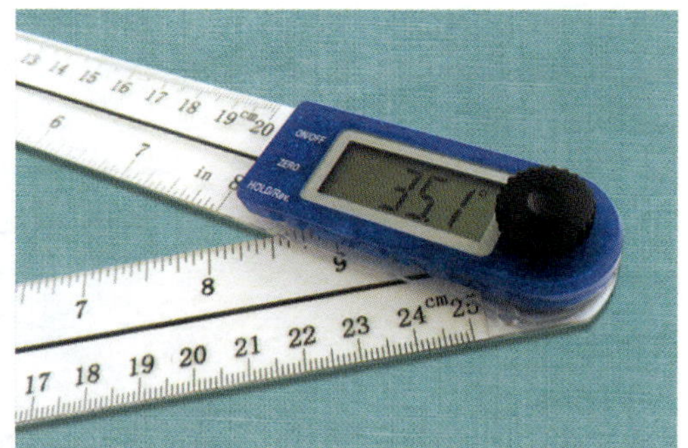


**Fig. 4.6:** Digital goniometer.

Some electrogoniometers are designed to measure motion at a single joint, such as the elbow or the hip, whereas others are designed to measure motion at a variety of joints (dynamic joint movements). Designs range from fairly cumbersome devices to more compact, portable systems. Although many electrogoniometers are capable of measuring motion in several planes simultaneously, the cost of these devices and the skill required for application have caused electrogoniometers to be used primarily in research applications.

### *Digital Goniometer*

A digital goniometer is a powerful tool in the hands of physiotherapists/clinicians to measure the joint range of motion precisely **(Fig. 4.6)**.

## Procedure/Principles of Goniometry

- ❖ The patient should be positioned in the relaxed manner and the joint to be measured should be free from any obstructions, such as pillow, couch, etc.
- ❖ The joint to be examined should be exposed properly by removing clothes from the site.
- ❖ Measurement should preferably be taken with the joint in neutral/0° position, except when fixed deformities in the joints exist.
- ❖ Total procedure should be explained to the patient.
- ❖ Therapist has to stand near to the patient facing the joint to be measured.
- ❖ Axis or the fulcrum of the goniometer is placed over the axis of the joint to be measured.
- ❖ Fixed arm and movable arm of the goniometer, should be aligned along the proximal and distal segments of the joint respectively, after establishing bony marks for measurement.
- ❖ Measurement of joint range of motion, should always be taken from the lateral aspect of the joint, in order to prevent obstruction.
- ❖ The clinician should support the goniometer in such a way that, it should not restrict the ROM.
- ❖ The clinician has to move the movable arm of the goniometer along the distal segment of the joint to measure the joint range (both AROM/PROM).
- ❖ The patient should be instructed to avoid trick movements, while measurement is performed.
- ❖ Measurement of degrees of movement produced, should be taken from the body/protractor of the goniometer.

## Factors Affecting the Joint Range of Motion

### *Soft Tissue Tightness*

Soft tissues, such as muscle, ligament, capsule, cartilage, synovial membrane tightness cause the reduction of range of motion of the joint. The soft tissue tightness may be due to the prolonged immobilization of the joint, injury around the joint or any joint diseases, such as osteoarthritis, rheumatoid arthritis, ankylosing spondylitis and TB arthritis, etc. Spasm of the muscles also contribute for joint stiffness.

If the joint structures are immobilized for prolonged period, it reduces the extensibility of soft tissues, forms adhesion with development of tightness of the soft tissue around the joint. There will be increased collagen fibers and reduction of the elasticity property of the fibers of the connective and soft tissues of the joint.

### *Adhesion Formation*

After resolution of inflammation, following injury and infection, the tenacious exudates form adhesion, binding the joint structures together, causing joint stiffness and reduction of joint range of motion. Lack of mobility of the joint leads to reduction in the flexibility and the nourishment (circulation) around the joint structures.

### *Injuries or Inflammation around the Joint*

Any recent injuries, inflammatory joint diseases, such as osteoarthritis, rheumatoid arthritis, ankylosing spondylitis and TB arthritis and psoriatic arthritis may cause severe pain around the joint. As the result of the pain patient may avoid performing the full range of movement. Sometimes due to fear of pain also patient may not perform any movement. So, as a result, there will be reduction in the active and passive range of movement.

### *Muscle Bulk*

Increased muscle bulk may cause the reduction of the active and passive range of motion due to soft tissue approximation. For example, for a common man the elbow flexion range of motion will be 125° to 135° but it is very much lower for the body-builders due to their huge biceps muscle bulk.

### *Gender*

The range of motion may vary with the gender. For example, females will be having less hip extension and hyper hip flexion after 25 years, but the same is reverse in males. Generally, females will be having the more flexible joints with increased range of motion than the males, due to excess relaxin hormone in females.

### *Age*

Individuals develop arthritic changes in the joints, due to aging process, leading to decreased joint space and ROM. The range of motion of joint will be more in the infant and childhood. Day-by-day the range of motion reduces as the age increases. While reaching the adulthood, the range of motion reduces while compared with the childhood and late childhood. The range of motion again bit increases in the old age due to the hypotonicity of the muscles and the reduction of the muscle bulk.

### *Bony Blocks/Loose Bodies*

Bony blocks/loose bodies in the joints affect the joint ROM greatly giving a hard end feel.

### *Nervous System Diseases/Disorders*

Sometimes the range of motion may be altered in diseases affecting the nervous system. Spasticity of the muscle, which is the result of the UMN lesion, will be reducing the range of motion and the joint becomes hypomobile. The LMN lesion, which causes the flaccidity, will result in hypermobile joint.

## Selection of the Goniometer

Selection of the goniometer is much more important factor while measuring the range of motion of the joint. If the bony segments of the joints are big, the bigger size, i.e., bigger length movable and stable armed goniometer has to be used and vice versa for joints with smaller segments. Normally, the inclinometer is mostly used to measure the pelvic motion, though, it can be used to measure ROM of the spine and certain peripheral joints.

## Measuring Procedures

### *Cervical Spine*

#### Flexion/Extension (Figs. 4.7A and B)

- **ROM**: Flexion: 0–45°, extension: 0–45°.
- **Position:** Sitting on a chair, thoracic and lumbar spine fully supported. A stick/ tongue depressor may be held between the teeth.
- **Fulcrum of goniometer**: Placed over the external auditory meatus.
- **Stationary arm**: Aligned in such a way that, it is perpendicular to the ground.
- **Moving arm:** Aligned parallel to the long axis of the stick/tongue depressor.
- **Tape measure for flexion/extension:** Distance between the chin and suprasternal notch is measured with an inch tape for documentation of flexion and extension **(Figs. 4.8A and B)**.

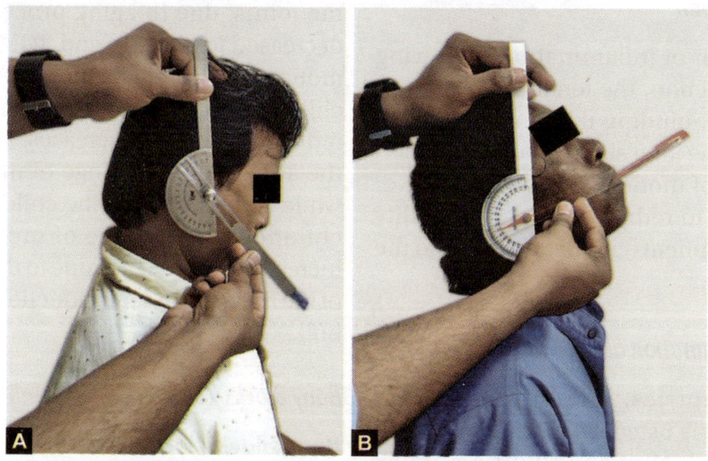


**Figs. 4.7A and B:** Measurement of cervical ROM: (A) Flexion; (B) Extension.

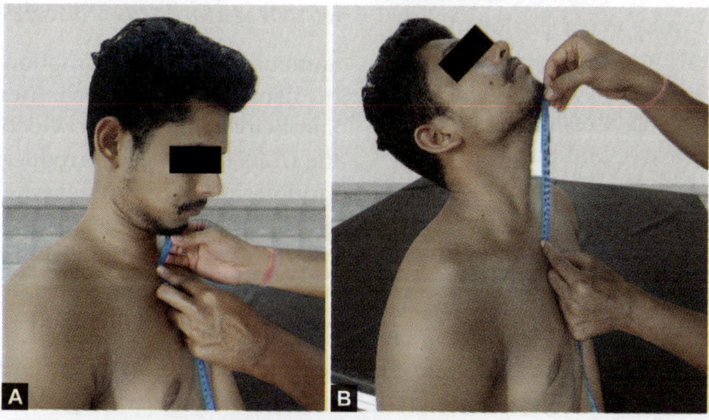


**Figs. 4.8A and B:** Measurement of cervical ROM, with measuring tape: (A) Flexion; (B) Extension.

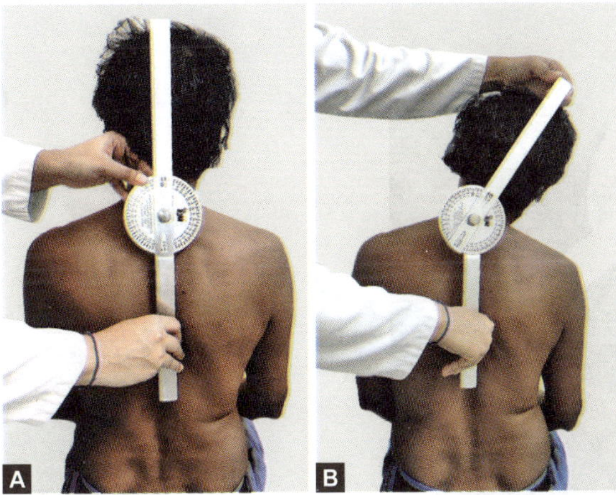

**Figs. 4.9A and B:** Goniometry for cervical lateral flexion: (A) Starting position; (B) Ending position.

### Lateral Flexion (Left/Right) (Figs. 4.9A and B)

- **ROM**: Lateral flexion to left and right: 0–45°.
- **Position:** Sitting on a chair/stool/bed, thoracic and lumbar spine fully supported and cervical spine is in vertical/neutral position.
- **Fulcrum of goniometer:** Placed over the spinous process of C7.
- **Stationary arm**: Aligned along the thoracic spine in such a way that, it is perpendicular to the ground.
- **Moving arm:** Aligned in line with the dorsal midline of head, using the occipital protuberance as reference.
- **Tape measure for lateral flexion:** Finding the distance between the mastoid process and tip of acromion with an inch tape can also be used to document lateral flexion **(Fig. 4.10)**.

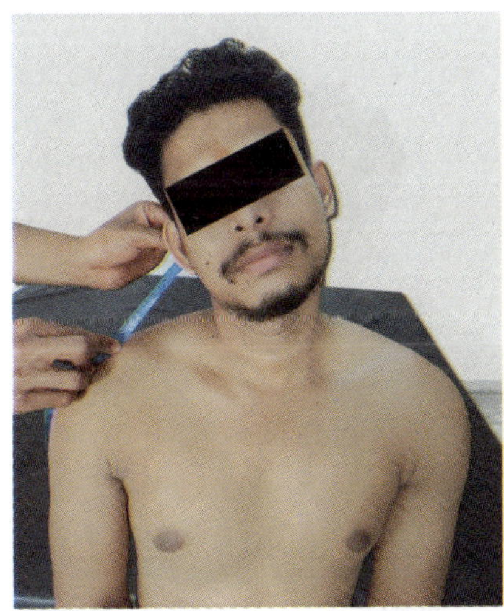

**Fig. 4.10:** Tape measure for cervical lateral flexion.

### Cervical Rotation (Left/Right) (Fig. 4.11)

- **ROM**: Rotation to left and right: 0–60°.
- **Position:** Sitting on a chair, thoracic and lumbar spine fully supported. A stick/tongue depressor may be held between the teeth for reference.
- **Fulcrum of goniometer**: Placed over the center of the cranial aspect of the head.
- **Stationary arm:** Aligned parallel to the imaginary line between the two acromial processes.
- **Moving arm:** Aligned parallel to the longitudinal axis of the tongue depressor/stick.

Tape measure for cervical rotation: Finding the distance between the center of chin and tip of acromion with an inch tape, as the patient rotates the neck, documents the rotation range of cervical spine **(Fig. 4.12)**.

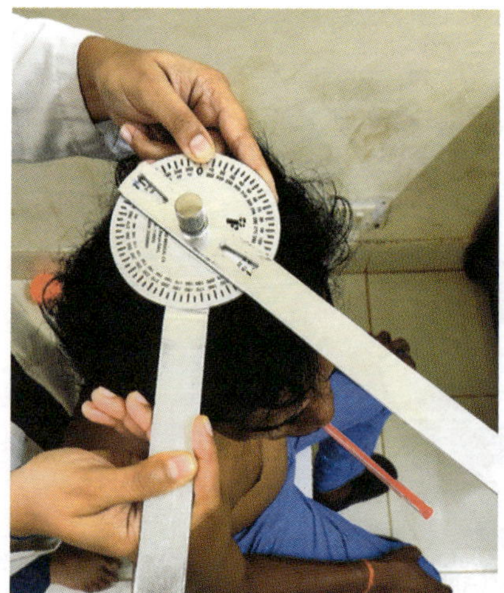

**Fig. 4.11:** Goniometry for cervical rotation.

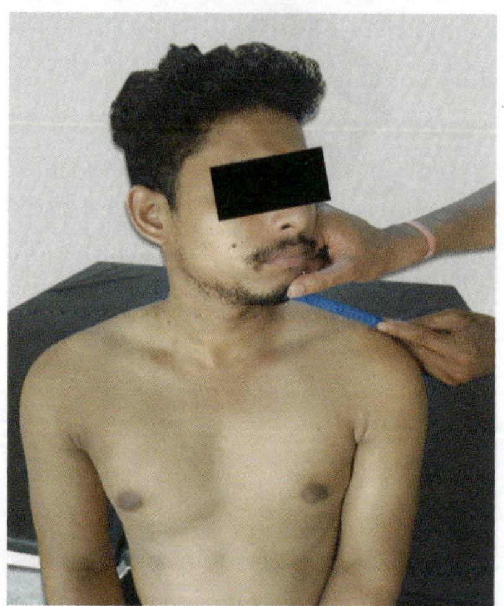

**Fig. 4.12:** Tape measure for cervical rotation.

### *Thoracolumbar Spine*

ROM: Flexion: 0–80°. Extension: 0–30°, lateral flexion (left and right): 0–35° (each), rotation (left and right): 0–45° (each).

**Measurement of Flexion/Extension**

ROM of flexion/extension is usually made through a measuring tape by using the following methods:

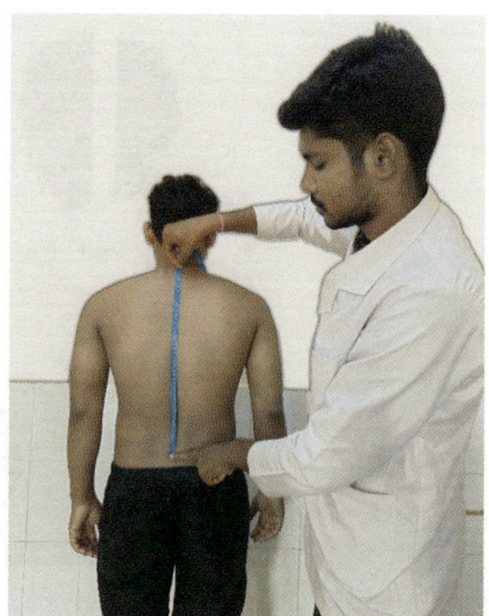

**Fig. 4.13:** Measurement of thoracolumbar flexion/ extension using an inch tape.

Patient standing, with the back exposed. The clinician marks the spinous processes of C7 and S1, puts a measuring tape on the spine extending from C7 to S1 and measures the distance between these two points in upright posture. Then the subject is asked to bend forward with the knees straight, and the distance between C7and S1 is again measured. The difference in measured values between second and first procedures gives the range of motion of thoracolumbar flexion. The same procedure is also followed to measure the extension ROM **(Fig. 4.13)**.

**Modified Schober's Method**

The patient standing with the back exposed, and feet 15 cm apart. Three marks as indicated below are made on the patient's spine with some erasable marker:

- ❖ One mark on the lumbosacral junction.
- ❖ Second mark on the spinous processes 10 cm above L-S junction.
- ❖ Third mark 5 cm below the first mark.

Measuring tape is aligned on the spine, one end of the tape on second mark and the other on third mark and the subject is asked to bend forward (flexion)/backward (extension). The distance between the second and third points

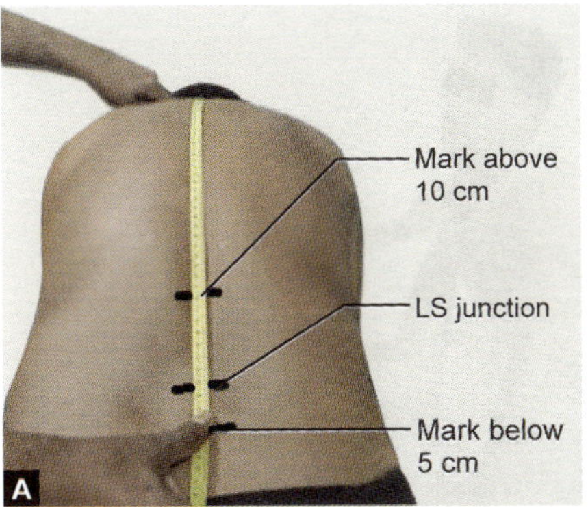

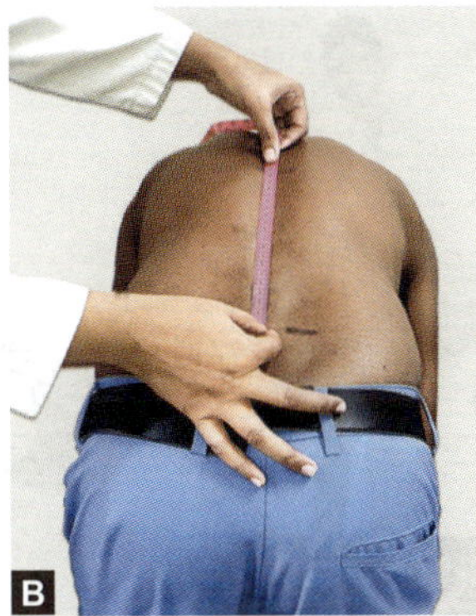

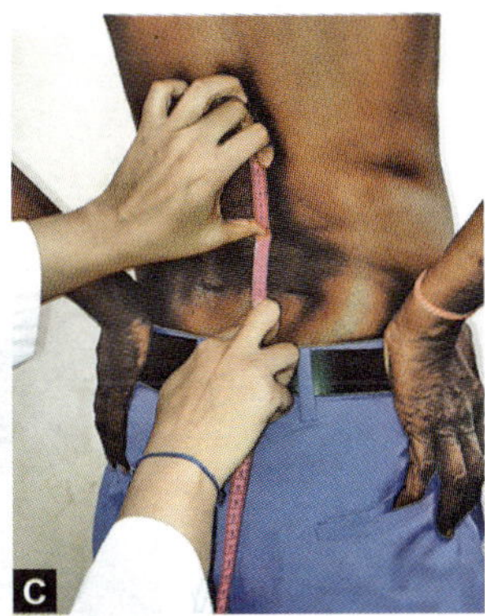


**Figs. 4.14A to C:** (A) Modified, modified Schober's test; (B) Modified, modified Schober's test for lumbar flexion; (C) Modified, modified Schober's test for lumbar extension.

are noted. This distance minus 15 cm is the ROM (for flexion and extension respectively) **(Fig. 4.14A)**.

The Modified, modified Schober's test (the Wolfson modified Schober test), where, instead of the L5-S1 junction as the 1st land mark, as described in the modified Schober's test, the spinal intersection of the left and right posterior superior iliac spines is taken as the 1st bony landmark and a point 15 cm above the 1st bony landmark is taken as the 2nd bony landmark. The measuring tape is placed between the first and second bony landmarks and the patient is asked to bend forward for flexion and backward for extension **(Figs. 4.14B and C)**. The change in length (total length—15 cm) indicates the amount of flexion/extension. As per evidence the normality MMST value for lumbar flexion in healthy adults is 6.85+/- 1.18 cm and for lumbar extension the value is: 2.42+/-0.74 cm This test is found more reliable as compared to modified Schober's test.

The third method of measurement of ROM of D-L spine flexion/extension is measuring the distance between floor and tip of middle fingers as the subject bends forward in standing with the knees straight for flexion range of motion and measuring the distance between the suprasternal notch and the floor/bed, as the subject extends the spine in prone, for extension range of motion **(Figs. 4.15A and B)**.

### Measurement of Lateral Flexion

The patient standing with back exposed. The fulcrum of the goniometer is aligned over the spinous process of S1, the stationary arm is aligned perpendicular to ground. The movable arm is aligned over the spine in line with C7. As the patient bends sideways the degree of lateral flexion is recorded from the body of the goniometer **(Fig. 4.16A)**.

The alternative method of measurement is measuring the distance between the patient's middle finger and floor, as he/she bends sideways **(Fig. 4.16B)**.

### Measurement of Rotation of D-L Spine

The subject sitting straight, so that the acromion processes are aligned directly over the iliac tubercles. The fulcrum of the goniometer is aligned over the center of the cranial aspects of head. The stationary and movable arms are aligned along the imaginary line joining both the acromion processes/iliac tubercles. As the subject rotates, the body with cervicothoracic spine as one unit, the angular displacement/measurement is taken from the body of the goniometer **(Fig. 4.17)**.

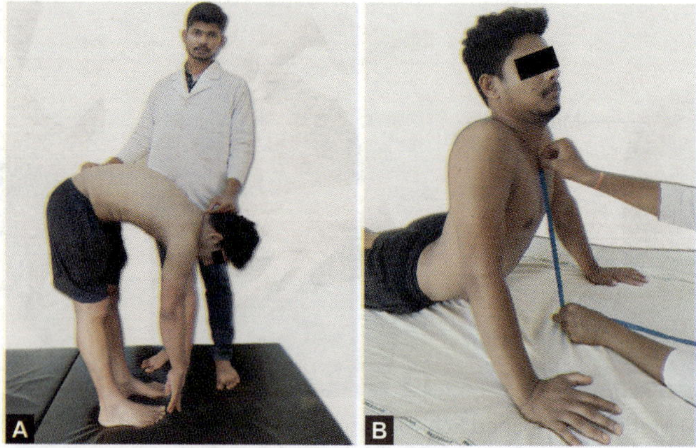

**Figs. 4.15A and B:** Tape measure for thoracolumbar ROM: (A) Flexion; (B) Extension.

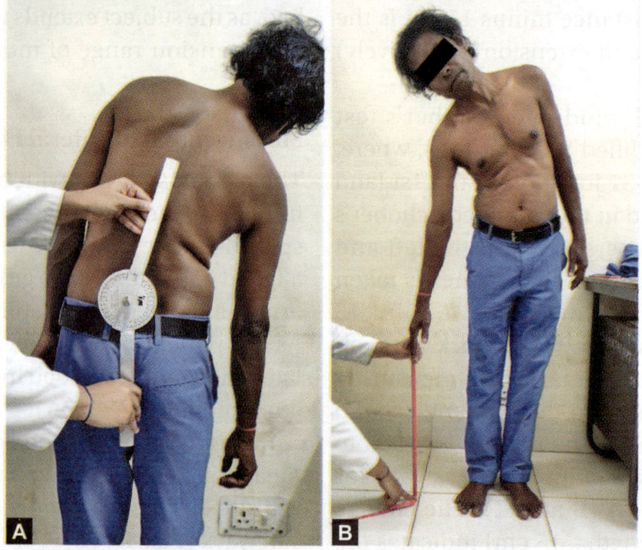

**Figs. 4.16A and B:** Measurement of lateral flexion of D-L spine: (A) Using goniometer; (B) Using inch tape.

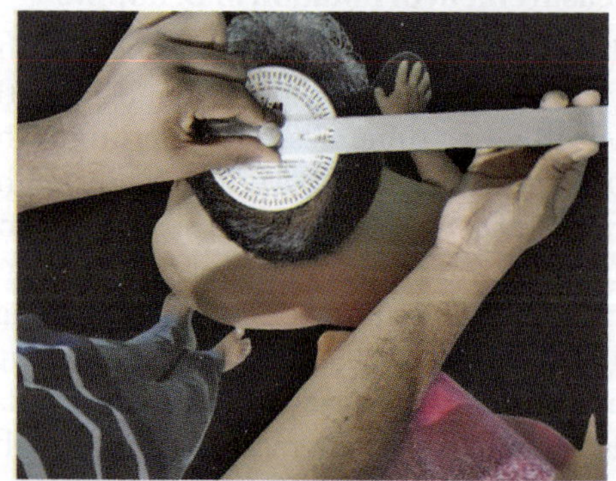

**Fig. 4.17:** Fixation of goniometer for D-L rotation.

## *Shoulder Joint*

### Flexion (Fig. 4.18A)

- **ROM:** 0–180°.
- **Position**: Supine lying.
- **Fulcrum of goniometer:** Close to the acromion process.
- **Stationary arm**: Along the mid axillary line of thorax.
- **Moving arm:** Along the lateral midline of humerus with reference to the lateral epicondyle.

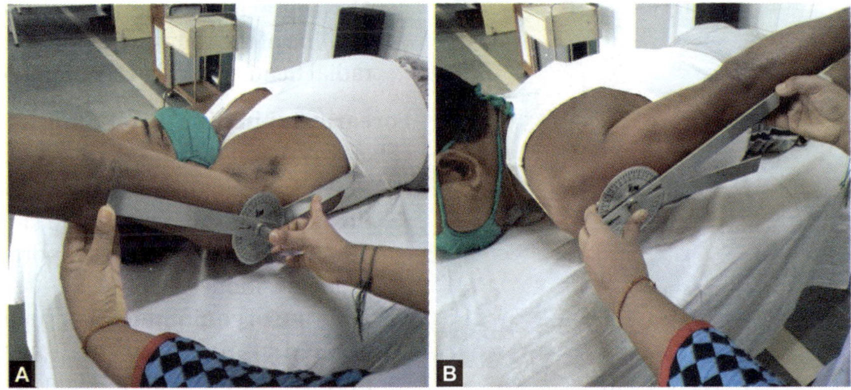

**Figs. 4.18A and B:** (A) Goniometry for shoulder flexion; (B) Goniometry for shoulder extension.

### Extension (Fig. 4.18B)

- **ROM:** 0–50/60°.
- **Position:** Prone lying.
- **Fulcrum of goniometer**: Close to the acromion process.
- **Stationary arm:** Along the mid axillary line of thorax.
- **Moving arm**: Along the lateral midline of humerus with reference to the lateral epicondyle.

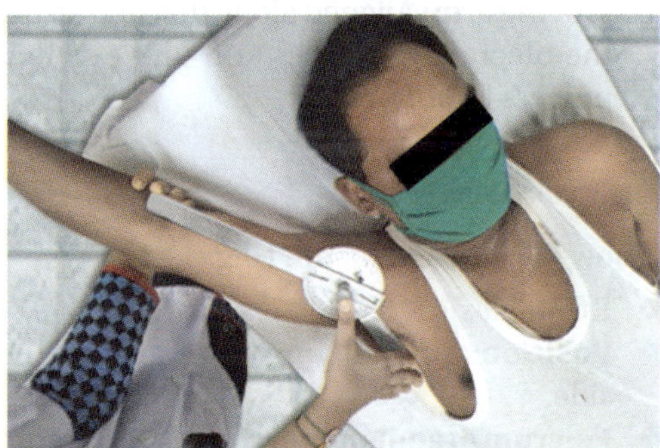
**Fig. 4.19:** Goniometry for shoulder abduction/adduction.

### Abduction/Adduction (Fig. 4.19)

- **ROM:** Abduction: 0–180°, adduction: 180–0°.
- **Position:** Supine lying.
- **Fulcrum of goniometer**: Close to the anterior aspect of acromion process.
- **Stationary arm:** Along the proximal arm, so that it is parallel to the midline of the anterior aspect of sternum.
- **Moving arm:** Along the medial midline of the humerus.

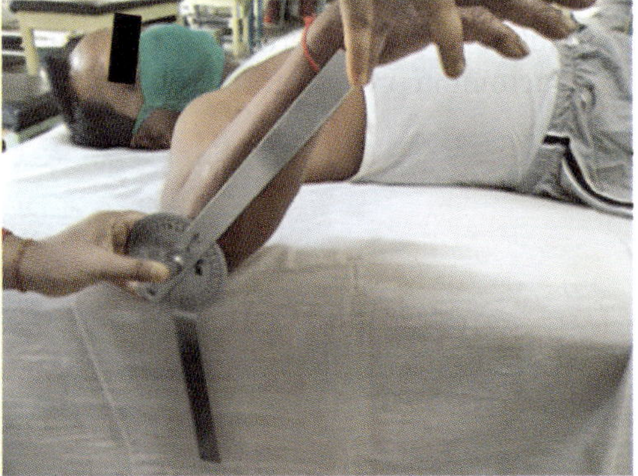
**Fig. 4.20:** Goniometry for—shoulder medial rotation/lateral rotation.

### Medial Rotation/Lateral Rotation (Fig. 4.20)

- **ROM:** Medial rotation: 0–70°, lateral rotation: 0–90°.
- **Position:** Supine lying, with shoulder in 90° of abduction, forearm perpendicular to the supporting surface with palm facing towards the feet. The elbow is at the edge of the couch.
- **Fulcrum of goniometer:** Center of the fulcrum of the goniometer is placed over the olecranon process of ulna.
- **Stationary arm:** The stationary arm is aligned perpendicular to the floor.

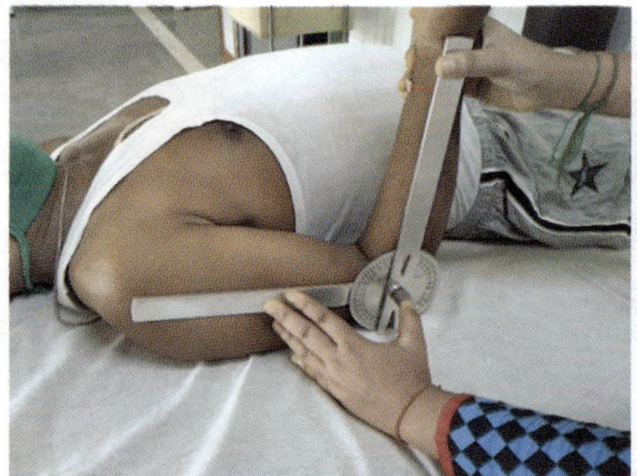

**Fig. 4.21:** Goniometry for elbow flexion/extension.

- **Moving arm:** Aligned along the ulna, using the olecranon process and ulnar styloid process for reference.

### *Elbow and Forearm*

#### Elbow Flexion/Extension (Fig. 4.21)

- **ROM:** Flexion: 0–150°, extension: 150–0°.
- **Position:** Supine lying, with arm by the side.
- **Fulcrum of goniometer:** Center of fulcrum of the goniometer is aligned over the lateral epicondyle of humerus.
- **Stationary arm:** Aligned along the lateral midline of the humerus, using the center of acromion process as reference.
- **Moving arm:** Aligned along the lateral midline of the radius with reference to the radial head and radial styloid process.

#### Forearm Supination/Pronation (Figs. 4.22A and B)

- **ROM**: Supination: 0–80°, pronation: 0–80°.
- **Position:** Sitting, arm by the side, elbow flexed to 90° and forearm supported in mid prone position.
- **Fulcrum of goniometer:** For supination—aligned at medial to the ulnar styloid process. For pronation—aligned at lateral to the ulnar styloid process.
- **Stationary arm:** For supination/pronation—aligned parallel to the anterior midline of the humerus.
- **Moving arm:** For supination—place across the ventral aspect of forearm, just proximal to the styloid processes. For pronation—place across the dorsal aspect of forearm, just proximal to the styloid processes of radius and ulna.

### *Wrist and Hand*

#### Wrist Flexion/Extension (Figs. 4.23A and B)

- **ROM**: Flexion: 0–80°, extension: 0–60°.
- **Position:** Sitting, shoulder abducted, elbow flexed to 90° and the pronated forearm resting on a pillow.

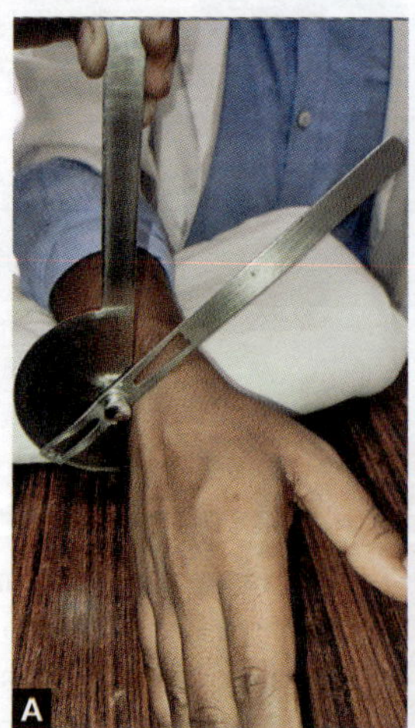

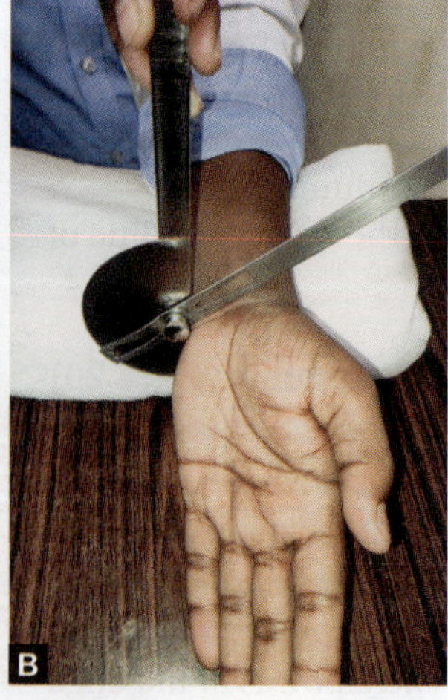

**Figs. 4.22A and B:** Goniometry for: (A) Forearm pronation; (B) Forearm supination.

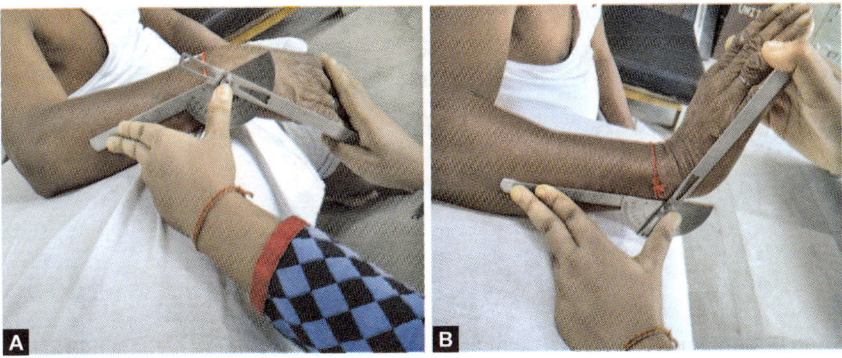

**Figs. 4.23A and B:** Goniometry for: (A) Wrist flexion; (B) Wrist extension.

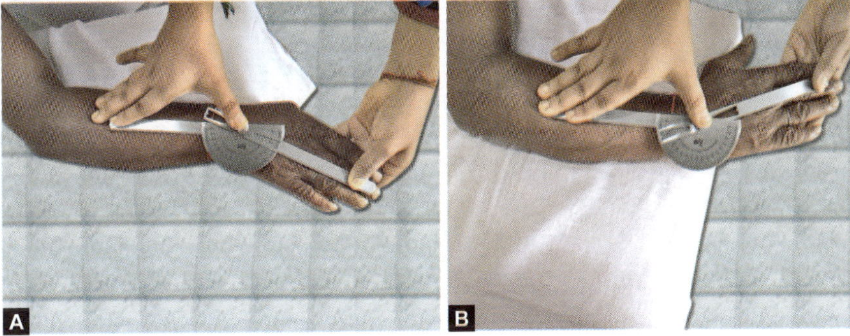

**Figs. 4.24A and B:** Goniometry for: (A) Wrist ulnar deviation; (B) Wrist radial deviation.

- **Fulcrum of goniometer:** For flexion/extension—place over the outer aspect of the wrist on the triquetrum.
- **Stationary arm:** For flexion/extension—align over the outer midline of ulna, using the olecranon and the ulnar styloid process as reference. Moving arm—align along the outer midline of the fifth metacarpal.

### Wrist Radial/Ulnar Deviation (Figs. 4.24A and B)

- **ROM**: Radial deviation: 0–20°, ulnar deviation: 0–30°.
- **Position:** Sitting, shoulder abducted, elbow flexed to 90° and the pronated forearm resting on a pillow.
- **Fulcrum of goniometer**: Center of fulcrum of the goniometer is aligned over the middle of the dorsal aspect of the wrist over the capitate.
- **Stationary arm:** Aligned along the dorsal midline of the forearm, using the lateral epicondyle of the humerus as reference.
- **Moving arm:** Aligned along the dorsal midline of the third meta carpal.

### *Thumb and Fingers (Figs. 4.25A to D)*

Measurement of ROM of small joints of the hand are made by using small goniometers made for the purpose. Examples of goniometry for the small joints, say PIP joint of finger, MCP and CMC joints of thumb are shown in **Figures 4.25A to D**. However, for complete goniometry of hand, the reader is advised to refer some books on goniometry.

## *Hip Joint*

### Flexion (Fig. 4.26)

- **ROM**: 0–120° (with knees flexed)
- **Position**: Supine

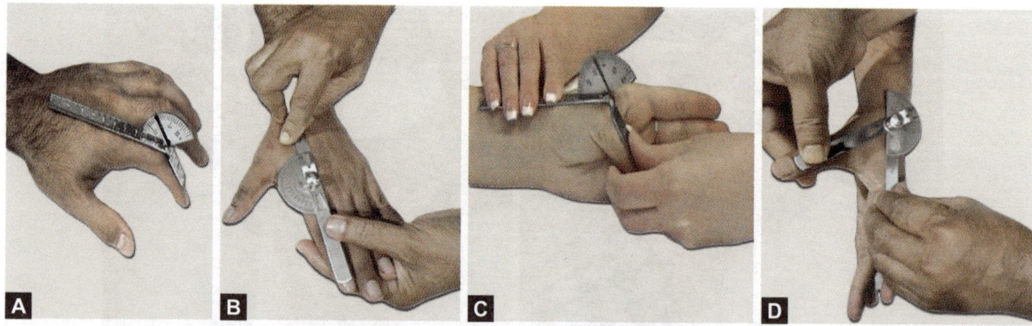

**Figs. 4.25A to D:** Goniometry for: (A) PIP joint flexion of fingers; (B) Abduction/adduction in MCP joint of fingers; (C) MCP flexion of thumb; (D) Palmar abduction in CMC joint of thumb.

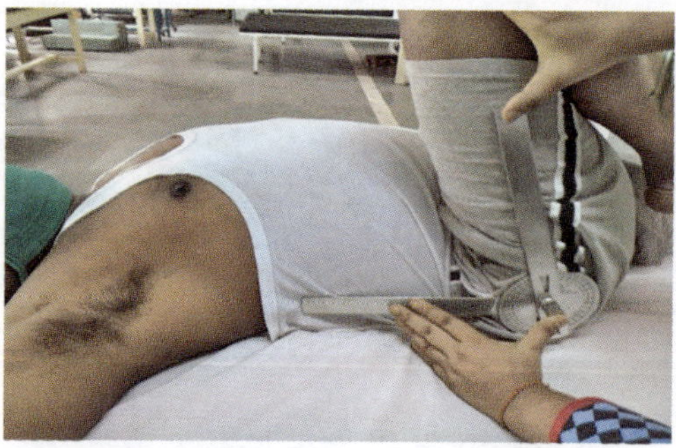

**Fig. 4.26:** Goniometry for hip flexion.

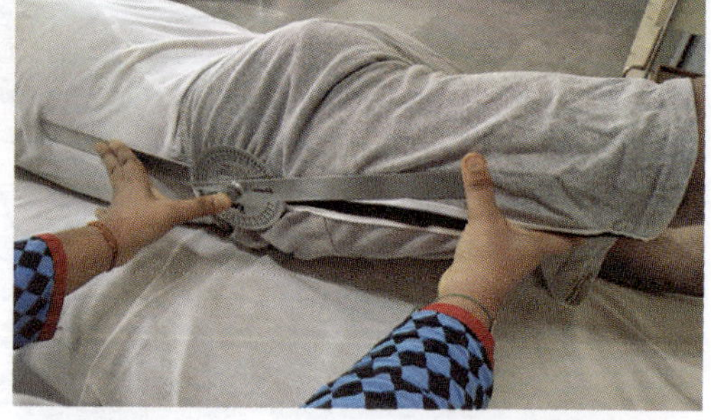

**Fig. 4.27:** Goniometry for hip extension.

- **Fulcrum of goniometer**: Lateral aspect of the hip joint over the greater trochanter.
- **Stationary arm:** Along the lateral midline of the pelvis and trunk.
- **Moving arm**: Along the lateral midline of femur using the lateral epicondyle as reference.

**Extension (Fig. 4.27)**

- **ROM**: 0–30°.
- **Position**: Prone lying
- **Fulcrum of goniometer**: Lateral aspect of the hip joint over the greater trochanter.
- **Stationary arm**: Along the lateral midline of the pelvis and trunk.
- **Moving arm:** Along the lateral midline of femur using the lateral epicondyle as reference.

**Abduction (Fig. 4.28)**

- **ROM**: 0–45°.
- **Position**: Supine lying

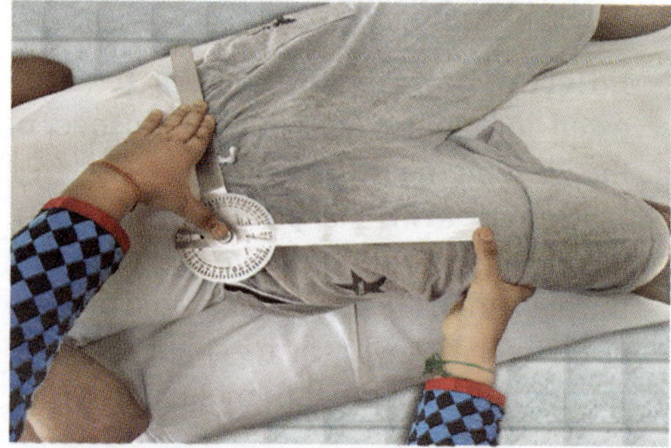

**Fig. 4.28:** Goniometry for hip abduction.

- **Fulcrum of goniometer**: Anterior superior iliac spine (ASIS).
- **Stationary arm:** Along the opposite ASIS
- **Moving arm:** Along the anterior midline of femur with reference to midline of patella.

**Adduction (Fig. 4.29)**

- **ROM:** 0–30°.

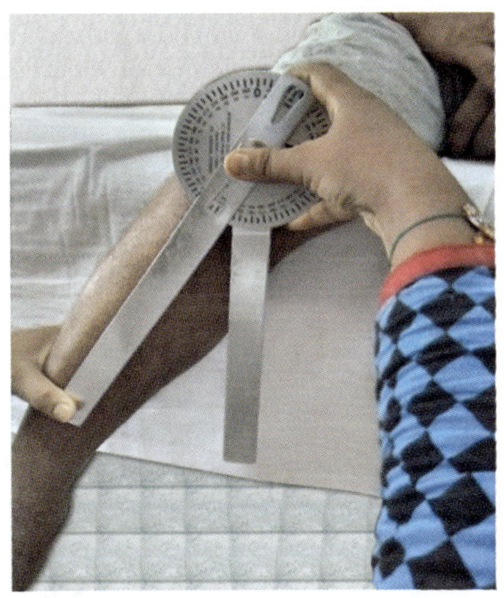

**Fig. 4.29:** Goniometry for hip medial rotation/ lateral rotation.

- **Position**: Position of patient and placement of goniometer is same as described for hip abduction.

### Medial/Lateral Rotation

- **ROM**: 0–45°.
- **Position**: Sitting on bed, with knees flexed to 90° at the edge of bed.
- **Fulcrum of goniometer**: Center of patella.
- **Stationary arm:** Perpendicular to the floor/parallel to the supporting surface.
- **Moving arm:** Along the anterior midline of the leg with reference to crest of tibia and midway between the two malleoli.

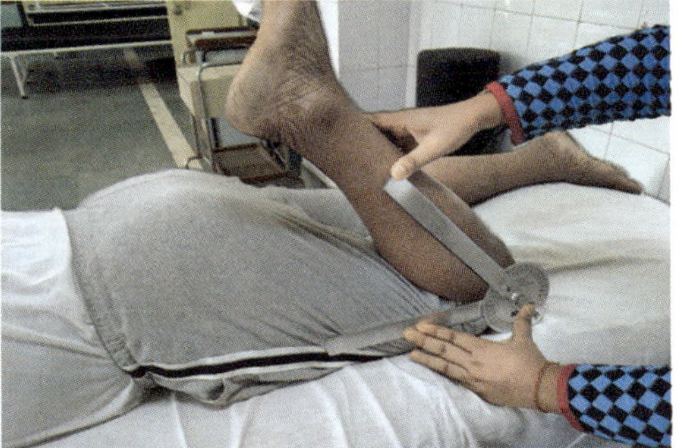

**Fig. 4.30:** Goniometry for knee flexion/extension.

## *Knee Joint*

### Knee Flexion/Extension (Fig. 4.30)

- **ROM:** Flexion: 0–135°, extension: 135–0°.
- **Position**: Prone lying
- **Fulcrum of goniometer**: Over the lateral epicondyle of femur
- **Stationary arm**: Lateral midline of femur using the greater trochanter as reference.
- **Moving arm:** Along the lateral midline of fibula with reference to the lateral malleolus.

## *Ankle and Foot (Figs. 4.31A and B)*

- **ROM**: Dorsiflexion: 0–20°, plantar flexion: 0–50°.
- **Position**: Sitting/supine with knee flexed
- **Fulcrum of goniometer:** Over the lateral aspect of the lateral malleolus.

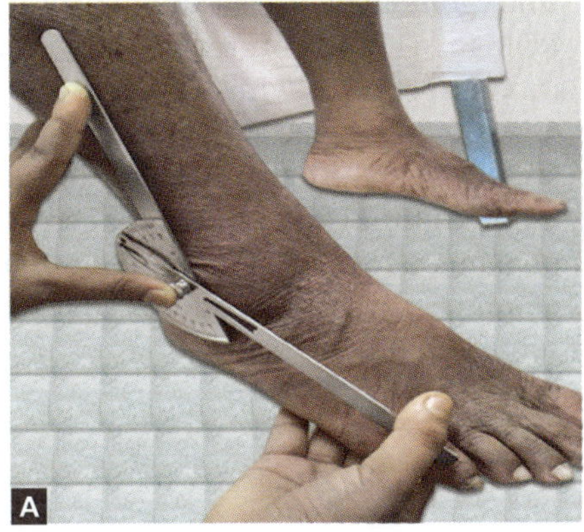



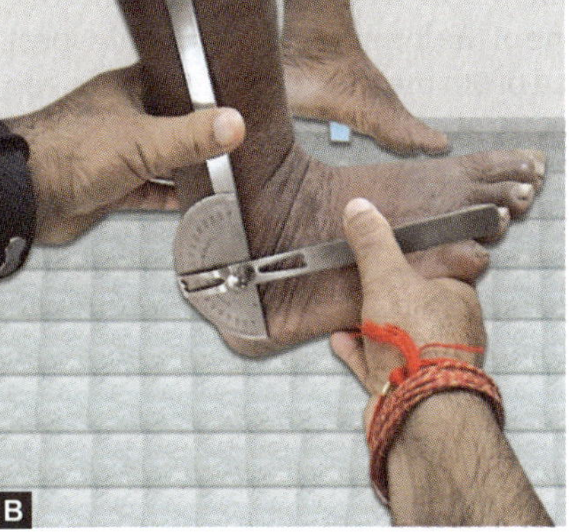



**Figs. 4.31A and B:** Goniometry for: (A) Ankle plantar flexion; (B) Ankle dorsiflexion.

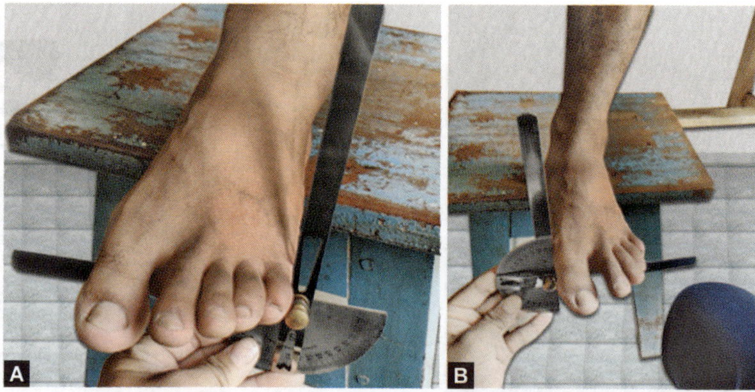

**Figs. 4.32A and B:** (A) Goniometry for inversion; (B) Goniometry for eversion.

- **Stationary arm**: Along the lateral midline of fibula using the head of fibula as reference.
- **Moving arm**: Aligned parallel to the lateral aspect of 5th metatarsal.

### Foot (Figs. 4.32A and B)

- **ROM**: Inversion: 0–30°, eversion: 0–20°.
- **Position**: Sitting on bed with flexed knee hanging at the edge and hind foot resting on the stool.
- **Fulcrum of goniometer**: For inversion—the fulcrum of the goniometer is aligned over lateral aspect of head of 5th metatarsal, and for eversion, the fulcrum is aligned over the medial aspect of head of first metatarsal.
- **Stationary arm:** For inversion, the stationary arm lies parallel to the anterior midline of the lower leg along lateral aspect of head of 5th metatarsal. For eversion, the stationary arm lies parallel to the anterior midline of the lower leg along the medial aspect of head of 1st metatarsal.
- **Moving arm:** For inversion and eversion—aligned along the plantar aspect 1st through the 5th metatarsal.

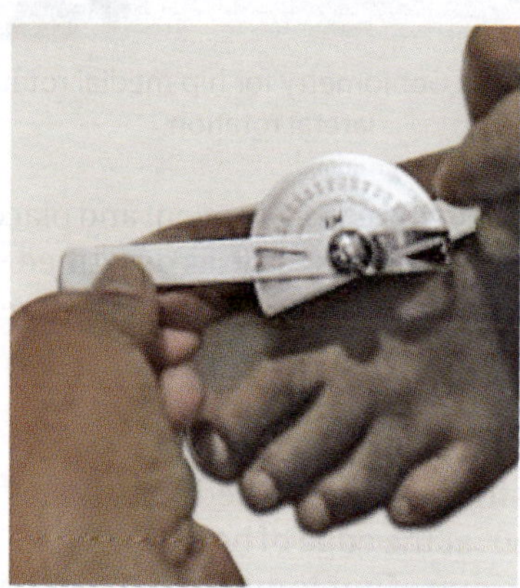

**Fig. 4.33:** Goniometry for abduction ROM of great toe.

## *Goniometry for Toes*

Goniometry for toes are performed by using small goniometers. Measurement of abduction ROM in MTP joint of great toe is demonstrated in **Figure 4.33**, where fulcrum is placed over the MTP joint of great toe, fixed arm is aligned over the long axis of the 1st metatarsal bone and movable arm is placed along the phalanges. However, for complete goniometry of joints of toes, the reader is advised to refer some goniometry book.

# 5 CHAPTER

# Posture and Balance

## POSTURE

Posture is the attitude assumed by the body either with support during muscular inactivity, or by means of coordinated action of many muscles working to maintain stability.

Every movement begins and ends in posture, as stated by Sherrington, that "posture follows movements like a shadow". All movements of the body are initiated from a posture, which is often used to describe both biomechanical alignment of the body and orientation of body in environment.

Postural stability, also referred to as balance, is the ability to control the center of mass in relationship to the base of support.

- Center of mass (COM), is defined as a point that is at the center of the total body mass **(Fig. 5.1A)**. For perfect balance of the body, the center of pressure is directly under the center of mass.
- The vertical projection of the COM is often defined as the center of gravity (COG).
- The base of support (BOS) is defined as the area of the body that is in contact with the support surface.
- The center of pressure (COP) is the center of the distribution of the total force applied to the supporting surface. The COP moves continuously around the COM to keep the COM within the support base (Benda et al., 1994; Winter, 1990). It is located at the point of application of the ground reaction force vector. The center of pressure is not a static entity. During human walking, the center of pressure is near the heel at the time of heel strike and moves anteriorly throughout the step, being located near the toes at toe-off. Accordingly, the ground reaction force acting on the surface also changes.
- **Ground reaction force:** The ground reaction force (GRF) is the force exerted by the ground on an object in contact with it. It is the force that opposes the force of gravity and allows the individual to stand upright, where the magnitude of the GRF is equal to the weight of the object and it acts perpendicular to the surface of the ground. During walking/running the ground reaction force changes it location of action, as per the contact of foot to the ground **(Fig. 5.1B)**.

In case of movement, say walking/running, the individual applies force on the ground, and the ground applies a force back on the individual, which helps in forward propulsion of the body. The ground reaction force has a component parallel to the ground, which is the frictional force. The coefficient of friction, is defined as the ratio of the frictional resistive force to the normal force, that pushes the objects/body together. It is expressed as: $\mu = F/N$, where $\mu$, is the coefficient of friction, F, is the frictional force, N is the normal force. A coefficient of friction >1, suggests a stronger frictional force, inhibiting displacement/movement. However, if the coefficient of friction is <1, it will result in propulsion.

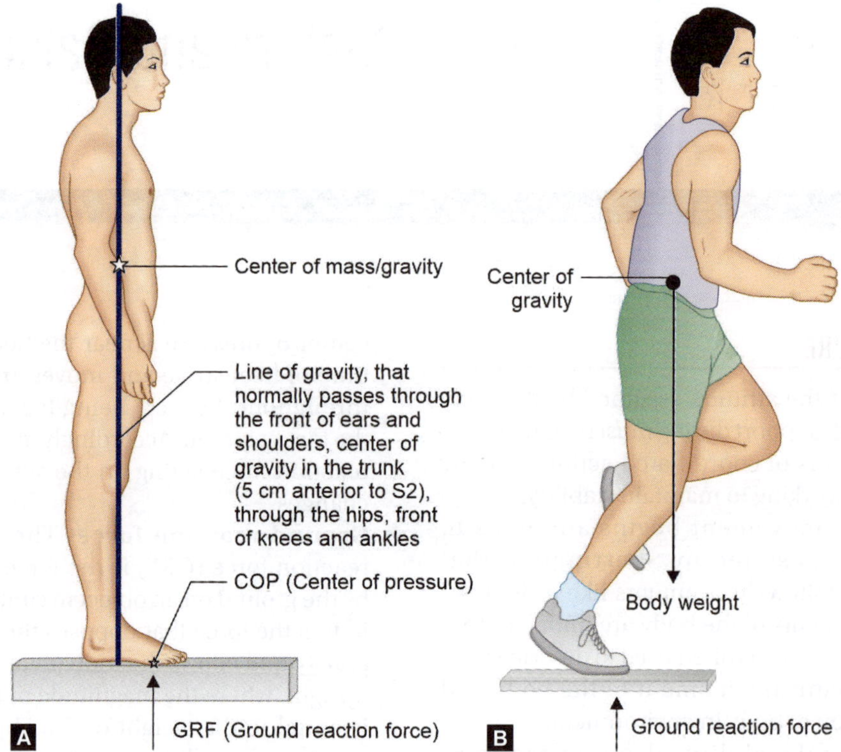


**Figs. 5.1A and B:** (A) Shows center of mass (COM), COP and GRF; (B) Shows the GRF acting at the ball of toes at push off phase, while walking/running.

## Postural Control

Postural control is a term used to describe the way the central nervous system (CNS) regulates sensory information from other systems in order to produce adequate motor output to maintain a controlled, upright posture. The visual, vestibular, and somatosensory systems are the main sensory systems involved in postural control and balance.

It is the person's ability to maintain stability of the body and body segments in space in response to forces that disturb body's structural equilibrium. It depends on the integrity of the central nervous system, visual, vestibular, and musculoskeletal system, that include information from receptors located in and around joints (i.e., joint capsule, tendons and ligaments) and from cutaneous receptors located in the sole of foot. It emerges from an interaction of the individual with the task and the environment.

Postural control for stability and orientation requires a complex interaction of musculoskeletal and neural components (systems).

### *Musculoskeletal Components*

It includes, joint range of motion, spinal flexibility, muscle properties, and biomechanical relationships among linked body segments.

### *Neural Components of Postural Control*

It includes the followings:

❖ **Sensory processes:** Organization and integration of visual, vestibular, somatosensory systems.

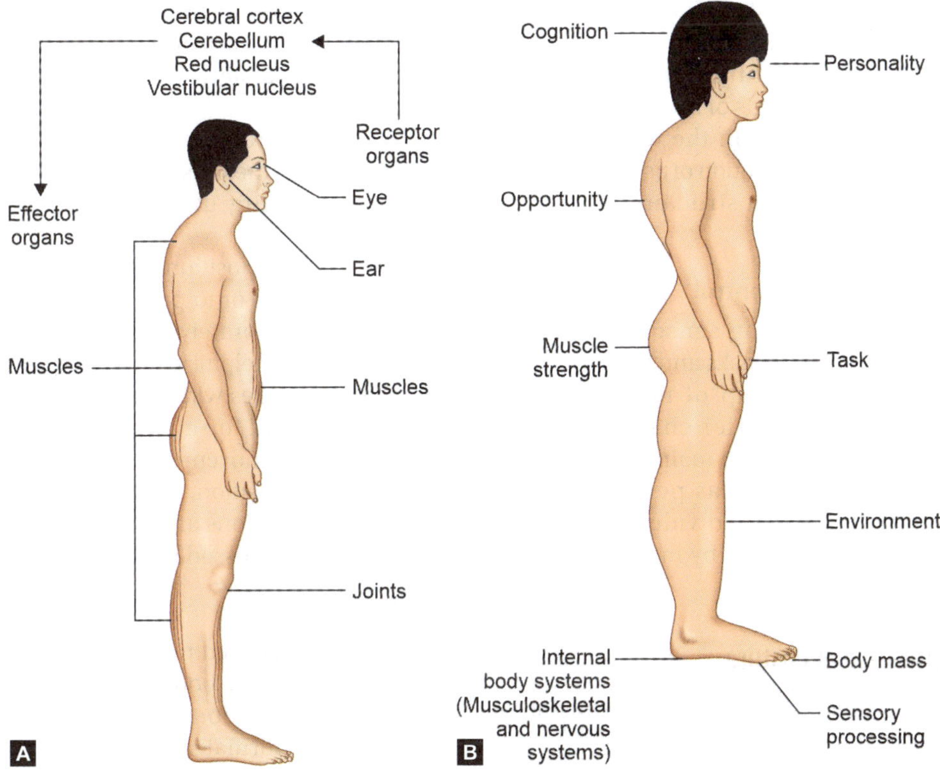


**Figs. 5.2A and B:** The postural control mechanism: (A) Postural reflex; (B) Adaptive postural control.

- **Central processing:** A higher-level integrative process, essential for mapping sensation to action, and ensuring anticipatory and adaptive aspects of postural control.
- **Effector component:** Sometimes referred to as the neuromuscular component which include organization of muscles throughout the body into neuromuscular synergies for postural alignment.

Postural control may develop by the postural reflex mechanism **(Fig. 5.2A)** or may develop voluntarily as per the imposed demands of the task, the individual is required to perform, called as adaptive postural control **(Fig. 5.2B)**.

### The Postural Reflex

- A reflex is by definition, an efferent response to an afferent stimulus. The afferent stimuli from variety of sources of the body such as muscles, eyes, ears and joint structures trigger the postural muscles to maintain postural tone for the development of the postures immediately during need. For example, when the legs slip on a slippery floor, and body tends to fall backwards, the afferent information from the different receptors stated above trigger the postural reflex, which maintain erect position of the body by moving the upper body forward so that the line of gravity falls within the supporting base. The receptors in the following organs provide the necessary afferent input.
- **Muscles:** Neuromuscular and neurotendinous spindles within the muscles record changing tension.
- **The eyes:** Visual sensation records any alteration in the position of the body with regard to the surroundings.

- **The ears:** Stimulation of the receptors of the vestibular nerve results from the movement of fluid contained in the semicircular canals of the internal ear.
- **Joint structures:** In the weight bearing position approximation of bones stimulates receptors in joint structures and elicits reflex reactions.

**Adaptive Postural Control**

It requires modifying sensory and motor systems to changing tasks and environmental demands. The group of muscles, most frequently the posterior chain antigravity muscles are recruited to maintain both static and dynamic posture as per the physical characteristic of the individual and nature of task to be performed by manipulating the environment.

## Classification of Posture

Posture, which is the basic prerequisite for movement are classified into:

### *Fundamental Postures*

These are the basic positions of body individuals adapt in their routine activities. There are five fundamental positions, as discussed below. Other postures individuals adapt, during functional activities are derived from the following fundamental postures:

- Standing
- Kneeling
- Sitting
- Lying
- Hanging

### *Derived Postures*

These are the positions, which are derived from the fundamental positions such as: standing, kneeling, sitting, lying, hanging. These are the postures, where the positions of the arms, leg or trunk may altered in the fundamental postures to modify the positions of the body, necessary to perform an activity/movement. The uses of derived positions are:

- To increase stability
- For relaxation
- To perform a particular exercise
- For reducing the muscle work
- For producing different functional activities.

These derived positions may be useful for our daily activities or to perform an exercise. This chapter elaborately explains about the position, which is helpful for an exercise and for day-to-day activities with relevant examples. The muscle work for a particular derived position and the movements, which occur in that particular position, are mentioned. The fundamental positions and positions derived from them are discussed below.

**Standing (Fig. 5.3)**

Standing, also referred to as orthostasis, is a position in which the body is held in an erect ("orthostatic") position and supported only by the feet. In normal standing, the base of support is about 5–10 cm, and the center of mass lies in front of the ankles. This is the most difficult position to hold, as the body need to be balanced on a narrow base, allowing minimal sway of body in anteroposterior and lateral directions. In erect standing posture the

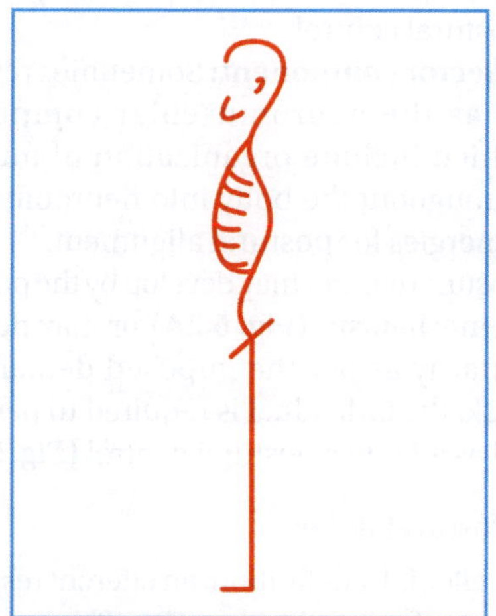

**Fig. 5.3:** Standing.

body undergoes a constant swaying motion called postural sway or sway envelope. The extent of the sway envelope for a normal individual standing with 4 inches between the feet can be as large as 12 degrees in the sagittal plane and 16 degrees in the frontal plane. In standing the whole body must be balanced and stabilized in correct alignment on feet with a small base of support by coordinated work of many muscle groups.

*Position of Body Segments*

- Feet are placed slightly apart with 2–4 inches distance between them.
- Knees are extended and aligned straight.
- Hip is in neutral position and slightly lateral rotated.
- Spine is erect.
- Shoulders down and back.
- Upper limb is hanging closely to the body.
- Palms facing inward towards the body.
- Neck is aligned straight.
- Head, thrusts upwards, ears levelled, and eyes look straight forward.

*Muscle Works in Standing (Fig. 5.4)*

Electromyography has detected slight activity in the muscles of the calf, hips, and lower back, and the core muscles play a significant role in maintaining stability in standing.

- Flexors and extensors of neck and trunk muscles counteract (co-contraction is present) and align the neck and trunk in straight position. Spinal extensors work more to stabilize the spine in erect position. The spinal flexor muscles counteracts and balances the spinal extensors. The core muscles play a role in maintaining stability. The core muscles are deep muscle layers that lie close to the spine and provide structural support. The transverse abdominals wrap around the spine and function as a compression corset. The multifidi are intersegmental muscles, that help to maintain stability.
- Elevators of the mandible closes the mouth.

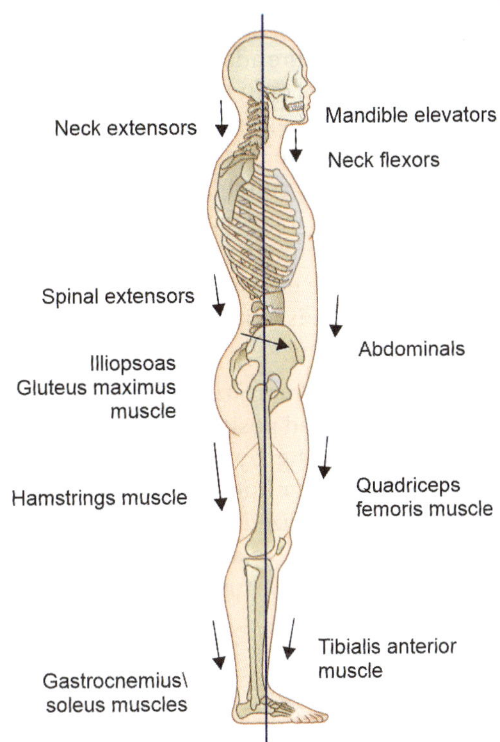


**Fig. 5.4:** Shows the muscles recruited in standing.

- Retractors of scapulae and adductors of the shoulder keep the shoulders in the adducted and slightly retracted position.
- Normally arms are relaxed or sometimes muscle work is minimal or nil.
- Hip extensors maintain the hip in neutral position and the flexors counteract on it for balancing the limb.
- The hip abductors maintain pelvic stability, which are more recruited in single leg standing.
- Hip lateral rotator keeps the hip in slightly rotated position.
- Ankle plantar and dorsiflexors counteract and keep the ankle in neutral position (plantigrade position).
- Toe flexors work more and make the ball of the toes grip with the floor.
- Intrinsic muscles of the foot stabilize the foot.

*Effect and Uses of Standing*

- ❖ This is the posture adapted for locomotion and majority of outdoor activities.
- ❖ Due to small base of support and high COG, the posture is less stable.
- ❖ This posture is suitable for persons who can maintain it correctly. If maintained correctly, it reduces muscle works and conditions the postural reflexes.
- ❖ This position is suitable for performing many exercises.

*Positions Derived from Standing*

Many of the derived positions can be derived from the standing by altering the arm, trunk and the lower limb alignments. These positions can be utilized for the different types of exercise regimen, relaxation, stability and accomplishing various functional tasks.

*Positions Derived by Altering Lower Limb Position*

- ❖ High standing
- ❖ Walk standing
- ❖ Stride standing
- ❖ Step standing
- ❖ Half-standing
- ❖ Toe standing
- ❖ Close standing
- ❖ Foot and on foot standing
- ❖ Cross standing.

High Standing

- ❖ Standing on the stool or in any raised platform **(Fig. 5.5)**.
- ❖ Movements of body segments are as mentioned above in standing.

**Muscle work:** Same as described for standing.

**Effect and uses:**

- ❖ To perform upper and lower limb exercises.
- ❖ To perform hanging, swinging of the arm and leg.
- ❖ To perform overhead activities.

**Examples:**

- ❖ To take some object from the height.
- ❖ Fitting the fan in the ceiling.

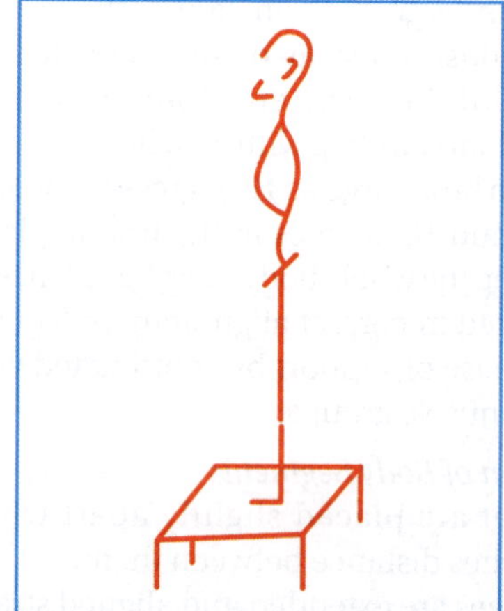

**Fig. 5.5:** High standing.

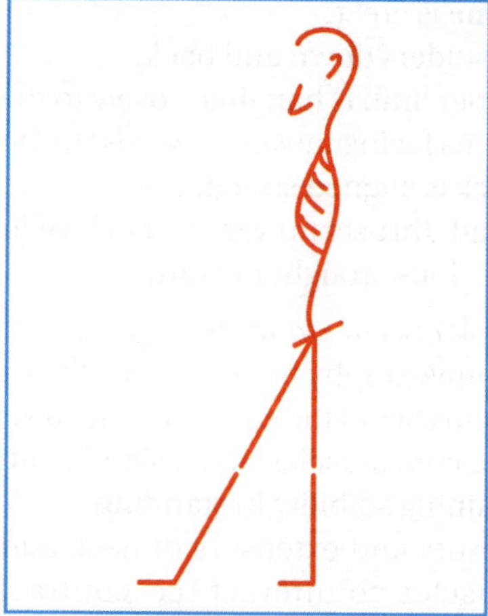

**Fig. 5.6:** Walk standing.

Walk Standing

- ❖ One leg is placed directly forwards, so that the heels are two feet-lengths apart and are on the same line. The body weight is equally distributed between them. Stability will be more in this position **(Fig. 5.6)**.

**Movements:**

- ❖ Hip—Flexion
- ❖ Knee—Extension
- ❖ Ankle—Mild plantar flexion.

**Muscle works:** The extensors of hip (eccentric contraction) and knee (concentric contraction) work strongly on the forward limb to maintain the position.

**Effect and uses:**

- The base is much enlarged in the antero-posterior direction, stabilizing the body for exercises in sagittal plane.
- Rotation of the pelvis towards the side of the forward leg is prevented by position of the back leg. This position can be used to localize rotation to spine.
- Tension of the hamstrings of the front leg, prevents anterior tilting of the pelvis while performing trunk flexion exercises.
- Starting position (position of readiness) for long distance running.
- Used to perform the hip, knee, ankle, and trunk muscles self-stretching.
- To achieve relaxation from the prolonged standing.
- Used as a posture for therapists to apply massage/mobilization exercises.

**Example:** Balancing on rope or rod.

### Stride Standing

This is achieved by abducting the legs, so that, the heels are 2 feet length apart and the angle between the feet remaining the same as in standing. The weight is equally distributed. The base is enlarged in a lateral direction, resulting in increase of steadiness in frontal plane **(Fig. 5.7)**.

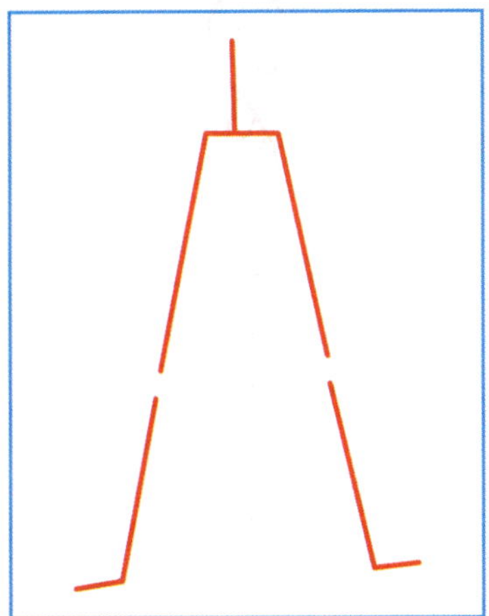

**Fig. 5.7:** Stride standing.

**Movements:**

- Hip abduction
- Knee extension.

**Muscle works:** The muscles of neck and trunk work in the similar manner as described for standing. Moreover the hip abductor muscles work to prevent sliding of the feet sideways.

**Uses in exercise therapy:**

- To perform the trunk, hip, knee exercises in the frontal plane.
- Used for stability, as the base is wider.
- Helps to stretch the hip adductors.
- Used by therapists while working on a heavy patient.

**Examples:**

- Sailors standing position.
- Standing posture while traveling in the bus.

### Step Standing

Standing with one foot on a higher level than the other. One foot is kept on the stool or on height. Hip and knee are flexed. This is also one of the stable postures **(Fig. 5.8)**.

**Movements:**

- Hip flexion.
- Knee flexion.
- Ankle plantigrade/dorsiflexion.

**Muscle works:** Besides the neck and trunk muscles, the muscles of the load bearing leg produce co-contraction to achieve stability.

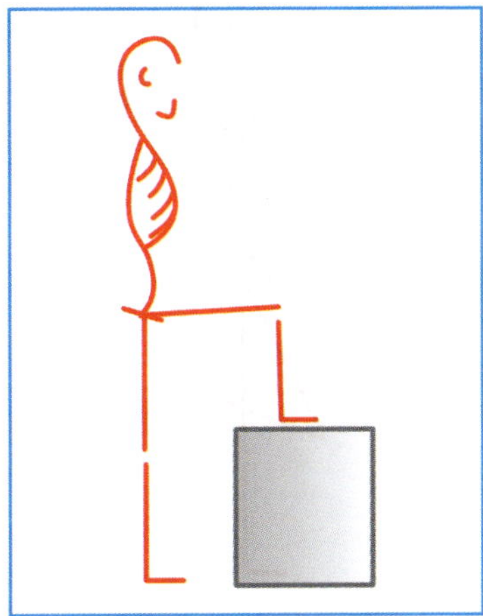

**Fig. 5.8:** Step standing.

The glutei muscles provide power to push off from the ground while stepping up onto a box/step and maintain the hip in flexion, the quadriceps help to stabilize the knee joint in flexion by eccentric contraction.

**Uses in exercise therapy:**

- For stretching the hip extensors, knee extensors and ankle plantar flexors.
- Mostly used for teaching weight transference before walking upstairs.
- Used for hemiplegic patients to promote weight bearing on the affected side.

**Examples:**

- Position adopted to tie the shoelace.
- Position adopted to cutting the toenails.

Half Standing

Standing with the one leg. One leg is flexed totally. It is the very difficult position to maintain for long period **(Fig. 5.9)**.

**Muscle works:**

- Abductors of the opposite side, i.e., supporting leg work to prevent downward tilt of pelvis.
- Spinal side flexors support the spine.
- Supporting leg muscles work strongly, by muscular co-contraction.

**Uses in exercise therapy:**

- Leg swinging exercise.
- Stretching the extensor muscles of hip and knee.

**Examples:**

- Used to pick-up some objects from the floor with the toes.
- Position adopted to remove the thorn in the sole of the foot.

Toe Standing

Standing on the toes and raising the body by ankle plantar flexion. This is also one of the unstable position because the COG rises and the BOS decreases in this position **(Fig. 5.10)**.

**Muscle works:**

- The plantar flexors of the ankle joint work strongly against gravity to keep the heels elevated.
- All other muscles of the lower limbs work more strongly than normal standing to maintain balance.

**Effect and uses:**

- The base of support is reduced and center of gravity is raised, compromising standing balance. Hence it can be used as a balancing strategy.
- Strong work of the foot muscles braces the longitudinal arches of feet, hence can be used as a therapeutic exercise for postural flat foot.

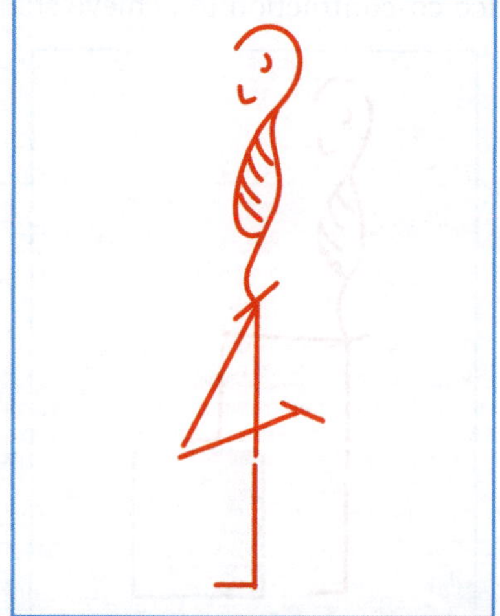

**Fig. 5.9:** Half-standing.

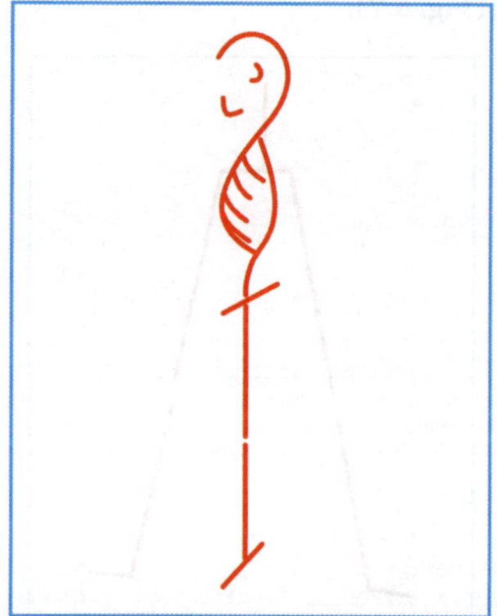

**Fig. 5.10:** Toe standing.

- There is a tendency for whole body to stretch, hence be used as a relaxation exercise.

**Uses in exercise therapy:**
- Strengthening the plantar flexors.
- Stretching the toe flexors and ankle dorsiflexors.
- As an exercise for postural flat foot.

**Example:** Raising the body by the toes to see the invisible things in the crowd.

Close Standing

Both the feet are kept closer and parallel to each other. It is difficult to maintain this posture due to the tension created in the leg muscles **(Fig. 5.11)**.

**Movement:** The movements that occur in close standing are same as standing, with the exception that the hips are internally rotated.

**Muscle works:** Same as normal fundamental standing, described earlier.

**Uses in exercise therapy:**
- To perform hip, trunk bending and rotational exercises.
- Arm swinging exercises.
- Starting position for sit-up exercises.
- To perform the upper and lower extremity exercises.

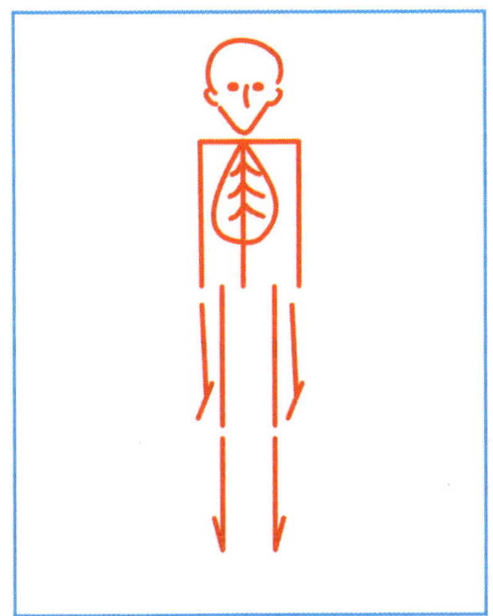

**Fig. 5.11:** Close standing.

**Examples:**
- Suriya namaskar position.
- Erect standing posture in military.
- Standing posture during the national anthem.

Lunge Standing

Standing in a split stance with one foot roughly 2–3 feet forward (forward lunge) or to the side (lateral lunge) of the other foot. Lunges are the great functional exercises that are performed to strengthen muscles of the lower limbs, which are of the following types:
- **Lateral lunge standing:** Standing in a split stance, with one leg abducted at the hip with knee in extension and ankle plantar flexion, and the other leg is abducted with knee in flexion and ankle in dorsiflexion. The trunk remains vertical **(Fig. 5.12A)**.
- **Forward lunge standing:** Standing in a split stance, where one leg is placed forward, with knee bent and foot flat on the ground, and other leg is placed behind. The trunk remains vertical **(Fig. 5.12B)**.

**Movements in lateral lunge standing:**
- Hip abduction and lateral rotation, knee extension on one side.
- Knee flexion of the relaxing leg.

**Movements in forward lunge standing:**
- Hip extension, and knee extension/partial flexion on one side.
- Hip and knee flexion of the relaxing leg.

**Muscle works:** In a lunge, many muscles work to both mobilize and stabilize the body. The muscles of the lower body, especially the quadriceps, glutei, and hamstrings—work both concentrically (shortening) and eccentrically (lengthening) during the lunge.

**Uses in exercise therapy:**
- Weight transmitting exercises.
- To perform balancing and coordination exercises.
- Lower limb stretching exercises.
- As warm up and cool down exercise.

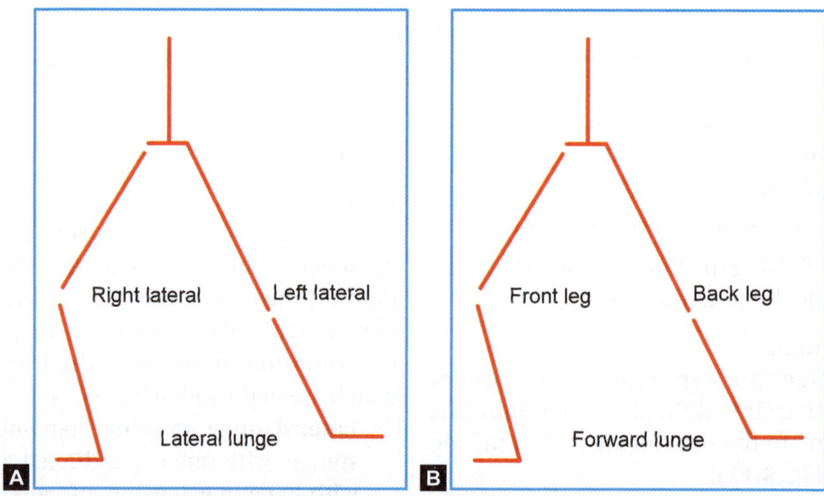


**Figs. 5.12A and B:** (A) Lateral lunge standing; (B) Forward lunge standing.

**Example:** Relaxed standing positions after prolong standing.

Cross Leg Standing

Legs are kept crossed. This is the unstable position due to the improper weight transmission. One leg is kept straight to bear weight and the other leg is rotated and kept across the supporting leg and the toes are placed on the floor **(Fig. 5.13)**.

**Movements (non-weight bearing leg):**

- ❖ Hip laterally rotated and slightly abducted.
- ❖ Knee flexed.
- ❖ Ankle slightly plantar flexed.

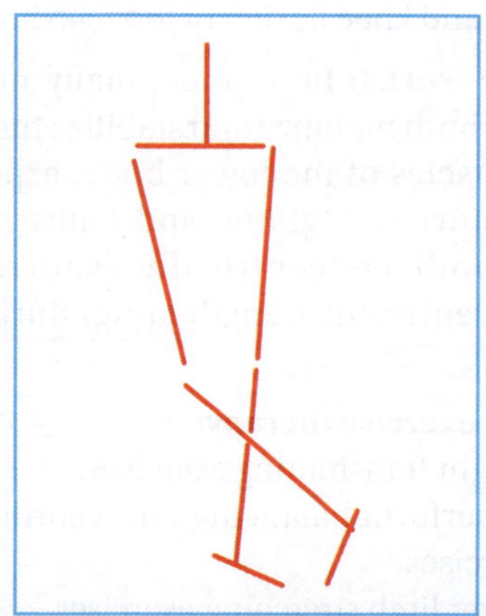

**Fig. 5.13:** Cross standing.

**Muscle works:**

- ❖ Muscles of the weight bearing leg produce co-contraction to make the limb rigid to bear weight.
- ❖ The hip internal rotators, quadriceps and ankle dorsiflexors of the non weight bearing leg contract eccentrically to maintain the posture of the leg.

**Uses in exercise therapy:**

- ❖ For relaxation.
- ❖ Weight transmission and balancing exercises.

**Example:** Stylish and casual relaxed standing position.

Foot and on foot Standing

One foot is kept on the dorsal surface of the other foot **(Fig. 5.14)**.

**Movements:**

- ❖ Hip flexed, adducted, and medially rotated.
- ❖ Knee flexion.
- ❖ Ankle plantar flexed.

**Muscle works:**

- ❖ Hip flexors, adductors and medial rotators of the upper leg contract concentrically.
- ❖ There is eccentric contraction of quadriceps and ankle dorsiflexors of the upper leg.

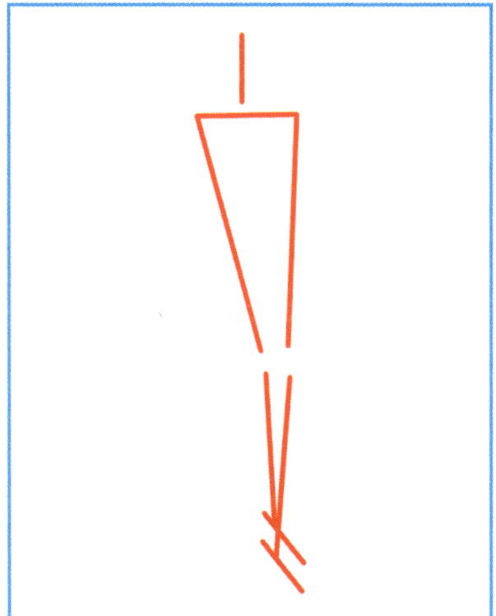

**Fig. 5.14:** Foot and on foot standing.

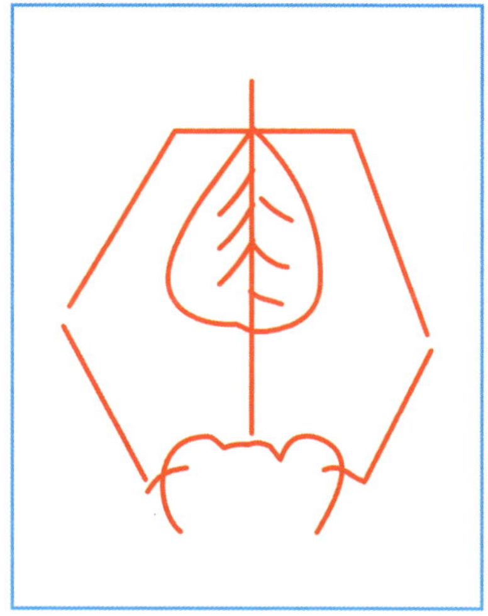

**Fig. 5.15:** Wing standing.

**Uses in exercise therapy:** Weight transmission and coordination exercises.

**Example:** The posture adopted while walking on hot surface.

### Positions Derived by Altering Arm Position

- Wing standing
- Bend standing
- Reach standing
- Stretch standing
- Yard standing
- Cross-arm standing
- Heave standing.

*Wing Standing*

This is used as a starting position for a number of standing exercises. Hands rest on the iliac crests, with the extended and adducted fingers placed anteriorly, and thumb placed posteriorly. The wrists are extended, forearms pronated, elbows flexed and shoulders adducted **(Fig. 5.15)**.

**Movements:**

- Shoulder adducted and medially rotated.
- Elbows flexed, and point straight sideways.
- Forearm pronated.
- Wrists extended.
- Thumb abducted.
- Fingers adducted and flexed.

**Muscle works:**

- The antigravity/postural muscles contract to keep the body upright over the feet.
- The adductors of shoulder joint (latissimus dorsi) contract sluggishly.
- Extensors of elbow contract eccentrically, to press the hand to the trunk/iliac crest.

**Effects and uses:**

- As the arms are held away from the trunk, from the axilla to the iliac crest, the posture allows the therapists to grasp the patient round the shoulder, during some trunk exercises.
- The fixed position of arm prevents their swinging, during trunk exercises.

**Uses in exercise therapy:**

- To perform trunk bending exercises.
- To perform neck exercises.
- To perform lower limb strengthening and stretching exercises.

**Example:** Relaxing position after prolonged walking or jogging.

*Bend Standing*

The shoulders are laterally rotated and strongly adducted, the elbows are flexed, the forearms are supinated with wrist and fingers flexed to rest above the lateral border of the

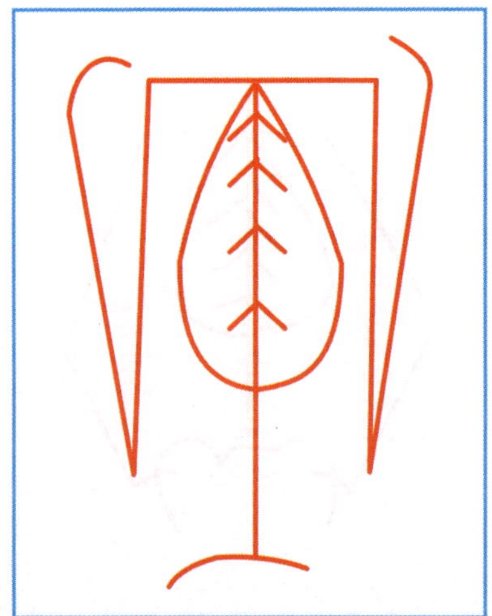

**Fig. 5.16:** Bend standing.

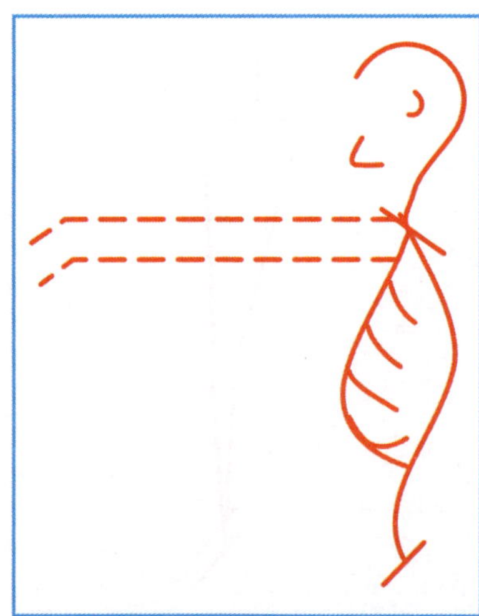

**Fig. 5.17:** Reach standing.

acromion process on the same side of the shoulder **(Fig. 5.16)**.

**Movements:**
- ❖ Shoulders adducted and laterally rotated.
- ❖ Elbow flexed.
- ❖ Forearm supinated.
- ❖ Fingers flexed.

**Muscle works:**
- ❖ The antigravity/postural muscles contract to keep the body upright over the feet.
- ❖ Lateral rotators and adductors of shoulder work strongly.
- ❖ The retractors and depressors of the scapulae work strongly as fixators.
- ❖ The flexors of elbow and supination of forearm work to maintain the position of forearm.
- ❖ The flexors of wrists and fingers may work slightly.

**Effect and uses:**
- ❖ This posture keeps the upper back in correct alignment.
- ❖ The thorax is expanded in this posture.
- ❖ As the full flexed elbows, reduces the weight arm/leverage, this posture is suitable for strengthening of weak shoulder abductors.

**Uses in exercise therapy:**
- ❖ Shoulder rotation exercises.
- ❖ Trunk bending exercises as well as neck exercises.

**Examples:**
- ❖ Policeman fixing the star on his shoulder.
- ❖ Removing dust from the shoulder.

### *Reach Standing*

It is used for performing and set up exercises by grasping bar with hand. The shoulders are flexed with elbows in extension, so that the upper limbs remain parallel to each other perpendicular to the body **(Fig. 5.17)**.

**Movements:**
- ❖ Shoulders flexed and elevated.
- ❖ Elbow extended.
- ❖ Forearm in supine/prone/mid prone position.
- ❖ Wrist extended, fingers slightly flexed, thumb slightly abducted and flexed.

**Muscle works:**
- ❖ The antigravity/postural muscles contract to keep the body upright over the feet.
- ❖ The shoulder flexors maintain the position against gravity.

- The scapular retractors, control the forward movement of scapulae through eccentric contraction.
- The extensors of elbows, work concentrically, and the wrist and finger extensors work eccentrically to hold the hand position.

**Uses in Exercise Therapy**

- To perform wrist exercise.
- Performing squatting, holding on a horizontal bar.

**Examples:**

- Position adopted to carry the child.
- Walking style in the dark place to avoid dashing on the objects.

*Yard Standing*

Upper limbs are abducted and kept in the sides and perpendicular to the body with palm facing up **(Fig. 5.18)**.

**Movements:**

- Shoulder abducted, laterally rotated, and extended.
- Elbow extended.
- Forearm supinated.
- Wrist extended, fingers slightly flexed, thumb abducted, and slightly flexed.

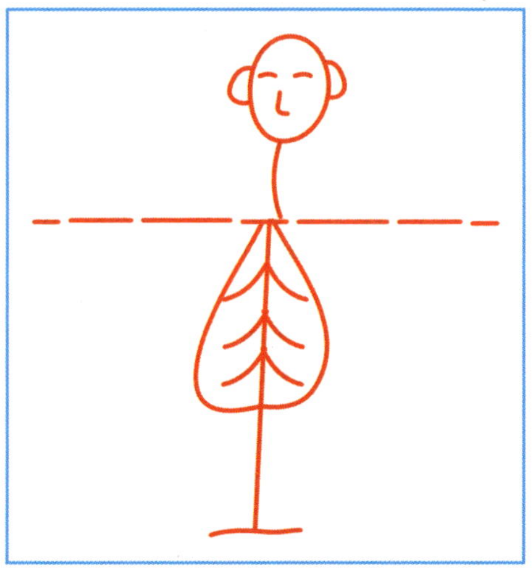

**Fig. 5.18:** Yard standing.

**Muscle works:**

- The antigravity/postural muscles contract to keep the body upright over the feet.
- The abductors, and lateral rotators of shoulders work concentrically, to hold arm at the sides.
- The extensors of elbows, wrists and fingers work to hold the limb in a straight line.
- The tendency to elevate the shoulder girdles is controlled by the scapulae depressors.

**Effect and uses:**

- The abductors of shoulders work at a marked mechanical disadvantage due to the longer weight arm.
- The position is corrective for postures of the upper back.

**Uses in exercise therapy:**

- To perform trunk rotation and bending exercises.
- To perform wrist, elbow, and finger exercises.
- To develop standing balance (high guard posture).

**Examples:**

- Balancing while walking on the rope or rod.
- Umpire's wide signaling in cricket.

*Stretch Standing*

The arms are fully elevated so that, they are in line with the body, parallel to each other and with palms facing each other **(Fig. 5.19)**.

**Movements:**

- Scapula elevated, shoulder flexed and medially rotated.
- Elbow extended.
- Wrist extended, fingers slightly flexed, thumb slightly abducted and flexed.

**Muscle work:**

- The antigravity/postural muscles contract to keep the body upright over the feet.
- The elevators of scapulae, along with upper trapezius and serratus anterior keep the arms elevated above the head.

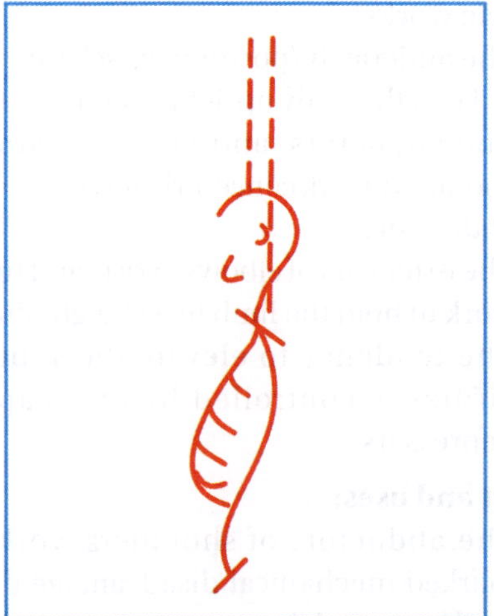

**Fig. 5.19:** Stretch standing.

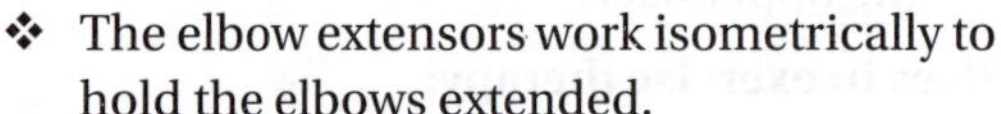

- ❖ The elbow extensors work isometrically to hold the elbows extended.
- ❖ The wrist extensors and finger flexors contract slowly.

**Uses in exercise therapy:**

- ❖ To perform arm swinging exercises.
- ❖ To perform trunk exercises.
- ❖ To facilitate high reach grasp standing in early stage of weight bearing.

**Examples:**

- ❖ Repairing the ceiling fan.
- ❖ Overhead activities.

**Cross-arm standing:** Elbows are flexed and hands are placed on the opposite side shoulder **(Fig. 5.20)**.

**Movements:**

- ❖ Shoulder adducted and medially rotated.
- ❖ Elbow flexed.
- ❖ Forearm pronated.
- ❖ Wrist and fingers in slight flexion.

**Muscle works:**

- ❖ The antigravity/postural muscles contract to keep the body upright over the feet.
- ❖ The shoulder adductors and medial rotators contract isometrically to keep the arms close to body.

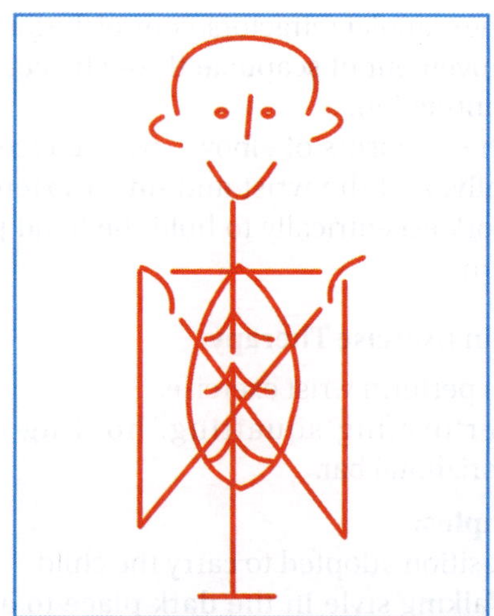

**Fig. 5.20:** Cross-arm standing.

- ❖ The elbow flexors and forearm pronators maintain elbows in flexion and forearms pronated.
- ❖ Wrist and finger flexors contract slightly.

**Uses in exercise therapy:**

- ❖ To perform trunk bending and rotation exercises.
- ❖ To maintain correction after shoulder dislocation.

**Example:** Waiters or slavery position.

*Heave Standing*

Arm and forearm kept at right angles and shoulders kept 90° abducted **(Fig. 5.21)**.

**Movements:**

- ❖ Shoulder abducted, and laterally rotated.
- ❖ Elbow flexed at 90°, forearms supinated.
- ❖ Wrist extended, fingers slightly flexed, thumb slightly flexed and abducted.

**Muscle works:**

- ❖ The antigravity postural muscles keep the body straight normally aligned over the feet.
- ❖ The abductors, and lateral rotators of shoulders work concentrically, to hold arm at the sides.
- ❖ The retractors and depressors of scapulae work strongly to act as fixators.

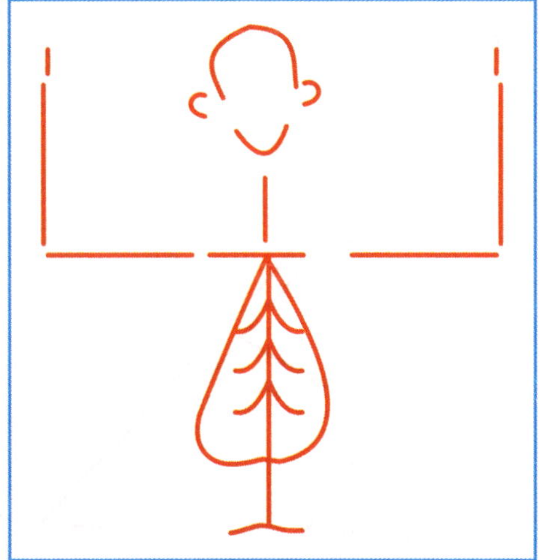

**Fig. 5.21:** Heave standing.

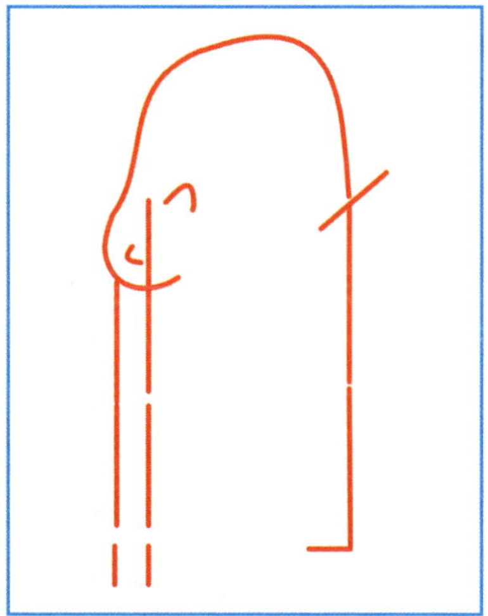

**Fig. 5.22:** Lax stoop standing.

- ❖ The elbow flexors and forearm supinator's work to keep the elbows flexed and forearms supinated.
- ❖ The wrist extensors and finger flexors may work slightly.

**Uses in exercise therapy:**

- ❖ Shoulder rotational movements.
- ❖ To perform forearm supination and pronation.

**Examples:**

- ❖ Position, adapted while dancing.
- ❖ Symbol of surrender.

### By Altering Position of Trunk

- ❖ Relaxed stoop standing/Lax stoop standing:
- ❖ Stoop standing.
- ❖ Fallout standing.

*Lax Stoop Standing*

The hips are flexed and the trunk, head and arms are relaxed, so that, they hang forwards and downwards. Balance is maintained by a slight plantar flexion of the ankle joints, causing a backward inclination of the leg **(Fig. 5.22)**.

**Movements:**

- ❖ Hip flexed.
- ❖ Trunk flexed.
- ❖ Upper limbs relaxed and kept hanging.

**Muscle works:**

- ❖ The intrinsic foot muscles grip the foot to floor.
- ❖ The ankle plantar flexors contract slightly to cause a posterior inclination of leg.
- ❖ The quadriceps femoris muscle contract to prevent buckling of the knees.
- ❖ The posterior cervical and back extensors undergo eccentric contraction.

**Uses in exercise therapy:**

- ❖ Trunk bending and stretching movement can be performed.
- ❖ Stretching the trunk and hip muscles.
- ❖ Balancing in standing.

**Examples:**

- ❖ Sweeping the floor.
- ❖ Position adopted while tying the lace or adjusting the shoes.

*Stoop Standing*

The hip joints are flexed, while the trunk, head and arms remain in alignment and are inclined. The trunk is inclined forward and upper limbs are placed parallel to the bodyline **(Fig. 5.23)**.

**Movements:**

- ❖ Hips are flexed.
- ❖ Shoulders adducted, extended and laterally rotated.

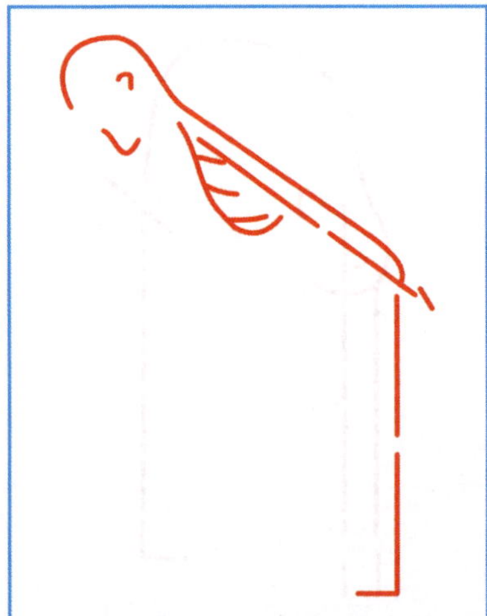

**Fig. 5.23:** Stoop standing.

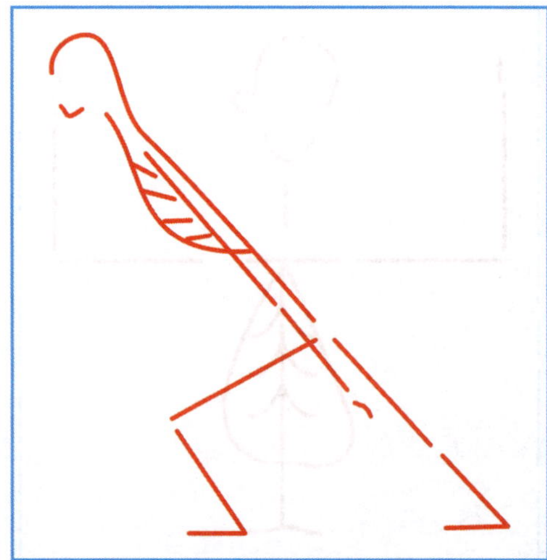

**Fig. 5.24:** Fall out standing.

- ❖ Elbows are extended.
- ❖ Wrists extended, fingers slightly flexed, thumbs slightly flexed and abducted.

**Muscle works:**

- ❖ Head is kept straight by the co-contraction of the prevertebral muscles and posterior cervical muscles.
- ❖ The back extensors and abdominals produce co-contraction to keep the trunk straight.
- ❖ The quadriceps contract strongly to counter act the action of hamstrings.
- ❖ Hip is flexed, causing the trunk inclined forward by the reverse action of psoas major.

**Uses in exercise therapy:**

- ❖ Position for pendular movements of the shoulder.
- ❖ Trunk bending and stretching exercises.
- ❖ Training balancing strategies such as hip strategy to maintain balance in standing.

**Example:** Rickshaw pulling position.

*Fallout Standing*

One leg is placed directly forwards to a distance of three feet-lengths with the knee bent. The back leg remains straight and the body (trunk) is inclined forwards in line with it **(Fig. 5.24)**.

**Movements:**

- ❖ Forward leg: Hip flexed and knee flexed.
- ❖ Backward leg: Hip extended, knee extended and ankle dorsiflexed.

**Muscle works:**

- ❖ Flexors of the hip of the forward leg, first contract concentrically and then statically.
- ❖ Neck flexors and extensors produce co-contraction to keep the head straight.
- ❖ Abdominal and back extensor muscles produce co-contraction to keep the trunk straight.

**Uses in exercise therapy:**

- ❖ Stretching the hip flexors.
- ❖ Strengthening exercises to the forward leg can be performed.
- ❖ Facilitating weight bearing/weight shifting onto the forward leg.

**Examples:**

- ❖ Pulling the loaded bullock cart.
- ❖ Position of readiness for running.

### *Sitting*

The position adopted while sitting on the stool or the chair is considered as the fundamental position of the sitting. The thighs and the legs are relaxed and the foot is resting on the floor/

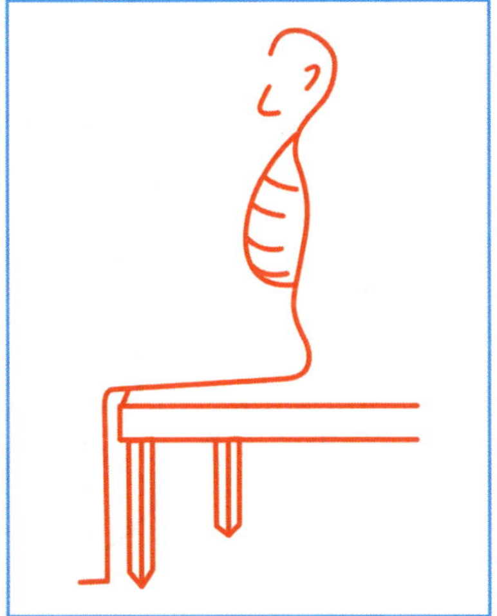

**Fig. 5.25:** Sitting.

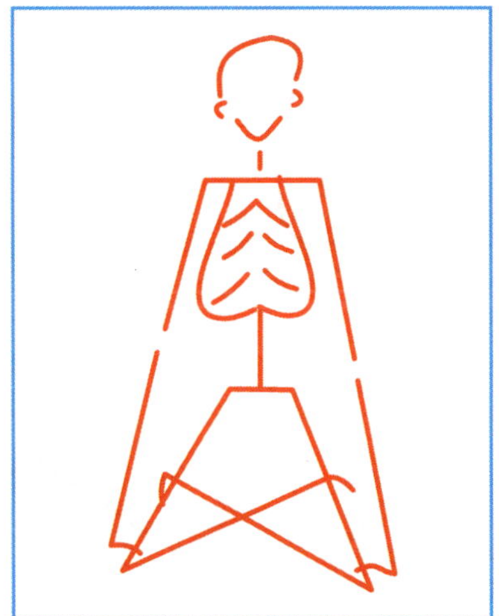

**Fig. 5.26:** Cross sitting.

hanging. From the trunk to head the position is same as said in standing posture. The base of support is more, so the COG lies down.

Due to the downward movement of the COG the position gets more stability than the standing and the muscle work required to hold the position is also less **(Fig. 5.25)**.

**Muscle works:** There is no muscle work in the lower limb because the stool supports thighs and legs, and the foot is resting on the floor. Remaining parts from the trunk to head the muscle work is same like the standing posture.

**Derived Positions from Sitting**

- Cross sitting
- Side sitting
- Crook sitting
- Long sitting
- Stoop sitting
- Stride sitting
- Ride sitting
- Foot sitting (squat sitting)
- Fallout sitting
- Crouch sitting

*Cross Sitting*

This involves sitting on the floor/bed, with the hips flexed, abducted and laterally rotated, knees flexed and ankles crossing each other. Both the legs are crossed and the weight is transmitted through both the hips **(Fig. 5.26)**.

**Movement:** Both the side hips are flexed, abducted, laterally rotated and knee flexed.

**Muscle works:** There is no muscle work in the lower limbs as the lower limbs are supported on bed/floor. Muscle works neck and trunk to maintain the position are same like muscle works needed to achieve sitting.

**Uses in exercise therapy:**

- Breathing exercise and reduce the respiratory distress
- Hip adductor stretching
- Trunk and neck exercise.

**Example:** Used for some floor level activities like eating, cutting vegetables, etc.

*Side Sitting*

This involves sitting on floor/bed, with one hip flexed, abducted with knee maximally flexed and ankle plantigrade and the other hip flexed, abducted and medially rotated with the knee partially flexed and the ankle plantigrade. For right side sitting, the right leg remains as in cross sitting and this hip supports the main weight of the trunk, while the left hip is abducted and medially rotated, so that

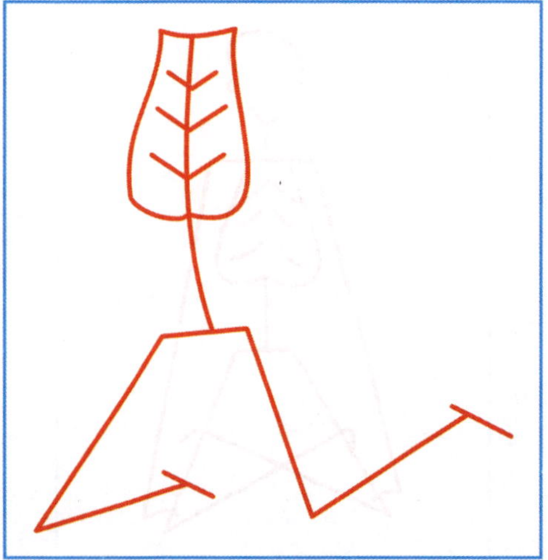

Fig. 5.27: Side sitting.

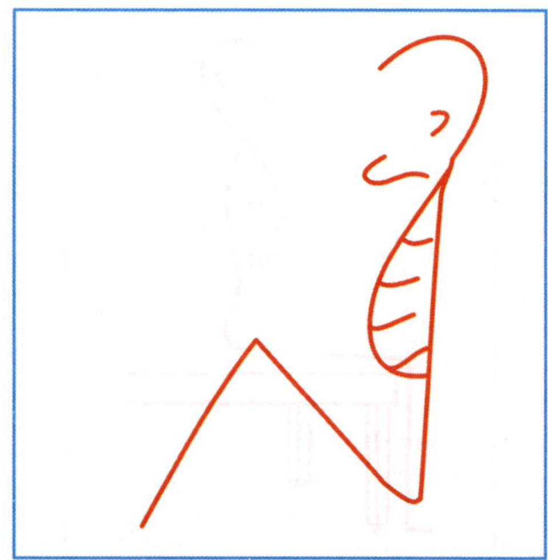

Fig. 5.28: Crook sitting.

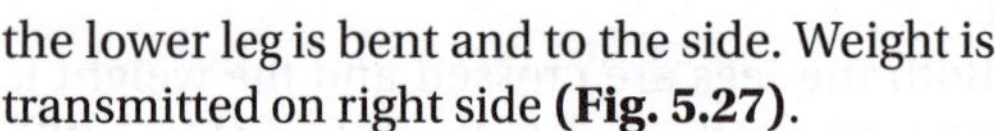

the lower leg is bent and to the side. Weight is transmitted on right side **(Fig. 5.27)**.

**Muscle works:** As in right side sitting, the pelvis is tilted laterally to right, the lateral flexors on left side contract to keep the trunk upright, and vice versa.

**Uses in exercise therapy:**
- Progression from prone to sitting in mat activity.
- To perform trunk exercises.

**Example:** All floor level activities like cutting vegetables and garland making.

*Crook Sitting*

This involves sitting on the floor with the hips and knees flexed, so that the feet are kept forward, while sitting on the floor **(Fig. 5.28)**.

**Movements:**
- Hips flexed.
- Knees flexed.
- Ankle in neutral position.

**Muscle works:**
- The neck muscles produce co-contraction, to hold the head in space.
- The trunk extensors undergo eccentric contraction to prevent excessive forward movement.
- The hip adductors and medial rotators contract eccentrically for prevention of sideways falling of the knees.

**Uses in exercise therapy:**
- To perform mat activities.
- To perform breathing exercises.
- To perform neck and ankle exercises.
- To correct kyphosis, as the movements can be localized to upper trunk.

**Example:** Relaxed wall sitting while watching TV.

*Long Sitting*

This involves sitting on the floor/bed with the hips flexed and the knees extended **(Fig. 5.29)**.

**Muscle works:**
- The neck muscles produce co-contraction to hold the head in space.
- Strong contraction of core muscles makes the trunk straight.
- The posterior pelvic tilt, results causing a tendency to fall backwards, is counteracted by contraction of the abdominals.

**Uses in exercise therapy:**
- To perform hip rotational movements.
- To perform ankle and knee exercises.
- To stretch hamstrings.
- To perform trunk exercises.

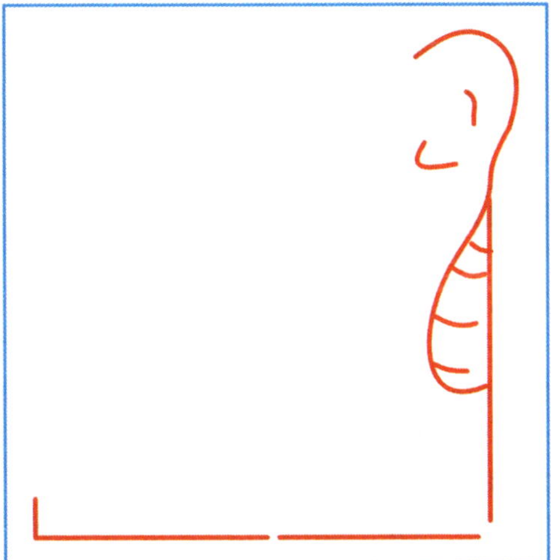

**Fig. 5.29:** Long sitting.

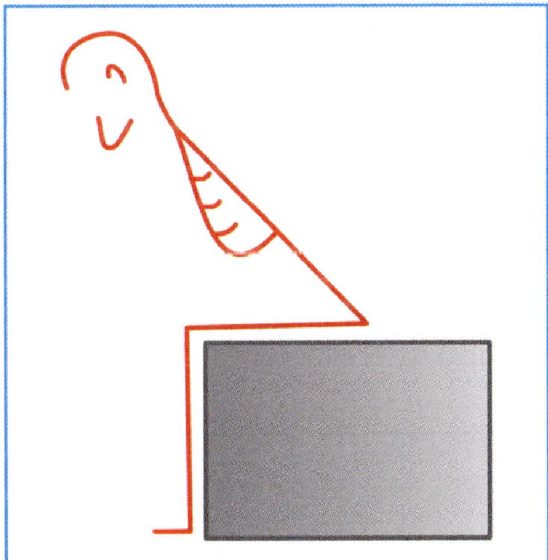

**Fig. 5.30:** Stoop sitting.

**Example:** Traditionally adopted position by the old age people for floor level activities.

*Stoop Sitting*

This involves sitting on a plinth/chair with the trunk inclined forwards from the hips and the feet resting on the floor. The head remains straight in line with the trunk **(Fig. 5.30)**.

**Movement:** Forward inclination of the trunk from the hips.

**Muscle works:**

- ❖ The hip flexors (psoas major) work with reverse origin and insertion, to bend the trunk forwards from the hips.
- ❖ Co-contraction of neck and trunk muscles keeps the head and trunk straight.

**Uses in exercise therapy:**

- ❖ Used for back and neck massage.
- ❖ Back muscles relaxation.
- ❖ To perform breathing exercises.
- ❖ Starting posture for training standing from sitting.

**Example:** Lazy sleeping position in the classroom.

*Stride Sitting*

This involves sitting with the hips abducted, so that the feet which usually rests on the floor, are usually two feet lengths apart **(Fig. 5.31)**.

**Movement:** Both hips remain abducted with the knees extended.

**Muscle works:**

- ❖ The neck and trunk muscles produce co-contraction, to keep the head and trunk vertical.
- ❖ The hip abductors contract to abduct the hips, so that wide base is maintained.

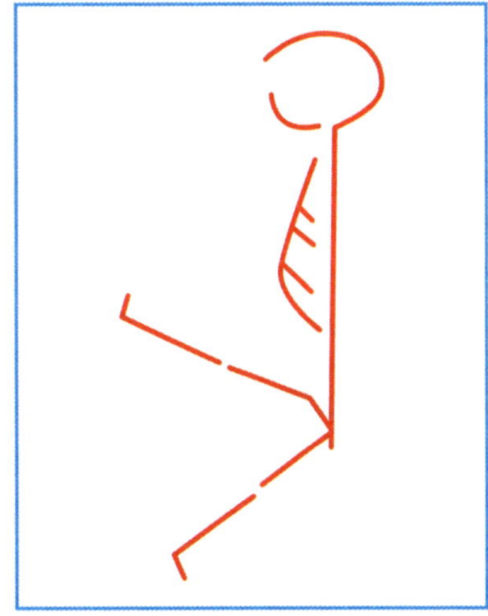

**Fig. 5.31:** Stride sitting.

**Uses in exercise therapy:**

- ❖ To develop sitting balance on mat.
- ❖ To perform neck and trunk exercises.
- ❖ To perform upper limb exercises.

**Example:** A common posture adapted by paraplegic patients to maintain sitting.

*Ride sitting*

This involves sitting on a table/gymnastic ball so that, the apparatus is gripped strongly between the knees by the hip adductors making the posture very stable. When sitting on a high plinth, both the thighs are strapped in abduction, and no muscle work in the legs are required to hold the position. When sitting on a stool/bench, both the hips are abducted and placed in either sides of the stool. If the foot rests on the floor, the position will be more stable **(Fig. 5.32)**.

**Movement:** Both the hips remain abducted with the knees flexed. A gymnastic ball may be placed between both the knees.

**Muscle works:**

- ❖ The neck and trunk muscles produce co-contraction, to keep the head and trunk vertical.
- ❖ If a gymnastic ball is placed between the knees, the hip adductors contract to hold the ball between the thighs.

**Uses in exercise therapy:**

- ❖ To perform leg swinging exercises.
- ❖ To perform neck and trunk exercises.
- ❖ To perform upper limb exercises.

**Examples:**

- ❖ Bike riding posture.
- ❖ Horse riding posture.

*Foot Sitting (Squat Sitting)*

Sitting on the feet **(Fig. 5.33)**.

**Movement:** Hips and knees are flexed and weight is transmitted through the feet.

**Muscle works:**

- ❖ Quadriceps and gluteus maximus work hardest (contract eccentrically) at the bottom of the squat.
- ❖ Neck and trunk flexors and extensors produce co-contraction to keep head and trunk straight.

**Uses in exercise therapy:**

- ❖ Starting position for stand-up exercises.
- ❖ Used for increasing mobility of hip and knees and to stretch tendo-Achilles.

**Examples:**

- ❖ The position adopted while washing clothes and cleaning vessels.
- ❖ Indian style toileting.

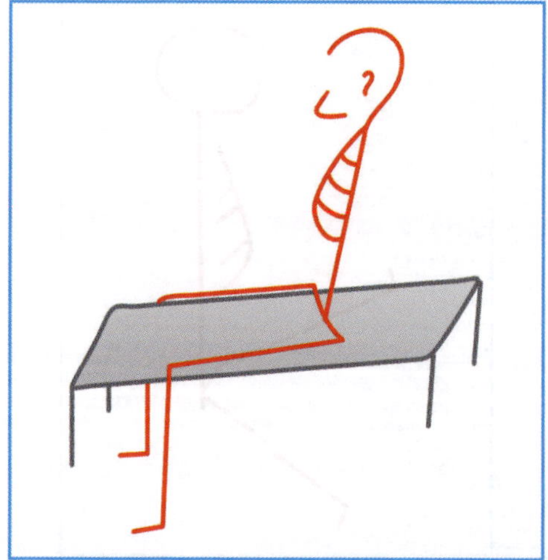

**Fig. 5.32:** Ride sitting.

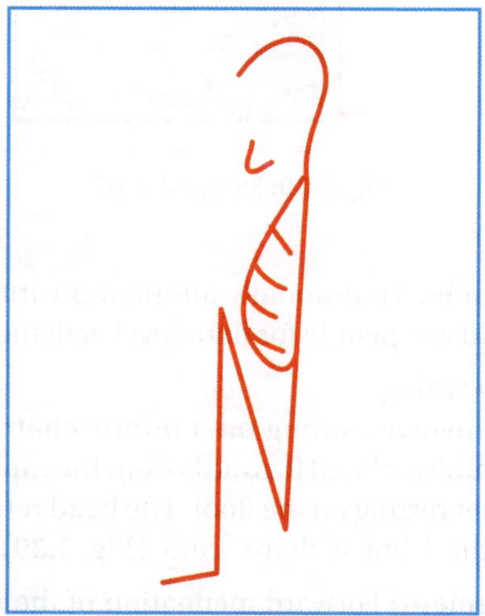

**Fig. 5.33:** Foot sitting.

*Fallout Sitting*

This involves sitting on a stool/plinth with the trunk inclined, so that, the forward leg is supported across the stool, and the backward leg is extending straight with the knee extended and ankle plantar flexed **(Fig. 5.34)**.

**Movements:**

- Hips and knees of the supported leg are flexed and weight is transmitted through the feet.
- Hip extension, knee extension and ankle plantar flexion occurs in the backwardly placed leg.

**Muscle works:**

- Flexors and extensors of neck and trunk produce co-contraction to remain straight in one line.
- The hip flexor of the supported leg work with reverse action, to incline the trunk forward.
- The hip and knee extensors and ankle plantar flexor of the unsupported leg, contract to maintain hip and knee extension and ankle plantar flexion.

**Uses in exercise therapy:**

- Stretch hip and knee extensors.
- Used to enhance pelvic stability and develop sitting balance.

**Example:** The position is generally not adapted in day-to-day life, however is selected for therapeutic purposes.

*Crouch Sitting*

The hips and knees are fully flexed, and the straight trunk is inclined forward to allow the hands to rest on the floor **(Fig. 5.35)**.

**Movements:**

- Hips and knees both the lower limbs are flexed, and ankles are dorsiflexed.
- Both the elbows and wrist, fingers and thumbs are extended.

**Muscle works:**

- Flexors and extensors of neck and trunk produce co-contraction to remain straight in one line.
- The hip flexors work with reverse action, to incline the trunk forward.
- Gluteus maximus and quadriceps undergo eccentric contraction for controlled hip and knee flexion.
- Muscles of shoulder girdle contract strongly to stabilize the scapulae and shoulders.
- Strong co-contraction of muscles of elbow, keep elbows straight.

**Uses in exercise therapy:**

- Stretch hip and knee extensors and tendo-Achilles.

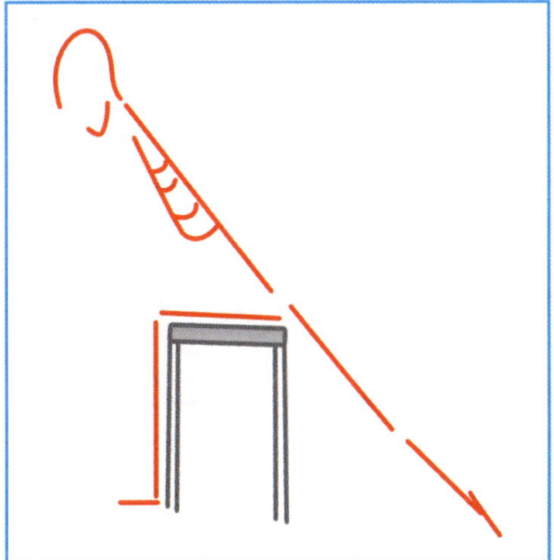

**Fig. 5.34:** Fallout sitting.

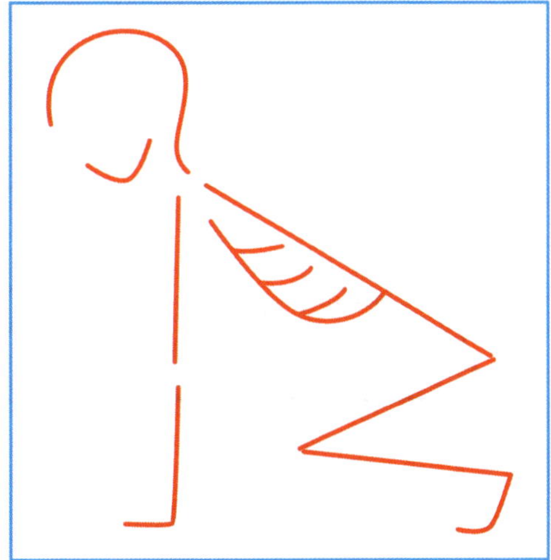

**Fig. 5.35:** Crouch sitting.

- Used to enhance weight bearing on hands.
- Used for hip and knee mobilization.

**Example:** The position is sometimes adapted by children with cerebral palsy for ambulation (Bunny hopping).

### Lying

*Starting Position/Fundamental Posture—Lying*

Lying on the floor or on the plinth, in supine position with arm by the side of the body and legs are kept straight. It is the most stable posture than any other fundamental starting position due to the lower placement of the COG and the broader base. This position can be adopted for prolonged period than any other starting position **(Fig. 5.36)**.

**Muscle works:**

In this posture the muscle work is minimal. Maximum muscles are relaxed except some muscles (discussed below):

- Neck side flexors counterbalanced to keep the head in neutral position.
- Flexors of the lumbar spine counteract with the spinal extensors to maintain the lumbar lordosis.
- Medial rotators of the hip produce slow eccentric contraction, to keep the hips in neutral position.

**Uses:** It is very much useful position to perform many of the upper limb, lower limb, trunk, neck exercises like strengthening, stretching, aerobic, anaerobic and breathing exercises.

**Derived Position from Lying**

- Prone lying
- Half-lying
- Crook lying
- Side lying.

### *Prone Lying*

Lying with face down and the body completely supported anteriorly on the plinth.

The anterior portion of the total body is turned towards the couch or floor. This position is inconvenient for maintaining for longer period. This position is very much difficult for the respiratory distress and elderly patients **(Fig. 5.37)**.

**Muscle works:** In relaxed prone lying, where the body is fully supported on plinth, there is no muscle work needed to hold the position. However, for active prone lying, used as static holding for postural training, or prior to exercises, the neck extensors and scapulae retractors and depressors work slowly to maintain slight neck extension to lift the

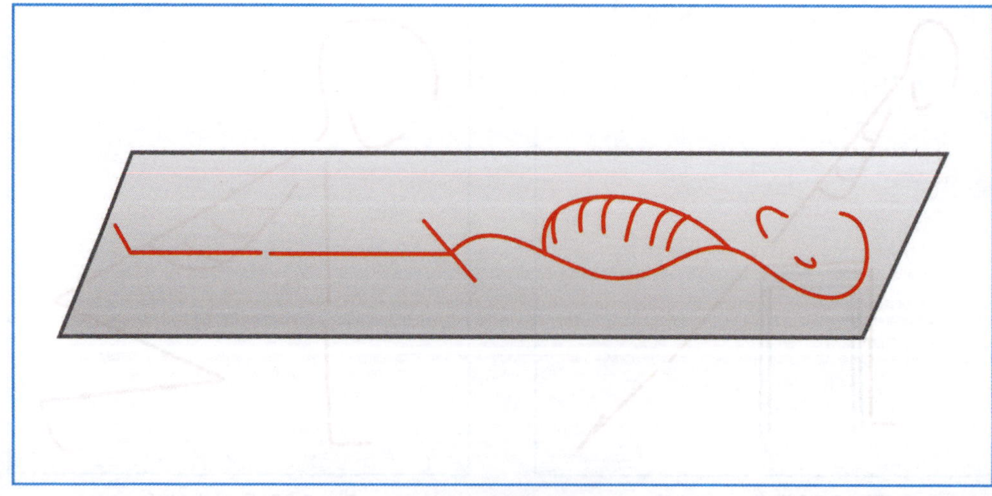

**Fig. 5.36:** Lying.

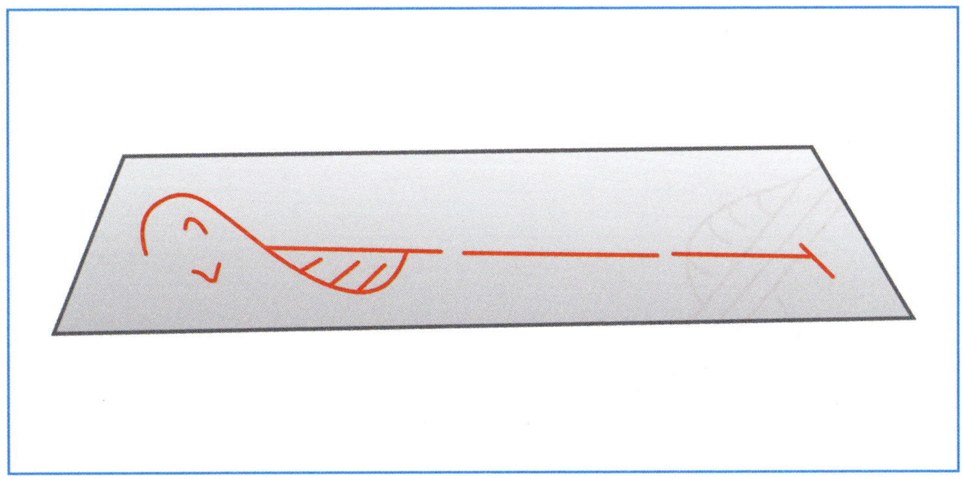

**Fig. 5.37:** Prone lying.

head from the supporting surface and to keep the shoulders backwards and downwards respectively.

**Uses in exercise therapy:**

- Spinal extensor and neck extensor exercises can be performed.
- This position can be used for back massage.
- Some of the upper and lower extremity exercises can be performed.

**Example:** Toppled position of getting blessing from the elders.

*Half Lying*

In supine, the trunk is raised forward from the hips at an angle of 45 degrees, either by pillow positioning or elevating the head end of the bed. The lower limbs are supported on the bed horizontally. Some amount of spinal muscle work may be present in this posture **(Fig. 5.38)**.

**Muscle works:** Very little muscle work is required to hold this position. There is slow contraction of neck extensors to prevent the head falling forward. The hip adductors and medial rotators contract slowly to prevent the knees falling to the sides, when knees are kept in flexion, without pillow support. Co-contraction between the left and right trunk lateral flexors are required to prevent falling to the sides.

**Uses in exercise therapy:**

- To practice breathing exercise and postural drainage.
- To perform Frenkel's exercise.
- To perform upper limb, lower limb, and trunk exercises.

**Example:** Relaxed position to adopt while reading book or watching TV.

*Crook Lying*

In supine, the hips and knees are flexed, so that the feet rest on the bed/ground.

Modifications are made in lower limb in the supine lying posture **(Fig. 5.39)**.

**Muscle works:** Very less muscle work is required to hold this position. The hip adductors and medial rotators produce slow eccentric contraction to prevent the knees falling to the sides.

**Uses in exercise therapy:**

- Abdominal muscle strengthening exercises can be performed.
- Pelvic bridging exercises can be performed.
- Position for breathing exercises, as it relaxes the abdominals.

**Example:** Relaxing position after yoga exercises.

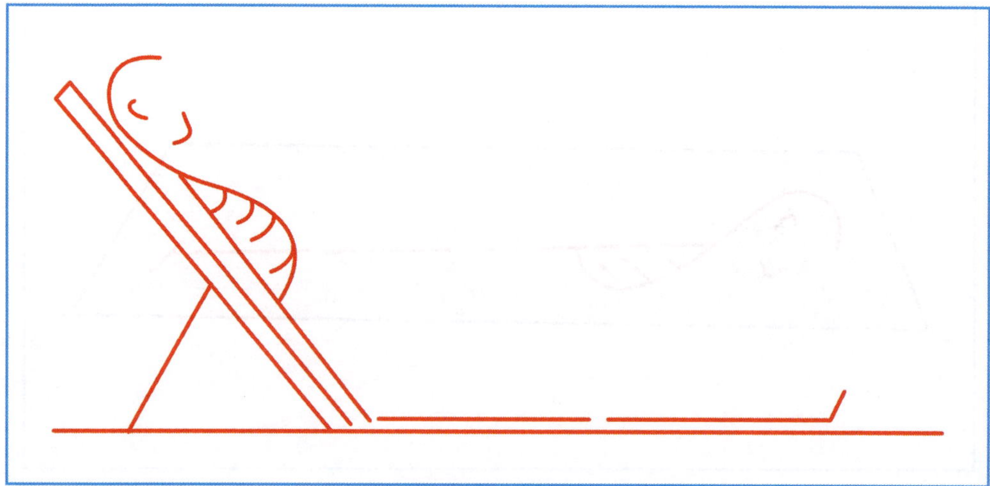

**Fig. 5.38:** Half lying.

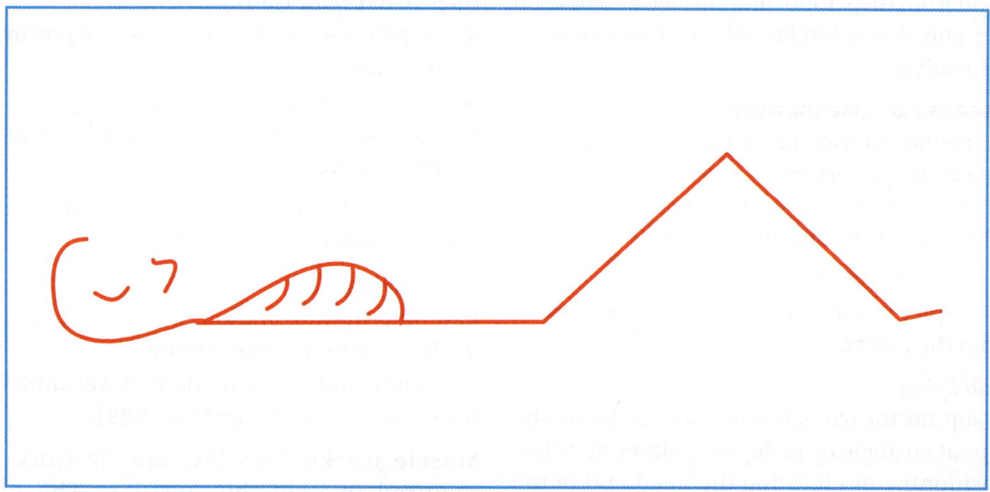

**Fig. 5.39:** Crook lying.

*Side Lying*

Lying on one side of the body. It is most inconvenient to maintain for longer period. The upper extremity which is placed under the body will be more painful and positioning the lower limb is also very much difficult. Upper extremity, which is below the body, is flexed and kept under the head, and the lower limb which is up to be placed forward to reduce the inconveniences. For relaxed side lying, 3 pillows are required, 1 each to support head, and upper most upper and lower limbs (**Fig. 5.40**).

**Muscle work:** When head and upper most limbs are supported on pillows, no muscle work is needed to hold the position.

**Uses in exercise therapy:**

- ❖ Many of the upper limb and lower limb exercises can be performed.
- ❖ Breathing exercises and postural drainage can be done.

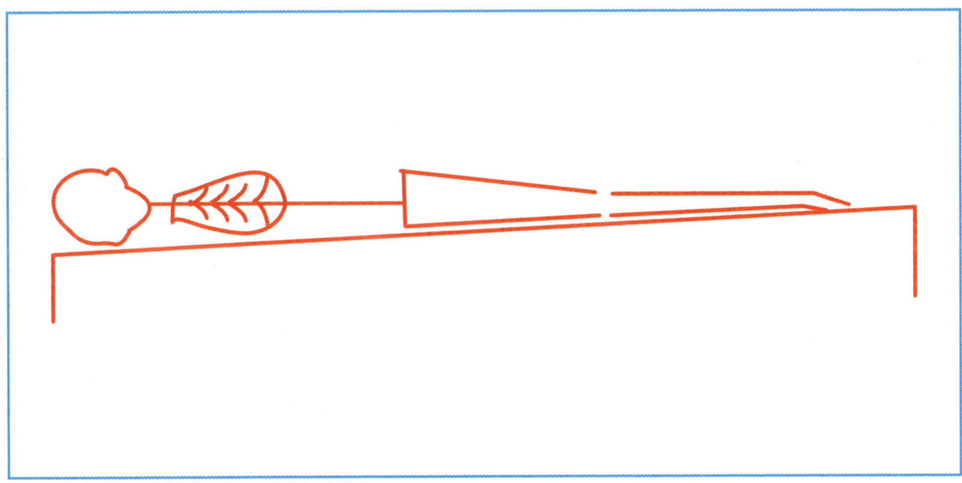

**Fig. 5.40:** Side lying.

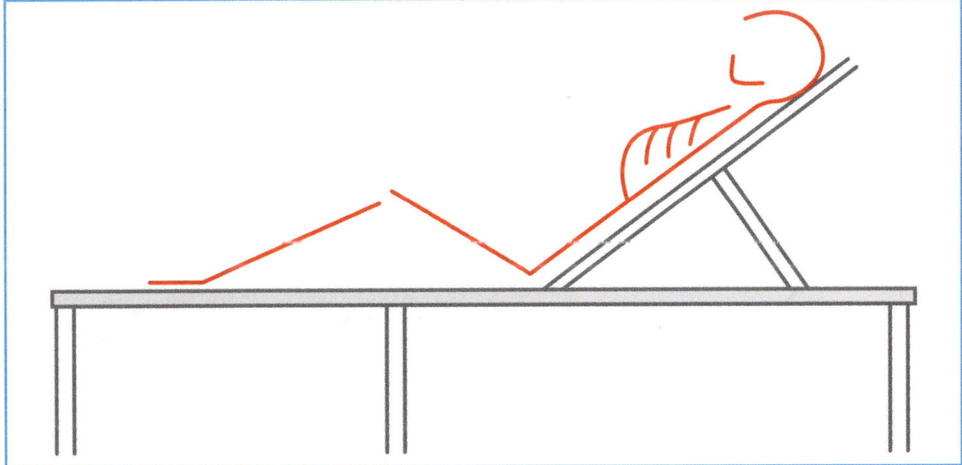

**Fig. 5.41:** Half crook lying.

- Frequent side lying is followed in patient's with spinal cord injury to prevent development of pressure ulcer.

**Example:** Talking to a friend, when bed ridden.

*Half Crook Lying*

In half lying, the knees are flexed and supported on pillows, so that the feet rest on the floor, to increase relaxation of the abdominals **(Fig. 5.41)**.

**Muscle works:** Very less muscle work is required to hold this position. The hip adductors and medial rotators produce slow eccentric contraction to prevent the knees falling to the sides, if not supported on pillows. Co-contraction between the left and right trunk lateral flexors are required to prevent falling to the sides.

**Uses in exercise therapy:**
- To practice breathing exercise and postural drainage.
- To perform Frenkel's exercise.

*Leg Prone Lying*

In prone lying, the lower limbs are supported on plinth and the trunk remains unsupported in space **(Fig. 5.42)**.

**Muscle works:** Strong eccentric contraction of the neck and trunk extensors are required to hold the position. Good strength of muscles of upper limbs is required to take hand support on the stool, placed on the ground, while performing exercises in this position.

**Uses in exercise therapy:**

- ❖ For strengthening of neck and back extensors.
- ❖ To teach protective extension reaction.

*Trunk Prone Lying*

In prone lying, the trunk is supported on plinth, and the lower limbs remain hanging, unsupported at the foot end of the bed **(Fig. 5.43)**.

**Muscle works:** As the head and trunk are fully supported on bed and the lower limbs remain hanging, no much muscle work is needed to hold the position.

**Uses in exercise therapy:** For strengthening of low back and hip extensors.

*Sit Lying*

In supine lying, the lower limbs remain flexed at the knees and hang downwards at the foot end of the bed **(Fig. 5.44)**.

**Muscle works:** As there is a tendency for lumbar extension, causing increased lumbar lordosis, due to tension (elongation) in the hip flexors, the abdominals and core muscles contract to minimize lumbar lordosis and keep the spine straight, as much as possible.

**Uses in exercise therapy:**

- ❖ For strengthening abdominal muscles.
- ❖ To train supine to sitting minimizing passive insufficiency of hamstrings.

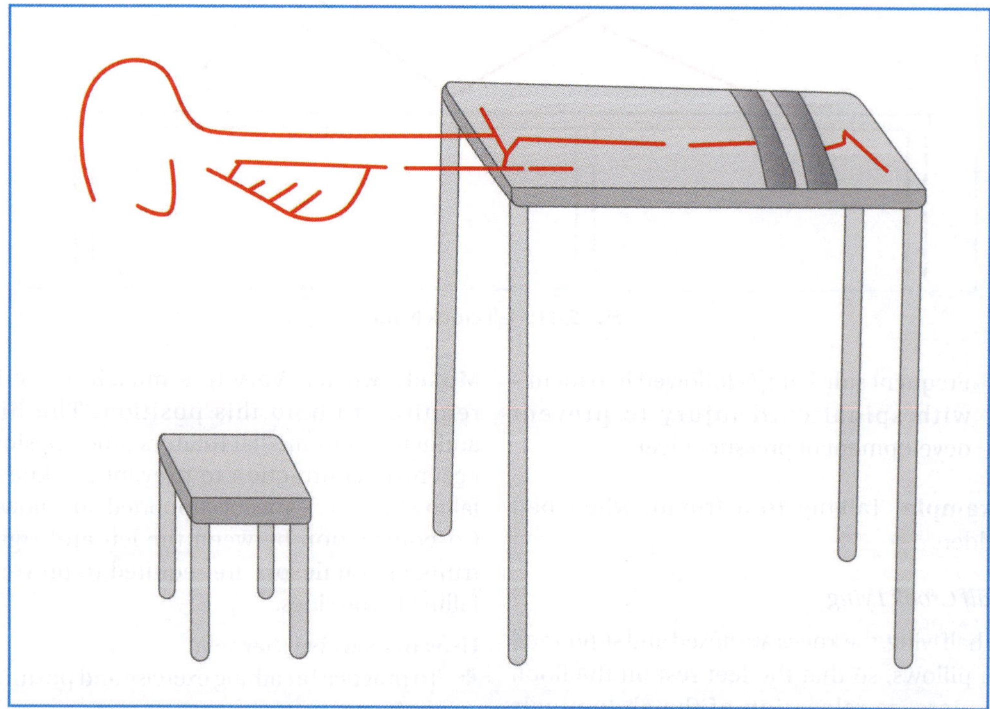

**Fig. 5.42:** The leg prone lying.

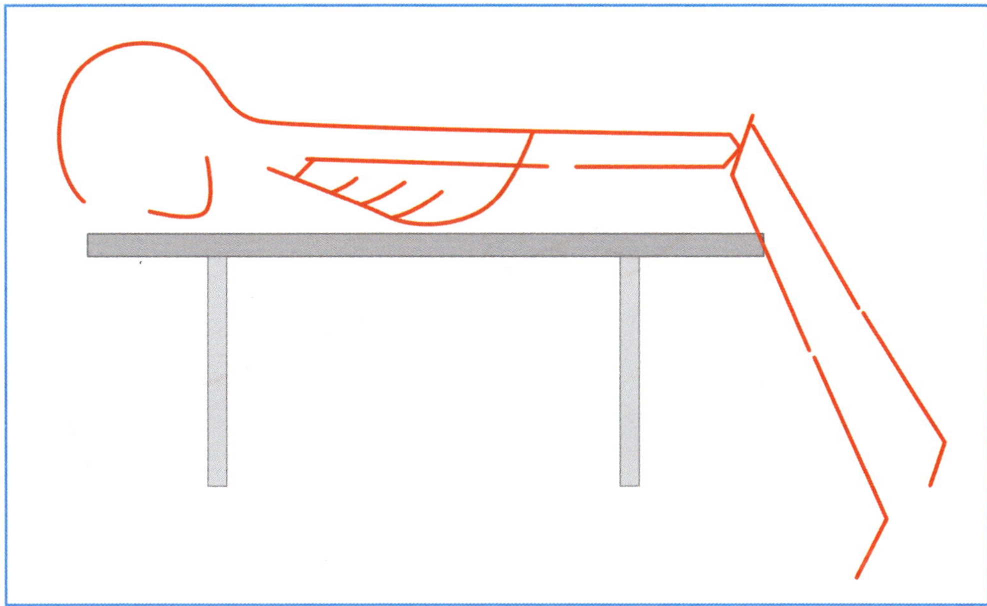

**Fig. 5.43:** The trunk prone lying.

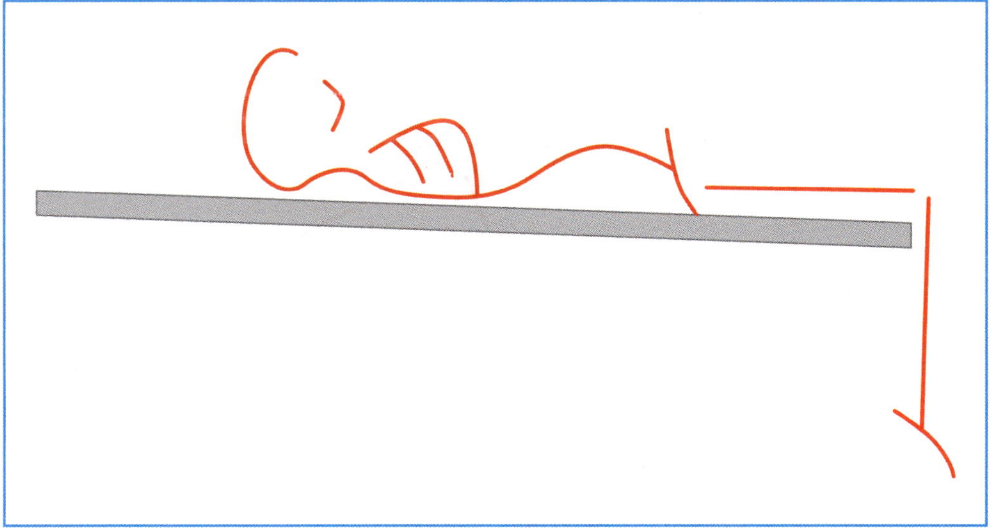

**Fig. 5.44:** Sit lying.

*Prone Falling*

From crouch sitting, the legs are extended in line with the trunk, so that the body is supported on the vertical arms and toes **(Fig. 5.45)**.

**Muscle works:**

- ❖ The extensors of elbow and all muscles of shoulder work strongly to support the weight of the body.

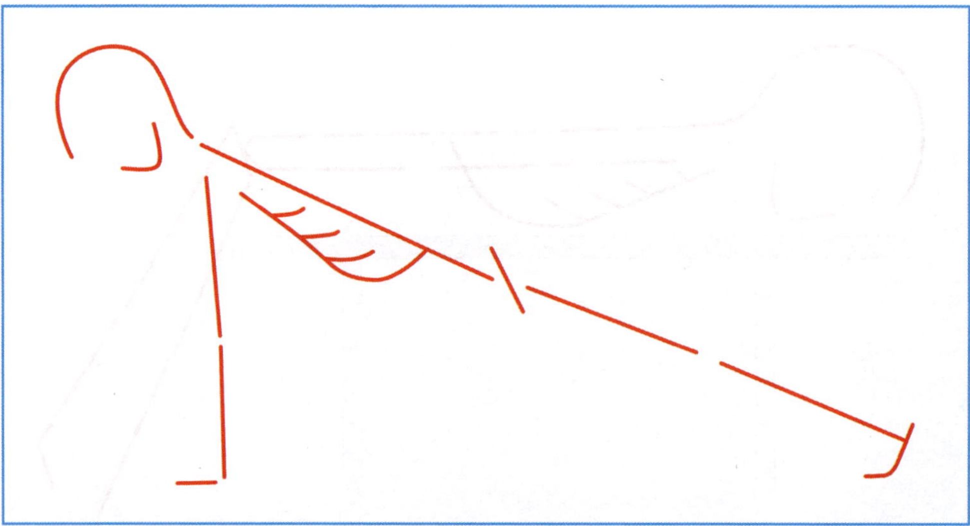

**Fig. 5.45:** Prone falling.

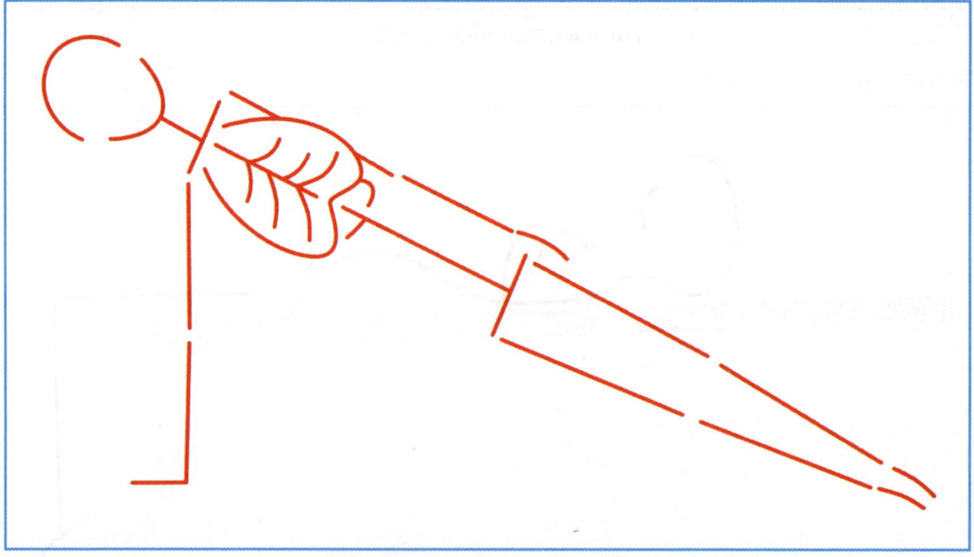

**Fig. 5.46:** The side falling posture.

- ❖ The serratus anterior muscle contracts to hold the scapulae firmly against the chest wall.
- ❖ The neck extensors and flexors produce co-contraction, to maintain position of head.

**Uses in exercise therapy:**

- ❖ To stretch hip flexors, elbow flexors.
- ❖ Promote weight bearing on the hands.

*Side Falling*

In side lying, the upper body is raised by pushing through the lower side arms so that, the body is in an inclined position, with weight on the lower side hand and foot **(Fig. 5.46)**.

**Muscle works:**

- ❖ The extensors of elbow and all muscles of shoulder on the supported side work strongly to support the weight of the body.

- Co-contraction of lateral flexors of trunk on both sides maintain trunk straight.
- Quadratus lumborum muscle on the lower side contracts to prevent sagging of the pelvis down.

**Uses in exercise therapy:**

- Used to stretch the convex side of a scoliotic curve.
- Used for strengthening the lateral flexors of trunk (the side plank exercise).

## Kneeling

This position is like the fundamental position of standing but the weight is transmitted through the knee joints due to the right-angle alignment of the knee to the body. The leg is resting on the floor and the ankle is plantar flexed. It is the very much difficult position to maintain for longer period **(Fig. 5.47)**.

Even though the COG falls down and the BOS is large, it is inconvenient to adopt due to the weight transmitted through the knee joint.

**Muscle works:**

- The leg is relaxed except the plantar flexors of the ankle, which keeps the ankle in plantar flexion state.
- Hip flexors, extensors counteracts with each other and keeps in vertical position and prevents the pelvic tilt.
- Quadriceps femoris undergoes eccentric contraction to prevent the knee flexing beyond 90°.
- Remaining muscle works are as said in standing posture.

**Uses in exercise therapy:**

- Many of the upper limb and trunk exercises can be performed.
- To perform the mat activities.
- To perform coordination and balancing exercises.

**Example:** Prayer position.

**Derived Position from Kneeling:**

- Half-kneeling
- Kneel sitting
- Prone kneeling
- Inclined prone kneeling.

*Half-kneeling*

One leg is bent at the knee, that supports most of the body weight, and the other leg is bent to a right angle at the hip, knee and ankle so that the foot is supported on the ground in a forward direction **(Fig. 5.48)**.

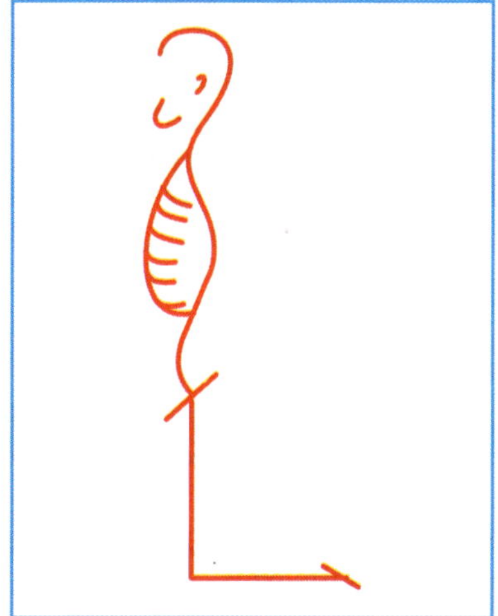

**Fig. 5.47:** Kneeling.

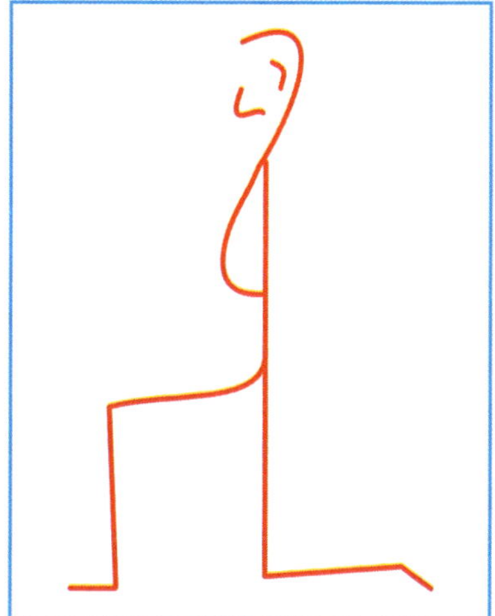

**Fig. 5.48:** Half-kneeling.

**Movements:**
- Forward lower limb: Hip flexed 90°, knee flexed 90°, ankle in plantigrade.
- Kneeling/supporting lower limb: Hip is in neutral position, knee flexed 90°, ankle plantar flexed.

**Muscle works:**
- The abductors of hip joint of the supporting leg and the lumbar side flexors of the opposite leg work to maintain trunk balance.
- There is muscular co-contraction of the supporting hip muscles for hip stability.
- The extensors of hip and knee of the forward leg work slightly to maintain balance.

**Uses in exercises therapy:**
- To perform the balancing and coordination exercises.
- To improve neck, trunk and pelvic control.
- To reduce spasticity through weight shifting.
- To mobilize hip, knee and ankle.
- To perform the mat activities for motor development.

**Example:** To practice some of yogic exercises.

### *Kneel Sitting*

Both the hips and knees are flexed so that the person sits over his heels **(Fig. 5.49)**.

**Movements:** Both the hips are partially flexed, knees fully flexed and ankles are plantar flexed.

**Muscle works:**
- Muscles of neck and trunk produce co-contraction to maintain neck and trunk stability.
- The hip extensors undergo eccentric contraction to maintain pelvic stability.

**Uses in exercise therapy:**
- To perform trunk stretching and strengthening exercises.
- To perform the stretching and strengthening exercises for the hip and knee muscles.

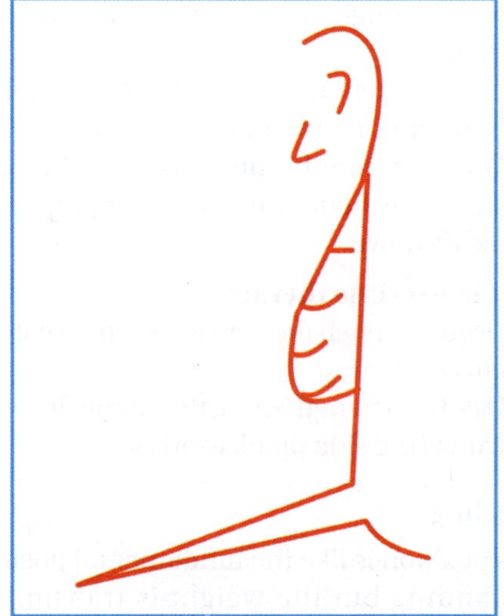

**Fig. 5.49:** Kneel sitting.

**Examples:**
- Playing posture adopted by the child.
- To perform some of the yogic exercises.

*Prone Kneeling*

The trunk is horizontal and the head is in line with the trunk. Body weight is supported both by the vertical arms with the elbow in extension and hands flat on the ground, as well as the thighs with hip and knees bent at right angles. It is otherwise called as quadruped position or animal position **(Fig. 5.50)**.

**Movements:**
- Trunk stabilized horizontally.
- Head is in line with the trunk.
- Shoulders flexed, elbows extended, wrist and fingers extended.
- Hips and knees flexed to right angels.
- Ankles plantar flexed.

**Muscle works:**
- Muscles of shoulder and pelvic girdles work with co-contraction to stabilize the supporting limb.
- Flexors of the lumbar spine prevent hollowing of the back.
- Co-contraction of muscles of elbows keep elbow straight.

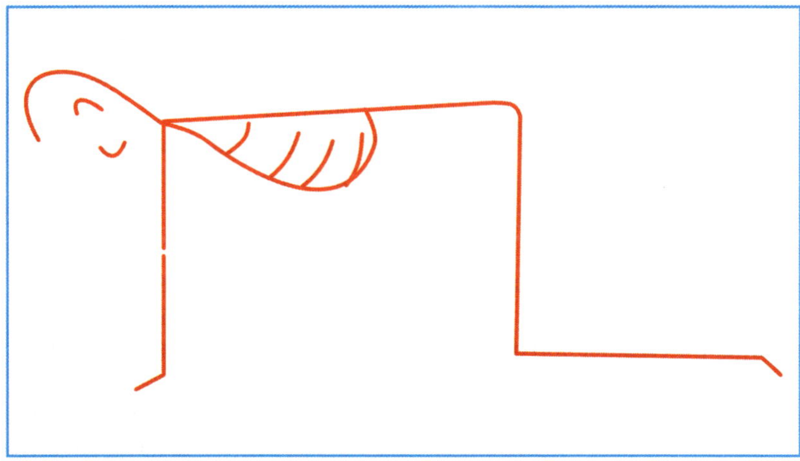

**Fig. 5.50:** Prone kneeling or quadruped position.

**Uses in exercise therapy:**

- To perform mat activity.
- To perform coordination exercises.
- Cat and camel exercises, for strengthening trunk muscles.
- To mobilize hip and knee joints.
- To reduce spasticity of elbow and wrist flexors.

**Example:** Child crawling position.

### *Inclined Prone Kneeling*

From prone kneeling, the trunk is inclined forward, so that, head rests on ground over clenched hands. This is the modified variety of quadruped/prone kneeling position **(Fig. 5.51)**.

**Movements:**

- Trunk forward bending.
- Shoulder abducted, flexed and medially rotated.
- Elbow flexed.
- Hips, knees flexed and ankles plantar flexed.

**Muscle works:**

- The neck extensors contract weakly to prevent neck flexion.

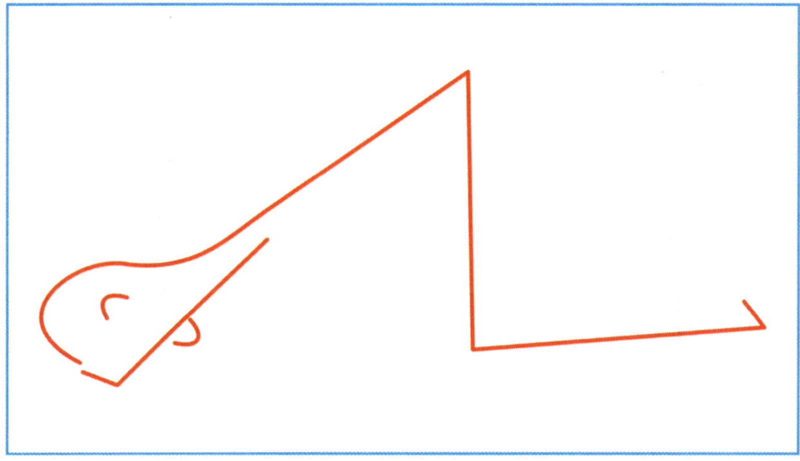

**Fig. 5.51:** Inclined prone kneeling.

- The core muscles of trunk work to keep the trunk straight.
- The hip and knee extensors work eccentrically to maintain the required hip and knee flexion.

**Uses in exercise therapy:**
- To perform breathing exercises and postural drainage technique.
- For stretching of hip and knee extensors.
- Can be considered as a position of ease in case of neurogenic claudication occurring in lumbar canal stenosis.

**Example:** Muslim *Namaz* position.

**Hanging**

Total body is suspended by grasping a horizontal bar with the hand **(Fig. 5.52)**.

**Movements:**
- Scapulae elevated, shoulders flexed, adducted and medially rotated.
- Elbow is extended.
- Fingers flexed and grasping the rod.

**Muscle works:**
- Adductor and medial rotators of the shoulder work strongly.
- Co-contraction of elbow flexors and extensors.
- Finger flexors work strongly and grasping the bar.
- Adductors of hip keep it in adducted posture.
- Plantar flexors keep the ankle in plantar flexed position.
- Trunk, knee and remaining muscles of the hip are free from the work and movement.

**Uses in exercise therapy:**
- To perform total body swinging movements.
- To perform upper limb strengthening and body-building exercises.
- To perform stretching exercises for spine (for correction of scoliosis), elbow flexors.

**Examples:**
- Mostly helpful in gymnastic activities.
- Bar exercises.

**Derived Position from Hanging**

*Half-hanging* ***(Fig. 5.53)***

Same like hanging, but the body is hanging with one side upper limb support. It is also a difficult posture to maintain for longer period. Total body weight is carried out by one side upper limb so that the shoulder, elbow and muscles are facing more strain.

**Muscle work:** Same like the muscles working during hanging.

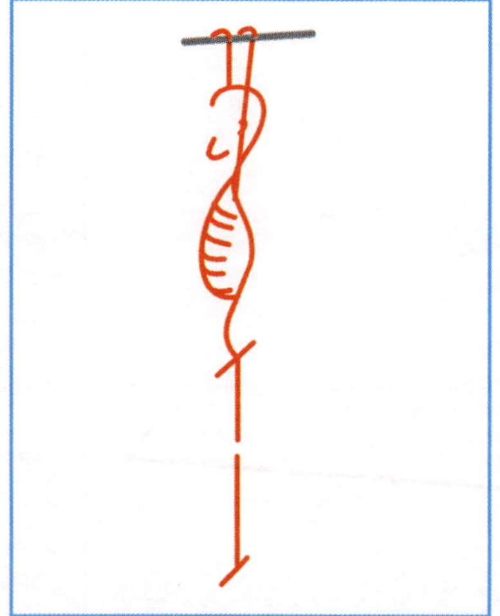

**Fig. 5.52:** Hanging.

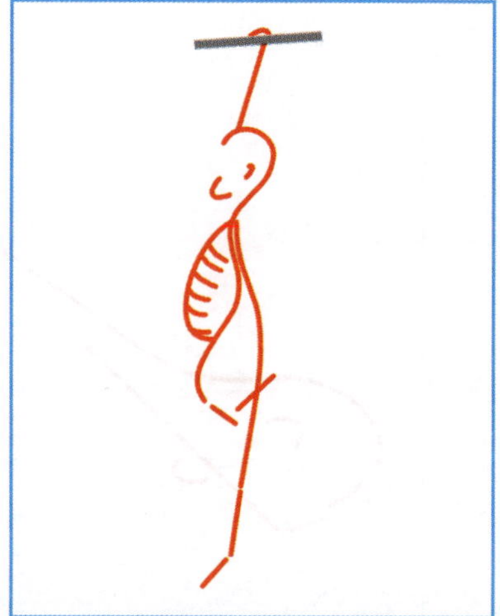

**Fig. 5.53:** Half-hanging.

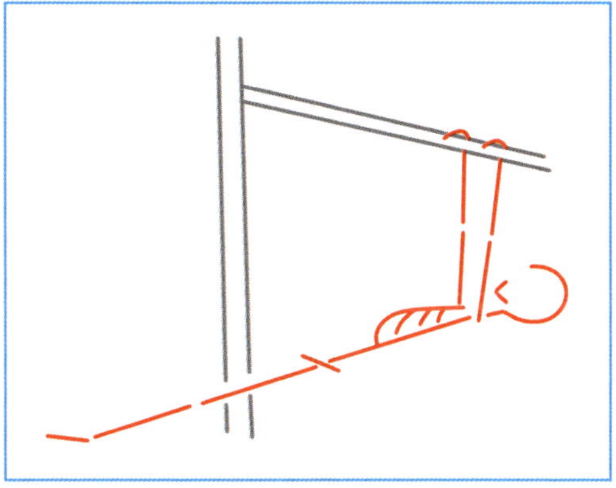

**Fig. 5.54:** Fall hanging.

**Uses in exercise therapy:** It is the most advanced strengthening program for the upper extremity. Generally, it is helpful for the body-builders and gymnastic peoples.

**Examples:**
Normally, it is used in gymnastic activities.

**Fall hanging:** The body is aligned in the oblique position by grasping a horizontal bar by the hands, and weight borne on the feet that rest on the floor **(Fig. 5.54)**.

**Muscle works:**
- Muscles of shoulder girdle contract strongly.
- Muscles of forearm (the finger and thumb flexors and opponens pollicis) contract strongly.
- The abdominals (rectus abdominis, internal and external obliques) contract strongly.
- Hip flexors and quadriceps strongly contract.

**Uses in exercise therapy:** It is the most advanced strengthening program for the upper and lower extremities and trunk. Generally, it is helpful for the body-builders and gymnastic peoples.

**The fundamental and derived postures are further classified into:**
- **Active postures:** These are the positions of the body, which are maintained by integrated action of many muscles. It could be static posture or dynamic posture:
  - **Static posture:** This is a constant pattern of posture, maintained by interaction of group of muscles that work more or less statically.
  - **Dynamic posture:** These are positions which are constantly modified and adjusted to meet the changing demands of body while performing movements for function.
- **Inactive posture:** These are attitudes assumed by the body while resting, where all the essential muscular activities required to maintain life are reduced to minimum.
- **Good posture/efficient posture**: Posture is said to be good, when it fulfils the purpose for which it is used with maximum efficiency and minimum effort.
  A good posture in lying, sitting and standing, where normal alignment of the body is maintained with minimal effort is essential for efficient movement performance as well as prevention of musculoskeletal complications. Development of good posture depends upon:
  - Intact/efficient Neuromusculoskeletal system.
  - Ergonomically designed working environment.
  - A stable psychological background.
  - Good hygienic conditions.
  - Opportunity of freedom for movement.
- **Poor posture/inefficient posture:** Posture is said to be poor or inefficient, when it fails to serve the purpose for which it is designed, or if unnecessary amount of muscular effort is used to maintain it.
  A poor posture, which is always inefficient, leads to unnecessary muscle contraction and energy consumption, leading to early fatigue, deformities, pain, abnormal gait etc. It develops due to:
  - Psychological stress and mental attitude.

- Poor ergonomics in workplace.
- Poor hygienic conditions.
- Prolonged fatigue.
- Pain.
- Muscle weakness.
- Occupational stress.

**Some of the faulty postures commonly seen in individuals causing musculoskeletal complications are:**

- **Lordotic posture (Fig. 5.55):** Lordosis refers to the normal inward curvature of the spine. When this curve is exaggerated with anterior pelvic tilt, it is referred to as hyper lordosis.
- **Sway back posture (Fig. 5.56):** This postural abnormality is associated with forward head, hyper-extended cervical spine, flexed thoracic spine, extended lumbar spine with posterior pelvic tilt and hyperextension of hips and knees and plantar flexed ankle.
- **Flat back posture (Fig. 5.57):** In this type of posture, there is forward head, extension of the cervical spine, extension of the thoracic spine, loss of lumbar lordosis and posterior pelvic tilt.
- **Forward head posture:** There is shift of the head forward with the chin poking out. It is caused by increased flexion of

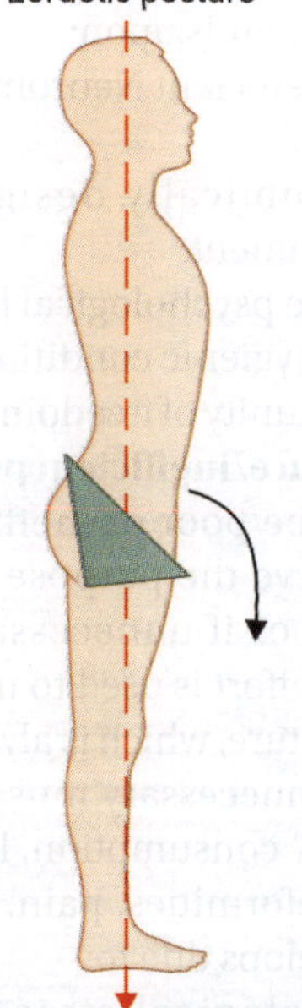

**Fig. 5.55:** Lordotic posture.

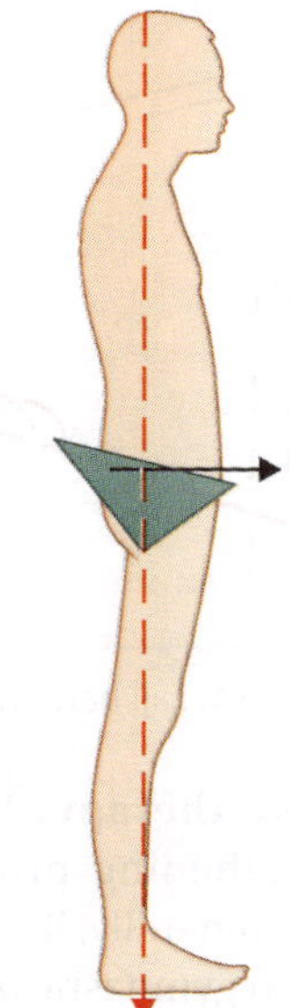

**Fig. 5.56:** Sway back posture.

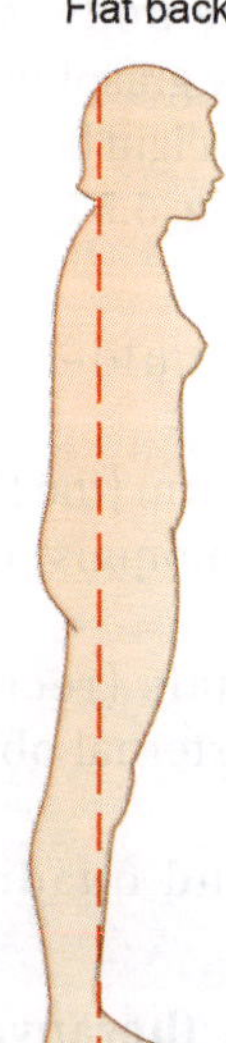

**Fig. 5.57:** Flat back posture.

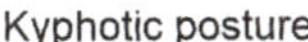


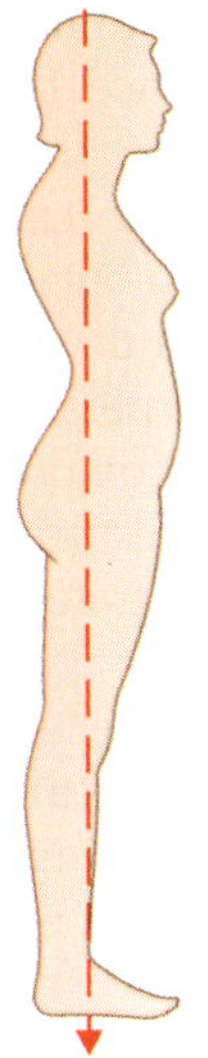

**Fig. 5.58:** Kyphotic posture.

the lower cervical and upper thoracic spine and increased extension of the upper cervical spine with extension of the occiput on C1.

- **Scoliosis:** This postural abnormality is associated with lateral bending of the spine (with lateral flexion of vertebrae towards the concave side and rotation of vertebrae towards the opposite side) from normal vertical line.
- **Kyphosis (Fig. 5.58):** This is the forward bending deformity of spine with increased posterior convexity of thoracic spine.

**Postural re-education:** As we know, posture precedes movement, hence a stable normal posture need to be developed for production of efficient functional movements. A postural re-education program consists of:

- Measures to reduce pain, fatigue, occupational and psychological stress.
- Creation of ergonomically designed working environment.
- Relaxation programs that include: Breathing exercises, Meditations, Music therapy, Relax passive exercises, low intensity aerobic exercises.
- Strengthening of weak postural muscles.
- Postural awareness training through bio-feedback devices such as postural mirror.

## Balance

Balance is the ability to maintain the line of gravity of the body within the base of support with minimal postural sway. Balance requires keeping the "Center of Mass" (COM) over the "Base of Support" (BOS) during static and dynamic situations.

- **Static balance/static postural control:** It is the ability to maintain stability and orientation with the center of mass (COM) over the base of support (BOS) with the body at rest.
- **Dynamic balance/dynamic postural control:** It is the ability to maintain stability and orientation with the center of mass (COM) over the base of support (BOS), while the body/parts of the body are in motion.

In-day-to day activities, individuals require to maintain stable steady posture, called static balance, where the center of mass is constantly kept over the base of support. However, in certain activities such as reaching forward in sitting or standing, the center of mass (COM), is made to move out of the base of support, still maintaining the body posture called dynamic balance.

Maintaining balance requires coordinated input from multiple sensory systems including the vestibular, somatosensory and visual systems as described below:

- **Vestibular system:** This sense organ regulates equilibrium through directional information as it relates to head position.
- **Somatosensory system:** The sensation of proprioception and kinesthesia of joints, information from skin and joints (pressure and vibratory senses), spatial position and movement relative to the support surface, movement and position of different body parts relative to each other, help in maintenance of postural tone retaining balance.

- **Visual system:** The perception of verticality of head and body motion, spatial location relative to objects help in maintenance of balance.

During perturbation of balance, where the center of mass is displaced, the interaction of various sensory systems allows the modifications needed to maintain stability in variety of environments.

During disturbance of balance:
- Adults rely on somatosensory inputs.
- Children rely more on visual input.

During quite stance, individuals have some displacement of center of mass within the limit of stability, where the balance is retained, even though the COM is displaced. Limit of stability is the maximum angle from vertical which can be tolerated. A cone of stability **(Fig. 5.59)**, which indicates the individual's ability to shift the COM of body from front to back and side to side without losing balance is exhibited by individuals during quite stance. This is manifested as postural sway.

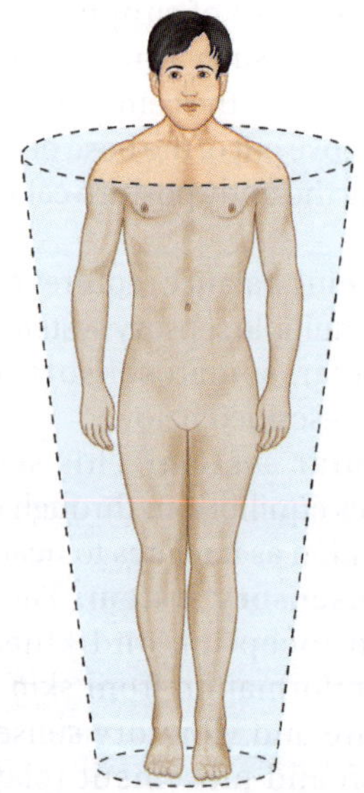

**Fig. 5.59:** Shows the cone of stability/postural sway in quiet stance.

- **A "Postural Sway"** refers to small postural shifts from front to back and side to side, during quiet stance. However while doing functional tasks, where there is shift in center of mass, normal individuals are able to maintain balance within the limit of stability. A "Limits of Stability" is defined as the distance a person can move, without losing balance or taking a step. When the balance is perturbed/lost individuals recruit different strategies described below to retain balance.
- **Ankle strategy:** The "ankle strategy" occurs with minimal perturbation of balance and involves shifting of COM at ankles **(Fig. 5.60)**. Control is distal-to-proximal. When perturbed from front to back, balance is retained by ankle dorsiflexion followed by knee extension and activation of abdominals. When perturbed from back to front, balance is retained by ankle plantar flexion, followed by knee flexion and activation of paraspinal muscles.
- **Hip strategy:** The hip strategy **(Fig. 5.61)** involves shifting of COM by flexing or extending at the hips and is recruited when the ankle strategy fails (i.e., to larger perturbations). It has proximal to distal pattern of activation of muscles. With forward sway abdominals are activated first followed by the quadriceps. With backward sway, paraspinal muscles are activated first followed by the hamstrings.
- **Stepping strategy:** This strategy is recruited to larger perturbations, when ankle and hip strategies fail to retain balance. It realigns the base of support under the center of mass (COM) by rapid steps **(Fig. 5.62)** or hops in the direction of the displacing force, thereby increasing the base of support and retaining balance.

Besides the training for development of strategies to maintain balance (ankle strategy

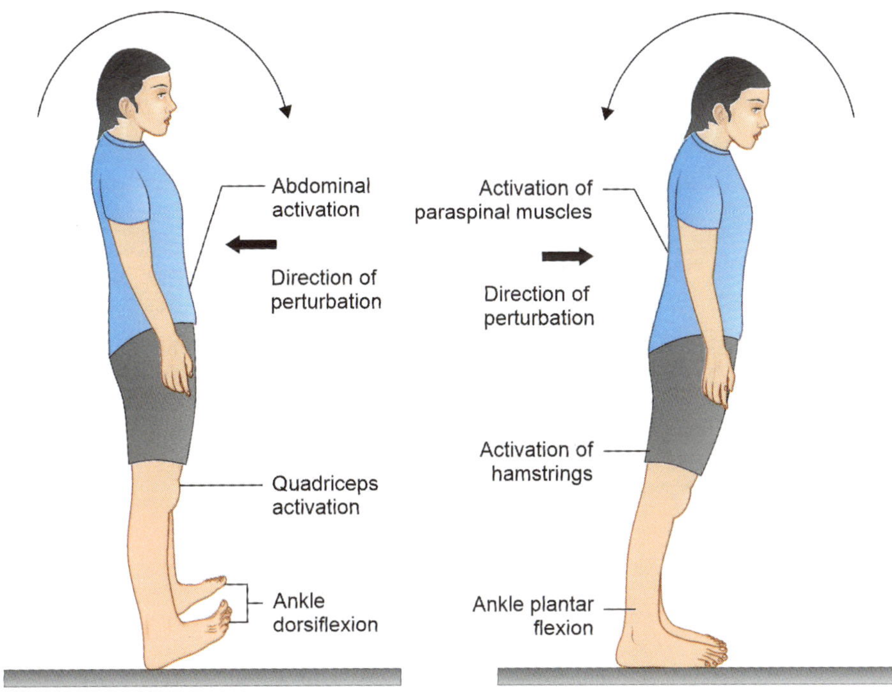


**Fig. 5.60:** The ankle strategy.

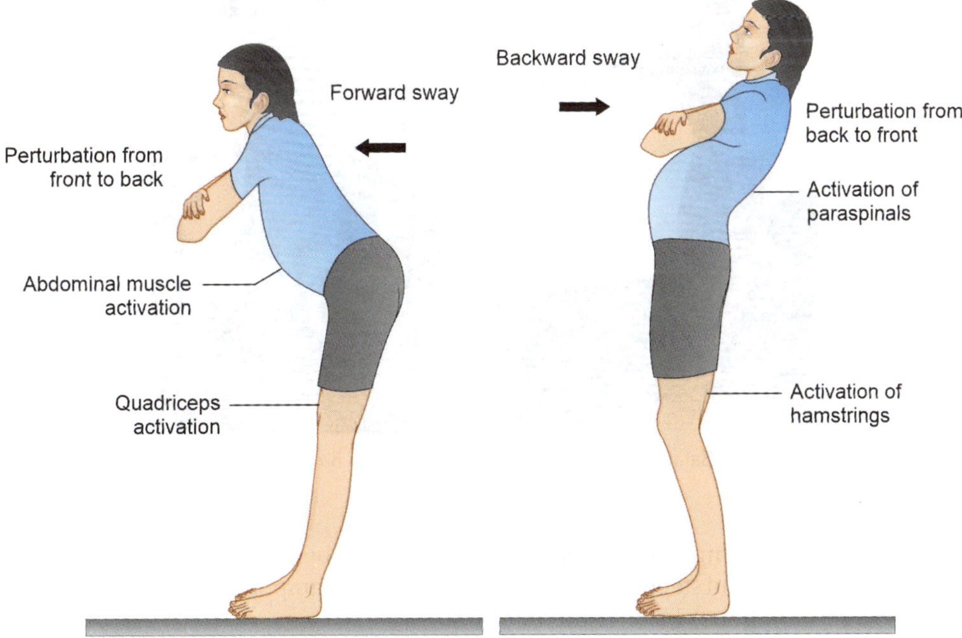


**Fig. 5.61:** The hip strategy.

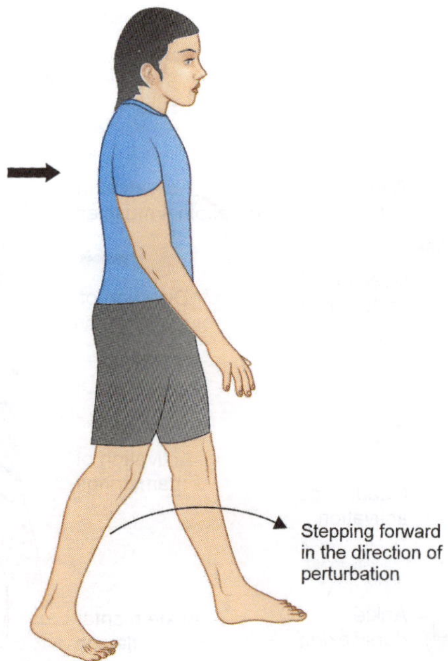


**Fig. 5.62:** The stepping strategy.

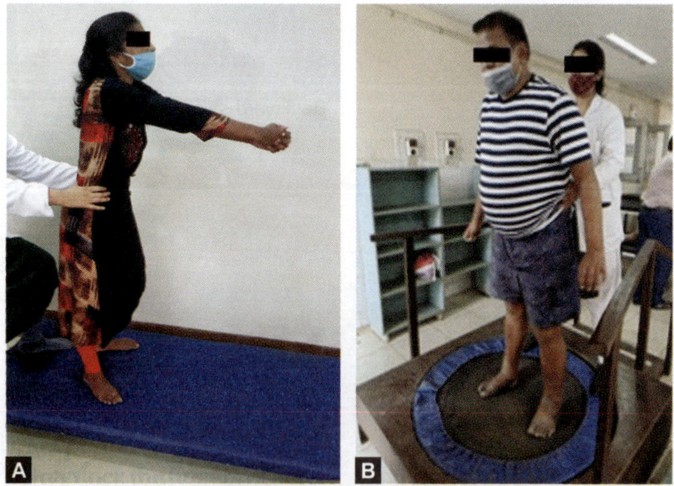


**Figs. 5.63A and B:** (A) Balance training on wobble board; (B) Balance training on trampoline.

for small perturbations, hip strategy for little stronger perturbations, and stepping strategies for very large perturbations), balance training should also be given on wobble board **(Fig. 5.63A)** and trampoline **(Fig. 5.63B)**.

# 6 CHAPTER Relaxation

## INTRODUCTION

Relaxation is a state of body and mind, which is free from tension resulting in freedom for exercising smooth decision making and execution of function and leading to a pain free and stress free living. It is a conscious effort to relieve excessive tension in the muscles and mind. Relaxation techniques reduce stress and help a person lead a better quality of life.

Our muscles develop tension as they contract during strenuous activities, as well as in certain pathological states, such as upper motor neuron disorders. The normal tension developed in muscles subsides, as the individual takes rest, and relaxes the body. Mental stress developed in individuals, also lead to physical tension, causing alteration of muscle tone and posture.

Relaxation of body and mind is very essential for efficient functional performance with less and less consumption of energy. Recognition of a state of tension followed by voluntary relaxation of the muscles and mind, provide a mean of helping the patient to consume less energy, as in the state of relaxation, there is increased mobility of joints and a bio mechanically efficient posture help in doing functional activities in an efficient way.

### Degrees of Relaxation

This implies, the degrees to which existing muscular and mental tension is alleviated. Physiotherapists play a great role in alleviating tension and inducing voluntary relaxation. A person, who is tensed can easily be recognized through the following features:

- Frowning
- Clenching of jaw and teeth
- Raised shoulders
- Clenched hands and tightly crossed legs
- Stooped posture
- Shallow breathing

### Benefits of Relaxation Therapy

Practicing relaxation techniques will result in the following health benefits:

- Relieves anxiety and depression/tension
- Reduces work-related stress
- Reduces the risk of cardiac complications
- Normalizes blood pressure and respiration
- Makes mind fresh and joyful
- Reduces insomnia and improves sleep

The procedures involved to induce relaxation include:

- Creation of a regulatory environment conducive to both physical and mental rest.
- Recognition of a state of tension
- Reassuring the patient and gaining confidence and cooperation
- Providing relaxation training/therapy

### Types of Relaxation

- Whole body/General relaxation
- Local relaxation
- Mental relaxation

### *I. Whole body or General relaxation:*

Support, comfort and a regulatory and restful atmosphere are essential requirements for general relaxation of the body, which are briefly discussed below.

A. **Support:** Proper support of the body contour and modifications of posture in lying and sitting are essential measures to induce relaxation. The weight of the body, when effectively counterbalanced, by the uniform upward pressure of a reciprocal surface, or by suspension, or by adapting a semi-flexed position of the lower limbs, eliminates mechanical tension in muscles and ligaments, helping in achieving relaxation. In lying or sitting, postural modifications need to be done as described here **(Figs. 6.1A to D)**.

   Whole body relaxation can be achieved by positioning the person in some resting position. Normally during the lying position, the postural tone of the muscles is less. Alternation is made in the lying posture to attain the maximum general body relaxation. All the derived positions from the lying are used for achieving the relaxation of an individual depending on the situation. The person has to be positioned preferably on the firm mattresses, with adequate pillow/sand bag support. In lying, postural modifications should be done as discussed below.

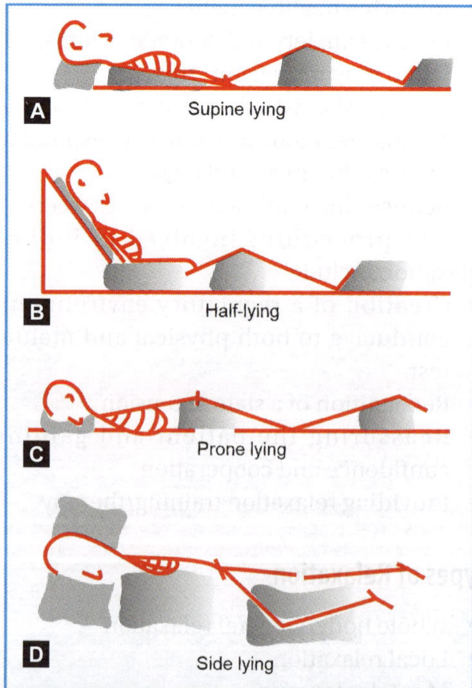


**Figs. 6.1A to D:** Relaxed positioning.

**Supine lying**

- The anterior portion of the body facing up or lying on the back.
- One pillow is placed under the head to prevent rotation to sides.
- One pillow under the knee, which prevents the hamstring tension, reduces the lordotic curvature over the lumbar region, reduce the abdominal muscle and iliofemoral ligament tension.
- Both the arms are abducted and placed on the pillows inside.
- Ankle is positioned in neutral position by placing sandbags.

**Half lying**

- This is similar like the supine lying and the head end is lifted up. This position is convenient for the respiratory distress patients and elderly patients because this position reduces the diaphragmatic tension by reducing the abdominal pressure.
- One pillow is placed under the head extended up to the thoracic region to support the upper trunk.
- One pillow is placed under the knee to reduce the hamstring, iliofemoral ligament and abdominal tension.
- Ankle is positioned in neutral position by placing the sandbags.

**Prone lying**

- Posterior portion of the body facing up or lying on the front portion of the body.
- This position will be difficult for the respiratory distress and elderly patients to maintain for longer period.

- One pillow is placed under the hips and the lower abdomen to reduce the abdominal pressure by which we reduce the diaphragmatic tension.
- A pillow under the leg and ankle is placed for comfortable alignment.

**Side lying**

- The person lying on his one side of the body.
- One pillow under head and neck, which supports and aligns with the body. The pillow should not be too high.
- Uppermost lower extremity hip and knee are flexed and placed on the pillow, which reduces the hip rotators and lower trunk muscular tension.
- Uppermost upper limb shoulder and elbow are flexed and placed over the pillow which reduces the tension of muscles of shoulder girdle and rotators of the shoulder.

B. **Comfort:** Besides adequate support to body parts, comfort in terms of freedom to breath deeply, mild warmth, relaxation of abdominals, minimal physical activity are essential components for achieving relaxation. The dresses worn should not be too tight, and the room should have circulation of free air. A light well balanced meal, timely voiding of bladder and bowel are conducive to achieve general relaxation.

C. **Restful atmosphere:** As relaxation of body and mind are interdependent, effort is essentially required to establish a state of mental rest. As many patients, such as cerebral palsy, head injury, stroke and cardiac patients, etc., are highly susceptible for disturbing influence of noise, the therapy/treatment room should be as quiet as possible. Bright lights and strong colors, such as red and bright yellow, are said to be stimulating, whereas a room with low well-diffused light with green and peach furnishings gives a soft and warm glow and provides an ideal setting for relaxation.

The behavior of the treating physician/physiotherapist plays a vital role in the creation of restful atmosphere. The voice of therapist should be low-pitched and clear.

**Additional Methods of Relaxation**

Even though, conditions favoring relaxation are provided, to the patient, sometimes tension persists and additional methods for relaxation should be followed, as described under:

i. **Conscious breathing exercises**

During rest, very often the person's mind remains active generating so many unwanted thoughts resulting in anxiety and tension. Breathing exercises with a slight pause at the end of expiration, may divert the attention of the person, making him concentrate on his own rhythm of breathing. During expiration,, which is a phase of relaxation a feeling of 'letting go' in the whole body should develop helping to eliminate anxiety and physical tension, there by inducing relaxation. The breathing exercises given are:

*Deep breathing exercises*

Deep breathing exercises, that involve taking slow, deep and even breaths help a person feel relaxed.

*Box breathing*

Box breathing is a powerful but simple relaxation technique that aims to return breathing to its normal rhythm after a stressful experience. It may help clear the mind, relax the body, and improves focus. It is also known as resetting the breath or four-square breathing, is easy to do, quick to learn, and can be highly effective in stressful situations. It is done through four steps, such as:

1. **Step 1:** Starting by breathing in through the nose for a count of 2–4 seconds.
2. **Step 2:** Holding the breath for a count of 2–4 seconds.

3. **Step 3:** Breathing out for a count of 2–4 seconds.
4. **Step 4:** Finally, holding breath again for another count of 2–4 seconds.

ii. **Relaxed passive movements:** Rhythmical passive movements of the limbs and head may assist in achieving relaxation. Mass movements of joints, e.g., flexion and extension of hip, knee and ankle, are preferable. The rhythm of small pendular movements is very effective in some cases.

iii. **Progressive relaxation:** Progressive muscle relaxation (PMR) is a deep relaxation technique that has been effectively used to control stress and anxiety, relieve insomnia, and reduce symptoms of certain types of chronic pain.

The technique of progressive muscle relaxation was described by Edmund Jacobson in the 1930s and is based upon his premise that mental calmness is a natural result of physical relaxation. This method is similar to the Yoga system and termed as "Savasana" or "Still Pose **(Fig. 6.2)**.

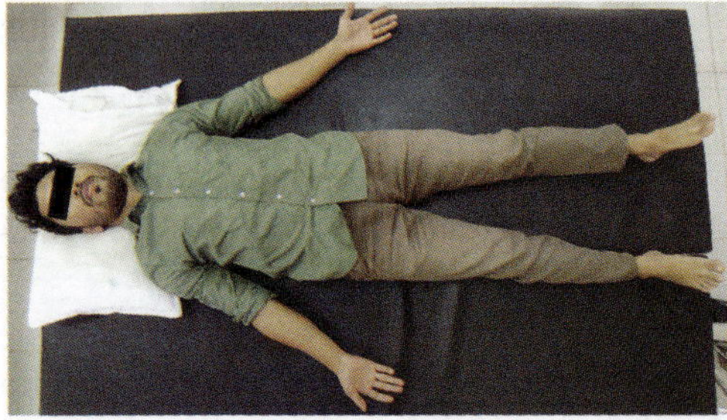

**Fig. 6.2:** The still pose.

It is based upon the simple practice of tensing, or tightening, one muscle group at a time followed by a relaxation phase with release of the tension **(Fig. 6.3)**. When the muscle tension is released, attention is directed towards the differences felt during tension and relaxation so that the patient learns to recognize the contrast between the two states.

It can be learned by nearly anyone and requires only 10 minutes to 20 minutes per day to practice.

The technique can be performed in, lying, sitting or standing. Breathing is included with tensing and relaxing the muscles, which involves breathing in with tensing (contracting the muscles), breathing out while relaxing. To begin the exercise, the individual slowly breathes in and tenses the first muscle group, then holds the breath and tension for 3–5 seconds. Next, the individual slowly breaths out while releasing the tension and relax the muscles for 10–15 seconds. The individual should try to visualize how the tension feels like and how it is slowly fading out of his/her body. Then, the individual breathes in and tenses the next muscle group, repeating this process for all of the muscle groups. The muscle groups commonly used in the technique are:

- Muscles of forehead
- Muscles of eyes/cheeks
- Muscles of lips/jaw

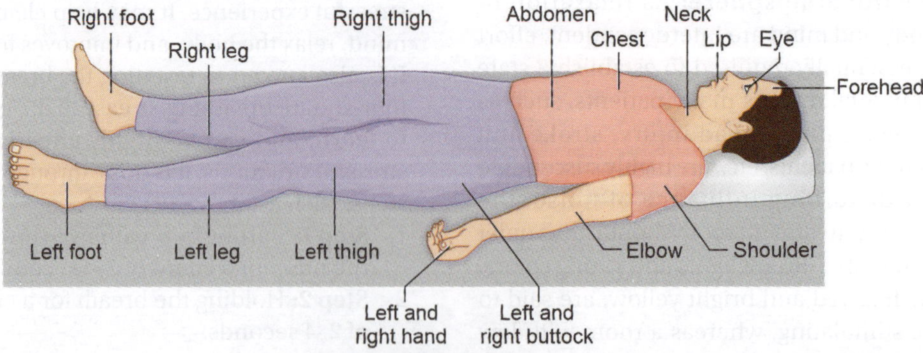


**Fig. 6.3:** Progressive relaxation.

- Muscles of neck
- Muscles of shoulders
- Muscles of back
- Muscles of chest
- Muscles of upper arms
- Muscles of hands/fists
- Abdominal muscles
- Muscles of hips/buttocks
- Muscles of thighs
- Muscles of calves/feet/toes

Sometimes progressive relaxation technique is used in combination with other techniques, such as guided imagery and deep breathing exercise. The technique has eight steps, briefly discussed below:

- **Step-1:** The patient should be made to lie/sit/stand comfortably in a room with minimal distraction.
- To start with, the muscles of feet are contracted for five seconds, followed by relaxation of the muscles for 10 seconds. Relief of tension and feeling of muscle relaxation stimulates calmness.
- Then the muscles of lower legs are contracted and relaxed for the same amount of time.
- Then the muscles of buttocks and hips are contracted and relaxed.
- Next, the abdominals chest muscles are contracted and relaxed.
- Then the muscles of shoulders are made to contract and relax.
- Next the facial muscles are made to contract and relax.
- At last, the muscles of hands are contracted (making a fist and holding for five seconds) and relaxed (for 10 seconds).

iv. **Contrast method:** In situations, where a patient is not able to feel the sensation of relaxation in tensed muscles, the contrast method, where the contrast between maximal muscle contraction and degree of relaxation which follows muscle contraction is demonstrated. The patient is told to contract any group or series of muscles, as strongly as possible and then to "let go" and "continue to let go".

v. **Physiological relaxation:** This method of relieving tension was devised by Laura Mitchell, in 1957, which is based on the physiological principle of reciprocal inhibition. The 'Mitchell Method' of physiological relaxation—often known as the 'simple method of relaxation'—is the name given to a technique of relaxing the whole, or parts of the body. Once learnt and practiced, it can be used easily and anywhere to relax and reduce the muscle tension produced by stress. The technique is based on:

- Reciprocal inhibition
- Diaphragmatic breathing
- A series of ordered isotonic contractions

**Principles of mitchell method of relaxation**

- Tightening or contracting muscles results in movement.
- Movement causes repositioning of the joints and limbs.
- When one is awake, the brain will register a change in body position through muscle, joint and skin sensation.
- The brain is only aware of the movement it causes. Movements are controlled by the nervous system; if one group of muscles is 'instructed' to tighten, the opposite group of muscles for that action receives an 'instruction' to relax. One can learn to recognize and be aware of tense muscles and joints. Instructing or 'ordering' the opposite muscle groups to tighten will automatically result in 'relax' messages being received by the tense muscles and joints. This new 'position of ease' can be learnt by registering the feeling in the muscles, joints and skin. Finding the position of ease of all the joints will result in relaxation.

**Technique**

The technique involves relaxing the whole body or part of body, by moving away from the position of stress and being aware of the new position. It helps to recognize and ease and physical symptoms of stress, and to maintain a good breathing pattern.

- Move away from the position of stress
- Stop
- Be aware of and feel the new position

For example:

- **For relaxing the shoulders:** The sitting patient is asked to pull the shoulders towards the feet, so the neck becomes longer. Then, he/she should stop and feel that the shoulders are down and relaxed.
- For relaxing the hips: The patient is asked to turn the hips outwards", then stop and feel that thighs and legs have rolled outwards.
- In the same manner, relaxation is achieved in the whole body.

Difference between Jacobson's relaxation and Mitchell relaxation technique:

| *Jacobson's relaxation technique* | *Mitchell's relaxation technique* |
|---|---|
| Diaphragmatic breathing with isometric contraction of muscles | Diaphragmatic breathing with isotonic contraction of muscles |

vi. **Autogenic training:** This relaxation technique used to alleviate many psychosomatic disorders was first described by German psychiatrist Johannes Heinrich Schultz in 1932. It is a system, that may stimulate psychological and physical calmness. It involves slowing and controlling the breath and teaching the body to respond to verbal instructions. During practice, a person concentrates on physical sensations of different parts of their body (inner sensations, rather than the environmental stimuli), by focusing on sensation of warmth, heaviness and relaxation.

The technique can be practiced in any comfortable posture. The main benefit of autogenic training is the autonomic self-regulation achieved by removing environmental distraction, training imagery that accompanies autonomic self-regulation, and providing a facilitative set of exercises that are easy to learn and remember The technique has six standard components, discussed below:

- Muscular relaxation by repetition of a verbal formula, "My right arm is heavy", emphasizing heaviness.
- Passive concentration focuses on feeling warm, initiated by the instruction "My right arm is warm".
- Initiation of cardiac activity using the formula "My heartbeat is calm and regular".
- Passive concentration on the respiratory mechanism with the formula "It breathes me".
- Concentration on the warmth in the abdominal region with "My solar plexus is warm".
- Passive concentration on coolness in the cranial region with the formula "My forehead is cool".

vii. **Guided imagery:** Guided imagery involves replacing negative or stressful feelings by visualizing pleasant and calming scenarios. It is a mind-body intervention by which a trained practitioner helps a patient to evoke and generate mental images that simulate or recreate the sensory perception of sights, sounds, tastes, smells, movements, and images associated with touch, such as texture, temperature, and pressure, as well as imaginative or mental content. It denotes the technique by which images are recalled from long-term or short-term memory, or created from fantasy, or a combination of both. The technique involves three steps, discussed below:

- **Step-1:** Patient sits/lies down in a comfortable position, in a room where distractions are negligible.
- **Step-2:** Patient visualizes a relaxing environment using sense of sight, sound, smell, taste and touch, by remembering one from memory or imagining a new environment.
- **Step-3:** Patient is asked to sustain the visualization, for as long as required, taking slow deep breaths and focusing on calm feelings.

viii. **Biofeedback:** This technique involves using electronic devices to measure different bodily functions, such as temperature of the skin, pulse rate, or tension in the muscles. Precise instruments measure physiological activity, such as brainwaves, heart function, breathing, muscle activity, and skin temperature. The therapy involves attaching sensors to a specific part of the body, which produce measurements as a person relaxes. A person can then use the feedback to help them make changes where necessary, such as relaxing a particular muscle.

**Body scan**

The body scan is a mindfulness meditation practice involving scanning the body for pain, tension, or anything out of the ordinary. It can help feel more connected to the physical and emotional self. This technique combines breathing with progressive muscle relaxation. After few minutes of deep breathing, the individual focuses on one part of the body or group of muscles at a time, and mentally releases physical tension felt (if any).

ix. **Mindfulness meditation:** This practice involves sitting comfortably, focussing on breathing and bringing the mind's attention to the present moment, without drifting into concerns about the past or the future. This is helpful for patients with anxiety, depression and pain.

x. **Practice of Yoga:** Yoga is a group of physical, mental, and spiritual practices or disciplines which originated in ancient India and aim to control and still the mind.

The ultimate goals of yoga are stilling the mind and gaining insight, resting in detached awareness, and liberation from saṃsāra and duḥkha, a process leading to unity with the divine or with one's self.

xi. **Repetitive prayer:** In this technique, the patient silently repeats a short prayer or a phrase from prayer as per his/her religion along with practice of breathing exercises.

### *II. Local Relaxation*

Relaxing the particular part or segment of the body is called as local relaxation As we know, general relaxation takes time and some times is not required, Effort should be made to achieve local relaxation by the following methods:

- **Massage:** Massage, such as light stroking, gentle effleurage, myofascial release help in inducing local relaxation by soothing effect, increased blood flow and increased venous and lymphatic return causing reduction of edema.
- **Passive stretching:** Gentle stretching of the spastic, spasmodic muscles help in relaxing the segment of the body over which the muscle works.
- **Contract-relax and pendular movements:** These start in the free range and gradually increase in amplitude may restore confidence and achieve relaxation.
- **In case of tightness and deformity:** Relaxation techniques for the shortened muscles and strengthening techniques for their antagonists, followed by integration of their reciprocal action into function,

to establish the increase in the range of movement.

❖ **In case of pain:** If the patient has pain over part or segment of the body, the pain relieving modalities, such as wax bath, hot water fermentation, IFT, TENS, SWD, and ultrasound can be used. Whenever the patient gets relief from the pain, he feels relaxation.

### *III. Mental Relaxation*

Mental relaxation plays the main role while treating the patient and to render the good service. The mental relaxation can be achieved with help of the above mentioned comfortable measures and also some other factors, such as:

❖ Alleviation of psychological fear to the treatment
❖ Coloring of the room
❖ Peaceful mentality

The coloring of the room has to be perfectly done, the selection of the color, place the main role in the alteration of the mind. Normally, mild/light colors give the mental peace, so the dark colors should be avoided. Not only the coloring of the wall but also the curtains, the clothes that we use in the clinic set-up also should be pleasant. The patient should have confident with the treatment, which he gets from the therapist. The therapist has to gain the confidence of the patient by explaining about the condition, treatment procedure, and effect of the treatment and necessity of treatment. The psychological state of the patient is much more important factor to treat an individual effectively. Health counseling may be effective and helps to gain the confidence of the patient. The noisy surrounding should be avoided because the louder sound may cause the mental alteration and may leads to frustration. The therapist's manner should be courteous, pleasant and his voice low-pitched and clear. The atmosphere of the room should be pleasant, sometimes low-pitched continuous "hum" can be used to smoothen the mind.

**Relaxation Training**

A relaxation training is selection and application of any method, process, procedure, or activity that helps a person to relax; attain a state of increased calmness; or otherwise reduce levels of pain, anxiety, stress or anger. Relaxation techniques are often employed as one element of a wider stress management program and can decrease muscle tension, normalize blood pressure, and normalize heart and respiratory rates, etc. Depending upon the need of the client the relaxation methods discussed above should be selected.

# 7 CHAPTER Pelvic Tilt

## DEFINITION

"Pelvic tilt is the angle created by a line running from the sacral endplate midpoint to the center of the bifemoral heads and the vertical axis". Simply speaking, it is the angular inclination of pelvis from its normal location. The average ranges of anterior and posterior pelvic tilting are 13.0 ± 4.9°, and 8.9 ± 4.5°, respectively.

The pelvic motion along with the hip and the vertebral column makes the normal sinusoidal curve in the gait cycle and these pelvic motions are called as "Pelvic tilt". These pelvic tilts may occur due to some pathological problems, such as abduction deformity of hips, that causes an infra/lateral pelvic tilt, or flexion contracture/deformity of hip, causing an anterior pelvic tilt. It is a common condition, that can cause bad posture, leading to problems with the spinal discs and increasing the risk of injury to spine. The normal pelvis and the deviations, such as anterior/posterior pelvic tilts are shown in **Figures 7.1 and 7.2**.

The pelvic may be inclined/tilted in below mentioned ways:

1. Anterior pelvic tilt
2. Posterior pelvic tilt
3. Lateral pelvic tilt
4. Pelvic drop
5. Pelvic rotation

### Anterior Pelvic Tilt

A forward tilt/rotation of pelvis is called an anterior pelvic tilt. It is caused by the shortening/contraction of the hip flexor and lumbar extensor muscles and the lengthening/weakness of the hip extensor and abdominal muscles. This increases the lumbar lordosis **(Fig. 7.3)**. Abdominal muscles and the hip extensors muscles are responsible for preventing the anterior pelvic tilt.

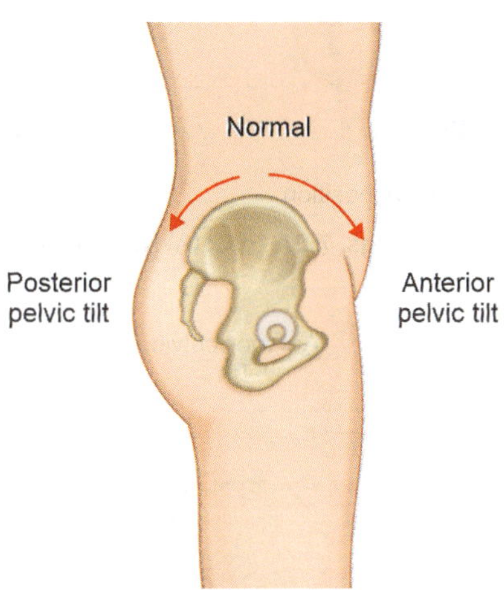


**Fig. 7.1:** Pelvis.

It leads to the following deviations in the pelvis:

- Anterior superior iliac spine (ASIS) moves anteroinferiorly.
- Pubic symphysis moves posteriorly and moves closure to the femur.
- ASIS is aligned horizontally with the posterior superior iliac spine (PSIS) and vertical line through the symphysis pubis changes in the anterior tilt.
- Sacral angle increases and the lumbar lordosis and thoracic kyphosis also increases.

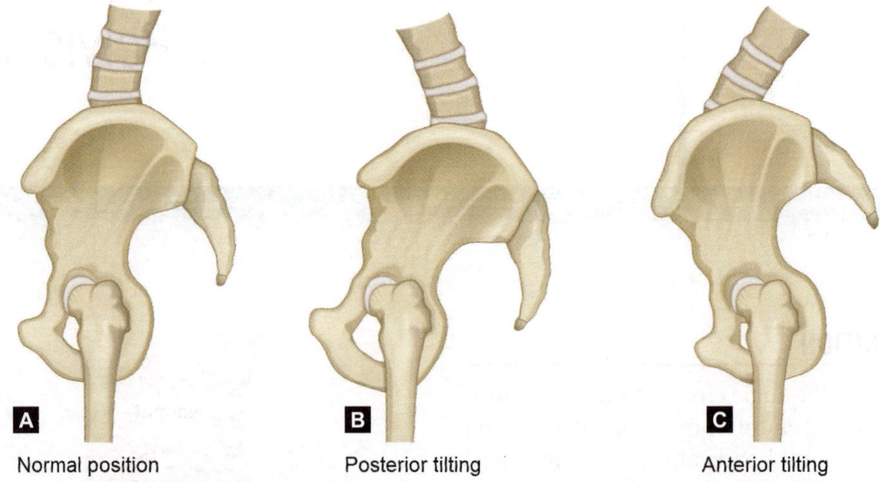


**Figs. 7.2A to C:** (A) Normal pelvis; (B) Posterior pelvic tilt; (C) Anterior pelvic tilt.

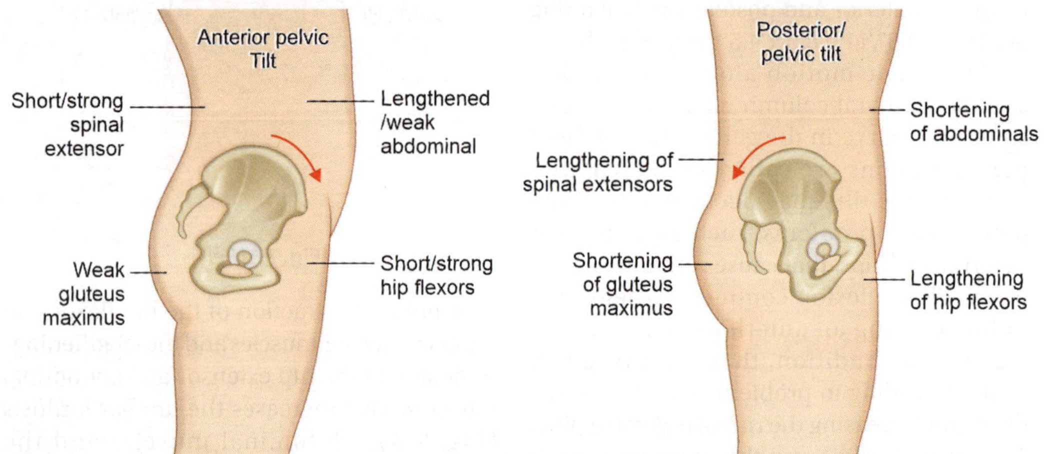


**Fig. 7.3:** Anterior pelvic tilt.

**Fig. 7.4:** Posterior pelvic tilt.

## Posterior Pelvic Tilt

It is a condition, where the pelvis has tilted/rotated excessively backwards. In this condition, the front of the pelvis rises and the back of the pelvis drops, while the pelvis rotates upwards. It is caused by an imbalance between the trunk and hip muscles. There occurs shortening/contraction of trunk flexors and hip extensors (gluteus maximus and hamstrings) and lengthening/weakness of hip flexors and lumbar extensors. Spinal extensors and hip flexors are responsible for preventing the posterior pelvic tilt. There is a decrease of lumbar lordosis **(Fig. 7.4)**. The following deviations occur in posterior pelvic tilt:

- ❖ ASIS moves posteriorly
- ❖ Pubic symphysis moves away from the femur
- ❖ Sacral angle decreases and the lumbar lordosis also decreases

**Figure 7.5** shows the muscles responsible for anterior and posterior pelvic tilts.

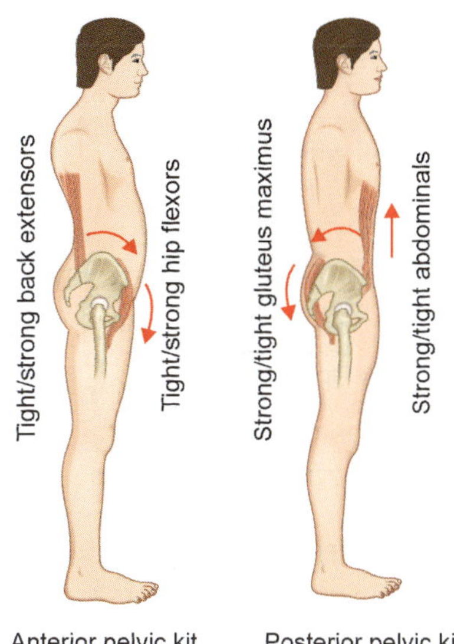


**Fig. 7.5:** Muscles involved in pelvic tilts.

## *Measurement of Anterior (AT) and Posterior (PT) Pelvic Tilts*

Anterior and posterior pelvic tilts occur in the sagittal plane and the coronal axis. Anterior and posterior pelvic tilts can be measured by the following ways:

### Measuring Lumbosacral Angle

The angle made by the line parallel to the ground and the line along the base of the sacrum makes the lumbosacral angle. Normal lumbosacral angle should be 30° **(Fig. 7.6)**. If it is increased said to be anterior pelvic tilt and if decreased called posterior pelvic tilts.

### Measurements using Pelvic Inclinometer

A pelvic inclinometer is a device used to measure the angle formed by the horizontal plane and a line passing through the midpoint of the posterior superior iliac spine (PSIS) and the midpoint of the anterior superior iliac spine (ASIS), which is known as pelvic tilt **(Fig. 7.7)**. Caliper-based inclinometers, described as pelvic inclinometers, have been developed to specifically assess pelvic tilt. Pelvic inclinometers have adjustable arms to facilitate direct contact with the bony landmarks in question. To assess pelvic tilt, the clinician aligns the adjustable arms with the ASIS and PSIS. This is most often described with the subject in a relaxed standing position. It is used to understand and measure the role of the pelvis in development of repetitive injury including lower back pain.

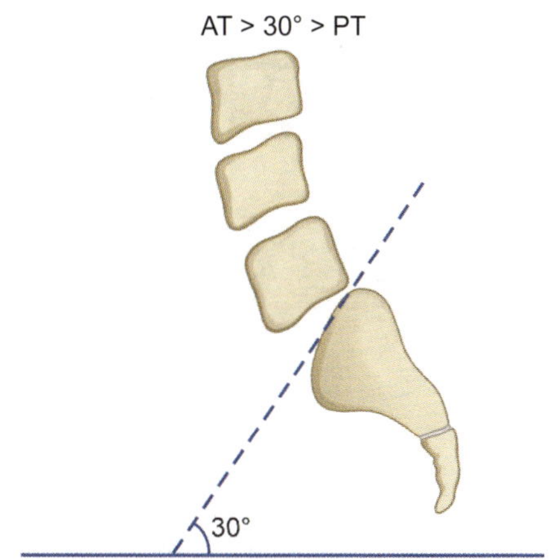


**Fig. 7.6:** Normal lumbosacral angle.

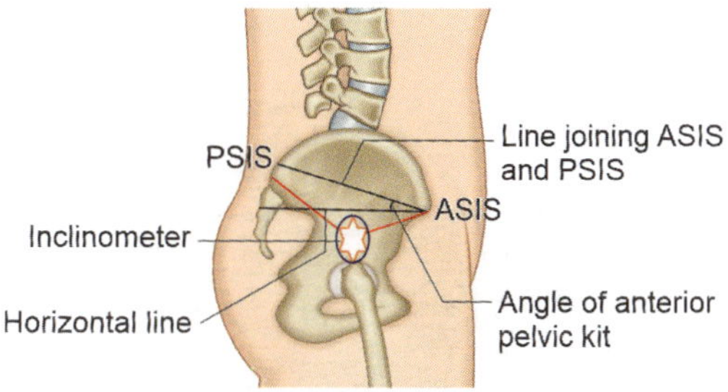


**Fig. 7.7:** Measurement of pelvic tilt.
(PSIS: posterior superior iliac spine; ASIS: anterior superior iliac spine)

**Smartphone applications:** More recently, applications that utilize the inclinometer functions within a smartphone have been developed and used to assess pelvic tilt.

## *Alternative Method of Measurement of Pelvic Tilt*

### Placement of Inclinometer between Pubis Symphysis (PS) and PSIS

One arm of the pelvic inclinometer is placed over the pubic symphysis and another over the PSIS **(Fig. 7.8)**. A neutral pelvis is slightly

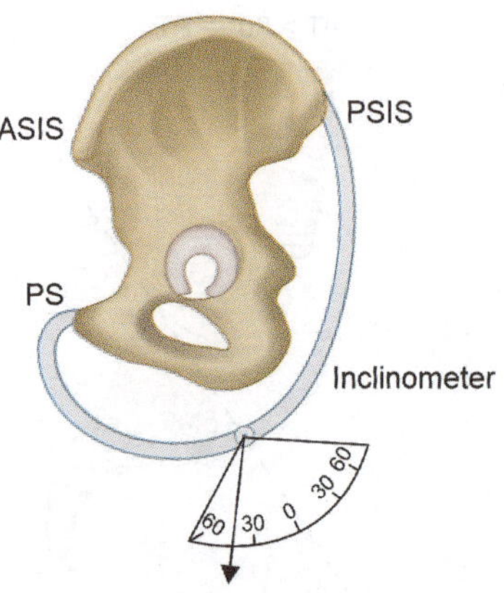


**Fig. 7.8:** Measurement of pelvic tilt.
(PSIS: posterior superior iliac spine; ASIS: anterior superior iliac spine; PS: pubis symphysis)

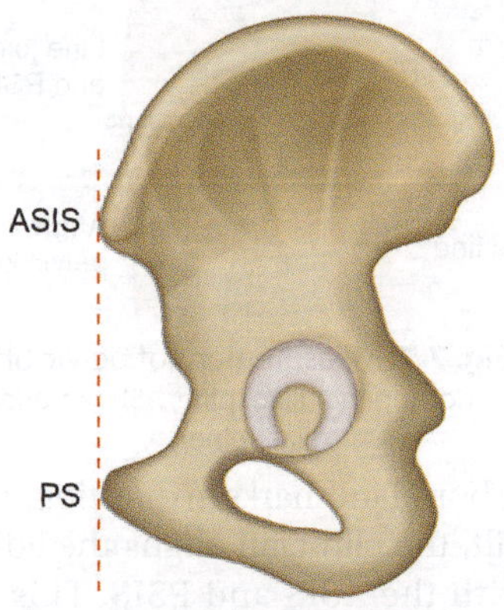


**Fig. 7.9:** The vertical line between ASIS and pubis symphysis.
(ASIS: anterior superior iliac spine; PS: pubis symphysis)

forward-tilted, perhaps 8–15 degrees for beginners, and by as much as 30 degrees for individuals with a greater range of motion and change in this angle, results in anterior (angle increased) or posterior pelvic tilt (angle decreased).

### Checking the Vertical line from ASIS to Symphysis Pubis

The line drawn from ASIS to pubic symphysis (PS) is normally a vertical line. The alternation of this line is an indication of anterior or posterior pelvic tilt **(Fig. 7.9)**.

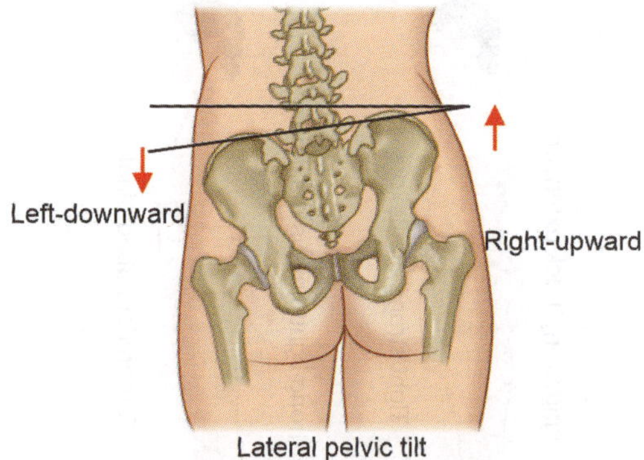


**Fig. 7.10:** Lateral pelvic tilt.

### Lateral Pelvic Tilt And Drop

A lateral pelvic tilt is the frontal plane motion of the entire pelvis around the anteroposterior axis **(Fig. 7.10)**. The pelvis shifts side to side, so much that one hip is higher than the other. This leads to unilateral muscle imbalances throughout the body. Imbalance of quadratus lumborum (tightening on elevated side and lengthening on the down side) and weakness of gluteus medius on the contralateral limb, is the main cause of uneven hips and lateral pelvic tilt.

- It occurs in the frontal plane and the AP axis.
- Both the ASIS are aligned in the horizontal line in the normal pelvic. If any changes occur in these alignment results in lateral tilt or drop.
- Possible during the unilateral as well as bilateral stances.
- In unilateral stance, one hip is fixed and another is freely moving and results in drop or hike.

### Hiking

During swing phase, a person with inadequate hip and knee flexion, hikes the pelvis to clear the ground. This is most common in patients with spastic hemiparesis. The following events occur during hiking:

- During hiking ASIS moves upwards and medially
- Spine goes for side flexion in the same side

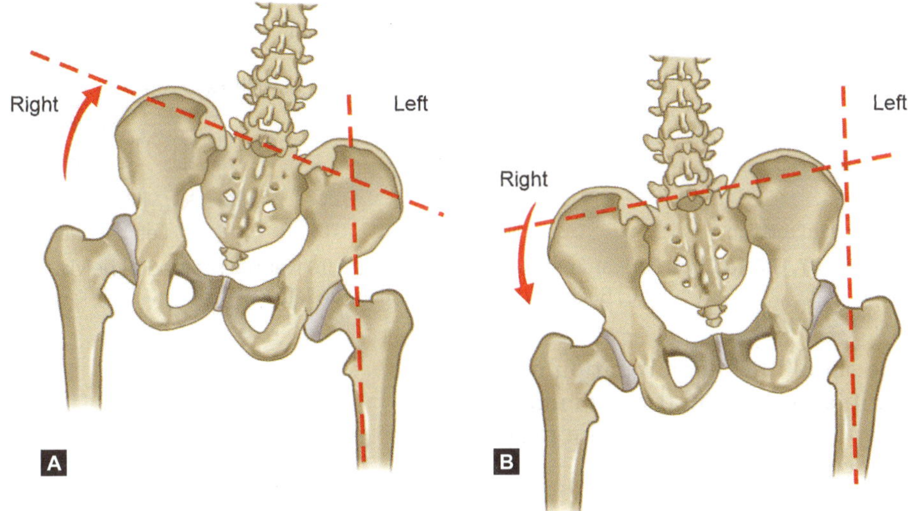


**Figs. 7.11A and B:** (A) Shows hiking of pelvis on right side; (B) Shows dropping of pelvis on right side.

- Hip goes for abduction in the hiking side
- Hiking occurs due to the contraction of the quadratus lumborum and the trunk side flexors **(Fig. 7.11A)**.

### Dropping of Pelvis

The pelvic drop, also called as hip drop, is lack of symmetry of pelvis leading to downward movement of one side of pelvis/hip than the other side hip/pelvis **(Fig. 7.11B)**. The following events occur during pelvic drop:

- ASIS moves inferiorly and medically.
- Spine goes for opposite side flexion.
- Hip goes for adduction in the drop side.
- Pelvic drop occurs due to the opposite hip abductors weakness. This sign is called as Trendelenburg's sign.
- Both the sides abductor paralysis leads to wadding type of gait otherwise called as "Duck walking".
- In the bilateral stance, if the weight is transferred to the right side, dropping occurs in the same side. During the right side dropping, the hip goes for adduction in the dropped side and abduction in the opposite side.

### Pelvic Rotation

- Pelvic rotation occurs in the transverse plane and the vertical axis.
- Pelvic rotation occurs when the swinging leg moves forward and backward on the supported or stance leg.

*Measurement of Pelvic Rotation*

"Supine pelvic tilt test," which involves asking the patient to lie supine with their knees bent and feet flat on the table. The examiner then observes the patient's pelvic position and notes any asymmetry or deviation from neutral position.

*Examples:*

- In normal walking, the forward motion in the right side leg results in the right side pelvic forward rotation, left side upper limb swings forward and the stance or weight-bearing hip goes for medial rotation.
- In case of backward motion of the right leg results in the backward rotation of the pelvic, right upper limb swings forward and the stance hip or weight-bearing hip goes for a lateral rotation **(Figs. 7.12A to C)**.

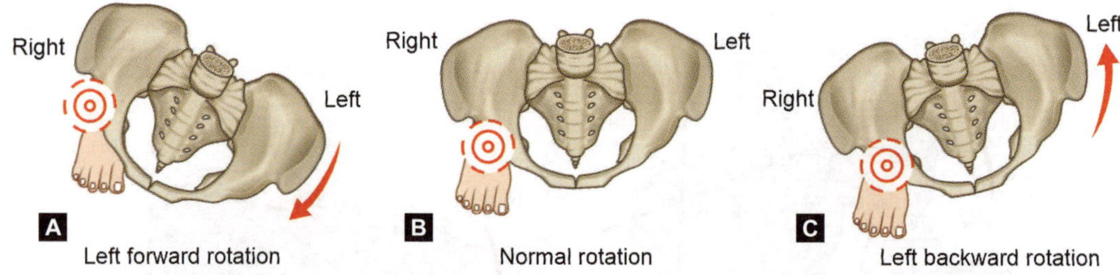


**Figs. 7.12A to C:** (A) Forward rotation of pelvis on left; (B) Neutral rotation of pelvis; (C) Backward rotation of pelvis on left.

There should be a combination of the pelvic, hip and the spinal movements to maintain the proper gait and the proper sinusoidal curve.

*Effect of Pelvic Tilt on Posture*

- **Anterior tilt of pelvis:** As the pelvis rotates forward, lumbar spine adopts a more extended (hyperlordotic) position, resulting in lordotic posture.
- **Posterior tilt of pelvis:** As the pelvis rotates backwards, lumbar spine adopts a more flexed (kyphotic) position, resulting in flat back posture. Swaying of the pelvis forward in relation to the feet, resulting in a posterior pelvic tilt, makes the lumbar spine flat with increased thoracic kyphosis resulting in sway-back posture **(Fig. 7.13)**.
- **Lateral tilt of pelvis:** In this postural misalignment one side of the pelvis is higher/lower than the other side. When the lateral tilt has resulted in a hike of pelvis, the trunk laterally flexes towards the tilted (same) side, whereas, if the lateral tilt has resulted in a drop of the pelvis, the trunk lateral flexes towards the opposite side **(Figs. 7.11A and B)**.

The types of pelvic tilts and their effects are summarized in the following table **(Table 7.1)**.

So, during the normal walking itself there is anterior tilt, posterior tilt, lateral tilt, drop and rotations present to propel the body forward. These tilts are altering the body segment during the normal walking and making convenient or easier the walking pattern and reducing the strain in the weight transmission. If any pathological disturbance occurs there will be marked and visible tilts seen. These pathological tilts or drops can be cured by the proper treatment that is by the regular strengthening or stretching program.

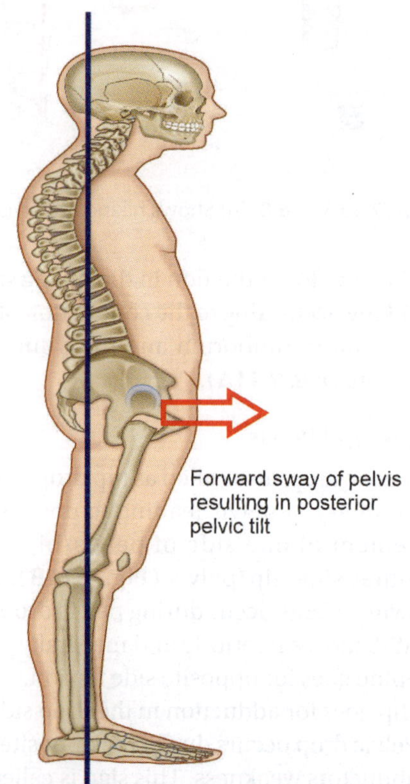


**Fig. 7.13:** Sway back posture.

**Table 7.1:** Pelvic tilt in short view.

| *Sr. No.* | *Pelvic* | *Vertebral column* | *Hip* | *Arm* |
|---|---|---|---|---|
| 1. | Anterior tilt | Hyperextension | Flexion | – |
| 2. | Posterior tilt | Flexion | Extension | – |
| 3. | Lateral tilt (hike) | Same side flexion | Abduction at the same side | – |
| 4. | Drop | Opposite side flexion | Adduction at the same side | – |
| 5. | Rotation (forward) | Opposite side | Medial rotation at opposite side or weight bearing side | Opposite side arm goes forward |
| 6. | Backward rotation | Opposite side | Lateral rotation at weight bearing side | Opposite side arm goes backwards |

# 8 CHAPTER

# Active and Passive Exercises (Movements)

## INTRODUCTION

The exercises which are needed for the assessment and treatment purposes, are called as therapeutic exercises. The person performing the exercises in gymnasium and jogging in the open field, does so to build the body and for healthy living. But the therapeutic exercises are the exercises, which are performed to come out from ones ailment or disease. These therapeutic exercises are totally different from the body-building exercises. The main goal of the therapeutic exercise is preparing or making the patient independent for performing symptom-free movements. It brings back the diseased or injured patient to the normal state, and it plays the major role in the rehabilitation of an individual. In the field of sports, exercises are advised for prevention of sports related injuries and to treat sports personnel, if they sustain any injury while playing. To perform the therapeutic exercise one should have thorough knowledge on anatomy, physiology, orthopedic, neurology, kinesiology, pathology, cardiopulmonary conditions and some of the physiotherapy related medical fields. Before advising exercises to the patient/ sport personnel, a thorough assessment of ROM, muscle power, exercise capacity of the individual are done by the physiotherapists/ clinicians. It is believed that the perfect assessment of the disease is the 75 percent of the treatment. Stretching, strengthening, coordination exercises, breathing exercises, mobilization and manipulation, gait correction are the some of the therapeutic exercises used for treating the ailment of the patient. Besides increase of flexibility and ROM, therapeutic exercises are given to increase strength, power and endurance, enabling the individual perform functional activities. Difference between muscle strength, power and endurance are shown in **Table 8.1**.

### Classification of Exercises

Exercises are classified into two types such as:

#### *A. Active Exercises*

These are exercises/movements performed by the individual by his own muscular efforts. Active movements are of two types:

1. Involuntary, where the movements are produced without the conscious control by the individual, e.g., reflex actions such as eye blinking to flash light).

**Table 8.1:** Difference between strength, power and endurance.

| *Muscle strength* | *Muscle power* | *Endurance* |
|---|---|---|
| Muscular strength is the ability to exert maximal force.<br>It is the greatest measurable force, that can be exerted by a muscle/ muscle groups to overcome resistance, during a single maximum effort. | Muscular power is the ability to exert maximal force quickly.<br>It is the work produced by the muscle per unit of time. | It is the ability to perform, low intensity, repetitive or sustained activities, over a prolonged period of time. |

2. Voluntary, where purposeful movements are made by the individual by the voluntary action of the muscles. Active (voluntary) exercises are classified into different types, depending upon the types of muscle contraction, as well as depending upon the assistance or resistance used to produce movements, which are briefly discussed below:

## I. Depending upon the Types of Muscle Contraction Exercises are Classified Into

i. *Isometric Exercise*

It is a form of exercise, involving the static contraction of muscle, without any visible movement in the angle of the joint. The term "isometric", combines the prefix "iso" (same) with "metric" (distance), meaning that, in this exercise the length of muscle does not change. In this type of exercise/muscle contraction, the force produced by the muscle is equal to the load lifted.

There are several forms of isometric exercises, such as:

**Muscle setting exercises:** Low intensity isometric exercises, performed against little or no resistance. These exercises are primarily used to maintain the bulk and strength of the muscles, in the acute stage of disease or injury, where either joint movement is not allowed, or severe pain retards the movement of joints. Isometric quadriceps **(Fig. 8.1)** and gluteal sets are the common examples of this types of exercise. Because muscle setting exercises are not performed, against any appreciable resistance, these exercises do not increase the muscle strength, except in very weak muscles.

**Stabilization exercise:** These exercises involve mid-range isometric contraction against resistance in antigravity positions and in weight bearing postures, if the same is permissible. It is performed in different forms, such as rhythmic stabilization/alternating isometrics.

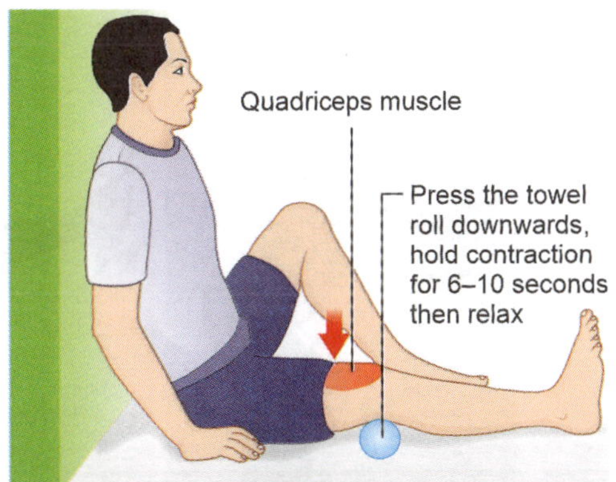


**Fig. 8.1:** Isometric quadriceps exercise/quadriceps muscle setting exercise.

**Multi-angle isometrics:** It is a system of isometric exercise, where resistance is added manually or mechanically, at multiple joint positions within the available range of motion. In situations, where dynamic resistance exercise is not permissible (full range joint motion is not permissible and strength gain is required throughout the range of motion) this exercise is prescribed **(Fig. 8.2)**.

**Factors to be considered for isometric training:**

- **Intensity:** The intensity (exercise load/resistance), must be progressively increased to progressively over load the muscle for a gain in strength. It is sufficient to use an exercise load of 60–80% of a muscle's force developing capacity to gain strength.
- **Duration:** The muscle contraction should be sustained for 6-10 seconds, which should be repeated 6-10 times in one set and the number of sets in one session and the number of sessions in a day depends on the patients condition and the effect required.
- **Joint angle:** The angle of joint at which strength gain is desired, exercise should be performed at that angle. Therefore, to achieve strength gain, muscle should be made to contract against a exercise load at 4-6 points in the range of motion.

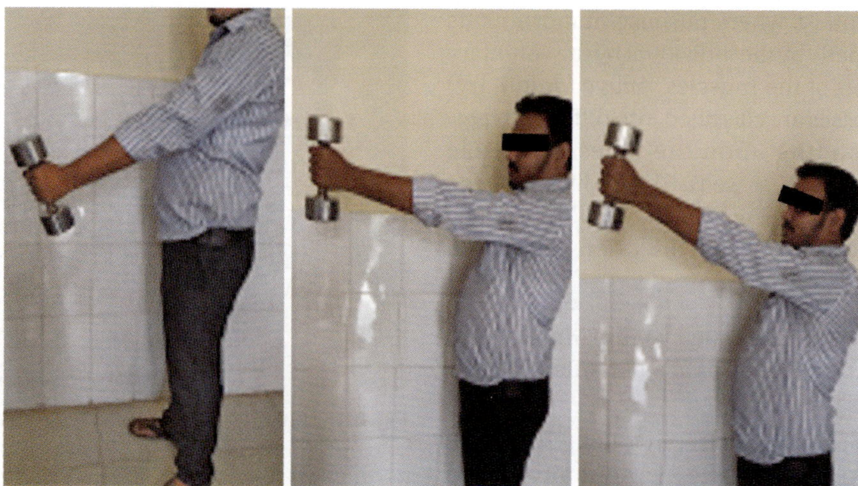

**Fig. 8.2:** Multi angle isometrics to shoulder flexors.

**Limitations of isometric exercise:** The gain in strength in such exercise is angle specific without much carryover into dynamic activities. Resisted isometric exercise is not as effective for developing muscle endurance as dynamic resistance exercise.

**Precaution of isometric exercise:**

- The exercise prescription requires great caution, because it causes a rise in heart rate (due to decreased vagal tone and increased discharge of cardiac sympathetic nerves).
- Within a few seconds of the start of the exercise, both systolic and diastolic blood pressure rises.
- As the exercise produces a tourniquet effect on the underlying blood vessels, increasing a great demand on the heart, great caution need to be taken while treating cardiac patients, and the duration of isometric contraction should not exceed beyond 6 seconds.

ii. *Isotonic/Dynamic Exercises*

The word isotonic is derived from: Iso-means same, tonic-means tension. Isotonic contraction/exercises are such exercises, where, when the muscles contract tension in the muscles remain the same, whilst the muscle's length changes. During an isotonic contraction, the force produced by the contracting muscle remains constant, while the velocity of movement changes.

There are two types of isotonic contractions/exercises, such as concentric contraction/exercise and eccentric contraction/exercise. In a concentric contraction, the muscle tension rises to meet the resistance, then remains the same as the muscle shortens. In eccentric contraction, the muscle lengthens due to the resistance being greater than the force the muscle produces.

As, actually the force/tension produced in the contracting muscles does not remain constant throughout the range of motion, the term "Isotonic" is not used now a days, and instead the term "Dynamic" exercise is currently used, in place of isotonic exercise. In dynamic exercises shortening or lengthening contraction of muscles occur producing intramuscular tension resulting in joint movements. As the dynamic contraction/exercise, produce, a near isotonic contraction, it is known as Auxotonic contraction/exercise.

The dynamic exercises are divided into:

- **Concentric exercises:** This exercise involve shortening contraction of the muscle producing joint movement, i.e., Muscles undergo physical shortening causing the joint motion and overcoming an external load. In this contraction the force generated by the muscles are greater than the weight of the part or resistance applied.

During a concentric contraction, a muscle is stimulated to contract according to the sliding filament mechanism. This occurs throughout the length of the muscle, generating force at the musculotendinous junction, causing the muscle to shorten, and changing the angle of the joint. For example in biceps curl in the upper limb, the biceps brachii muscle undergo shortening, causing elbow flexion **(Fig. 8.3)**.

- **Eccentric contraction/exercise:** During an eccentric contraction/exercise, the muscles undergo lengthening contraction (sarcomere lengthens) producing movement in the joint **(Fig. 8.4)**. During this contraction, the force (load) opposing the contraction of the muscle is greater than the force produced by the muscle, causing physical lengthening of the muscle as it controls the load. Rather than, working to pull a joint in the direction of muscle contraction, the muscle acts as brake and slow the movement of joint and lengthens while generating force.

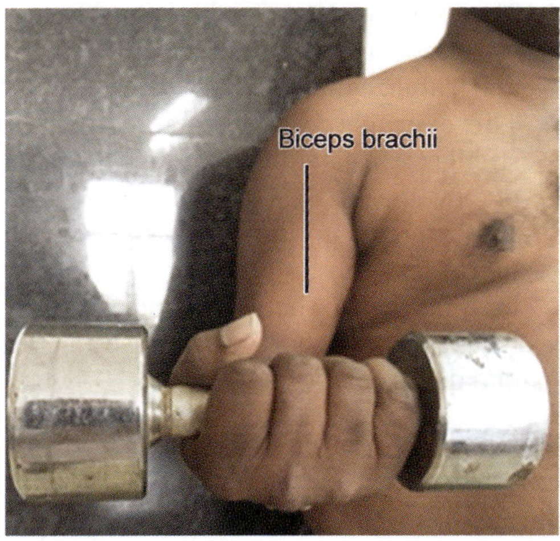


**Fig. 8.3:** Concentric resisted exercise to biceps brachii.

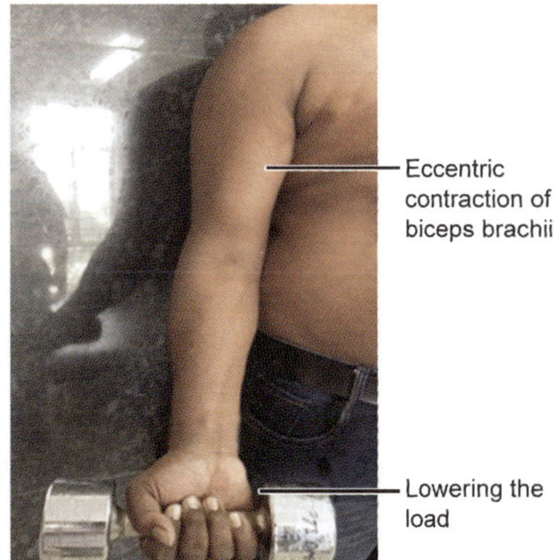


**Fig. 8.4:** Demonstrates eccentric contraction of biceps brachii.

The typical features of eccentric exercise include:

- It produce high muscle force.
- It has lower metabolic demand as compared to concentric and isometric exercises, resulting in less fatigue, low cardiovascular demand.
- It involves fewer motor unit recruitment as compared to other types of contractions.
- It produces greater neural adaptations. Exercise featuring a heavy eccentric load can actually support a greater weight (muscles are approximately 10% stronger during eccentric contraction than during concentric contraction). This type of muscle contraction/ exercise results in greater muscular damage and results in delayed onset muscle soreness (DOMS), one to two days after training.

- **Auxotonic contraction/exercise:** This is almost an isotonic contraction because there is some fluctuation towards the end of the contraction. For example, during biceps curl, muscular tension to overcome resistance does not remain the same through the exercise. Tension is highest at

**Table 8.2:** Difference between isometric and dynamic exercises.

| *Isometric exercise* | *Dynamic (isotonic exercise)* |
|---|---|
| Tension in the muscle rises markedly | Tension in the muscle is either constant, or variable |
| Length of the muscle remains unchanged | The muscle either shortens/lengthens |
| Produces no external work | Produces external work |
| More energy expenditure | Less energy expenditure |

a point parallel to the floor level, and eases off above and below this point. Therefore, tension in the muscle changes as the length of muscle changes.

Differences between isometric and dynamic (isotonic) exercises are shown in **Table 8.2**.

Expenditure of energy in various exercises are:

Eccentric exercise < concentric exercise < isometric exercise.

Muscular tension produced in various types of contractions are:

Dynamic (concentric) < isometric < dynamic (eccentric).

iii. *Isokinetic Exercise*

Isokinetic refers to "iso"- means same and "kinetic" means motion. This exercise was first introduced by J J Pemine in 1968. Isokinetic exercise is a form of resistance training that involves moving at a constant speed with varying resistance. It puts a consistent tension on the muscles, while moving them through a full range of motion at a constant speed. It can help to increase muscle strength, flexibility, balance and coordination. The isokinetic dynamometers **(Fig. 8.5)** currently in use, have the facility for testing and training of concentric, eccentric muscle work along with multi angle isometric and passive ROM exercises. These types of movements are usually applied in water sports, skating, climbing, running etc.

This velocity spectrum rehabilitation program, that provides speed specific strength training is typically performed at medium or fast velocities. Initially the angular velocity is kept low (15–30 degrees/second), which is gradually progressed to medium (60–90 degrees to 180 degrees/second) or high velocities (180 degrees to 360 degrees/second).

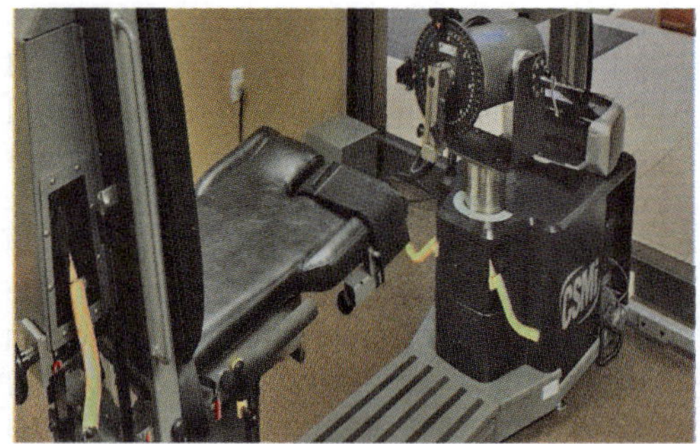

**Fig. 8.5:** Isokinetic dynamometer.

**Benefits of isokinetic exercise:**

- Isokinetic exercises are used for rehabilitation and recovery since it is a controlled form of exercise.
- Being able to control the resistance and speed it helps to prevent injury, increases muscle flexibility and controls muscle development.
- It is a form of strength training that can increase muscle tone, strength, and endurance. It can also help improve balance and coordination, and boost metabolism.
- The exercise also has a beneficial impact on the core muscles that support the spine and stabilize the body.
- The exercise allows muscles to gain strength consistently all through the range of movement.
- This exercise improves muscle strength, increases lean body mass, and reduces body fat, there by helps in reducing obesity.
- It has a positive effect on cognitive function and quality of life.

## II. Open and Closed Kinematic Chain Exercises

**The dynamic exercises are further typed into:**

- **Open kinematic chain exercises:** In open kinetic chain exercises, the segment

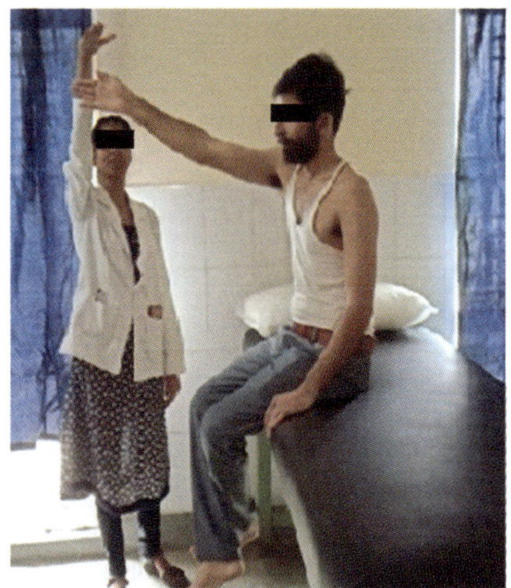

**Fig. 8.6:** Open kinematic chain exercise.

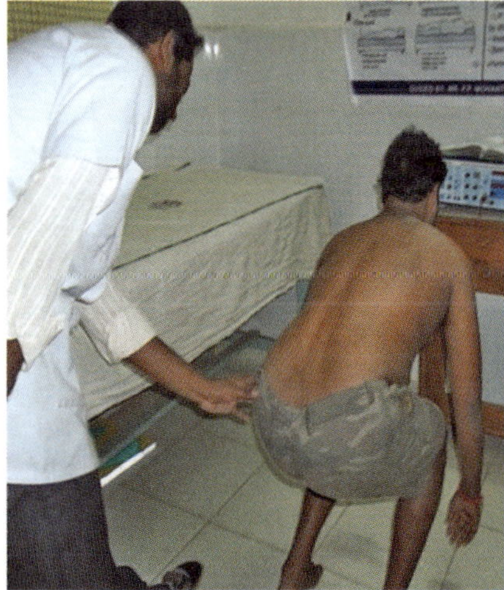

**Fig. 8.7:** Closed kinematic chain exercise.

furthest away from the body, known as the distal aspect, usually the hand or foot is free and not fixed to an object.

**For example:** Sitting, raising the arm upward is an open kinematic chain exercise **(Fig. 8.6)**.

- **Closed kinematic chain exercise:** In these types of exercises, the distal ends of the limbs are fixed, and movement of any joint brings about movement of other joints of the chain. For example: Squatting, where the distal lower limbs, i.e., feet are fixed on the ground **(Fig. 8.7)**.

*Plyometric Exercises*

Plyometrics is defined as the exercises that enable a muscle to reach maximum force in a short period of time, through a series of explosive body weight resistance exercises using the stretch-shortening cycle (eccentric followed by concentric contraction) of the muscle, to enhance physical capacity.

This training focuses on learning to move from a muscle extension (stretch/eccentric contraction) to a contraction (shortening/concentric contraction) in a rapid or "explosive" manner, such as in specialized repeated jumping **(Fig. 8.8)**.

This exercise is a popular form of training used to improve athletic performance. These exercises are primarily used by athletes, especially martial artists, sprinters and high jumpers.

### III. Depending upon the Assistance and Resistance Used, Active Exercises are Classified into:

- Active assisted exercise.
- Active free exercise.
- Active assisted/resisted exercise.
- Active resisted exercise.

i. *Active Assisted Exercise*

This is the exercise, where assistance is provided by an outside force, either manual or mechanical when muscle strength is inadequate to complete the motion, i.e., when the voluntary contraction of the muscle is insufficient to produce movement, needing the addition of an external force to the complete range. The assistance should be controlled/applied in such a way that, it does not substitute for the muscle action, or else, the movement becomes passive. As stated, the assistance given could be of the following types:

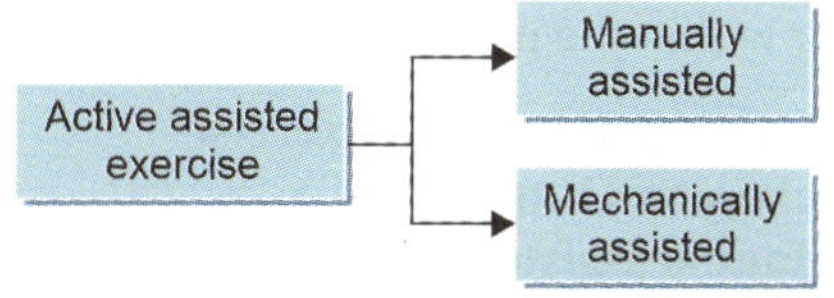

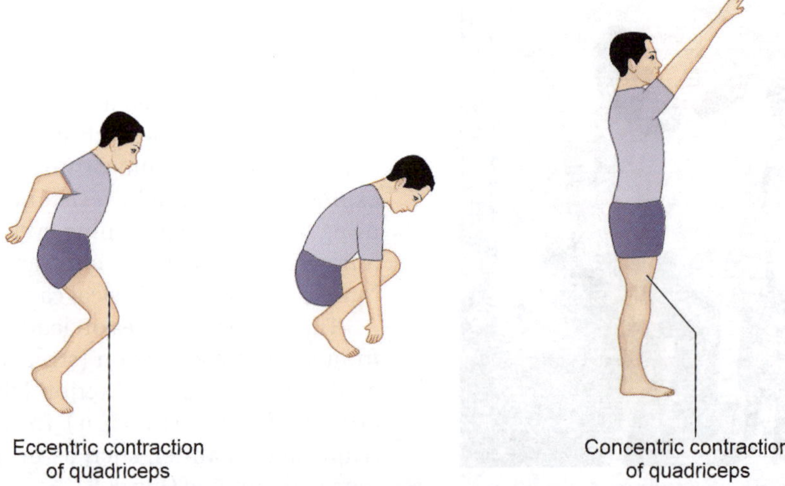


**Fig. 8.8:** Plyometric exercises.

**Types of Assisted Exercises:** The assisted exercises can be performed manually and mechanically. The manual assisted exercise having the two divisions, i.e., auto assisted and assisted by external agent, which are discussed below:

**Auto assisted exercise:** The patient himself can assist with his opposite extremity to perform the assisted exercise.

**For example:**
- The opposite leg is used by the patient to increase the flexion movement of the knee in prone lying.
- Upper limbs are used to move the lower limb **(Fig. 8.9)** or opposite side upper limb.

This type of active assisted exercise is very much helpful for the home programming exercise. The main advantage of this exercise is that, the patient can perform the exercise conveniently within the limit of pain, as he/she knows, when pain appears during movement and further movement through the pain may cause more damage to the soft tissues/joint structures, there by limiting movement to occur within the pain free range.

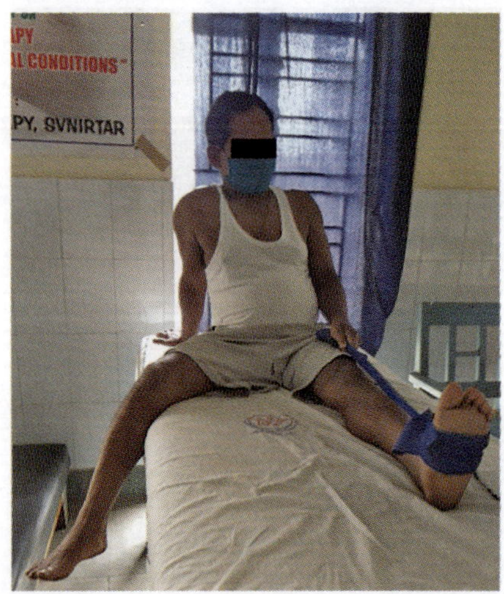

**Fig. 8.9:** Auto assisted exercise (Movement of lower limb, by own upper limb).

**External agent assisted exercise**
**It is classified into:**
- **Manual assisted exercise:** The assistance may be given by the therapist or by any of the medical professionals or sometimes by the patient's relatives and friends. The patient has to try to perform the movement up to his ability.
- **Mechanical assisted exercise:** The assisted exercise done with the help of the mechanical devices are called mechanical assisted exercises. Suspension therapy, pulleys and springs, therabands, buoyancy of water etc., are some of the examples for the mechanical assistance.

**Principles of active assisted exercise:**

- **Position:** The body segment to move should be positioned with muscles in the partial state of shortening, gravity either assisting or eliminated, and in a pain free position.
- **Range:** The assistance given is changeable depending on the range. Normally, in the beginning and end range, the muscles strength will be less while compared with the middle range. So, that the assistance provided should be more in the beginning and end range than the middle range.
- **Command:** Some command is needed to activate the patient and perform the effective movement. The command gives perfect guideline to the patient to practice an activity.
- **Concentration:** Concentration of the patient is most contributing in the performance of assisted exercises, otherwise the movements will be passive in character. Therapist has to make the patient to concentrate on the treatment well, for effective performance of the assisted exercises.
- **Speed:** Speed of the movement should be low, allowing the patient to recruit the existing motor units to perform the movement. If the speed is increased the patient cannot cope up with the movement.
- **Repetition:** The movement has to be repeated, so that the joint range and the muscle power can be improved. However, appearance of fatigue, should be taken into consideration, while repeating the movements.

**Techniques of active assisted exercise:**

- The patient should be explained about the procedure and Dos and Don'ts.
- The part to be treated should be supported to minimize the effects of friction and gravity.
- A quick stretch should be given to the muscle to be facilitated.
- Verbal command to move in the direction of action of the muscle should be given.
- The patient should be assisted to complete the movement by the combined action of his muscular effort and therapist's assistance.
- The assistance should be given in such a way that, it should not be a substitute for patient's action, rather an augmentation for movement.
- Repetition should be done as needed, without inducing fatigue.

**Effects and uses of active assisted exercise:**

- **Builds confidence:** It helps to build confidence of the patient in his/her ability to move, helping him/her to cooperate more and more to produce movement.
- **Maintains and increases ROM:** The exercises (particularly the auto assisted types) help to maintain and increase the ROM of the joints in pathological states (traumatic and arthritic conditions), by preventing and breaking adhesions (if any).
- **Maintains muscles properties:** In states of immobility on bed, these exercises, help to maintain the elasticity and contractility properties of muscles, promoting gradual recovery and restoration of function.
- **Strengthens weak muscles and develops endurance:** When the patient has weak muscles (a grade of 2-, in the MRC grading system), active assisted exercises are used to provide enough assistance to strengthen the weak muscles and develops muscular endurance.
- **Prevents osteoporosis/Maintains bone integrity:** As the nonambulatory patient periodically performs the movements by auto assistance, the bone metabolism is maintained, by pulling of the muscle (tendon) on bone, there by preventing osteoporosis.

- **Prevents tightness/contracture/deformity:** As the joints are periodically moves with assistance, soft tissue tightness is prevented to develop, hence soft tissue contracture and joint deformation are prevented.
- **Increases circulation of blood:** The exercises, performed at regular intervals, help for increase of blood flow to tissues (muscles, joints, bone etc.), there by supplies nutrition and oxygen maintaining tissue metabolism.
- **Increases venous and lymphatic return:** During states of immobility, when the patient is confined to bed, active assisted exercises, performed at regular interval, helps to increase venous and lymphatic return, by exerting a pumping action on the circulatory system, due to alternate muscle contraction and relaxation, there preventing oedema and DVT.
- **Improves neuromuscular co-ordination**: The exercises performed repeatedly by the patient using own assistance/assistance by the clinician, help him to learn the correct pattern of movement, receiving proper sensory feedback from the contracting muscles and moving joints, developing neuromuscular co-ordination.
- **Improves motor control:** Repeated practice of the movement with assistance helps to learn and produce movement required for function, there by promoting recovery.

ii. *Active Free Exercise*

Active free exercises are those which are performed by the patient's own muscular efforts without the assistance or resistance of any external force, other than that of the gravity.

These are bodily movements that improve and maintain the physical fitness level of the individual. There will not be any application of manual or mechanical assistance or resistance in this type of exercise **(Fig. 8.10)**.

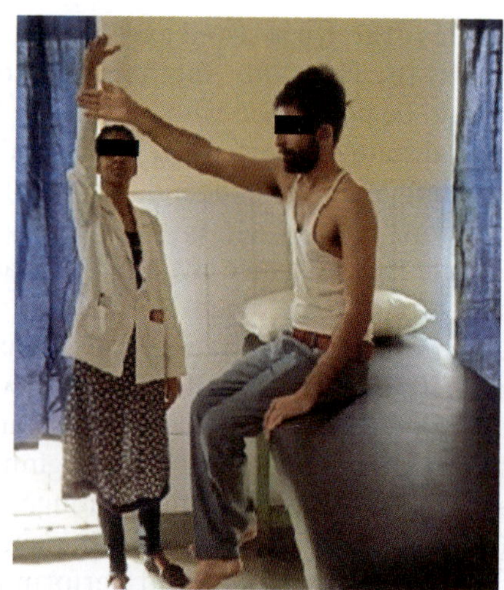

**Fig. 8.10:** Active free exercise to shoulder flexors.

These exercises are indicated when the power of muscle is 2 or more as per MRC grading.

- **Advantage of free exercise:** It helps in maintaining range of motion and muscle properties by the patient himself/herself without relying on others for this purpose. It is much useful as home exercise program.
- **Disadvantage of free exercise:** It frequently makes insufficient demands on neuromuscular system to elicit the maximal response required for redevelopment of weak muscles. There is also possibility to perform irrelevant and trick movements, which may train performance of wrong patterns.

  The free exercises are classified, into the following types according to the extent of area involved such as:
- **Localized:** Localized exercises are designed to produce some local and specific effect, for example to mobilize a specific joint, say elbow joint following post fracture immobilization, or strengthening of a specific muscle say quadriceps in high sitting when the power of muscle is between grade 2–3, as per MRC grading.
- **Generalized:** Generalized exercise are designed to produce movement in

multiple joints of the body, such as walking, running etc.

**The character of free exercise may be:**

- **Subjective:** These are the exercises, where the attention of the performer is focused on the form and pattern of exercise to ensure accuracy of performance. These exercises consist of more or less anatomical movements performed in full range. Example: Hopping, jugging, dancing.
- **Objective:** In this exercise, the patient's attention is concentrated on achievement of a particular goal such as arm stretching upwards to hold a ball.

**Techniques of free exercise:**

- The patient should be explained about the procedure and Dos and Don'ts.
- The starting position should be selected as per requirement/goal.
- Verbal command should be given to move in the desired direction.
- The speed of the movement should be selected as per the effect required. Usually, the speed is kept low during learning period, slowly increasing as the strength and co-ordination increases.
- The duration and frequency of the exercise depends on the patient's capacity. Usually three repetitions of practice of each exercise, with short rest periods or change of activity in between, ensure sufficient practice without undue fatigue.

**Effect and uses of active free exercise:** The effect and consequent uses of any particular free exercise depend on the nature of the exercise, its extent and the intensity and duration of its performance. The common effects and uses are:

- **Increases confidence:** The achievement of coordinated and purposeful movement in an efficient way, assures the patient of his/her ability to gain cognitive control of his body, giving him confidence to attempt other and new activities which are complex in nature. Objective exercises are used for this purpose.
- **Induces relaxation:** The exercises performed in rhythmical and swinging manner, which are pendular in character, helps for relaxation of the hypertonic muscles in the region of the joint moved. The alternating and reciprocal contraction and relaxation of the opposite muscle groups, which is required to sustained the movement, helps to restore the normal state of relaxation which follows contraction. This type of exercise is used in conjunction with other methods which induce relaxation to reduce a state of wasteful tension in muscles, which limits the range of joint movement and reduces the efficiency of neuromuscular coordination.
  As the patient is able to perform free movements required for indoor games, the pleasure so derived from the games, stimulate mind inducing relaxation.
- **Increases joint mobility:** The normal range of motion is maintained by exercises performed in full range. When the range of movement is limited, rhythmical swinging pendular exercises incorporating overpressure at the limit of the free range may serve to increase ROM, by breaking adhesion and loosening tight soft tissues.
- **Maintenance and increase of strength, power and endurance of muscles:** The strength, power and endurance of the working muscles are maintained or increased in response to the tension created in them. A high degree of tension, resulting in increase in power can be developed by free exercises when the muscles work against the resistance offered by the body weight, or against the mechanical disadvantage of an adverse leverage provided by a long and heavy limb.
- **Increases the efficiency of cardiovascular and respiratory system:** During vigorous

or prolonged exercise the rate and depth of respiration is increased supplying more oxygen to the tissues for metabolic function. The heart rate also increases, to provide more blood flow to the peripheral organs, and there is production of mild warmth in the tissues, due to increased, blood flow. Muscular contraction increases both the carbon dioxide content and the temperature of the blood, and both these factors stimulate the circulatory and respiratory systems to further activity. The rise in temperature of the body is kept within normal limits by dilation of the skin capillaries and stimulation of the sweat glands, thus enabling heat to be lost from the surface. Cerebral cortex, respiratory, cardiac and vasomotor centers which are part of autonomic nervous system, cause release of adrenaline in the blood stream, which increases heart rate and blood pressure. The pressure variation in abdominal and thoracic cavities, due to increased respiratory movements, results in increased venous return to heart as well as increased cardiac output.

- **Increases lymphatic and venous return and prevents DVT:** Repeated active free exercises, in the form of functional and sports activities are helpful for increasing venous and lymphatic return, thereby helping for prevention of oedema and formation of DVT. However, if a patient is confined to bed, repeated free exercises performed at regular intervals, helps to achieve such effects also.
- **Increases neuromuscular coordination:** Repeated exercises performed at regular intervals, improves coordination, resulting in decreased concentration, and increased automaticity (enhancing performance of movements like a habit).

  Activities, that require concentration or much effort become easy with passage of time, i.e., playing piano.
- **Improves motor control:** Repeated active free exercises, helps to enhance motor control due to the effects of motor learning.

iii. *Active Assisted, Resisted Exercise*

In this exercise, the muscle work is resisted through the initial part of the range and assisted through the remaining part of the range **(Fig. 8.11)**. For example, a patient with a power of quadriceps more than a grade of 3 with a quadriceps lag, is resisted through the initial part of range and assisted through the remaining part of the range, to make the muscle work through full range of knee extension. The techniques and effects and uses of this exercise is as applicable to assisted and resisted exercises.

iv. *Resisted Exercise*

Resisted exercise is an essential element of Rehabilitation programs, for persons with impaired functions and for those, who wish to promote and maintain health and physical wellbeing.

It can be defined as, a form of active exercise in which dynamic or static muscle contraction is resisted by an outside force, either applied manually by the therapist/caregiver or mechanically, to increase strength, power and endurance of the muscle.

Dynamic resistance exercise involve movements (concentric/eccentric) with resistance.

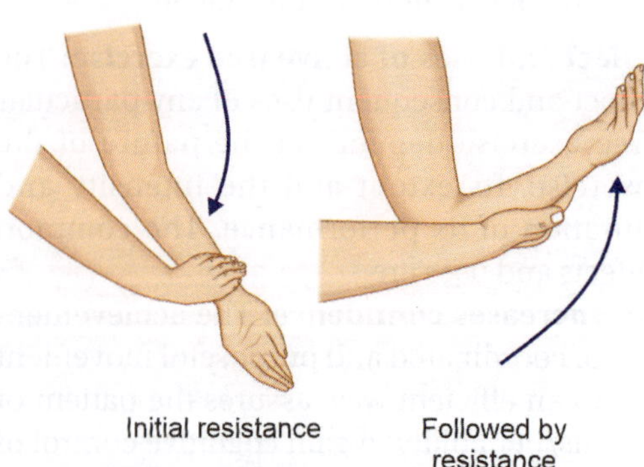


**Fig. 8.11:** Active assisted, resisted exercise to elbow flexors.

**Types of resisted exercises:** Resisted exercises are of two types namely:

1. **Manual resisted exercises:** In the manual resisted exercise, the resistance can be given by therapists, some other medical professionals and relatives or friends. The resistance also can be applied by the patient himself with his opposite extremity. These exercises can be operated by the following individuals:
   - ❖ The therapist/clinician.
   - ❖ Patient himself.
   - ❖ Relatives and friends.
2. **Mechanical resisted exercise:** It is the active resisted exercise, in which, the resistance is provided by equipments to either a dynamic or isometric muscle contraction. A variety of mechanical equipments are available, ranging from simple to complex, small to large, expensive to nonexpensive. The choice to select one depends on the patient's need and ability, goal of the exercise and availability of the apparatus.

   Mechanical resisted exercises can be performed by the followings **(Figs. 8.12A to F):**
   - ❖ Free Weights.
   - ❖ Springs.
   - ❖ Therabands.
   - ❖ Exercise bicycle.
   - ❖ Gymnasium equipments like quadriceps table.
   - ❖ Pulley and weights.
   - ❖ Water (Buoyancy of water in hydrotherapy).

   The following figure **(Fig. 8.13)**, shows, resisted exercise to quadriceps using spring.

   The resisted exercise increases the muscle strength and the muscle bulk earlier than any other exercise program. These resisted exercises can be stated when the muscle power is 2, i.e., from gravity eliminated position.

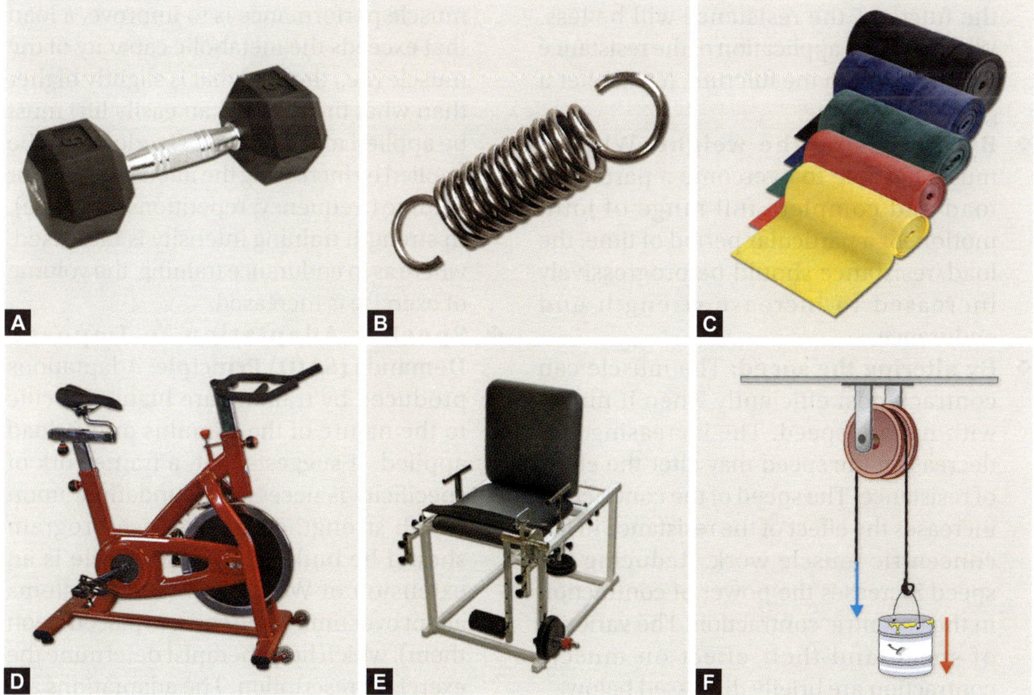


**Figs. 8.12A to F:** Mechanical equipments for resisted exercise: (A) Free weight (dumbbell); (B) Spring; (C) Therabands; (D) Static cycle; (E) Quadriceps table; (F) Pulley and weight.

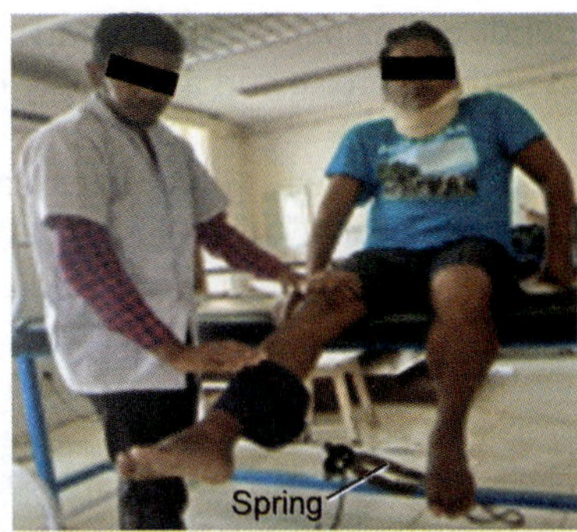


**Fig. 8.13:** Resisted exercise to quadriceps using spring.

The resistance can be changed by altering the below mentioned factors.

- **By positioning against gravity**: When the joint is positioned in a way, where the distal segment moves against gravity, gravity will offer resistance to the muscles moving the distal segment.
- **By altering the leverage:** When the application of the resistance is near from the fulcrum, the resistance will be less. Whereas if the application of the resistance is far away from the fulcrum, it will offer a greater resistance.
- **By increasing the weight:** When a muscle is able to overcome a particular load and complete full range of joint motion for a particular period of time, the load/resistance should be progressively increased to increase strength and endurance.
- **By altering the speed:** The muscle can contract most efficiently when it moves with natural speed. The increasing and decreasing the speed may alter the effect of resistance. The speed of the contraction increases the effect of the resistance in the concentric muscle work. Reducing the speed increases the power of contraction in the eccentric contraction. The varieties of speed and their effect on muscle contraction are briefly discussed below:
  - **Natural speed:** Movements performed in the natural speed require less effort of the muscle, and also it may vary with the individuals. Generally, all the exercises performed at the natural speed are beneficial and effective.
  - **Reduced speed:** If the speed is decreased the greater muscle work is required to perform the full ROM. When exercises are performed at reduced speed, the gravity exerts more resistance on the muscles.
  - **Increased speed:** Exercises performed at increased speed, need greater muscular effort. If the speed of exercise is more, it may lead to inaccurate/trick movements.

**Principles of strength training (resistance training):**

- **Overload principle:** This is used for increasing muscle performance. This guiding principle of exercise prescription for resisted exercise to improve muscle performance (strength) states that, if muscle performance is to improve, a load that exceeds the metabolic capacity of the muscle (i.e., the load that is slightly higher than what the muscle can easily lift) must be applied to the muscle. Overload can be applied by increasing the intensity (load) or volume (frequency, repetitions and time). In strength training intensity is increased, where as in endurance training, the volume of exercise is increased.
- **Specific Adaptation to Imposed Demands (SAID) Principle:** Adaptations produced by training are highly specific to the nature of the stimulus or overload applied. It suggests that, a framework of specificity is necessary foundation, upon which strengthening exercise program should be built up. This principle is an extension of Wolff's law (body systems adapt over time to the stresses placed upon them), which help therapist determine the exercise prescription. The adaptations are specific to strength, power, endurance, functional activity, joint angle, sequence

of muscle activations, energy systems and virtually all other variables present. As per the principle, if the functional activity requires strength, rather than endurance, then the intensity and duration of exercise should be designed to improve strength. The principle, also guides about the mode (type of contraction), velocity and limb position (joint angle) to be selected for specific therapeutic benefit. For example, if quadriceps is weak in the terminal part of knee extension, the resistance (as per overload principle) should be applied at that range in which the muscle is weak.

- **Transfer of training:** This principle, which is contrary to the SAID principle, speaks about carry over of training effects from one variation of exercise or task to another. For example, strength training in one speed of exercise has been shown to provide some improvement in strength at higher or lower speeds of exercise. Similarly, cross training effect is found to occur, when strength is built up in one limb, where strength training is given to the contra lateral limb. Even though, small degree of transference of training occurs in strength training, it is advisable to design exercise programs, that resemble the movement patterns required for the functional activities.
- **Reversibility principle:** The adaptations achieved through resistance exercise persist as long as the resistance exercise is performed regularly and go back gradually to the pre-exercise levels once the training is stopped. This means the effects of resistance training are reversible. The adaptive changes such as gain in strength and endurance, obtained in strength training is gradually lost, if the individual does not maintain the practice by performing regular activities or exercise programs. This detraining effect, which is reflected by a gradual reduction in muscle performance begins within a week or two of cessation of resisted exercise and continues until the training effects are lost. It is therefore recommended that to maintain strength and endurance after strength training, the individual should engage himself for routine functional activities or should perform regular resisted exercise.
- **Inter individual variability:** Every individual responds to resistance exercise in different way. Similar stimuli may bring about lot of changes in one person, but not in another.

**Guidelines for Prescription of Resisted Exercise**

- **Examination and evaluation:**
  - Determine the base line:
    - General physical examination.
    - Find the muscle strength: Manual muscle testing, Dynamometry, Repetition maximum (RM).
    - Find the ROM by Goniometry.
    - Assess the functional performance.
    - Periodic reassessment.
- **Preparation:**
  - Plan the regime according to the need and equipments available.
  - Explanation and demonstration.
  - Ensure proper clothing, diet, hydration.
- **Application:**
  - Warm-up: Light repetitive dynamic exercise for the muscles to be exercised.
  - Placement of resistance distally.
  - Decide the direction of movement (concentric/eccentric).
  - Stabilize the proximal segment.
  - Cooldown.

**Techniques of Resisted Exercise:**

- Explain the patient about the procedure and Dos and Don'ts.
- Select the starting position as per requirement of the goal.
- Give verbal command to move in the desired direction.
- Stabilize the proximal or distal joint to prevent substitution.

- Select the determinants of resisted exercise such as: **mode** [manual/mechanical, types of muscle contraction (isometric, dynamic, isokinetic), **position during exercise** (weight bearing/non-weight bearing)], **intensity** (amount of resistance/ load), **volume** (total number of repetitions and sets of a particular exercise during a particular exercise session), **frequency** (number of exercise sessions per day/ week), **duration** (total number of weeks or months, during which resistance exercise program is carried out—6–12 weeks of resistance training is ideal achieving muscle hypertrophy and increased vascularization of muscle), **rest interval** [dependent on intensity or volume of exercise—for example between sets of moderate intensity and volume exercise (8–12 RM levels), a 30–60 seconds rest period is selected, and for higher intensity exercises (at a 3–5 RM level) a longer rest period is selected before performing another set of same exercise], **speed of exercise** [(for concentric exercises, the speed is kept low to have higher force generation, and for eccentric exercises, it is found that initially, the force production in the muscle increases in proportion to the speed of muscle lengthening and subsequently it levels off), the training speeds should be geared to match the demands of desired functional activities], **periodization protocol** (systematic variation in exercise intensity and volume at regular intervals over a specific periods of time).
- Follow a warm-up protocol before starting moderate to high intensity exercise, and a cool down protocol at the end of the program
- Integrate resistance training into functional activities to maintain carry over and prevent de-training effect.

**Effect and Uses/Benefits of Resisted Exercises**

- **Increases muscle strength, power and endurance:** Resisted exercises increases the strength of the muscles through increase of muscle tension, as Strength $\alpha$ Tension. Strength of the muscle is directly proportional to the tension created inside the muscle. The exercise increases the muscle bulk and muscular power. Power is related to the strength of the muscle and the speed. The greater the intensity of exercise and shorter the time period taken to generate force, the greater is the muscle power.

  Power = Force × Distance/Time

  The force creating the particular motion or the movement of the body lever for the particular duration is meant as power.
  The force or tension created inside the muscle is high in resisted exercise. Some theories explain about the power, which is the high intensity of muscle activity. High intensity exercise carried out over a short period of time called as anaerobic exercise, where as lower intensity exercise carried out for a longer period of time is called as aerobic exercise.
  The exercise can be started from the muscle power 2 onwards as per MRC grading, where resistance can be applied to the muscle contracting in horizontal plane, though mostly resisted exercises are performed, when the power of the muscle is grade 3 or more as per MRC grading, where weak muscles are made to contract against gravity and resistance.
  Low resistance, high repetition exercises increase endurance of muscles.

  The gain in strength and endurance in resisted exercise is said to occur due to:
  - *Neural adaptations:* Starts after 4 weeks of regular training, due to decreased inhibition by CNS, decreased sensitivity of GTO, and increased firing at neuromuscular junction, and increased recruitment of motor units.
  - Skeletal muscle adaptations: Starts between 4–8 weeks of resistance training. Hypertrophy of muscles occur

due to increased myofibril volume. There is increased protein synthesis and decreased protein degradation. Maximum hypertrophy occurs in high volume moderate intensity exercise, performed eccentrically. Tensile strength of connective tissues in muscles increases due to the skeletal muscle adaptations.

- Increases strength of connective tissues such as ligaments and tendons, by increasing their tensile strength, due to adaptation in connective tissues.
- Increases muscle mass through hypertrophy of individual muscle fibers, due to adaptations in skeletal muscles discussed above (causes muscle hypertrophy), and reduces, body fat.
- Increases bone mineral density, preventing the risk of osteoporosis. This is due to the adaptations of resisted exercise on bones, where there is reduction of loss of minerals from the bones.
- Improves co-ordination and balance.
- Increases blood flow to the working muscles, provides more nutrition and $O_2$, promoting repair of injured tissues.
- It increases body temperature.
- Decreases stress on the joints and reduces the risk of soft tissue injuries during functional activities, and improves posture.
- Helps for prevention or control of chronic conditions (back pain, heart disease, arthritis, obesity and depression).
- Improves sense of wellbeing, boosts confidence and self-esteem.

**Progressive Resisted Exercise**

Progressive resisted exercise is a dynamic resistance training in which a constant external load is applied to the contracting muscle by some mechanical means, which is incrementally increased. This is performed to increase strength and endurance of muscle groups.

While performing the resisted exercise with the weights, it is very much difficult to find out how much weight has to be used and how many repetitions to be done by the injured patients after recovering. At the same time, if the more weight is lifted more times, the muscle gets fatigue or sometime there is possibility for microtears. To come out of this situation De Lorme and Watkins have formed one exercise regimen in 1945 to improve the muscle strength, power and endurance. As per this regimen the weight is gradually increased and also he explained about how many repetition to be practiced. One should know about repetition maximum (RM) before entering into the exercise regimen.

Repetition Maximum

Repetition maximum (RM), is a method of quantifying exercise intensity given by Delorme.

A (RM) is defined as, the greatest amount of weight a muscle can move through the available range of motion for a specific number of times.

1 RM for a muscle is the maximum weight (resistance), with which the muscle can contract through full/available ROM, for one time without fatigue. The muscle will be unable to perform the repetition for the second time.

10 RM for a muscle is the maximum weight (resistance), with which the muscle can contract through full/available ROM, for 10 times without fatigue. The muscle will be unable to perform the repetition for 11th time.

**Uses of Repetition Maximum (RM):**

- To document a baseline measurement of dynamic strength of a muscle.
- To identify an exercise load to be used during exercise.
- To find out prognosis in reassessment and alter the exercise regime accordingly.

**Training zone using RM:** The amount of resistance used in the training program is usually a percentage of 1 RM, which varies from individual to individual, such as:

- ❖ For sedentary people: 30–40% of 1 RM.
- ❖ For untrained healthy individual: 60–70% of 1 RM.
- ❖ For highly trained individuals: 80–95% of 1 RM.

A exercise session may have a single set or multiple sets. Single set exercises are used with low intensity, in early phase of rehabilitation. For gain of strength and endurance, multiple sets are recommended. For strength gain, low repetition high resistance exercises, and for endurance, high repetition, low resistance exercises are performed.

The exercise regimens may vary depending on the condition or the disease and from one patient to another. At present 4 types of progressive resisted exercise regimens are available.

1. De Lorme and Watkins
2. MacQueen
3. Zinovieff (Oxford technique).
4. DAPRE technique.

1. *De Lorme and Watkins Technique:*

- ❖ 10 times with 1/2 10 RM.
- ❖ 10 times with 3/4 10 RM.
- ❖ 10 times with 10 RM.

**Progression:**

- ❖ 30 times weekly 4 sessions
- ❖ Every week 10 RM progression.

**For example:** Consider 10 RM—1 kg.

**First week:**

- ❖ 1/2 of 10 RM—1/2 kg.
- ❖ 3/4 of 10 RM—3/4 kg
- ❖ Full of 10 RM—1 kg

**Exercise regimen is**

- ❖ 10 times with 1/2 kg
- ❖ 10 times with 3/4 kg
- ❖ 10 times with 1 kg

**Second week:**

Progression 10 RM
= 10 RM + 10 RM
= 1 kg +1 kg
= 2 kg

**Exercise Regimen is**

- ❖ 10 times with 1 kg
- ❖ 10 times with 1.5 kg
- ❖ 10 times with 2 kg

**Third week program:** 10 RM added in the second week weight.

- ❖ In this exercise regimen, the weight is increased, i.e., first with 1/2 kg followed by 3/4 kg and 1 kg.
- ❖ Each and every session the patient has to lift the above said three types of weights 10 times each. So, that daily 30 times lifting been done.
- ❖ In each and every session 30 times the exercise should be done with 2 breaks by the patient.
  i.e., 10 times 1/2 10 RM (1/2 kg) → Break → 10 times with 3/4 10 RM (3/4 kg) → Break → 10 times 10 RM (1 kg)
- ❖ Weekly 4 sessions the exercise has to be practiced. *For example*, Monday, Wednesday, Friday, Sunday (i.e., every alternative day's) exercise has to be practiced and remaining days, i.e., Tuesday, Thursday, Saturday given rest.

2. *MacQueen Technique:*

- ❖ 10 times with 10 RM
- ❖ 10 times with 10 RM
- ❖ 10 times with 10 RM
- ❖ 10 times with 10 RM

**Progression:**

- ❖ 40 times 3 sessions weekly.
- ❖ Every 1–2 weeks progression 10 RM

*For example:*
Consider 10 RM = 1 kg

**First week**

- ❖ 10 times with 1 kg
- ❖ 10 times with 1 kg
- ❖ 10 times with 1 kg
- ❖ 10 times with 1 kg

**Second week:**

Progression 10 RM
Second week 10 RM = 10 RM + 10 RM
= 1 kg + 1 kg

Second week 10 RM = 2 kg

**Third week:** progression 10 RM from the second week weight.

- ❖ 1 kg weight is lifted 40 times with 3 breaks per each session. In this regimen no change of weight between each and every breaks. Same weight is used throughout one session.
  10 times with 1 kg → break → 10 times with 1 kg → break → 10 times with 1 kg → break → 10 times with 1 kg.
- ❖ The exercise has to be carried out 3 sessions weekly. *For example,* Monday, Thursday, Sunday (with a gap of two days) with rest for the remaining four days rest.

3. *Zinovieff (Oxford Technique)*

- ❖ 10 times with 10 RM
- ❖ 10 times with 10 RM minus 1 lb
- ❖ 10 times with 10 RM minus 2 lb
- ❖ 10 times with 10 RM minus 3 lb
- ❖ 10 times with 10 RM minus 4 lb
- ❖ 10 times with 10 RM minus 5 lb
- ❖ 10 times with 10 RM minus 6 lb
- ❖ 10 times with 10 RM minus 7 lb
- ❖ 10 times with 10 RM minus 8 lb
- ❖ 10 times with 10 RM minus 9 lb

*Progression:*

- ❖ 100 times 5 sessions weekly
- ❖ 10 RM progression daily.

*For example:*

- ❖ Consider 10 RM = 20 lb
- ❖ 10 times with 20 lb
- ❖ 10 times with 19 lb
- ❖ 10 times with 18 lb
- ❖ 10 times with 17 lb
- ❖ 10 times with 16 lb
- ❖ 10 times with 15 lb
- ❖ 10 times with 14 lb
- ❖ 10 times with 13 lb
- ❖ 10 times with 12 lb
- ❖ 10 times with 11 lb

**Second day:**

Progression 10 RM daily

Second day 10 RM = 10 RM + 10 RM
= 20 lb + 20 lb
= 40 lb

- ❖ 10 times lift with 40 lb
- ❖ 10 times lift with 39 lb
- ❖ 10 times lift with 38 lb
- ❖ 10 times lift with 37 lb
- ❖ 10 times lift with 36 lb
- ❖ 10 times lift with 35 lb
- ❖ 10 times lift with 34 lb
- ❖ 10 times lift with 33 lb
- ❖ 10 times lift with 32 lb
- ❖ 10 times lift with 31 lb

Third day progression 10 RM from the second day weight.

- ❖ Each and every 10 lifts break has to be given the 1 lb also reduced for each 10 lifts. Finally, the patient will be performing 100 lifts per session.
  10 lifts with 20 lb→ break→ 10 lifts with 19 lb→ break → 10 lifts with 18 lb → break → 10 lifts 17 lb → break →10 lifts with 16 lb→ break→ 10 lifts with 15 lb→ break → 10 lifts with 14 lb → break → 10 lifts with 13 lb → break → 10 lifts with 12 lb→ break→ 10 lifts with 11 lb.
- ❖ Every week 5 sessions of exercises are carried out. For *example,* Monday to Friday the exercises will be performed and remaining two days given rest before starting next week exercise regimen.

4. *Daily Adjusted Progressive Resisted Exercise (DAPRE) Technique*

It is based on 6 RM working weight. It is more systematic and takes into account the different rates at which individuals progress during rehabilitation or conditioning program. The protocol includes the following **(Table 8.3)**.

The key to the DAPRE technique is that on the third and fourth sets of exercise the patient performs as many repetitions as possible. The number of repetitions performed during the third and fourth sets is used to determine the amount of weight that is added to (or sometimes removed from) the working weight for the next set and session, respectively. The number of repetitions performed during the 3rd set, is used to determine the adjusted working weight for the 4th set. The number

**Table 8.3:** The DAPRE protocol.

| *Sets* | *Repetitions* | *Amount of resistance* |
|---|---|---|
| 1 | 10 | 50% of 6 RM |
| 2 | 6 | 75% of 6 RM |
| 3 | Maximum possible | 100% of 6 RM |
| 4 | Maximum possible | 100% of adjustable working weight |

of repetitions performed during the 4th set, is used to determine the adjusted working weight for the next day.

**Example:** Let's take 6 RM as 8 kg for a patient.

- ❖ For set 1: 10 repetitions @ 50% of 6 RM=4 kg.
- ❖ For set 2: 6 repetitions @ 75% of 6 RM=6 kg.
- ❖ For set 3: Maximum repetitions @ 100% of 6 RM, i.e., repetitions can be adjusted according to patient lifting 8 kg of weight.
- ❖ For set 4: Maximum repetitions @ 100% with adjusted working weight, i.e., repetition and weight both can be adjusted according to patient.

Adjustment of working weight calculation **(Table 8.4)**.

The number of repetitions completed in set 3 is used with **Table 8.4**, to determine the adjusted working weight for set-4. The number of repetitions completed during the 4th set, is used to determine the working weight for the next session.

**Table 8.4:** Calculation of adjusted working weight using DAPRE protocol.

| *Repetition in set-3* | *Adjusted working weight for set-4* | *Adjusted working weight for next session* |
|---|---|---|
| 0–2 | Decrease weight by: 5–10 lbs (2.3–4.5 kg) | Decrease the weight by: 5–10 lbs (2.3–4.5 kg) |
| 3–4 | Decrease weight by: 0–5 lbs (0–2.3 kg) | Keep the weight same |
| 5–6 | Keep the weight same | Increase the weight by: 5–10 lbs (2.3–4.5 kg) |
| 7–10 | Increase the weight by: 5–10 lbs (2.3–4.5 kg) | Increase the weight by: 5–15 lbs (2.3–6.8 kg) |
| 11 or more | Increase the weight by: 10–15 lbs (4.5–6.8 kg) | Increase the weight by 10–20 lbs (4.5–9 kg) |

**Other methods of resistance training:**

- ❖ **Circuit training:** It is primarily a resistance based workout, that proceeds through a group of strengthening exercises, targeting different muscle groups. The technique involves a pre-established sequence of continuous exercise, performed for major muscle groups, as an aspect of total body conditioning. Each resistance exercise is performed at an exercise station for a specified number of sets and repetitions, without any rest between movements. The exercise keeps the heart work at a steady pace, enhancing both aerobic and strength gain benefits. The exercise builds lean muscle mass, and reduces body fat, hence can be considered as an important component of weight management program. An example of circuit training workout is given below:

  Squats for 60 seconds → Push-ups for 60 seconds → Jumping jacks for 30 seconds → Lunges on each side for 45 seconds → Plank for 30 seconds → Side lifts on each side for 30 seconds.
- ❖ **Interval training:** This is a type of exercise, that involves, alternating periods of high intensity exercise, with periods of rest or low intensity exercise. This is a work out for improving cardiac function (endurance), where alternate short, high intensity bursts of activity (running, jogging, swimming, cycling, rowing etc.) are performed with rest or a low intensity exercise between them.

This exercise is a best method to increase endurance, as it leads the heart and lungs to adapt to the increasing load of high intensity exercise.

## *B. Passive Exercises*

Passive movements are movements produced by an external force during muscular inactivity or when muscular activity is voluntarily reduced significantly to permit movements.

These are the movement, which are performed with the help of the external force whenever the muscles fail to perform the movement by its own. In clinical conditions, where active movements by the patient is not possible due to muscular inactivity/pain, or when active movement produced by the patient is insufficient to mobilize a stiff joint, the body segments need to be moved by an external system, and the resulting movement is called passive movement (exercise).

The force/external agent used to produce movement could be:

- ❖ Manual force used by therapists/care giver or patient through use of the intact limb.
- ❖ Mechanical force, such as a continuous passive motion (CPM) exerciser **(Figs. 8.14A and B)**.

**Classification of passive movements:** Passive movements are classified into:

- ❖ Relaxed passive movements including accessory movements.
- ❖ Passive manual mobilization techniques, that include:
  - ▪ Mobilization of joints.
  - ▪ Manipulation of joints.
  - ▪ Controlled sustained stretching of tight structures.

**Relaxed Passive Movements**

*I. Physiological Movements*

These are bodily movements/exercises performed smoothly and accurately by the physiotherapist/clinician within the pain free available range and in a direction same as the direction of active movements.

Principles of Relaxed Passive Exercise

- ❖ The patient is made fully relaxed during the procedure, and explained about the requirements and benefits.
- ❖ Fixation of the proximal segment should be done to localize the movement to the desired joint and to avoid compensatory movements.
- ❖ The moving part is supported comfortably and fully, to develop confidence and promote relaxation.
- ❖ Traction in the long axis of the joint is given to reduce intra articular friction, there by promoting greater excursion of the joint.

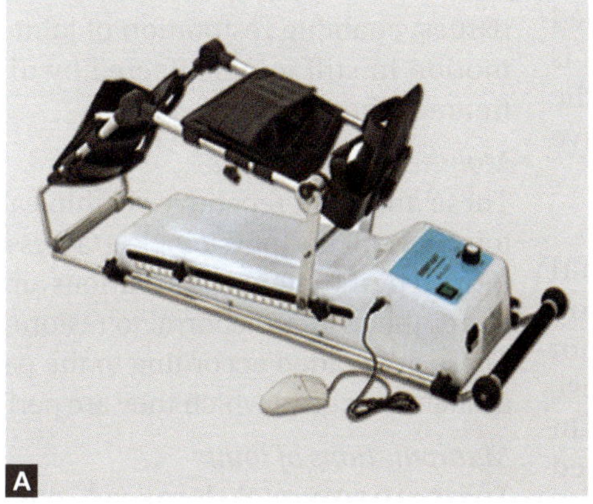
A

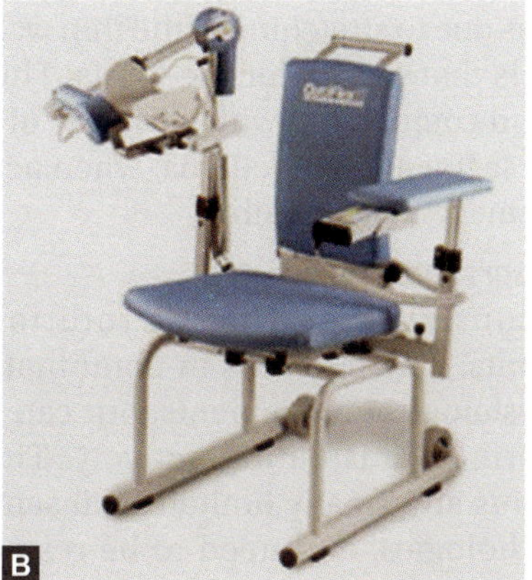
B

**Figs. 8.14A and B:** (A) CPM machine for knee joint; (B) CPM machine for shoulder.

- Range of movement is as full as possible and no pain and spasm should be induced during the movement.
- Speed of the movement performed should be uniform, slow and rhythmical to achieve relaxation.
- Duration/number of repetitions of movement performed depends on the purpose for which the movement is performed.

Effects and Uses of Relaxed Passive Exercise:

- Induces relaxation of the segment/whole body due to the soothing effects produced by continuous rhythmical movements, hence used before mobilization/ stretching/strengthening exercises.
- Maintains available ROM and extensibility of soft tissues and prevents adhesion formation, tightness (adaptive shortening), contracture and deformities in joints. One passive movement given to the joints at frequent intervals are sufficient for the purpose, however two movements to each joint performed twice daily is also adequate.
- Helps to preserve the memory of movements by stimulating the kinesthetic receptors during the periods when active movements are not possible.
- Assist in venous and lymphatic return and prevent formation of deep vein thrombosis (DVT), due to mechanical pressure created due to movement, as well as due to stretching of the thin walled vessels that cross over the joints. This is used in conjunction with elevation of the body segment with oedema, when active movement is not possible.

*II. Accessory movements*

These consist of gliding or rotational movements, which occurs in combination with physiological movements, but can not be performed in isolation actively. These movements are usually limited or absent in joint pathologies, and need to be restored by the therapists through mobilization techniques.

Principles of giving accessory movements:

- Position the patient in a position as appropriate for restoration of movement.
- Ensure that the patient is fully relaxed and the part is fully supported.
- Fix the proximal segment.
- Perform small amplitude gliding and rotational movements in a graded manner, comparing with such movements found on the sound side without traumatizing the joint.
- Follow direction of movement as appropriate, i.e., when concave surface is made to glide over convex surface, the gliding is done in the direction of rolling of the distal segment of the joint **(Fig. 8.15A)**, and when convex surface is moved over concave surface, gliding is given in the opposite direction of rolling of the distal segment of the joint **(Fig. 8.15B)**.

Effects and Uses of Accessory Movements:

- Enhances joint play, hence beneficial for restoration of physiological movements of joints.
- In stiffness of joints, accessory movements to joints are given before physiological movements.

### Passive Manual Mobilization Techniques

These are passive movements where controlled forces are applied either manually, or mechanically to stretch/mobilize soft tissues, enabling restoration of joint range of motion in stiff joints affected by disease or trauma. These include:

*Mobilizations of Joints*

These are small repetitive rhythmical oscillatory movements (physiological/accessory) performed by the clinicians in various amplitudes under the patient's control to restore mobility These are graded according to the part of the available range in which they are performed.

*Manipulations of Joints*

These are accurately localized, single, quick decisive movements of small amplitude

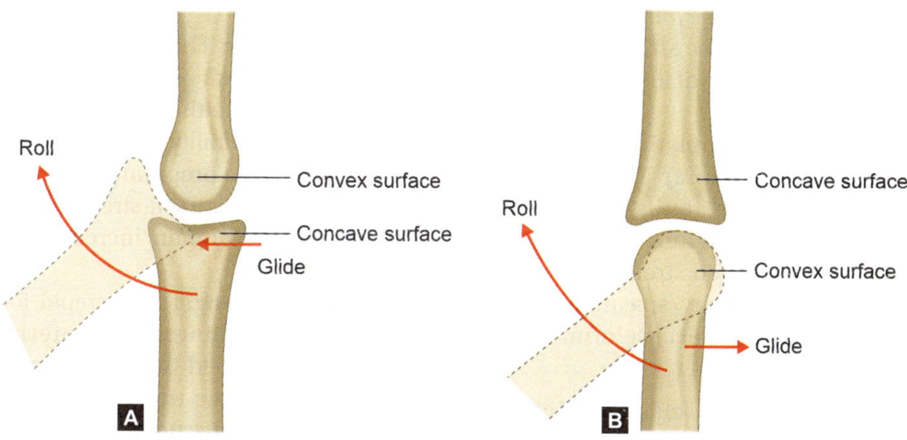


**Figs. 8.15A and B:** (A) Concave surface moving over convex surface; (B) Convex surface moving over concave surface.

and high velocity applied by the clinicians and are completed before the patient can stop it. These movements are done either by the Physiotherapists in a therapeutic environment or by the Orthopedic surgeon under general anesthesia. After the joint is manipulated by the Surgeon, the mobility is maintained and increased by the Physiotherapist either manually or by using CPM device.

*Controlled Sustained Stretching of Tightened Structures/Passive Stretching*

These are forceful passive movements, where sustained stretching force is applied to tight soft tissues either manually or mechanically by therapists using weight and pulley, weight cuffs, or devices like dynamometers etc. to elongate tight structures to correct deformities, improve joint range of motion and to restore function. Before passive stretching is performed, the differentiation between tightness (a state of shortening of soft tissues, which can be elongated by passive force) and contracture (a state of shortening of soft tissues, which cannot be elongated by passive force) should be made.

*Principles of Passive Manual Mobilization and Stretching*

- Make an initial assessment of joint, that includes ROM, joint play, end feel.
- Decide the position of the patient and the joint (loose pack position), technique (Maitland, Kaltenborn, Cyriax, etc.) and grades of mobilization/manipulation as appropriate.
- Stabilize the proximal segment to localize the force at the affected joint.
- For passive stretching, the patient should remain relaxed and the sustained stretching force should be applied for a minimum of 30 seconds. Repetition of stretches depends upon the tolerance of the patient and the effects required.
- The stretch/elongation should be maintained by suitable positional devices/orthoses to achieve permanent deformation/elongation (creep).
- Evaluate each joint mobilized/manipulated at the end of each session as well as at periodic intervals.
- Any gain in range of motion and flexibility need to be maintained by regular exercises and functional integration.

*Effects and Uses of Passive Joint Mobilization/ Manipulation and Passive Stretching*

- Mobilization of joints at low grades help in reduction of pain'
- Mobilization/manipulation breaks intra articular/periarticular adhesions and corrects positional faults in joints and restores mobility and function.
- Steady and sustained stretching helps in reduction of spasticity/spasm, elongates tight soft tissues, corrects deformities.

*Types of Stretching Exercises*

Stretching exercises are classified into the following types, depending upon the mode of their performance, such as passive or active, manual or mechanical.

**Passive Stretching**

- **Static stretching:** This is the most commonly performed stretching exercise, where the tight soft tissues are lengthened past the point of tissue resistance and held in the lengthened position for an extended period of time preferably 30 seconds or more with a maintained stretch force. It is done manually by therapists or mechanically.
- **Static progressive stretching:** In this type of stretching exercise, the tight soft tissues are held in the lengthened position, until a degree of relaxation is achieved. Then the shortened structured are further lengthened and held in the new lengthened position for some time.
- **Cyclic stretching/intermittent stretching:** In this type of stretching, a relatively short duration stretch force is applied repeatedly and gradually with intermittent release to cause elongation of tight tissues.
- **Mechanical stretching:** In this type of stretching, devices like orthotics, weights (weight cuffs/sand bags), therabands, weight and pulley circuits, traction devices, automated devices such as CPM, Dynamometers, etc. are used to apply a sustained stretch to elongate tight soft tissues.

**Active stretching**

- **Self-stretching:** This stretching exercise is carried out independently by a patient as advised by the therapists, to maintain/ increase the flexibility of the tight tissues, as a home exercise program. For example: A straight leg raise is a self-stretching done by the patient to maintain/increase flexibility of hamstrings.
- **Ballistic stretching:** This is a rapid, forceful, high speed, high intensity intermittent stretch, performed by the patient as per instruction of the therapist to increase flexibility of soft tissues and increase joint range of motion. The Codman's exercise used to mobilize shoulder joint, uses ballistic stretching **(Fig. 8.16)**.
- **Neuromuscular inhibition techniques/ PNF stretching:** These procedures reflexively relax tension in shortened muscles prior to or during stretching. These include:
  - **Hold and relax:** The tight muscle is kept in a comfortably lengthened position and the patient is asked to isometrically contract the muscle against the resistance given by the therapist, and subsequently to relax the muscle voluntarily. As the patient

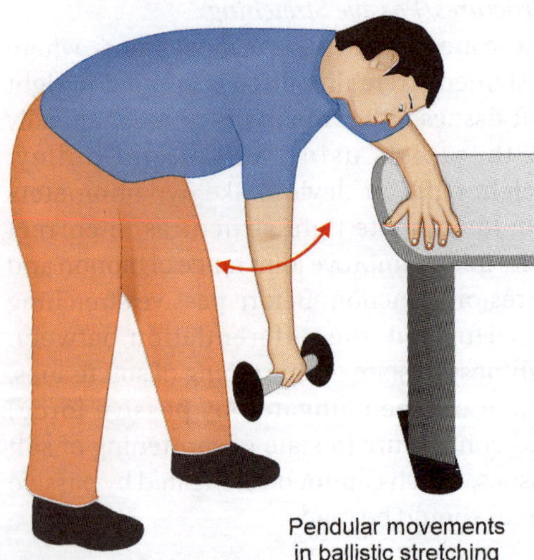


**Fig. 8.16:** Ballistic stretching.

relaxes, the therapist moves the extremity through the gained range. The procedure is repeated several times.

- **Hold relax with agonist contraction:** The same procedures as done for hold and relax are followed. After the patient contracts the tight muscle, have him/her contract the agonist (opposite of tight muscle) concentrically to achieve elongation of the tight muscle.
- **Agonist contraction:** The tight muscle is passively lengthened to a comfortable position, and subsequently the patient is asked to contract the agonist muscle (opposite of tight muscle) concentrically. The therapist applies mild resistance to the contracting muscle. The tight muscle will relax and lengthen as a result of reciprocal inhibition.

### Determinants of Stretching Exercises

- **Intensity:** The lower the intensity, the longer the time the patient will tolerate stretching and soft tissues can be held in a lengthened position. The higher the intensity, the less frequently the stretching intervention can be applied.
- **Duration:** Stretch duration of 15, 30, 45, or 60 seconds or 2 minutes are effective, however, studies reveal that a long duration stretch (say for 60 seconds) is no way more beneficial than a 30 second stretch. Most stretch durations are maintained at 30 seconds.
- **Frequency:** For a general fitness program, the American College of Sports Medicine recommends static stretching for most individuals that is preceded by an active warm-up, at least 2–3 days per week. Each stretch should be held 15–30 seconds and repeated 2–4 times. The frequency of stretch depends upon the degree of tightness and functional integration of the affected segment.

### Contraindications for Passive Stretching

- Acute inflammation.
- Recent fracture.
- Hyper mobility.
- Severe osteoporosis.
- Loose body in joint.
- Hemophilic arthritis.
- Early tendon repair/transfer.

# 9 CHAPTER Relaxed Passive Movement

## INTRODUCTION

### Definition

These are movements performed accurately, rhythmically and smoothly by the physiotherapists/clinicians through available range of motion (according to anatomy of joints) within the limits of pain. The pain free movements are performed in the same range and direction as active movements.

### Principles of Relaxed Passive Movement

- **Relaxation:** Patient has to be positioned in relaxed manner before starting the treatment procedure. The starting position should be so selected, that it should provide adequate support and comfort to both patient and the therapist throughout the movement. The therapist has to adopt the walk standing/stride standing position while treating the patient.
- **Fixation:** The proximal segment of the joint to be moved, should be fixed by the therapist to ensure, localization of the movement to the moving joint and to prevent unnecessary movements in the proximal joints.
- **Support:** Full and comfortable support to the moving segment by the therapist is essential to make the patient confident and relaxed.
- **Traction:** Long axis traction is given to increase the space between the articular surfaces. It reduces the intra-articular friction as well as breaks the adhesion formation in the joint. Free passive movement can be performed due to the less friction effect done by the long axis traction.
- **Range of movement:** Range of movement of the joint should be pain free, to avoid spasm of the surrounding muscles.
- **Speed of movement:** As, it is essential that, relaxation is maintained throughout the movement, the speed of movement should be slow, and the movement should be done in rhythmical manner without inducing jerk with suitable repetitions.
- **Stance of physiotherapist/clinician:** The physiotherapist should stand either in walk standing/stride standing in the direction of line of movement.
- **Repetitions:** 8–10 repetitions of movements should be given in a session performed twice in a day.
- **Sequence of movement:** Neuromotor disorders—proximal to distal for flaccid muscles and distal to proximal for spastic muscles. For relief of oedema the sequence should be distal to proximal.

### Effect and Uses of Relaxed Passive Exercises

- Maintains range of motion and prevents formation of adhesions and joint stiffness.
- Maintains the physiological properties of muscles (elasticity, extensibility etc.) and prevents tightness and contracture.
- Helps in preserving and maintaining the memory of the movement pattern through stimulation of kinesthetic receptors.

- Assists in venous and lymphatic return and increases arterial blood flow, due to the mechanical force acting on the thin-walled vessels, and interstitial spaces of tissues.
- Prevents deep vein thrombosis, due to enhancement of venous return.
- Induces local and general relaxation, due to the soothing effects of repetitive rhythmical movements.
- Enhances joint sensation, i.e., sense of joint position and movements.

## Indications of Use of Relaxed Passive Exercises

- Patients in the state of coma, to maintain physiological properties of muscles and prevent joint stiffness, soft tissue tightness and deep vein thrombosis.
- Inflammatory lesion to joints, where active movement is painful.
- Paralytic conditions, where active movement is not possible.
- In edematous limb, such as oedema in upper limb after radical mastectomy.
- To induce relaxation in patients with muscle spasm.
- To promote motor control, during inactivity by enabling the patient remember the pattern of movement.

## Contraindications of Relaxed Passive Exercise

- Recent/unhealed fracture.
- Acute inflammation, causing joint effusion.
- Immediate post operative surgical procedures, like tendon repair/transfer.
- Recent burns.
- Recent sprain/strain.
- Development of myositis ossificans/heterotrophic ossification.
- Presence of signs of DVT.
- Malignant lesions.
- Active infection to bone (osteomyelitis) and joints.
- Hemarthrosis.
- Hemophilic arthritis with bleeding into joints.
- Recent plaster.

## Procedure of Relaxed Passive Movement

The therapist has to adopt the walk stand position and should face the patient's face, so, that he/she can observe the patient's reaction (for any pain) while performing movement.

Right side is taken as an example and explained in detail about the procedures followed for different joints of the body.

## A. Upper Limb

### *Shoulder Joint*

**Flexion (Fig. 9.1)**

- **Position of the patient:** Supine lying.
- **Position of the therapist:** Standing beside the patient and facing the patient's face.

**Grasps**

- Left hand of the therapist restricts the wrist and carpometacarpal movement of the patient.
- Therapist's right hand should grasp the lower part of the arm of the patient.

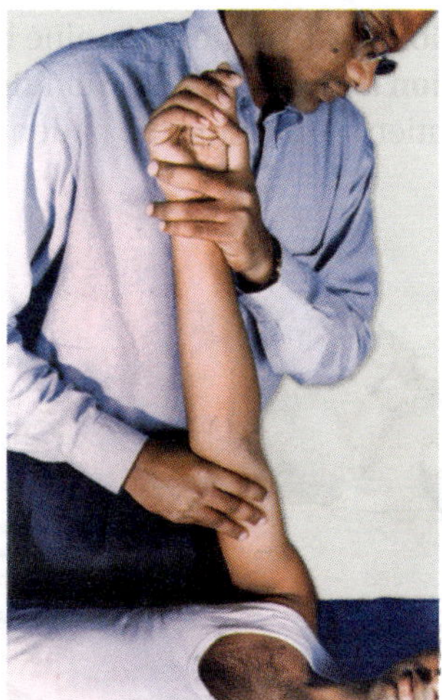

**Fig. 9.1:** Relaxed passive movement for flexion of shoulder.

**Procedure:** The patient is asked to remain relaxed and report, if any pain/discomfort is felt. Mild long axial traction is given and the movement is performed. The traction should be maintained throughout the movement. To start with, traction is applied by the right hand and above 90° the traction is maintained by the left hand of the therapist. Movement is performed within the available range, and repeated for desired number of times.

**Extension (Fig. 9.2)**

- ***Position of the patient:*** Side lying.
- **Position of the therapist:** Standing back to the patient and facing the shoulder joint.

**Grasp**

- Forearm and elbow is placed over the right side forearm of the therapist by flexing the elbow of the patient and wrist movement is restricted by the therapist's hand.
- Left hand of the therapist stabilizes the scapula of the patient.

**Procedure:** It is not possible to apply the long axial traction. Therapist's right hand performs the extension movement of the shoulder.

**Abduction (Figs. 9.3 and 9.4):**

- **Position of the patient:** Supine lying:
- **Position of the therapist:** Standing beside the patient and facing the patient's face.

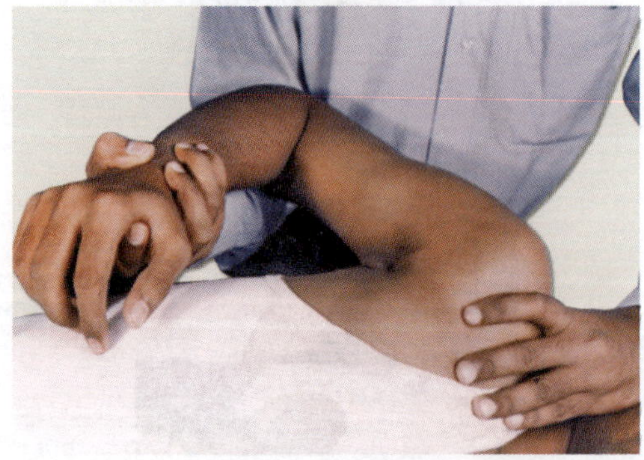

**Fig. 9.2:** Relaxed passive movement for extension of shoulder.

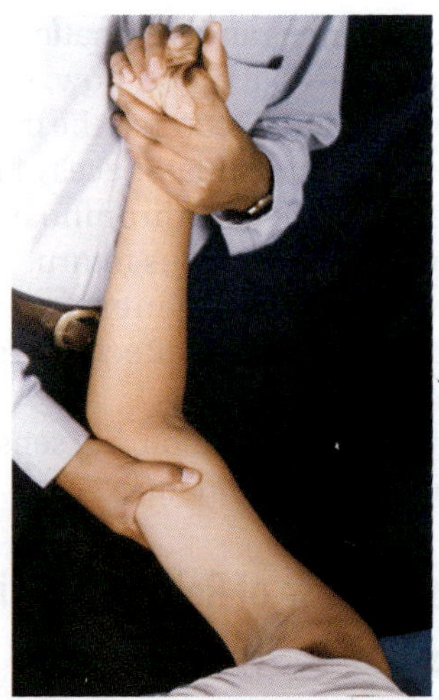

**Fig. 9.3:** Relaxed passive movement of abduction of shoulder (starting stage).

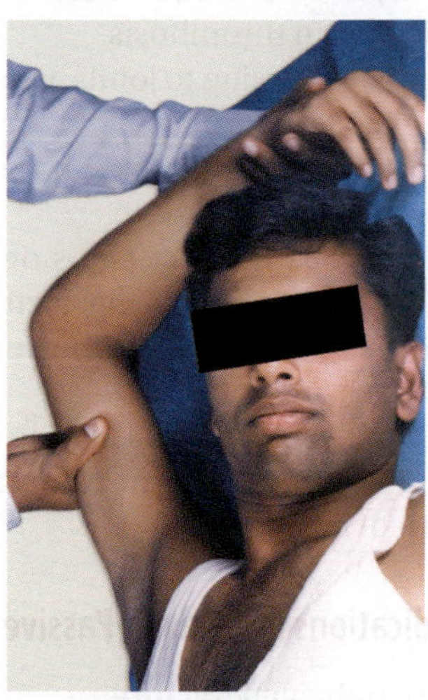

**Fig. 9.4:** Relaxed passive movement for abduction of shoulder (end stage).

**Grasp**

- Patient's elbow is flexed (90°).
- Patient's wrist is grasped by the left hand of the therapist.
- The lower part of the arm is grasped by the therapist's right hand **(Fig. 9.4)**.

**Procedure:** Therapist applies long axis traction to the arm with his/her right hand and performs shoulder abduction. In the

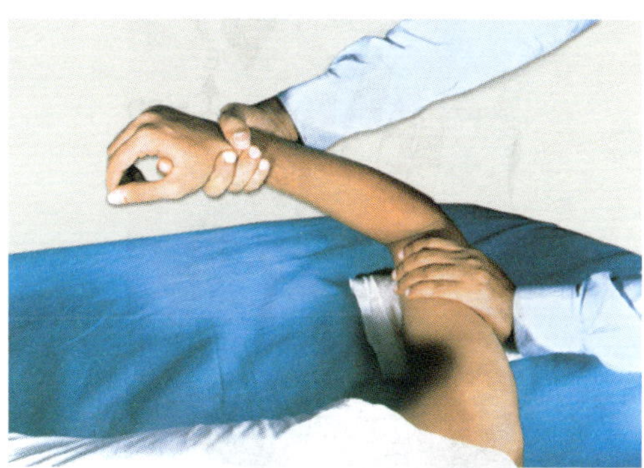

**Fig. 9.5:** Relaxed passive movement for medial rotation of shoulder.

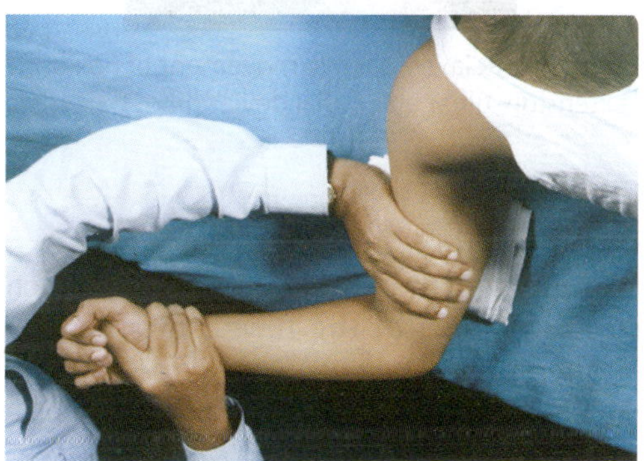

**Fig. 9.6:** Relaxed passive movement for lateral rotation of shoulder.

final range to gain the maximum abduction range, the lateral rotation of the shoulder is done.

**Medial and lateral rotation (Figs. 9.5 and 9.6):**

- **Position of the patient:** Supine lying.
- **Position of the therapist:** Standing beside the patient and facing the patient's shoulder.

**Grasp**

- Patient's shoulder is abducted to 90° with the elbow in 90° of flexion.
- Therapist's left hand grasps the lower end of the arm and right hand grasps the wrist and hand of the patient.

**Procedure:** Long axis traction is applied and the medial and lateral rotation movement of the shoulder is performed by the therapist.

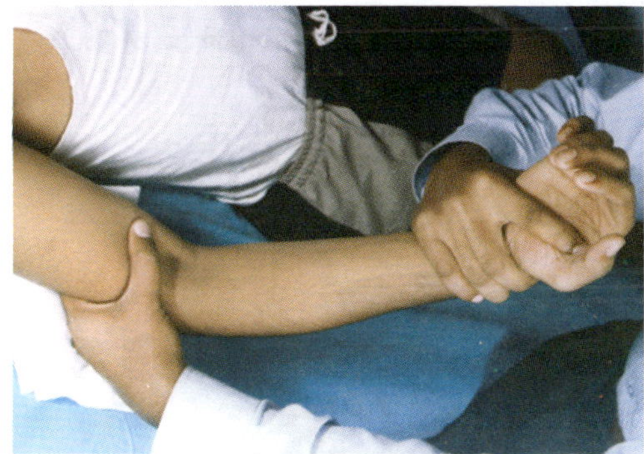

**Fig. 9.7:** Relaxed passive movement for flexion and extension of elbow.

### *Elbow Joint*

**Flexion and extension (Fig. 9.7):**

- **Position of the patient:** Supine lying:
- ***Position of the therapist*:** Standing beside the patient and facing the patient's elbow.

**Grasp**

- Therapist grasps the lower arm of the patient with his/her left hand and fixes to the couch.
- Therapist's right hand grasps the wrist and hand of the patient.

**Procedure:** Therapist applies gentle long axis traction to the forearm with the right hand and performs elbow flexion and extension.

### *Forearm (Radio Ulnar Joints)*

**Supination and pronation (Fig. 9.8):**

- **Position of the patient:** Supine lying.
- **Position of the therapist:** Standing beside the patient and facing him.

**Grasp**

- Elbow is flexed to 90°.
- Arm is fixed with the couch by the therapist's left hand.
- Wrist and hand are grasped by the therapist's right hand.

**Procedure:** It is not possible to apply traction to radio ulnar joint in this technique.

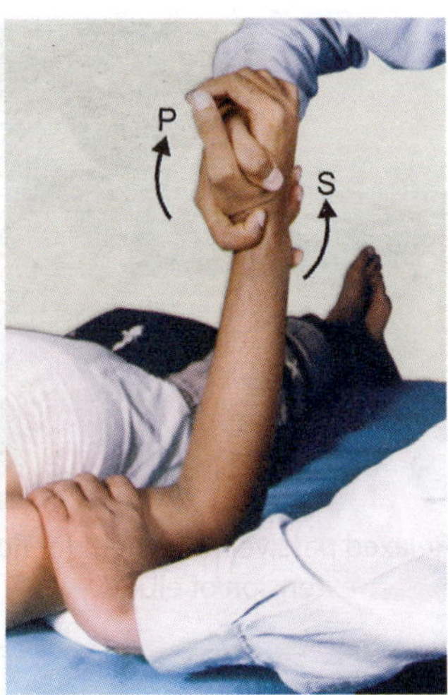

**Fig. 9.8:** Relaxed passive movement for supination and pronation of forearm.

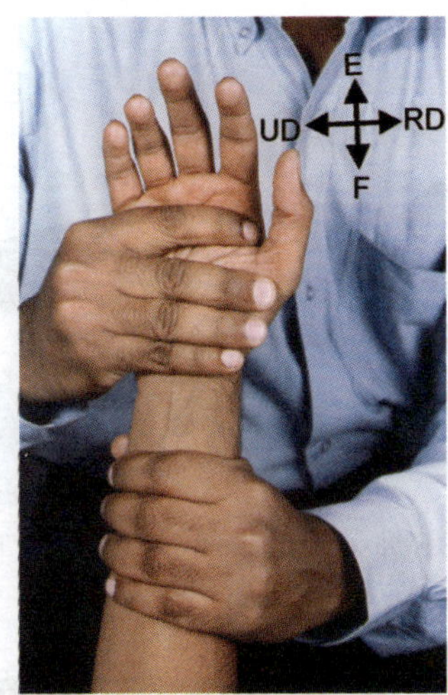

**Fig. 9.9:** Relaxed passive movement of flexion, extension, ulnar and radial deviation of the wrist.

Therapist's right hand performs the supination and pronation movement in the available range.

### *Wrist Joint*

**Flexion and extension (Fig. 9.9):**

- **Position of the patient:** Supine lying.
- **Position of the therapist:** Standing beside the patient and facing him.

**Grasp**

- Elbow flexed near to 90°, and arm supported by a pad of towel on the couch.
- Lower part of the forearm is held by therapist's left hand.
- Right hand of the therapist grasps the carpals and MCP joints.

**Procedure:** With mild long axial traction, flexion and extension movements are performed by the therapist's right hand in available range.

**Ulnar and radial deviations (Fig. 9.9)**

- **Position of the patient:** Supine lying.
- **Position of the therapist:** Standing beside the patient and facing him.

**Grasp**

- Elbow flexed near to 90°, and arm supported by a pad of towel on the couch.
- Lower part of the forearm is held by therapist's left hand.
- Right hand of the therapist grasps the carpals and MCP joints.

**Procedure:** With mild long axial traction, the ulnar and radial deviation movements are performed by the therapist's right hand in available range.

### *Thumb Joint (Carpometacarpal Joint)*

**Flexion, extension, abduction, adduction, opposition (Fig. 9.10):**

- **Position of the patient:** Supine lying.
- **Position of the therapist:** Standing beside the patient and facing him.

**Grasp**

- Therapist's right hand grasps the palm of the patient.
- Left hand of therapist grasps the thumb of the patient.

**Procedure:** With mild long axis traction all the thumb movements can be performed with

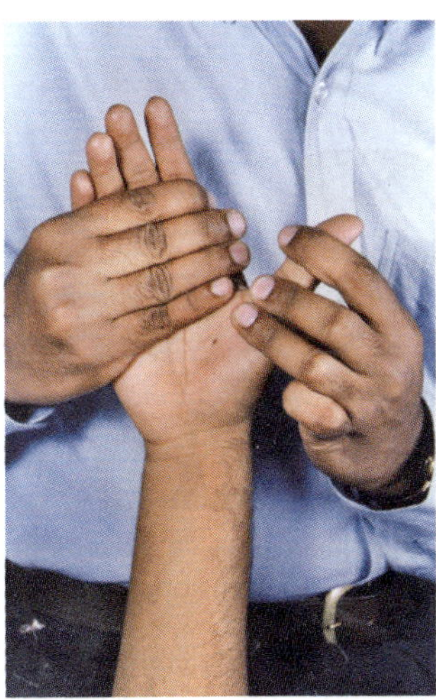

**Fig. 9.10:** Relaxed passive movement of flexion, extension, abduction, adduction and opposition movement of the thumb.

the therapist's left hand (flexion, extension, abduction, adduction, opposition).

### *Metacarpophalangeal Joint of Fingers (Fig. 9.11)*

**Flexion, extension, abduction, adduction:**

- **Position of the patient:** Supine lying.
- **Position of the therapist:** Standing beside the patient and facing him.

**Grasp**

- Therapist's right hand grasps the palm of the patient without covering the MCP joint.

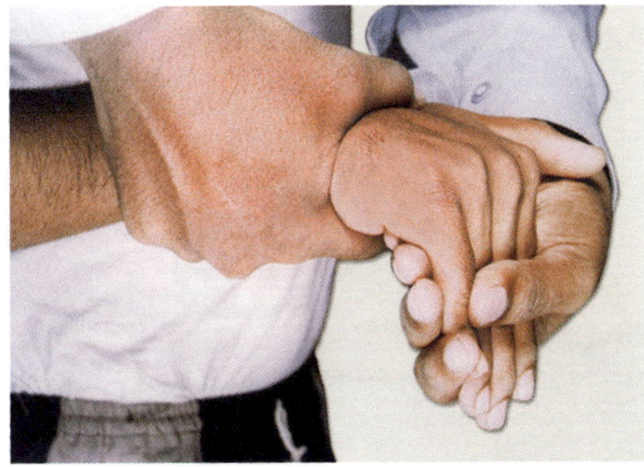

**Fig. 9.11:** Relaxed passive movement of flexion, extension, abduction and adduction of MCP joint of fingers.

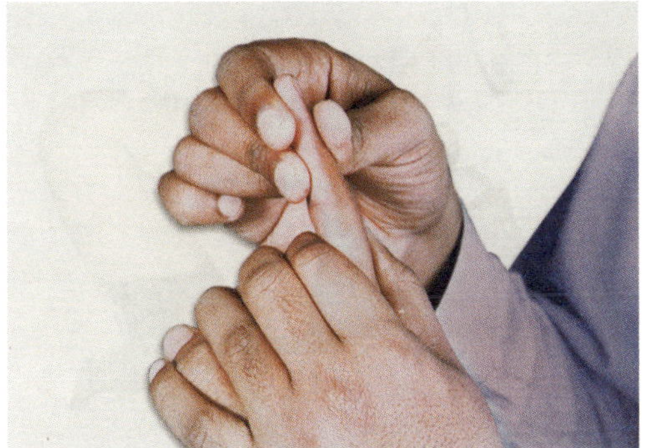

**Fig. 9.12:** Relaxed passive movement of flexion and extension of interphalangeal joint.

- Left hand of the therapist grasps the fingers of the patient in extension.

**Procedure:** With mild long axis traction flexion and extension, abduction, adduction of the metacarpophalangeal joints are performed by the left hand of the therapist.

### *Interphalangeal Joint of Fingers and Thumb (Fig. 9.12)*

**Flexion and extension of fingers and thumb:**

- **Position of the patient:** Supine lying.
- **Position of the therapist:** Standing beside the patient and facing him.

**Grasp**

- Left hand fingers of the therapist stabilize the proximal part of the joint.
- Distal part of the joint is grasped by the right hand fingers.

**Procedure:** With mild traction flexion and extension movements of PIP and DIP joints of fingers and IP joint of thumb are performed in available range by the therapist's right hand.

## B. Lower Limb

### *Hip Joint (Fig. 9.13)*

**Flexion**

- **Position of the patient:** Supine lying.
- **Position of the therapist:** Standing beside the patient and facing him.

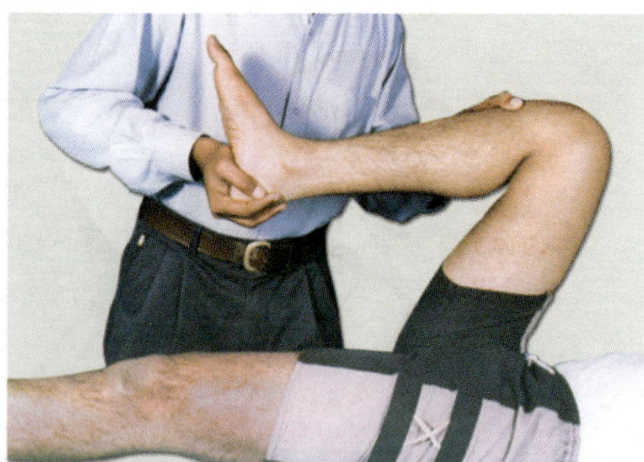

**Fig. 9.13:** Relaxed passive movement of flexion of hip.

### Grasp

- ❖ Therapist's right hand grasps the heel of the patient.
- ❖ Therapist's left hand grasps the posterior part of knee with the thumb kept over lateral side of the knee.

**Procedure:** It is impossible to apply long axial traction for this movement. Knee and hip flexion movements performed together to achieve full range of hip flexion by reducing the hamstring and rectus femoris tension. While performing movement the therapist's left hand from the posterior part of the knee gradually moved and comes to anterior side of the knee. While returning to neutral, the left hand should again move to posterior aspect of knee to prevent thrusts.

### Extension (Fig. 9.14)

- ❖ **Position of the patient:** Side lying.
- ❖ **Position of the therapist:** Standing at the back side of the patient.

### Grasp

- ❖ Patient's knee is flexed to 90°.
- ❖ The therapist's right forearm, supports the patient' leg, with the hand grasping the front of the knee joint.
- ❖ Therapist's left hand stabilize the pelvic of the patient.

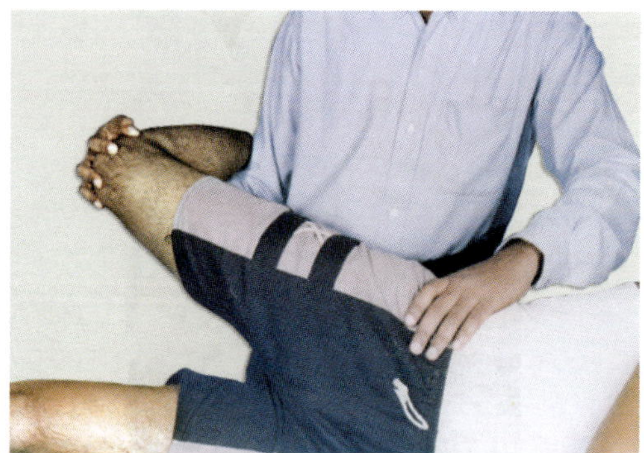

**Fig. 9.14:** Relaxed passive movement for hip extension.

**Procedure:** Therapist's right hand performs extension movement of the hip.

### Abduction and Adduction (Fig. 9.15)

- ❖ **Position of the patient:** Supine lying.
- ❖ **Position of the therapist:** Standing beside the patient and facing him.

### Grasp

- ❖ Right hand of the therapist grasps the lower part of leg.
- ❖ Therapist's left hand grasps the posterior part of the knee joint.
- ❖ Pelvis is stabilized by body weight.

**Procedure:** Without traction the abduction and adduction movement is performed within the available range by the therapist's both hands.

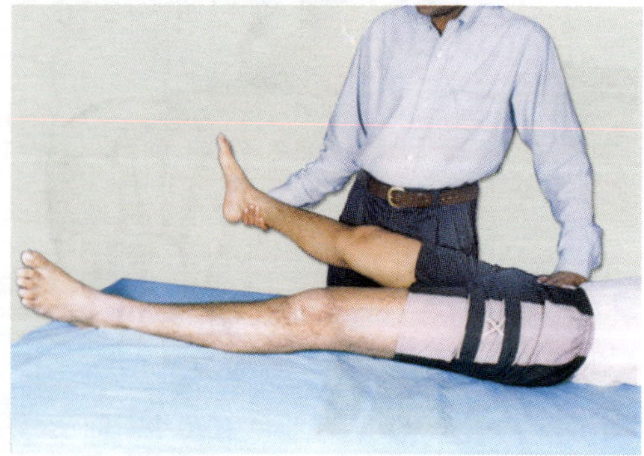

**Fig. 9.15:** Relaxed passive movement for hip abduction and adduction.

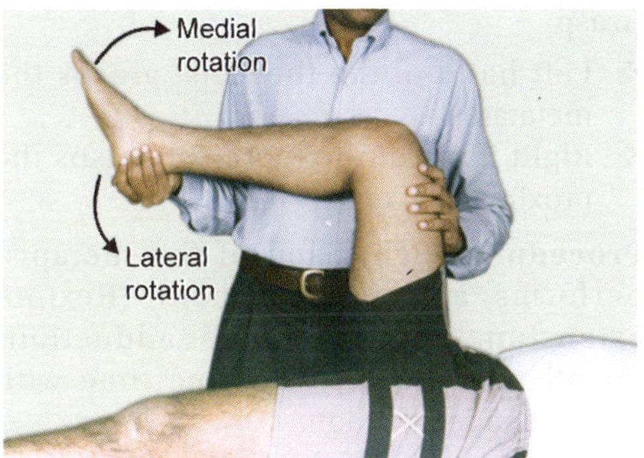


**Fig. 9.16:** Relaxed passive movement of hip medial and lateral rotation.

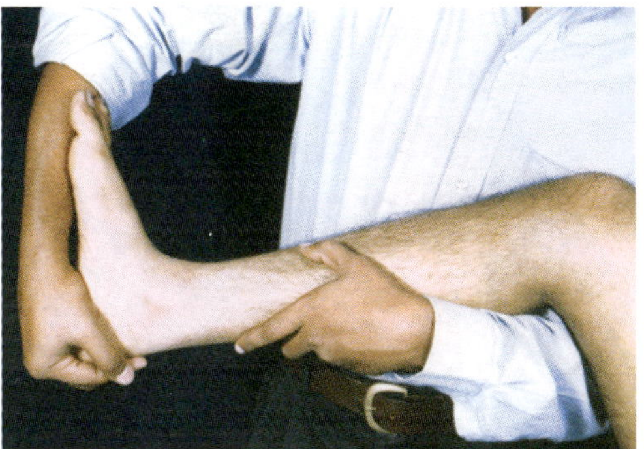

**Fig. 9.17:** Relaxed passive movement of ankle plantar and dorsiflexion.

### Medial and Lateral Rotation (Fig. 9.16)

- **Position of the patient:** Supine lying.
- **Position of the therapist:** Standing beside the patient and facing the hip joint of the patient.

### Grasp

- Patient's knee and hip are kept in 90° flexed position.
- Left hand of the therapist grasps the lower part of thigh.
- Right hand grasps the heel and lower part of the leg of the patient.

**Procedure:** Medial and lateral rotation within the available range is performed by movement of the leg inwards (lateral rotation) and outwards (medial rotation) without any traction by the therapist's right hand.

## *Knee Joint*

### Flexion and Extension

Combined knee and hip flexion and extension are done as shown in **Figure 9.13**. However, if combined movement is painful, isolated knee flexion and extension can be done in side lying, with the thigh supported on pillows. One hand of therapist stabilizes thigh, and the other hand, holding the ankle, moves the knee into flexion and extension.

### Patellofemoral Joint

The lateral to medial and superior to inferior glides are discussed in the chapter on joint mobilization.

## *Ankle Joint*

### Plantar and Dorsiflexion (Fig. 9.17)

- **Position of the patient:** Supine lying.
- **Position of the therapist:** Standing beside the patient and facing the ankle joint of the patient.

### Grasp

- Patient's knee joint is flexed.
- Patient's leg is supported by the therapist's left side forearm and the same side hand grasps the lower part of the leg.
- Right hand of the therapist grasps the calcaneum of the patient with the forearm supporting the sole of the moving foot.

**Procedure:** The therapist's right hand and the forearm perform the plantarflexion and dorsiflexion movement. Knee joint is flexed for reducing tension in the gastrocnemius muscle (i.e., to overcome passive insufficiency of gastrocnemius).

## *Midtarsal Joint*

### Inversion and eversion of foot (Fig. 9.18)

- **Position of the patient:** Supine lying.

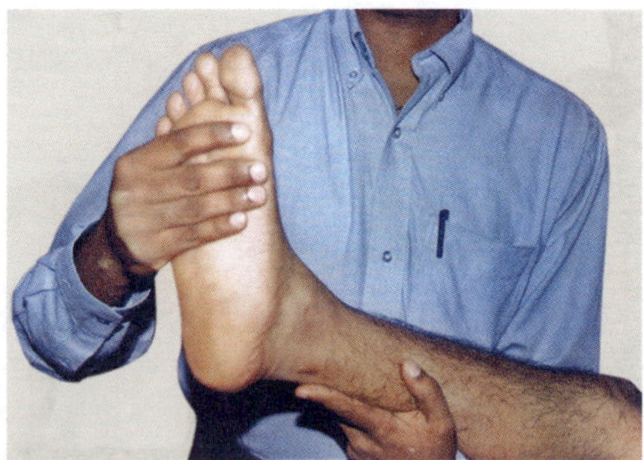

**Fig. 9.18:** Relaxed passive movement for midtarsal inversion and eversion.

- **Position of the therapist:** Standing beside the patient and facing the foot of the patient.

**Grasp**

- Therapist's left forearm supports the lower leg, with the hand grasping the calcaneum.
- Right hand of the therapist grasps the forefoot over the metatarsals.

**Procedure:** Therapist's right hand performs the inversion and eversion movement.

### *Metatarsophalangeal Joint of Toes and Great Toe (Fig. 9.19)*

**Flexion and extension**

- **Position of the patient:** Supine lying.
- **Position of the therapist:** Standing beside the patient and facing the foot of the patient.

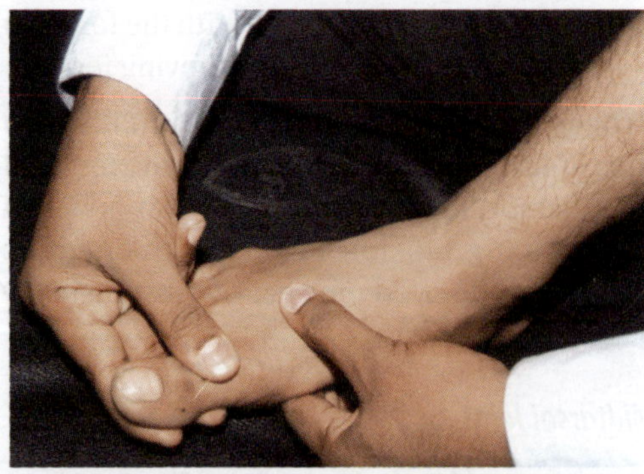

**Fig. 9.19:** Relaxed passive movement for metatarsophalangeal flexion and extension.

**Grasp**

- Left hand of the therapist grasps the metatarsals.
- Right hand of the therapist grasps the proximal phalanx.

**Procedure:** Right hand of the therapist performs all the movement (flexion, extension, abduction and adduction) for all toes together in same time with recommended traction.

### *Interphalangeal Joint*

**Flexion and Extension**

- **Position of the patient:** Supine lying.
- **Position of the therapist:** Standing beside the patient and facing the interphalangeal joint of the patient.

**Grasp**

- Left hand of the therapist grasps the proximal articular segment.
- Right hand grasps the distal articular segment.

**Procedure:** Therapist's right hand is performs flexion and extension movement of the interphalangeal joints.

### *Neck/Cervical Spine (Fig. 9.20)*

**Flexion/extension, lateral flexion and rotation:**

- **Position of the patient:** Supine lying. The head of patient supported by the therapist at the edge of head end of bed.
- **Position of the therapist:** Standing back to the patient's head.

**Grasp**

Therapist grasps the occipital region of the patient with both the hands with thumbs in abduction.

**Procedure:** With mild traction flexion, extension, side flexion and rotational movements are performed by therapist's both hands.

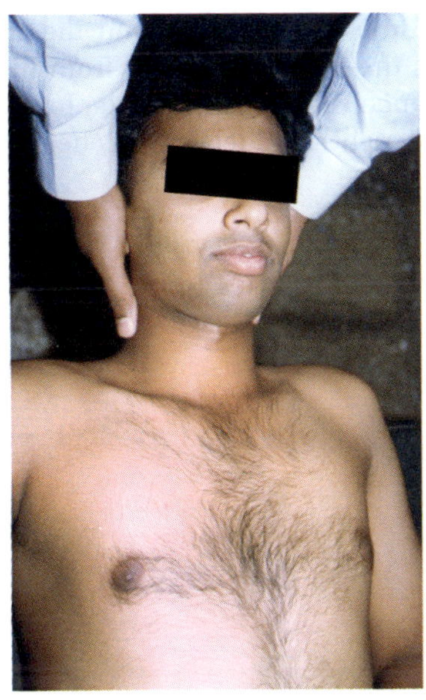

**Fig. 9.20:** Relaxed passive movement of neck.

### *Lumbar Spine*

#### Lumbar Flexion (Fig. 9.21)

- **Position of the patient:** Crook lying.
- **Position of the therapist:** Standing besides the patient.

#### Grasp

- Left hand of the therapist grasps the front of upper legs.
- Right hand of the therapist is placed on the sacrum.

**Procedure:** The therapist lifts the patient's heel off the bed and pushes the knees towards the chest to achieve maximum lumbar flexion, followed by lowering the feet to the bed. The movements are repeated several times as per need.

#### Lumbar Extension (Fig. 9.22)

- **Position of the patient:** Prone lying.
- **Position of the therapist:** Standing besides the patient.

#### Grasp

- Patient's knee joints are flexed and held by therapist's right forearm.
- Therapist's right hand grasp the thighs of the patient.
- Therapist's left hand stabilizes the upper trunk.

**Procedure:** Both the thighs are lifted up until the anterior rotation of the pelvic occurs.

#### Lumbar Rotation (Fig. 9.23)

- **Position of the patient:** Crook lying.
- **Position of the therapist:** Standing beside the patient.

#### Grasp

- Therapist's right hand is placed over the right thigh of the patient.
- Left hand prevents the upper trunk motion by applying the counter force over the right shoulder region.

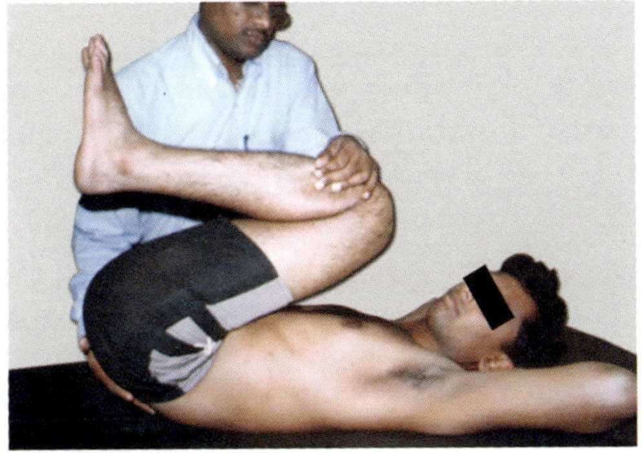

**Fig. 9.21:** Relaxed passive movement for lumbar flexion.

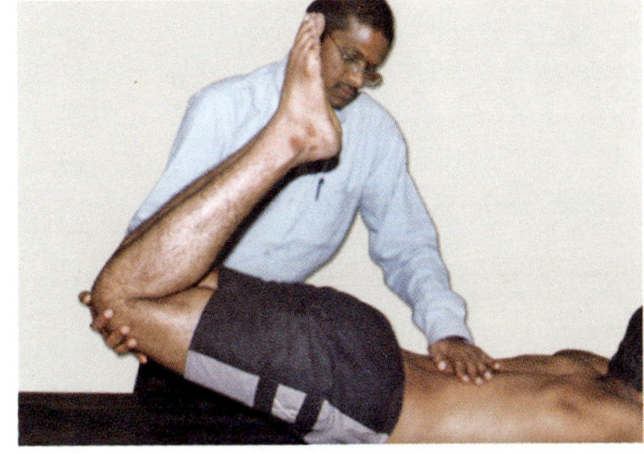

**Fig. 9.22:** Relaxed passive movement of lumbar extension.

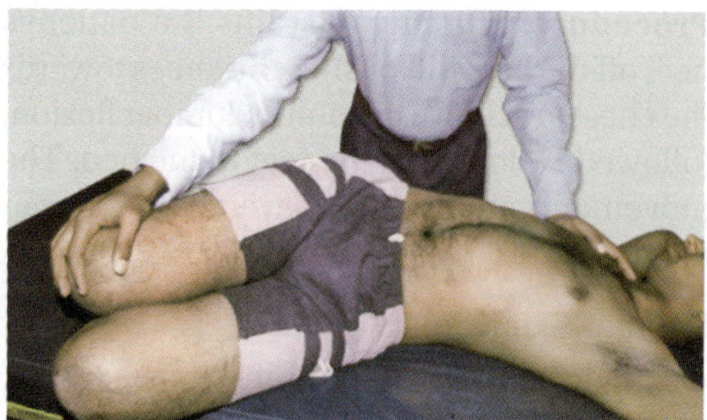

**Fig. 9.23:** Relaxed passive movement of lumbar rotation.

**Procedure:** With the right hand, the therapist pushes the right thigh away from him/her, simultaneously applying counter force on the patient's right shoulder with his/ her left hand.

# 10 CHAPTER Peripheral Joint Mobilization

## INTRODUCTION

The contribution of physiotherapy, in the field of orthopedic medicine is highly commendable. The biomechanical treatment frame/approach applied for neuromuscular and musculoskeletal disorders gives emphasis on stretching tight soft tissues, strengthening weak muscles, and at the same time mobilization of stiff joints to restore function. Healing touch to mobilize soft tissues and stiff joints have been described by many pioneers of orthopedics and physiotherapy such as Geoffrey D Maitland, Australian physiothcrapist, New Zealand physiotherapist Robin McKenzie, Freddy Kaltenborn and Olaf Evjenth, James Henry Cyriax (called as father of orthopedic medicine), John Mennel, etc. When the orthopedic examination reveals the joint hypomobility or decreased ROM, there the mobilization plays its major role. There are two types of mobilizations: (a) Joint mobilization (b) Soft tissue mobilization.

### Definition

A joint mobilization is a manual (hands-on) therapy/treatment meant to help decrease pain, improve range of motion and increase function. It is a "a manual therapy technique comprising a continuum of skilled passive movements that are applied at varying speeds and amplitudes to joints, muscles or nerves with the intent to restore optimal motion, function, and/or to reduce pain.

It is a slow, repetitive, rhythmical, oscillatory arthrokinematic and osteokinematics movement done by a therapist within the available range and using various gradings under the patient's control.

This chapter discusses about the joint mobilization techniques in the introductory level. The therapist should have the knowledge about the anatomy, kinematics, and ortho, neuro, and musculoskeletal disorders to perform the effective mobilization techniques. A knowledge of different types of joints in human body is essential to diagnose joint dysfunctions and plan mobilization. **Table 10.1** shows the different types of joints in human body.

### Kinematics

The branch of mechanics concerned with the motion of objects without reference to the forces which cause the motion. It is the descriptions of motion and includes the time, space and mass aspects of a moving object. It is of two types:

1. Arthrokinematics
2. Osteokinematics.

#### *Arthrokinematics*

'Arthrokinematics refers to the movement of joint surfaces.

It is derived from: Arthro—joint, kinematics—motion.

The movement, which occurs in the joint surface, between the articulating ends of bones that form the joint is called as an "arthrokinematics".

**Table 10.1:** Types of joints.

| *Types of joints* | *Examples* | *Functions* |
|---|---|---|
| Synarthroses/ fibrous (immovable) | • Sutures: Sutures of skull.<br>• Syndesmoses (held by bands)—mid-radioulnar, mid-tibiofibular, coracoacromial, inferior tibiofibular. | These fibrous joints can absorb shock and produce little or no movements of the articulating bones. |
| Amphiarthroses/ cartilaginous (slightly movable) | • Synchondroses (held by cartilage)—sternocostal joint.<br>• Symphyses (a disc of fibrocartilage separates the bones): Vertebral joints, symphysis pubis. | These cartilaginous joints attenuate the applied force and permit, more movements of the articulating bones, as compared to synarthrodial movements. |
| Diarthroses/ synovial (freely movable) | • Plain type joint: These joints permit some gliding movements, e.g., intermetacarpal/ intertarsal/intercarpal joints, facet joints.<br>• Hinged joints: These are uniaxial joints, such as ulnohumeral joint, interphalangeal joint.<br>• Pivot joints: These joints allow rotation around the joint axis, e.g., atlantoaxial joint, superior and inferior radioulnar joint.<br>• Condyloid: radiocarpal (wrist) joint.<br>• Saddle joint: Carpometacarpal joint of thumb.<br>• Ball and socket joints: These joints permit movements in all the three planes, e.g., shoulder joint, hip joint. | These joints have articular cartilages covering the articulating ends of the bones. The synovial membrane, that lines the capsule, secrets the synovial fluid, which acts as the joint lubricant. These joints are freely mobile, and produce movements in different directions. |

- ❖ The articular surface undergoes for movement and the other remains stable.
- ❖ These arthrokinematic movements are called as "joint play movements".

**Types of arthrokinematics movements**

It is of the following types:

1. Rolling
2. Sliding (gliding)
3. Spinning
4. Traction
5. Compression.

### 1. Rolling

Rolling is a type of motion that combines rotation and translation of the bony segments with respect to a surface. Rolling is when a joint surface moves in relation to the other surface during angular motion. The roll happens in the direction of the osteokinematic movement. New points on the rolling surface will contact new points on the other surface as rolling occurs. It occurs between the flat and curved surface. For example, ball rolling on the floor **(Figs. 10.1A to C)**. Convex surface moving on concave surface or vice versa, is the rolling motion. Rolling is combined with the gliding, spinning during the physiological movements.

### 2. Gliding

Gliding/sliding is the translation movement of one joint surface on another joint surface. Gliding occurs when the surfaces of bones slide past one another in a linear direction, but without significant rotary or angular movement. Gliding occurs between either the flat or curved surfaces. For example, square box is moving on oblique floor **(Fig. 10.2)**.

- ❖ Joint surfaces are congruent.
- ❖ Pure gliding is impossible in human joints because there are no complete congruent surface joints.
- ❖ Direction of gliding depends on whether the moving surface is concave or convex.

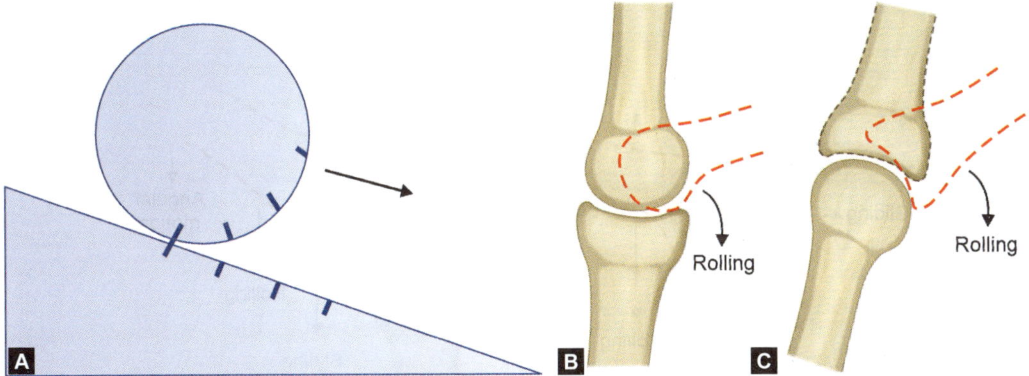


**Figs. 10.1A to C:** (A) Ball is moving on flat surface; (B) Convex surface is moving on concave surface; (C) Concave surface is moving on convex surface.

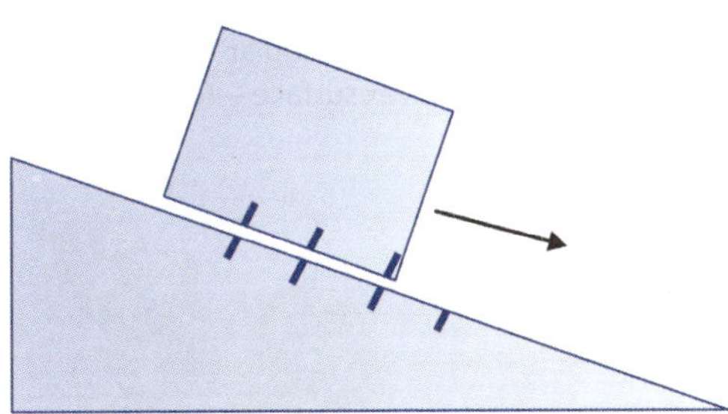

**Fig. 10.2:** Square box is moving on flat surface.

- Direction of gliding will be towards the physiological movement if the concave surface moves on the convex surface (concave-convex rule).
- Direction of gliding will be opposite to the physiological movement if the convex surface moves on the concave surface.

*Convex-concave Rule*

- More the congruent surface, more the sliding occurs and more the incongruent surface, more the rolling occurs.
- While concave surface moves on convex surface gliding rolling occurs towards the angular movement.
- While convex surface moves on concave surface rolling occurs towards the angular movement and gliding occurs opposite to that **(Figs. 10.3A and B)**.

*Note:* While practicing mobilization technique gliding movement has to be selected, based on the physiological movement.

1. In a joint if upward movement is restricted and the moving bone surface is convex then the treatment direction is downward **(Fig. 10.4)**.
2. In a joint if upward movement is restricted and the moving bone surface is concave then the treatment direction is upward **(Fig. 10.5)**.

### 3. Spinning

Spinning is a pure rotational movement. During spinning, multiple points of the moving joint surface comes in contact with one point on the stationary joint surface. In this motion, moving surface rotates on the stable surface **(Fig. 10.6A)**.

- Rotational movement of the articulating surface occurs around its axis **(Fig. 10.6B)**
- Rotation occurs in the stationary mechanical axis.
- It combines with the rolling and gliding and results in rotatory type of physiological movements.

*Example:* Spinning of the head of humerus in glenoid cavity of scapula in shoulder movements. Radiohumeral joint pronation and supination movement.

### 4. Traction and Distraction

Traction is the longitudinal pull on the long axis of a bone to cause separation of the

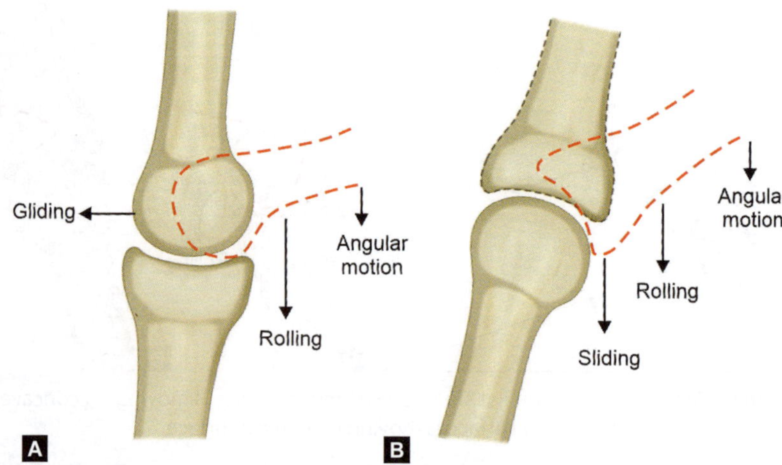


**Figs. 10.3A and B:** (A) Convex surface is moving on concave surface—rolling, angular motion in one direction and the sliding in another side; (B) Concave surface is moving on convex surface—rolling, angular motion, sliding occurs in the same direction.

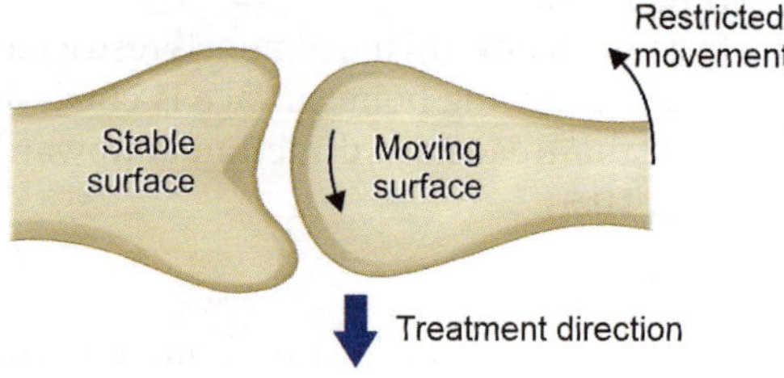


**Fig. 10.4:** Treatment direction.

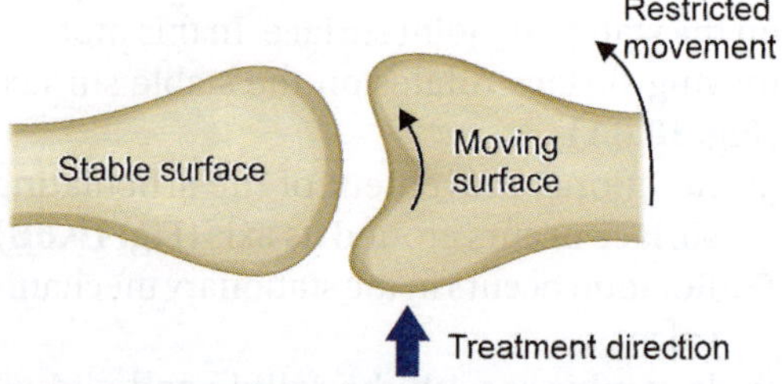


**Fig. 10.5:** Treatment direction.

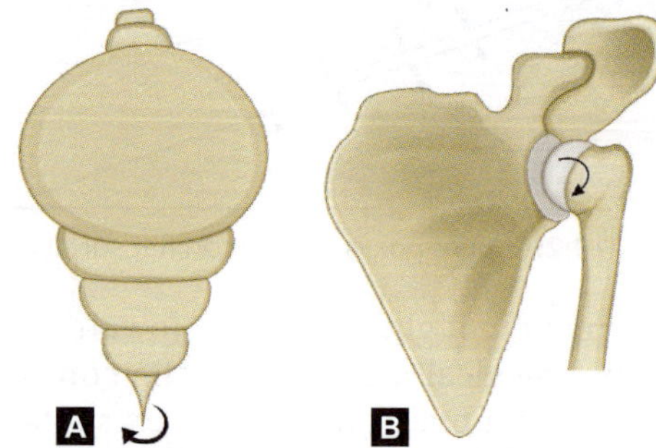


**Figs. 10.6A and B:** (A) Top is spinning on the floor; (B) Head of the humerus spinning on the glenoid cavity of the scapula.

articulating surfaces **(Fig. 10.7A)**, whereas distraction is the separation or pulling apart of the joint surfaces, where the distal articulating surface moves at right angles to the proximal articulating surface/treatment plane **(Fig. 10.7B)**.

- ❖ The joint space increases during traction and distraction.
- ❖ It reduces the joint friction.
- ❖ It enhances the joint play movement.

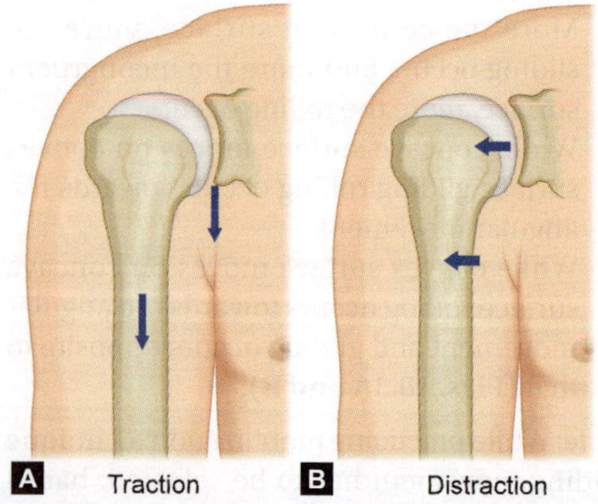


**Figs. 10.7A and B:** (A) Traction; (B) Distraction.

**5. Compression**

- ❖ Joint compression are sensory processing activities that, provide input to the joint by squeezing/compressing.
- ❖ Articular parts are pushed towards each other.
- ❖ Distal articular bone surface moves towards the proximal articular bone surface.
- ❖ Movement is perpendicular to and towards the treatment plane.
- ❖ More common in the weight-bearing joints.
- ❖ Articular surface will be having more contact with each other.
- ❖ Squeezing of the synovial fluid takes place during compression.
- ❖ Over compression leads to joint structure deterioration **(Fig. 10.8)**.

### *Osteokinematics*

Osteokinematics describes clear movements of bones which are visible from the outside. They are the gross physiological movements that occur between two bones. They arise from rotation around the joint axis.

**It is derived from:** Osteo—bone, kinematics—movements.

The angular movement of bones in the human body, called as physiological movements, occur as a result of a combination of rolls, spins, and slides (arthrokinematics). Normally, particular joint ROM is mentioned as physiological ROM. The physiological movement may differ from one joint to another due to the structure of the bony alignment and the structure of the soft tissues around the joint. Some joint has uniaxial movement, some has biaxial and some has triaxial. Due to some pathological disturbance some joints may have more mobility called "hypermobile joints". It is due to the laxity of the ligaments, reduced tension in the joint capsule and the soft tissues around the joint. Mobilization techniques are totally contraindicated for the hypermobile joints. The joints, which have less mobility, are called "hypomobile joints". It is due to spasm of the muscles, tightness of ligaments and capsule or any other soft tissues around the joint and sometime may be due to adhesion formation. This type of joints need mobilization exercises.

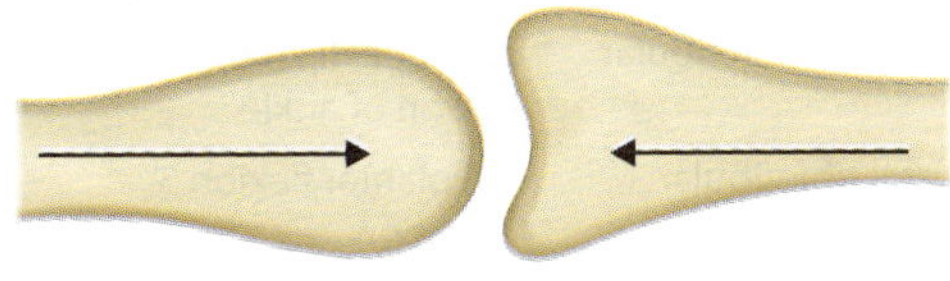

**Fig. 10.8:** Compression.

These osteokinematics movements are the visible movements and are determined by the invisible arthrokinematics movements. It is believed that the arthrokinematic movements are very much needed for the effective osteokinematic movements. Where the joint play movements are lacking the joints said to be hypomobile. The reduction of joint play in articular surface reduces the physiological movement (hypomobile joint) and vice versa occurs in the hypermobile states.

#### Manual Grading of Movement

The joint movement can be graded in the following manner, depending on the movement that take place in a particular joint. Amount of the motion from the resting position can be measured by the goniometer. If the joints are hypermobile or hypomobile there shall be some change of normal joint ROM.

Grade 0—No movement (stiff joint).
Grade 1—Considerable limited movement.
Grade 2—Slightly limited movement.
Grade 3—Normal
Grade 4—Slightly increased movement.
Grade 5—Considerable increased movement.
Grade 6—Unstable (or) flail joint.

Joints can be categorized into three categories, based on the above grades:

1. Hypomobile: Grades: 0, 1, 2.
2. Normal: Grade: 3.
3. Hypermobile: Grades: 4, 5, 6.

Flexion/extension, abduction/adduction. Lateral rotation/medial rotation, inversion/

eversion, supination/pronation are the osteokinematic movements in the limbs, where as flexion/extension, lateral flexion and rotation are the osteokinematic movement of the spine.

## Position of Joints

The tension in the joint varies from one position to another, the knowledge of which is essentially required by the therapist for positioning the joints in a state of relaxation and positioning for mobilization. The therapist uses some position for examination, some for relaxation, and some for treatment purposes. The difference between loosed packed and closed packed positions are shown in **Table 10.2.** The joint positions are typed into three types, which are briefly discussed below:

1. Loose packed position
2. Zero position.
3. Close packed position (tightly packed position).

### *1. Loose Packed Position/Resting Position*

The loose-packed position **(Table 10.3)** is also called the open packed-position, where the contact between the articulating surfaces are minimum. A joint's loose-packed position is the position with the least amount of congruency where the capsule and ligaments are lax and joint play (accessory movement) is optimized.

**Table 10.2:** Difference between close packed and loose packed position.

| *Close packed position* | *Loose packed position* |
|---|---|
| Position with the most amount of joint congruency | Position with the least amount of joint surface congruency |
| Capsule and supporting ligaments are maximally tight | Capsule and supporting ligaments are lax |
| Accessory movement/ joint play is minimum | Accessory movement/ joint play is maximum |

### *2. Zero Position (Starting Position)*

This is the starting position of the joint. While measuring the ROM by the goniometer, the zero position is taken as starting point of the measurement. For example, to measure the shoulder joint movements like flexion, extension, adduction, abduction with goniometer, the zero position we adopt is the arm kept by the side of the chest wall, and for the medial and lateral rotations the adopted

**Table 10.3:** Resting position (loose packed position).

| *Joints* | *Position* |
|---|---|
| Shoulder | Slightly abduction of the shoulder 35–55° |
| Sternoclavicular joint | Clavicle is horizontal position |
| Acromioclavicular joint | Clavicle is in horizontal position |
| Scapulothoracic joint | Clavicle is in horizontal position and scapula is positioned from 2 to 7 ribs |
| Humeroulnar | 70° flexion of elbow, 10° supination |
| Humeroradial | Full extension of elbow, supination |
| Proximal radiaoulnar joint | 35° supination 70° flexion of elbow |
| Distal radioulnar joint | 10° supination |
| Wrist | Neutral with slight ulnar deviation |
| 1st carpometacarpal joint | Midway between the flexion extension abduction and adduction |
| Metacarpophalangeal joint | Slight flexion |
| Interphalangeal joint | PIP 10° flexion, DIP 30° flexion |
| Hip | 30° flexion 30° abduction slight external rotation |
| Knee | 25° flexion |
| Patellofemoral | Full extension of knee |
| Proximal tibiofibular | 25° knee flexion 10° plantar flexion of ankle |
| Distal tibiofibular | 10° plantar flexion 5° inversion |

*Contd...*

*Contd...*

| *Joints* | *Position* |
|---|---|
| Ankle | 10° plantar flexion midway between inversion and eversion |
| Subtalar | Midway between inversion eversion with 10° plantar flexion of ankle |
| Midtarsal | Midway between supination pronation with 10° plantar flexion of ankle |
| Tarsometatarsal | Midway between supination and pronation |
| Metatarsophalangeal | Midway between supination and pronation abduction and adduction |
| Interphalangeal joint | Slight flexion |

position is the shoulder in 90° abduction with elbow in 90° flexion.

### *3. Close Packed Position (Tightly Packed Position)*

In this position that joint stability and congruency is the greatest. The contact of joint surfaces are maximum in this position. In this position, the capsules and ligaments are maximally tight and there is limited accessory movement. It is essential for the therapist, to have a sound knowledge about the close packed position of all the joint to avoid any of the mobilization techniques in this position **(Table 10.4)**.

Besides, the loose packed and close packed, position, the therapist/clinician, should have knowledge of movement limitation in capsular pattern, so as to cause stretching of the joint capsule, to achieve joint mobility. **Table 10.5** shows movement limitation of various joints of the body occurring in a capsular pattern.

**Table 10.4:** Close packed position

| *Joints* | *Position* |
|---|---|
| Shoulder | Maximum abduction and external rotation |
| Sternoclavicular joint | Arm maximum elevated |
| Acromioclavicular joint | Shoulder 90° abduction |
| Scapulothoracic joint | None |
| Humeroulnar | Full extension, supination |
| Humeroradial | 90° flexion, 5° supination |
| Proximal radioulnar joint | Full extension and 5°supination |
| Distal radioulnar joint | 5° supination |
| Wrist | Full extension and radial deviation |
| 1st carpometacarpal joint | Full opposition |
| Carpometacarpal (2nd–5th) | Full flexion |
| Metacarpophalangeal | 1st—maximum extension 2nd–5th—maximum flexion |
| Interphalangeal joint | Maximum extension |
| Hip | Maximum extension, medial rotation and abduction |
| Knee | Maximum extension and external rotation |
| Patellofemoral | 60–90 degrees of knee flexion |
| Proximal tibiofibular | Maximum dorsiflexion of ankle |
| Distal tibiofibular | Maximum dorsiflexion of ankle |
| Ankle | Maximum dorsiflexion |
| Subtalar | Full inversion |
| Midtarsal | Full supination |
| Tarsometatarsal | Full supination |
| Metatarsophalangeal | Full extension |
| Interphalangeal joint | Full extension |

## Physiology of Joint Motion

### *Nutrition*

Joint articular surfaces are avascular and it receives the nutrition from synovial fluid. The synovial fluid circulates inside the capsule to supply the nutrition to the articular surfaces. The synovial fluid movement occurs by the compression of the articular cartilage and

**Table 10.5:** Capsular pattern of limitation of various joints of human body.

| *Joints* | *Capsular pattern of movement limitation (from most limited to least limited)* |
|---|---|
| Temporomandibular joint | Opening of jaw |
| Cervical spine | Equal limitation of side flexion and rotation, extension |
| Thoracic spine | Equal limitation of side flexion and rotation, extension |
| Lumbar spine | Extension, equal limitation of side flexion and rotation |
| SI joint | Pain when joint is stressed |
| Shoulder | Lateral rotation, abduction, medial rotation |
| Sternoclavicular joint | Pain at extreme range of movement |
| Acromioclavicular joint | Pain at extreme range of movement |
| Humeroulnar (elbow) joint | Flexion, extension |
| Proximal radiaoulnar joint | Supination, pronation |
| Distal radioulnar joint | Pain at extremes of rotation |
| Wrist | Flexion and extension equally limited |
| 1st carpometacarpal joint | Abduction, extension |
| Carpometacarpal joint: 2–5 | Movement limitation in all directions |
| Metacarpophalangeal joints | Flexion, extension |
| Interphalangeal joints | Flexion, extension |
| Hip joint | Flexion, internal rotation, abduction |
| Knee joint | Flexion, extension |
| Ankle joint | Plantar flexion, dorsiflexion |
| Subtalar joint | Inversion |
| Midtarsal joint | Dorsiflexion. Plantar flexion, adduction, medial rotation |
| 1st MTP joint | Extension, flexion |
| 2nd–5th MTP | Flexion, extension |
| IP joint of toes | Flexion, extension |

capsule. During loading and unloading as well as the motion of the joint, the synovial fluid movement inside the synovial cavity is facilitated.

The joint mobilization techniques promote good nutrition supply to the joints. Immobilization of the joint may result in atrophy of the articular cartilage, synovial membrane, and formation of adhesion. This can be corrected by the mobilization techniques.

### *Extensibility*

Joint mobility maintains the extensibility and tensile strength of the articular tissues. If the joint is immobilized, the ligaments, tendons and cartilages loose its extensibility property, which leads to joint stiffness and hypomobility. Normal joint movement prevents the contracture, shortening, and thickening of the tissues. The mobilization techniques are also helpful to prevent the contracture and thickening of the soft tissues and improve the extensibility property of the soft tissues.

### *Stimulation of Joint Receptors*

Joint receptors transmit the impulses to the afferent nervous system from the joint. The joint receptors give the awareness of the position and movement of the joints. Injury, disease or immobilization of the joint may cause the lack of functioning of the joint receptors. There are four types of joint receptors **(Table 10.6)**.

## Effect of Pathological Changes of the Joint

Each and every structure of the joint is much more important for the total functioning of the joint. Defect in any of the structure leads to improper functioning of the joint. The various factors leading to joint pathology are briefly discussed below.

**Table 10.6:** Different types of joint receptors.

| *Type I* | |
|---|---|
| Name: | Ruffini |
| Quality: | Postural |
| Stimulus: | Activated by the postural faults |
| | Activated by the stress of the joint capsule |
| | Activated by traction and oscillatory techniques |
| Characteristics: | Low threshold and slow adaptive |
| | Located mainly around the knee, hip, and shoulder |
| Location: | Superficial joint capsule, periosteum, ligaments and tendons |
| Response: | It provides static position, speed and velocity of the movement |
| *Type II* | |
| Name: | Pacini or paciniform |
| Quality: | Dynamic |
| Stimulus: | Activated by the changes in joint motion |
| | Activated more with oscillatory techniques than traction |
| Characteristics: | Low threshold, rapid adaptive |
| Location: | Deep layer of capsule |
| | Mainly in lumbar spine, hand, foot, jaw |
| Response: | Provides joint motion sense |
| *Type III* | |
| Name: | Golgi or Golgi Mazzoni |
| Quality: | Inhibitive |
| Stimulus: | During end range stretch |
| Characteristics: | High threshold, very slow adaptive |
| | Activated by joint mobilization technique |
| Location: | Inner layer of joints, ligaments and tendons |
| Response: | Sense of direction of movement |
| | Regulation of muscle tone |
| *Type IV* | |
| Name: | Non-myelinated free nerve endings |
| Quality: | Nociceptive |
| Stimulus: | Noxious mechanical stress or biomechanical stress |
| Characteristics: | High threshold and non-adaptive |
| Response: | Produces tonic contraction |
| Location: | Located in most tissues like blood vessels, synovial layer of the capsule, fat pads, ligaments, tendons and periosteum |

## Disease

Joint diseases like rheumatoid arthritis, osteoarthritis, TB arthritis, psoriatic arthritis, ankylosing spondylitis, etc., may cause some deformation of the some joint structures resulting in the improper, imperfect movement of the joint. For example, in RA the synovial membrane gets affected, so that there is alteration in the synovial fluid secretion. Joint lubrication is altered and the joint structures may not get proper nutrition. Lack of nutrition may cause deformation of the joint structures. In osteoarthritis erosion or degeneration of the cartilages occurs. So, there will be restricted movement and painful movement. If the disease progresses, it results in contracture and weakness of the muscles, ligament tightness, osteophyte formation over the articular surfaces, osteoporotic changes in the articular surface, etc., making the joints immovable.

## Injury

Injury of the joint structure causes improper movement and improper gait pattern. Loading and unloading of the joint will be painful. If the synovial membrane is injured, it secretes more synovium. Lacking of the stability comes due to the ligament injury. Injury of capsules and cartilages results in lacking of loading and unloading. Any tendon injury may cause the lack of movement over the joint. So, depending on the structures injured, the outcome of the effect on joints may differ. But the net result will be improper or lack of movement of the joint.

### Immobilization

Immobilization may be imposed by the plaster cast, bedrest, and fear of pain. Due to the non-mobility of the joint, many changes over the joint structures occur. The effects of immobilization are discussed in **Table 10.7**.

Normally, after immobilization, tightness of soft tissues develop, which if not corrected, leads to contracture of the soft tissues. Hence proper positioning, stretching and mobilization exercises should be performed to prevent development of contracture and maintain joint mobility.

### Overuse

Prolonged standing, sitting or attaining one particular posture or performing one particular movement may create some strain and stress of the surrounding structures of the joint. Continuous loading of a joint tissue that is deformed earlier may not get the time to recover. So the joint structures may be more prone to get overuse injury or syndrome. Normally, the cartilages, which is the most important connective tissue for loading of a joint, if undergoes deformation and degeneration due to overuse, may result in joint osteoarthritis.

**Table 10.7:** Effects of immobilization.

| Sl. No | Structure | Changes |
|---|---|---|
| 1. | Bone | Osteoporosis |
| 2. | Ligaments | Osteoclastic activity leads to weakness of the ligaments. Decreased matrix compound and degenerative changes in the ligaments lead to deterioration of biomechanical activities |
| 3. | Cartilage | Decreased proteoglycans, decreased water content, decreased thickness, increased stiffness |
| 4. | Capsule | Decreased proteoglycans, increased water content, atrophy of the capsule |
| 5. | Tendon | Decreased collagen content, atrophy, size of the collagen fiber decreases |
| 6. | Synovium | Proliferation of fibro-fatty connective tissue and formation of adhesion |

### Indications of Joint Mobilization

- Post-traumatic stiffness of the joint.
- Postoperative stiffness of the joint.
- Post-immobilization stiffness of the joint.
- Adhesion formation around the joint.
- Atrophy and tightness of the capsule.
- Atrophy of the synovial membrane.
- Disuse atrophy of the joint structures.

### Contraindications of Joint Mobilization

- Synovial effusion/hemarthrosis.
- Recent fractures around the joint. Dislocation.
- Recent injuries around the joints.
- Acute rheumatoid arthritis/psoriatic arthritis/TB arthritis.
- Flail joint.
- Malignant tumors.
- Severe osteoporosis.
- Prolonged intake of steroids.
- Immediately after surgery around the joint such as arthroplasty/arthrodesis.
- Scoliotic spine (where spine can be mobilized after the deformity is corrected).
- Spondylolisthesis (where the affected segments are not mobilized).

Before mobilization of joint, the clinician should give passive movements to the joints, and feel the tissue resistance at the end of range of motion, called as end feel. End feel is a type of sensation or feeling, which the examiner experiences, when the joint is at the end of its available passive range of motion. Depending on the end feel, joint mobilization exercises are planned. The normal and pathological end feels are discussed in **Tables 10.8A and B.**

**Table 10.8A:** Normal end feel.

| *Type of end feel* | *Structures involved* |
|---|---|
| Soft | Approximation of soft tissues, e.g., knee flexion, where calf muscles and hamstrings approximate |
| Firm | Muscular stretch, e.g., hip flexion with knee straight.<br>Capsular stretch, e.g., hyperextension of MCP joints of fingers.<br>Ligamentous stretch, e.g., forearm supination, where tension develops in the palmar radioulnar ligament of the inferior radioulnar joint |
| Hard | Bone contacting bone, e.g., elbow extension |

**Table 10.8B:** Pathological end feels.

| *Type of end feel* | *Examples* |
|---|---|
| Soft: Feels boggy with fluid shift in a joint, that has a firm or hard end feel | Synovitis/edema |
| Firm: Occurs in a joint, that normally has a soft or hard end feel | Increased muscular tone/tightness of capsule |
| Hard: Grating or bony block present, sooner or later in the ROM of a joint, that normally has a soft or firm end feel | Loose body in a joint, myositis ossificans |
| Empty: Pain and muscle spasm restricts movements. No resistance is felt, except the patient's protective muscle splinting or muscle spasm | Bursitis, acute inflammation, abscess |

While mobilizing the stiff joint the therapist may feel the restrictions of movements caused by different joint structures. Limitations may be due to capsule, ligaments, muscle, skin, fascia, cartilages or adhesions. The limitations or restrictions of movement, which is felt by the therapist, is called as first tissue stop (pathological limit). Normally, the passive movements can cross the first tissue stop. If the therapist adds more force after reaching first tissue stop, he may feel again the restriction of movement by some structures called as second tissue stop (anatomical limit). If a force more than required to cross the first tissue stop is applied, the tissue will be moving into the plastic range, where deformation of tissues occur. If the therapist crosses the second tissue stop, the tissue may be separated or teared. So, the joint mobilization techniques should be performed within the second tissue stop **(Figs. 10.9A and B)**.

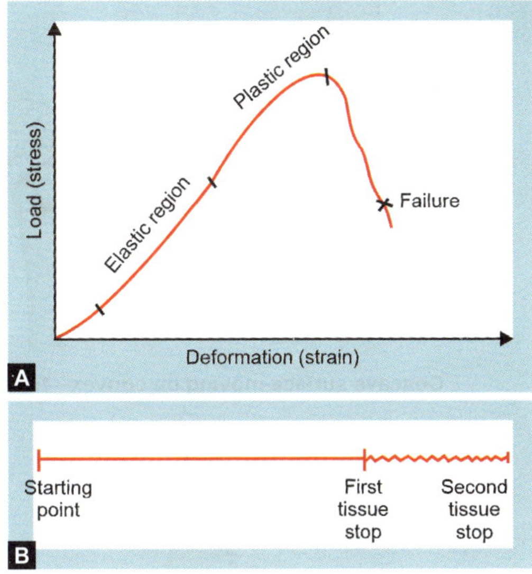


**Figs. 10.9A and B:** (A) Stress-strain curve; (B) Tissue restriction on passive joint play test.

One more factor such as rapid mobilization technique, also influences the joint extensibility. Joint extensibility can be gained by the rapid mobilization technique, which may increase the extensibility of the tissue than the slow techniques. So the stretch administered up to the plastic phase or attaining about to the second tissue stop may give good result with rapid mobilization technique than the medium mobilization technique.

## Treatment Plane

It lies over the concave surface of the articular surface. The treatment plane moves with the

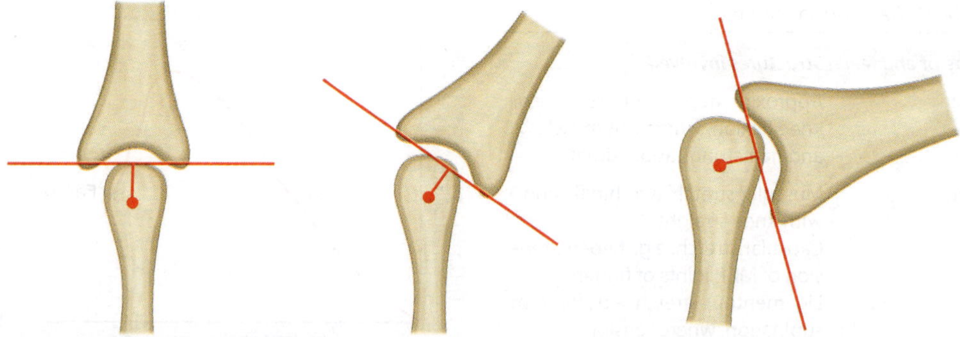

Concave surface moving on convex—treatment plane moves with the concave surface

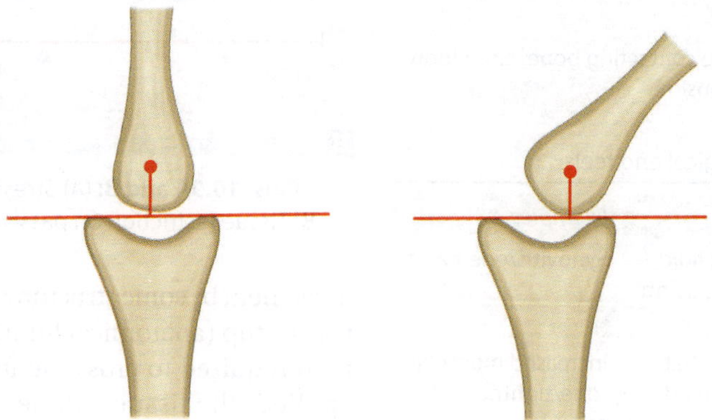

Convex surface move on concave—stationary treatment plane

**Fig. 10.10:** Treatment plane.

movement of the concave surface. It will be constant or stable while the convex surface moves. The treatment plane is perpendicular to the axis of the rotation. The joint distraction is given perpendicular to the treatment plane **(Fig. 10.10)**.

While assessing a joint movement or joint play, movement parallel (traction) or perpendicular to the treatment (distraction) plane should be performed. The gliding or rolling tests are done parallel to the treatment plane.

Traction and distraction can be performed parallel or perpendicular to the treatment plane respectively. This joint play movement decides the grade of the joint movement.

## *Principles of Joint Mobilization*

### Relaxation

Patient has to be positioned in relaxed manner before starting the treatment procedure, to get cooperation from him/her. During the relaxed state there will not be any muscle work and the total body part will be fully relaxed. The therapist's position also plays an important role to treat the patient. The therapist has to adopt the walk standing position while treating the patient.

### Fixation

The joint/segment, which is proximal to the mobilizing joint, should be fixed to avoid trick/vicarious movement, so that the accessory movements may not occur in that joint which may reduce the ROM of the mobilizing joint and also the movement can be localized to one particular joint.

**Support**

The distal part of the joint being moved should be supported fully by the therapist, to localize the movement to the moving joint. The therapist should grasp firmly which may stimulate the nerve endings and improve the condition, and provide psychological support of the patient.

**Treatment Direction**

The treatment direction may be parallel or perpendicular to the treatment plane. Distraction may be applied perpendicular to the treatment plane. The oscillatory technique and traction may be performed parallel to the treatment plane.

**Treatment Force and Range**

The treatment force depends on the grade of the movement of the joint; which may be gentle or forcible. The treatment force is given within the second tissue stop or within the plastic range or sometime about to reach the breaking point of the tissue.

## *Treatment Techniques*

Treatment is graded according to the amount of the motion and the joint play movement of the joint. There are two systems of grading of the mobilization.

1. Traction/distraction technique
2. Oscillatory technique.

**1. Traction/Distraction Technique (Fig. 10.11A)**

**Grade I:** Slow, small amplitude perpendicular movement (distraction) to the concave joint surface performed within the first tissue stop.

**Grade II:** Slow, large amplitude perpendicular movement (distraction) to the concave joint surface done up to the first tissue stop.

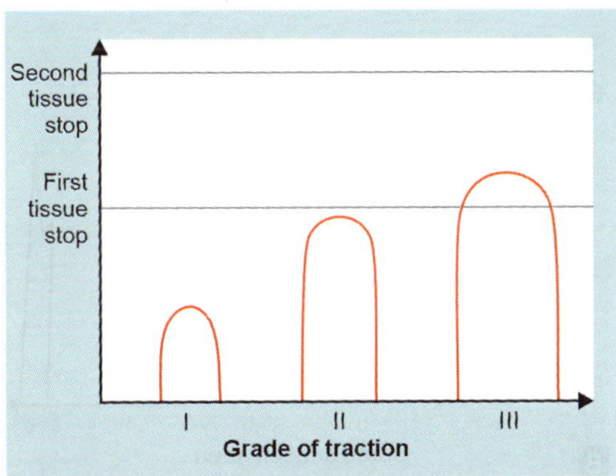


**Fig. 10.11A:** Traction joint mobilization with gradings.

**Grade III:** Slow, large amplitude perpendicular movement (distraction) to the concave joint surface performed up to the level of crossing the first tissue stop, but without reaching the second tissue stop.

*Uses*

**Grade I:** Used for reducing the pain.

**Grade II:** Used for pain reduction and increases the periarticular extensibility.

**Grade III:** Used for periarticular extensibility, to correct the positional fault and reduces the spinal disc herniation.

**2. Oscillatory Technique (Maitland Grades) (Fig. 10.11B)**

**Grade I:** Slow, small amplitude oscillatory movement parallel to the concave joint surface performed within the beginning range.

**Grade II:** Slow, large amplitude oscillatory movement parallel to the concave joint surface performed within the first tissue stop.

**Grade III:** Slow, large amplitude oscillatory movement parallel to the concave joint surface performed up to reaching the first tissue stop.

**Grade IV:** Slow, small amplitude oscillatory movement parallel to the concave joint surface performed slightly through the first tissue stop (pathological limit).

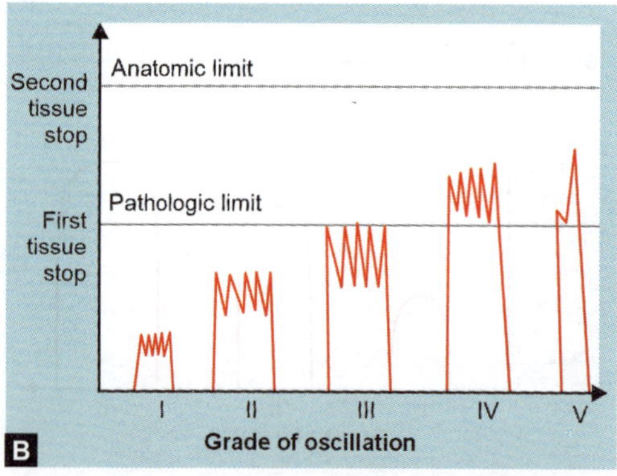


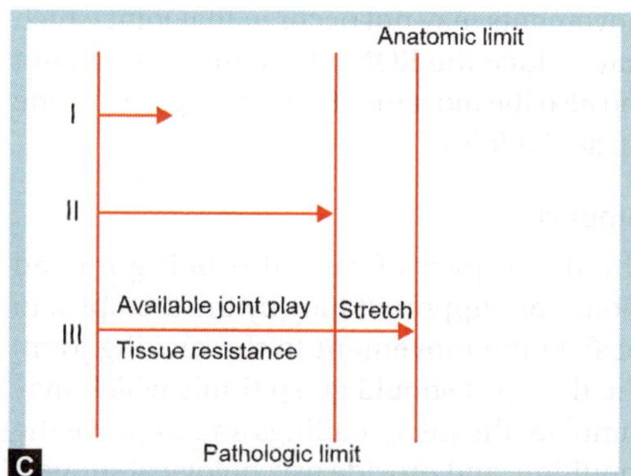


**Figs. 10.11B and C:** (B) Oscillatory joint mobilization with gradings (Maitland grades); (C) Sustained stretch mobilization (Kaltenborn's grades).

**Grade V:** Slow, small amplitude, large velocity, thrust movement parallel to the concave joint surface performed to snap the adhesion and up to about to reach the second tissue stop (anatomical limit).

**Uses of Grades of Mobilization**

**Grades I and II:** Reduce pain.

**Grades III and IV:** Reduce the pain, increases the periarticular extensibility, correct the postural faults, breaks the adhesion.

**Grade V:** Reduces the locked facets and breaks the adhesion.

The rhythmical oscillatory movements are categorized into three types such as:

1. Slow: 1 oscillation for 2 seconds, i.e., 30 oscillations per minute are given. This is selected for more acute conditions.
2. Medium: 1 oscillation per second, i.e., 60 oscillations per minute.
3. Fast: In this 2 oscillations are given in a second, for about 1 minute, which are used for more chronic conditions.

Traction mobilization is given for 10 seconds followed by rest period of several seconds. Normally, the mobilization can be performed combined with the other modalities like wax bath, hot water fomentation, massage, Infrared, ultrasound, etc.

### *3. Sustained Stretch Mobilization (Kaltenborn's Technique) (Fig. 10.11C)*

The three grades described by Kaltenborn are:

**Grade I (Loosen):** Small amplitude at the beginning of the ROM. Neutralizes pressure in joint without actual joint surface separation. Helps to reduce pain.

**Grade II (Tighten/taking up the slack):** Large amplitude movement up to tissue resistance. Separates articulating surfaces, taking up the slack. Used initially to determine joint sensitivity.

**Grade III (Stretch):** Large amplitude movement, into resistance. Stretches the soft tissues surrounding joints. Increases mobility in hypomobile joints.

**Clinical reasoning for joint dysfunction:** Identification, classification of joint dysfunction and selection of intervention are shown in **Table 10.9**.

## Mobilization Procedures for Individual Joints

### *Sternoclavicular Joint (Fig. 10.12)*

**Type**

Synovial joint.

**Variety**

Saddle variety.

**Table 10.9:** Clinical reasoning for joint dysfunction.

| *Cause of limited motion* | *Identification* | *Treatment intervention* |
|---|---|---|
| Intra-articular adhesion/ pericapsular stiffness | • ROM unaffected by proximal or distal joint positioning<br>• Capsular end feel | Graded mobilization |
| Shortened extra-articular muscle groups | ROM affected by proximal or distal joint positioning | Stretching |
| Muscle weakness | ROM affected by gravity | Strengthening |
| Pain | Empty end feel | Modalities<br>Grades: I, II mobilization |
| Nerve root adhesion | Neural tension test | Neural mobilization |
| Soft tissue restriction | Palpation | Soft tissue mobilization |

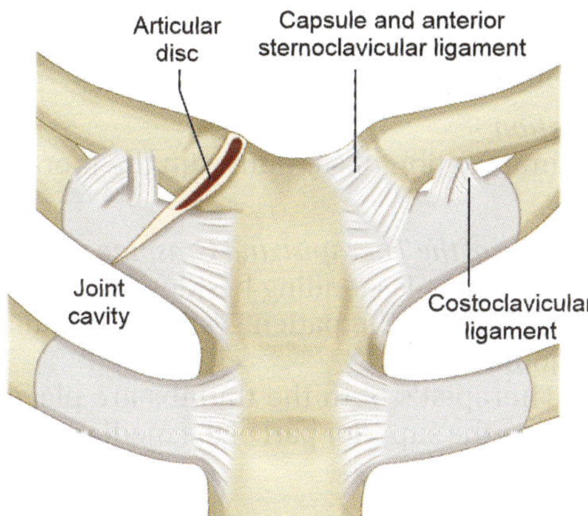


**Fig. 10.12:** Sternoclavicular joint.

## Articular Surface

- ❖ Medial end of clavicle (concavoconvex)
- ❖ Clavicular notch of the manubrium sternum)

*Ligaments*

- ❖ Anterior sternoclavicular ligament.
- ❖ Posterior sternoclavicular ligament.
- ❖ Interclavicular ligament
- ❖ Costoclavicular ligament.

*Osteokinematics*

- ❖ Elevation of the shoulders—shrugging the shoulders or abducting the arm over 90°
- ❖ Depression of the shoulders—drooping the shoulders or extending the arm at the shoulder behind the body
- ❖ Protraction—the lateral end of the clavicle moves anteriorly
- ❖ Retraction—the lateral end of the clavicle moves posteriorly

## Muscles Responsible

*Elevation*

- ❖ Trapezius (middle fibers)
- ❖ Levator scapulae
- ❖ Rhomboidus major, minor.

*Depression*

- ❖ Latissimus dorsi, pectoralis major
- ❖ Serratus anterior, pectoralis minor
- ❖ Subclavius.

*Protraction*

Serratus anterior, pectoralic major and minor.

*Retraction*

Trapezius, rhomboidus major, minor.

*Arthrokinematics*

Arthrokinematics relations with the osteokinematics movements are:

- ❖ Elevation—caudal gliding
- ❖ Depression—cranial gliding
- ❖ Protraction—ventral gliding
- ❖ Retraction—dorsal gliding.

## Positions

*Starting position*

Clavicle lies in horizontal position.

*Resting positing*

Clavicle lies in horizontal position.

*Close packed position*

Full elevated position.

*Capsular pattern*

In full elevation it is restricted.

**Cranial Gliding (Fig. 10.13)**

*Goal*

- ❖ To increase the joint play movement of the sternoclavicular joint.
- ❖ To reduce the pain around the sternoclavicular joint.
- ❖ To increase the depression movement of the shoulder.

*Position of the Patient*

Supine lying.

*Fixation*

Natural fixation of sternum with the thoracic cage.

*Position of the Therapist and Grasping*

- ❖ Therapist is standing besides the patient and facing the patient's sternoclavicular joint.
- ❖ Therapist's both the thumbs are placed below the medial end of the clavicle.

*Procedure*

Therapist's both the thumbs are gliding the clavicle in the cranial direction.

**Caudal Gliding (Fig. 10.14)**

*Goal*

- ❖ To increase the joint play movement of the sternoclavicular joint.
- ❖ To reduce the pain around the sternoclavicular joint.

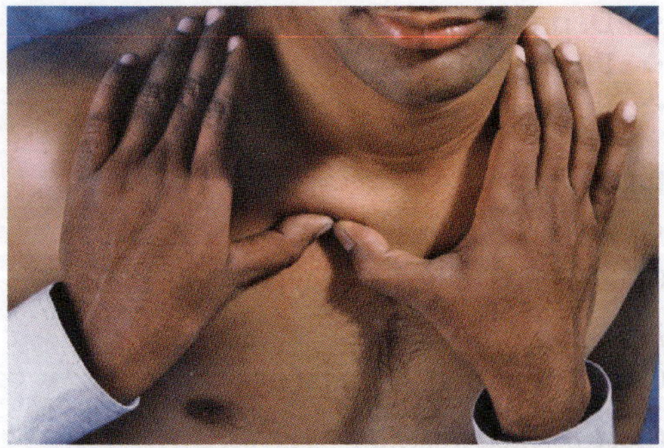

**Fig. 10.13:** Sternoclavicular joint cranial gliding.

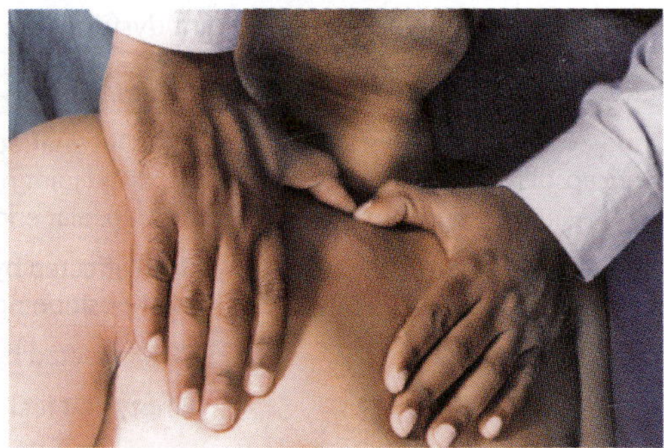

**Fig. 10.14:** Sternoclavicular joint caudal gliding.

- ❖ To increase the elevation movement of the shoulder.

*Position of the Patient*

Supine lying.

*Fixation*

Natural fixation of sternum with the thoracic cage.

*Position of the Therapist and Grasping*

- ❖ Therapist is standing besides the patient and facing the patient's sternoclavicular joint.
- ❖ Therapist's both the thumbs are placed over the superior part of the medial end of the clavicle.

*Procedure*

Therapist's both the thumbs glide the clavicle in the caudal direction.

**Ventral Gliding (Fig. 10.15)**

*Goal*

- ❖ To increase the joint play movement of the sternoclavicular joint.
- ❖ To reduce the pain around the sternoclavicular joint.
- ❖ To increase the protraction movement of the shoulder.

*Position of the Patient*

Supine lying.

*Fixation*

Therapist's right hand fixes the sternum.

*Position of the Therapist and Grasping*

- ❖ Therapist is stands besides the patient and faces the patient's sternoclavicular joint.

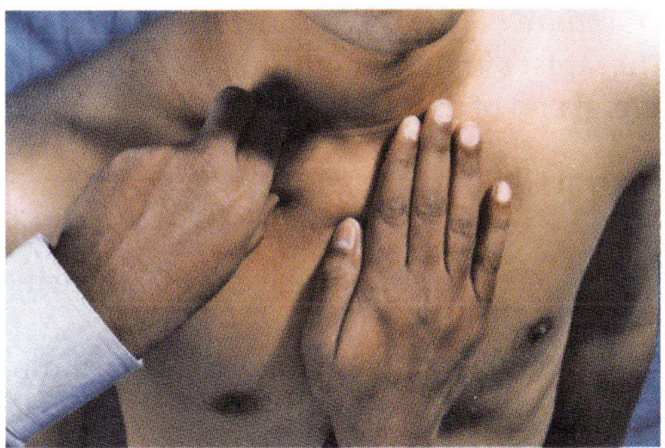

Fig. 10.15: Sternoclavicular joint ventral gliding.

- Therapist's left hand is grasps the medial two-thirds of clavicle with the thumb below and the fingers up.

*Procedure*

Therapist's left hand pulls the clavicle up and glides anteriorly.

### Dorsal Gliding (Fig. 10.16)

*Goal*

- To increase the joint play movement of the sternoclavicular joint.
- To reduce the pain around the sternoclavicular joint.
- To increase the retraction movement of the shoulder girdle.

*Position of the Patient*

Supine lying.

*Fixation*

Natural fixation of sternum with the thoracic cage.

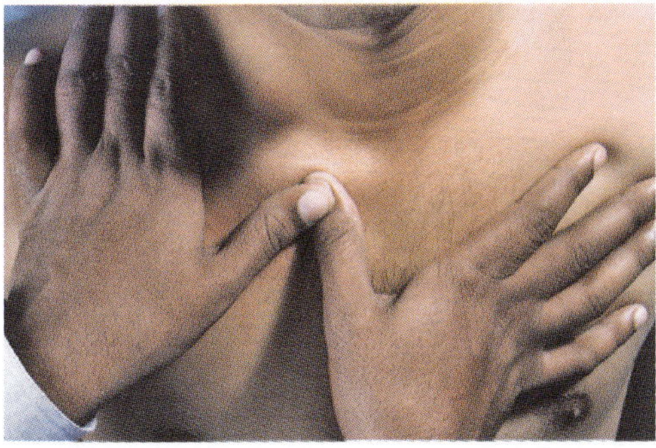

Fig. 10.16: Sternoclavicular joint dorsal gliding.

*Position of the Therapist and Grasping*

- Therapist stands besides the patient and faces the patient's sternoclavicular joint.
- Therapist's both the thumbs are placed over the anterior part of the medial end of the clavicle.

*Procedure*

Therapist's thumbs apply pressure over the anterior part of the medial end of the clavicle and posteriorly glide the clavicle.

## *Acromioclavicular Joint (Fig. 10.17)*

**Type:** Plane type of synovial joint.

### Articular surfaces

- Lateral end of clavicle (flat)
- Medial margin of the acromion process of scapula (flat).

### Ligaments

- Acromioclavicular ligament
- Coracoclavicular ligament.

### Movements

- **Osteokinematics:** As said in sternoclavicular joint.
- **Arthrokinematics:** Arthrokinematics relation with the osteokinematics.
- Elevation—dorsal gliding
- Depression—ventral gliding

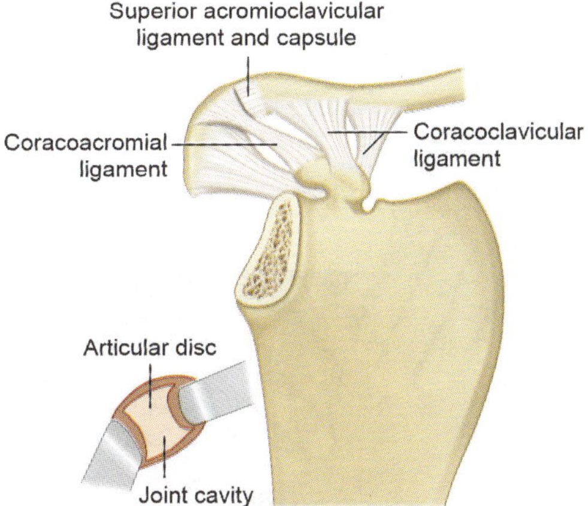


Fig. 10.17: Acromioclavicular joint.

**Position**

- **Starting position:** Clavicle lies in horizontal position.
- **Resting position:** Clavicle lies in horizontal position.
- **Close packed position:** 90° abduction of the shoulder.
- **Capsular pattern of limitation:** Full elevation of shoulder girdle is limited.

**Dorsal Gliding (Fig. 10.18)**

*Goal*

- To increase the joint play movement of the acromioclavicular joint.
- To reduce the pain around the acromio-clavicular joint.
- To increase the elevation movement of the shoulder.

*Position of the Patient*

Sitting.

*Fixation*

Therapist's left hand grasps the shoulder and the acromion process with thumb anteriorly and the fingers posteriorly.

*Position of the Therapist and Grasping*

- Therapist is standing in front of the patient and facing the patient's acromioclavicular joint.
- Therapist's right hand thumb is placed over the lateral end of the anterolateral aspect of the clavicle.

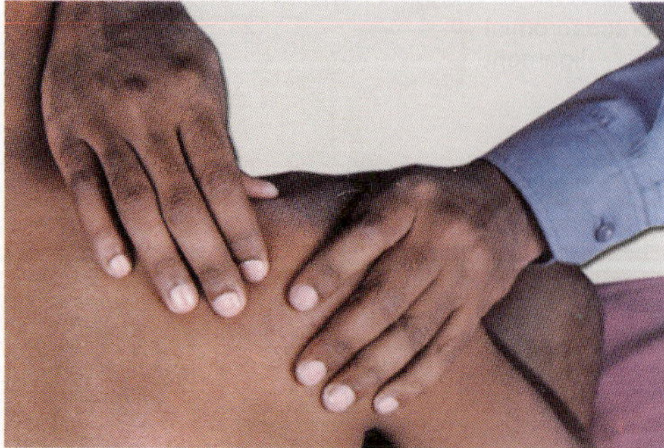

**Fig. 10.18:** Acromioclavicular joint dorsal gliding.

*Procedure*

Therapist's right hand thumb is gliding the lateral end of the clavicle posteriorly.

**Ventral Gliding (Fig. 10.19)**

*Goal*

- To increase the joint play movement of the acromioclavicular joint.
- To reduce the pain around the acromio-clavicular joint.
- To increase the depression movement of the shoulder.

*Position of the Patient*

Sitting.

*Fixation*

Therapist's right hand grasps the shoulder and the acromion process.

*Position of the Therapist and Grasping*

- Therapist is stands back to the patient and faces the patient's acromioclavicular joint.
- Therapist's left hand thumb is placed over the later end of the posterior aspect of the clavicle with the fingers in the anterior grasping.

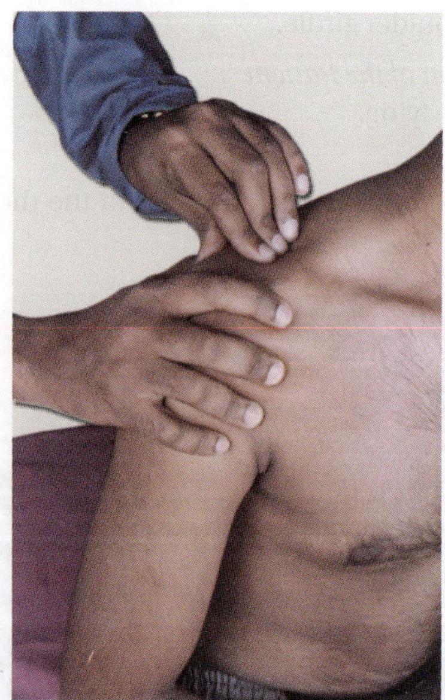

**Fig. 10.19:** Acromioclavicular joint ventral gliding.

*Procedure*
Therapist's left hand thumb glides the lateral end of the clavicle anteriorly.

## *Scapulothoracic Joint*

### Type

Fibrous joint

### Articular surface

- ❖ Anterior surface of the scapula.
- ❖ Posterior portion of the ribs.

### Ligaments

None.

### Movements

**Osteokinematics:** As said in sternoclavicular joint.

### Arthrokinematics

- ❖ Elevation—cranial gliding, lateral gliding
- ❖ Depression—caudal gliding, medial gliding
- ❖ Protraction—lateral gliding
- ❖ Retraction—medial gliding
- ❖ Medial rotation—caudal gliding, medial gliding
- ❖ Lateral rotation—cranial gliding, lateral gliding.

### Position

- ❖ **Starting position:** Clavicle is in horizontal position.
- ❖ **Resting position:** Clavicle is in horizontal position and scapula is positioned from 2 to 7 ribs.
- ❖ **Close packed position:** None.
- ❖ **Capsular pattern:** None.

### Distraction (Fig. 10.20)

*Goal*
- ❖ To increase the joint play movement of the scapulothoracic joint.
- ❖ To reduce the pain around the scapulothoracic joint.

*Position of the Patient*
Side lying, facing the therapist.

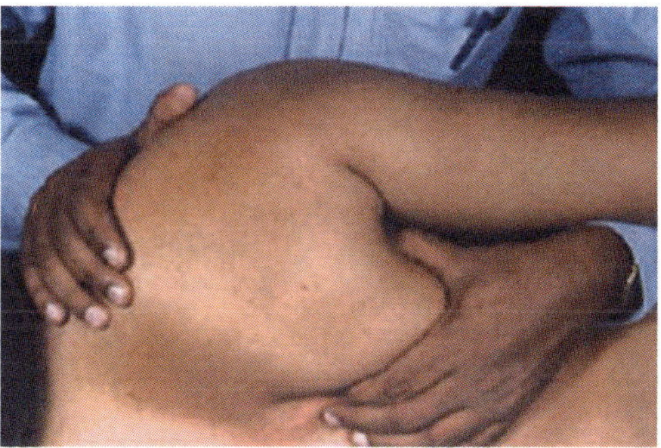

**Fig. 10.20:** Scapulothoracic joint distraction.

*Fixation*
Therapist's right hand fixes the acromioclavicular joint.

*Support*
Patient's upper limb rests on the therapist's left forearm.

*Position of the Therapist and Grasping*
- ❖ Therapist is stands in front of the patient and faces the scapulothoracic joint.
- ❖ Therapist's right hand fixes the acromioclavicular joint.
- ❖ Therapist's right hand grasps the inferior angle of the scapula.

*Procedure*
Therapist's left hand pulls the scapula from the rib.

### Cranial Gliding (Fig. 10.21)

*Goal*
- ❖ To increase the joint play movement of the scapulothoracic joint.
- ❖ To reduce the pain around the scapulothoracic joint.
- ❖ To increase the scapular elevation and lateral rotation.

*Position of the Patient*
Side lying.

*Fixation*
Therapist's left hand fixing the acromioclavicular joint.

*Support*
Patient's upper limb is resting on the therapist's left forearm.

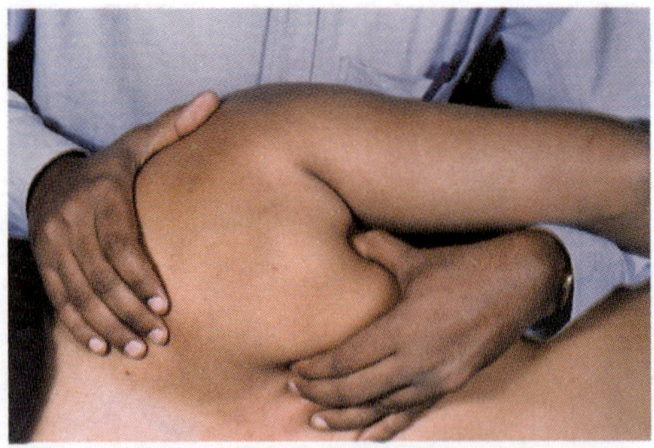

**Fig. 10.21:** Scapulothoracic joint cranial gliding.

*Position of the Therapist and Grasping*

- ❖ Therapist stands in front of the patient and facing the scapulothoracic joint.
- ❖ Therapist's right hand fixies the acromio-clavicular joint.
- ❖ Therapist's left hand grasps the inferior angle of the scapula.

*Procedure*

Therapist's left hand performs the cranial gliding with the distraction.

**Caudal Gliding (Fig. 10.22)**

*Goal*

- ❖ To increase the joint play movement of the scapulothoracic joint.
- ❖ To reduce the pain around the scapulo-thoracic joint.
- ❖ To increase the scapular depression and medial rotation.

*Position of the Patient*

Side lying.

*Fixation*

Therapist's left hand fixes the acromioclavicular joint.

*Support*

Patient's upper limb rests on the therapist's left forearm.

*Position of the Therapist and Grasping*

- ❖ Therapist is stands in front of the patient and faces the scapulothoracic joint.
- ❖ Therapist's right hand fixes the acromio-clavicular joint.
- ❖ Therapist's left hand grasps the inferior angle of the scapula.

*Procedure*

Therapist's right hand performs the caudal gliding of the scapulothoracic joint.

**Medial Gliding (Fig. 10.23)**

*Goal*

- ❖ To increase the joint play movement of the scapulothoracic joint.
- ❖ To reduce the pain around the scapulo-thoracic joint.
- ❖ To increase the scapular retraction, medial rotation and depression.

*Position of the Patient*

Side lying.

*Fixation*

No need of the fixation for this technique.

*Support*

Patient's upper limb rests on the therapist's left forearm.

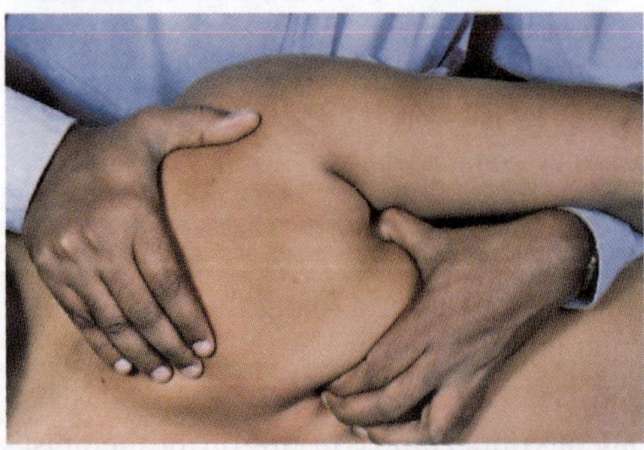

**Fig. 10.22:** Scapulothoracic joint caudal gliding.

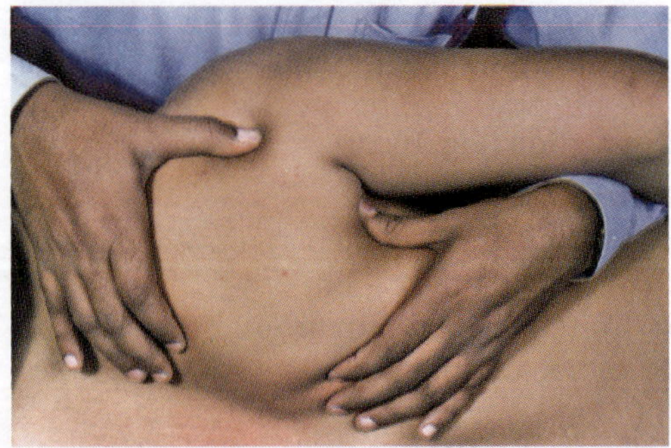

**Fig. 10.23:** Scapulothoracic joint medial gliding.

*Position of the Therapist and Grasping*

Therapist's both the hands are placed over the lateral border of the scapula one over the acromion process and another over the inferior angle of the scapula.

*Procedure*

Therapist's both hands glide the scapula in medial direction.

**Lateral Gliding (Fig. 10.24)**

*Goal*

- ❖ To increase the joint play movement of the scapulothoracic joint.
- ❖ To reduce the pain around the scapulothoracic joint.
- ❖ To increase the scapular protraction, elevation and lateral rotation.

*Position of the Patient*

Side lying.

*Fixation*

No need of the fixation for this technique.

*Support*

Patient's upper limb is resting on the therapist's left forearm.

*Position of the Therapist and Grasping*

- ❖ Therapist stands in front of the patient facing the scapulothoracic joint.
- ❖ Therapist's both hands and fingers are placed over the medial border of the scapula in spreader manner and the thumbs are placed over the lateral border.

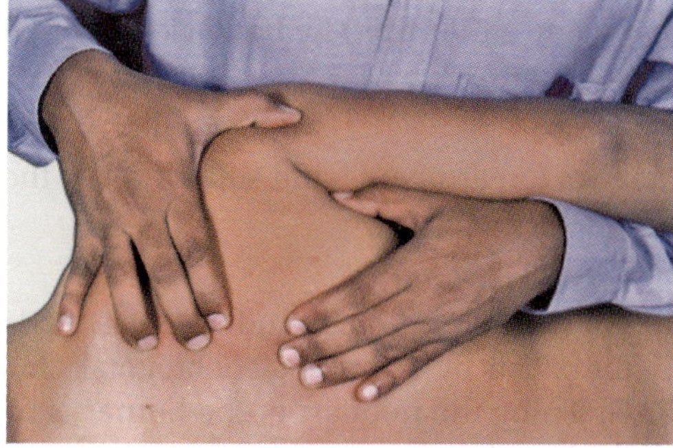

**Fig. 10.24:** Scapulothoracic joint lateral gliding.

*Procedure*

Therapist's both the hands glide the scapula in lateral direction.

### *Shoulder Joint (Figs. 10.25A and B)*

**Type**

Synovial joint—ball and socket type (spheroid).

**Articular surfaces:**

- ❖ Glenoid cavity of scapula (concave)
- ❖ Head of humerus (convex).

**Ligaments:**

- ❖ Superior glenohumeral ligament
- ❖ Middle glenohumeral ligament
- ❖ Inferior glenohumeral ligament
- ❖ Coracohumeral ligament
- ❖ Transverse humeral ligament
- ❖ Coracoacromial ligament.

**Arthrokinematic:** Arthrokinematic relations with the osteokinematics movements are:

- ❖ Abduction—inferior gliding, superior rolling
- ❖ Flexion—posterior gliding, anterior rolling
- ❖ Extension—anterior gliding, posterior rolling
- ❖ Adduction—superior gliding, interior rolling.

While convex surface moves on concave surface, rolling occurs towards the angular movements and the gliding will be opposite to the angular motion.

**Range of Motion (ROM)**

Refer **Table 10.10**.

*Positions*

I. **Starting position:** Upper limb hanging parallel to the trunk with elbow in extension.
   **Movements and muscles responsible (Table 10.11)**
   **Osteokinematics:**
II. **Resting/loose packed position:** Slightly abduction of the shoulder (35–55°).
III. **Close packed position:** Extreme abduction and lateral rotation.

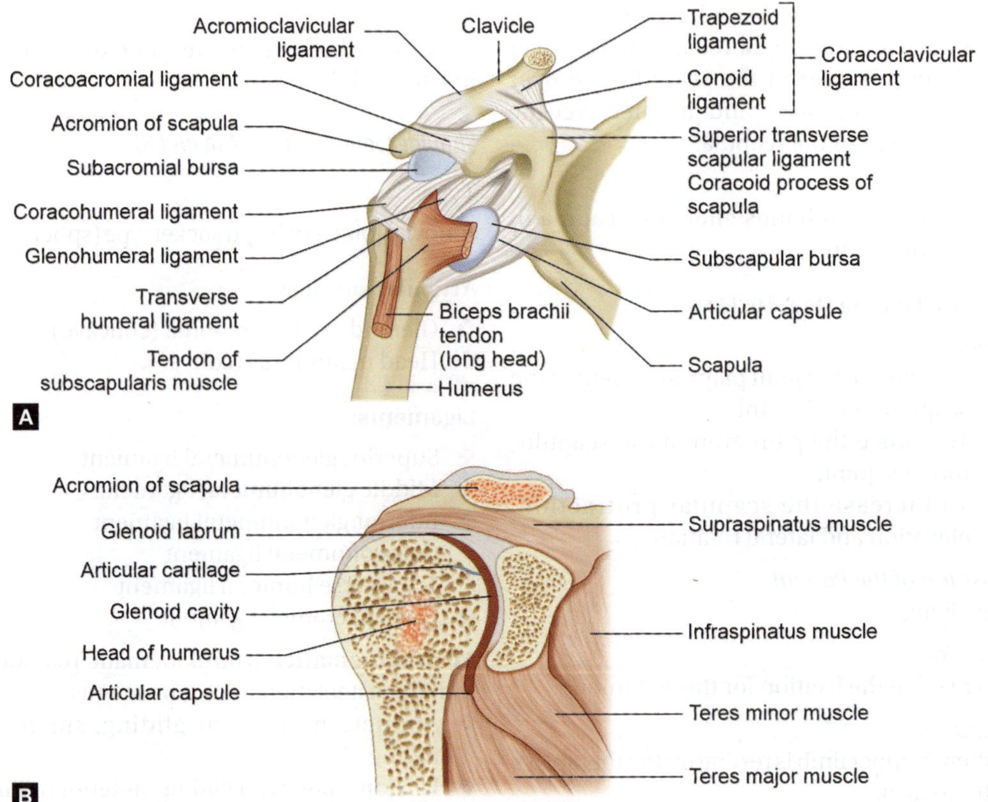


**Figs. 10.25A and B:** Shoulder joint. joint: (A) Diagram of shoulder joint anterior view; (B) Sagittal section of shoulder joint.

**Table 10.10:** Shows the ROM of shoulder joint.

| | |
|---|---|
| Flexion | 0–180° (150–180°) |
| Extension | 0–45° (40–60°) |
| Abduction | 0–180° (150–180°) |
| Adduction | 0° |
| Hyperadduction | 0–35° (25–35°) |
| Internal rotation | 0–90° (70–90°) |
| External rotation | 0–90° (80–90°) |

**IV. Capsular pattern:** Lateral rotation → abduction → medial rotation.

### Distraction of Shoulder (Fig. 10.26)

*Goal*

- ❖ To increase the joint play movements in the glenohumeral joint.
- ❖ To break the adhesion formation.
- ❖ To increase the joint space to improve joint play.

*Position of the Patient*

Supine lying with shoulder adducted.

*Fixation*

Scapula is either fixed by body weight or by an assistant.

*Support*

Patient's forearm and hand supported by the therapist's forearm.

*Therapist's Position*

- ❖ Walk standing position and standing beside the patient by facing the glenohumeral joint.
- ❖ Grasping the midpart of the humerus by the both hands.

**Table 10.11:** Muscles responsible for shoulder movement.

| Sl. No | Movement | Muscle responsible for |
|---|---|---|
| 1. | Flexion | • Clavicular head of pectorals major<br>• Anterior fibers of deltoid<br>• Biceps<br>• Coracobrachialis |
| 2. | Extension | • Latissimus dorsi<br>• Teres major<br>• Triceps<br>• Posterior fibers of deltoid |
| 3. | Abduction | • Supraspinatus (initiations of abduction 0–15°)<br>• Middle fibers of deltoid (15–90°)<br>• Upper trapezius and serratus anterior for final degree of abduction (90–180°) |
| 4. | Adduction | • Latissimus dorsi<br>• Teres major<br>• Coracobrachialis<br>• Pectoralis major<br>• Subscapularis |
| 5. | Medial rotation | • Anterior fibers of deltoid<br>• Teres major<br>• Pectoralis major<br>• Subscapularis<br>• Latissimus dorsi |
| 6. | Lateral rotation | • Posterior fibers of deltoid<br>• Teres minor<br>• Infraspinatus |
| 7. | Circumduction | Combination of all the muscle |

- ❖ Therapist's right hand placed up and the left hand down.

*Procedure*

Articular surfaces are pulled apart by the therapist's right hand.

**Caudal Gliding/Traction (Fig. 10.27)**

*Goal*

- ❖ To increase joint play movements.
- ❖ To improve the abduction ROM.

*Position of the Patient*

Supine lying and the shoulder in adducted position.

*Fixation*

Scapula is fixed by body weight or some assistant.

*Support*

Distal part to the mobilizing joint is supported by the therapist's forearm or positioning the patient's forearm and hand between the therapist's upper arm and trunk.

*Therapist's Position*

- ❖ Standing side to the patient, facing the glenohumeral joint.
- ❖ Grasping the upper part of the humerus by both the hands.

*Procedure*

Therapist's right hand performing traction and the caudal gliding.

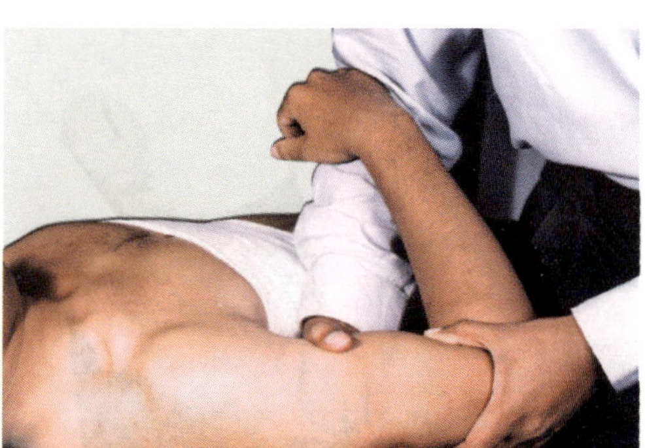

**Fig. 10.26:** Shoulder joint distraction.

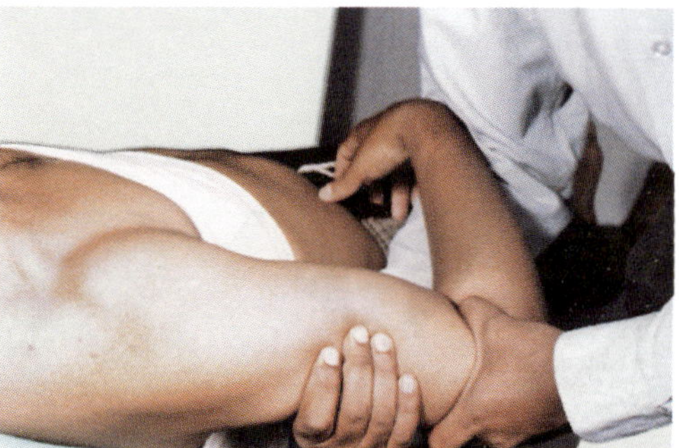

**Fig. 10.27:** Shoulder joint caudal gliding/traction.

## Caudal Gliding (Progression) (Fig. 10.28)

*Goal*

- To improve joint play movements.
- To increase abduction ROM from the available range.

*Position of the Patient*

Supine lying and the mobilizing glenohumeral joint kept in available abduction range.

*Fixation*

Scapular movement is restricted by the body weight or by some assistant.

*Support*

The patient's forearm and the hand is placed between the therapist's upper arm and trunk.

*Therapist's position*

- Therapist standing behind the abducted or mobilizing glenohumeral joint.
- Therapist's left hand with the web space, positioned over the patient's upper part of the humerus.
- Therapist's right hand is placed over the distal part of the humerus.

*Mobilizing Force*

- Traction applied by the right hand of the therapist.
- Caudal gliding is done by the web space of the left hand of the therapist.

*Note:* Progression is achieved by the mobilizing (gliding) the joint in the available range.

## Dorsal Gliding (Fig. 10.29)

*Goal*

- To improve joint play movements.
- To increase the flexion and internal rotation ROM of the glenohumeral joint.

*Position of the Patient*

Supine lying with the mobilized glenohumeral joint is slightly abducted and placed in the end of the couch. A pad of towel is placed under the scapula.

*Fixation*

Scapular movements are restricted by body weight or by one assistant.

*Support*

The patient's forearm and hand rests on the therapist's forearm.

*Therapist's Position and Grasp*

- Therapist stands beside the patient by facing the glenohumeral joint.
- Therapist's right palm of the hand is positioned on the upper part of the humerus.
- Therapist's left hand grasps the distal part of the humerus.

*Procedure*

- Traction applied by the therapist's left hand.
- Therapist's right hand glides the humerus in the dorsal direction.

## Dorsal Gliding (Progression) (Fig. 10.30)

*Goal*

- To improve joint play movements.

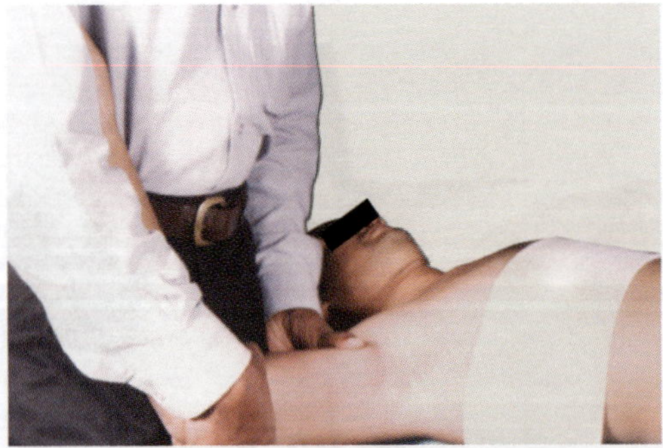

**Fig. 10.28:** Shoulder joint caudal gliding progression.

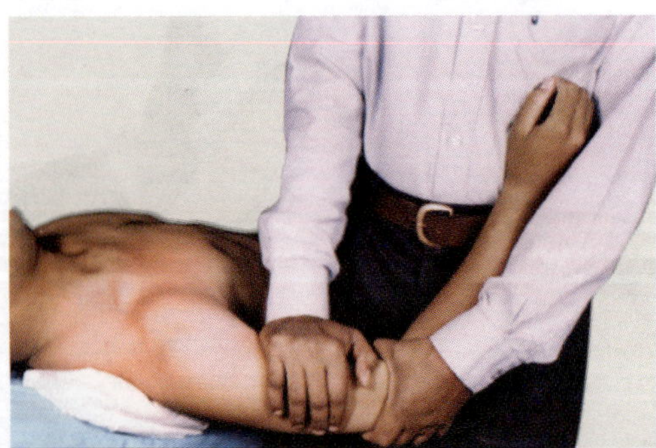

**Fig. 10.29:** Shoulder joint dorsal gliding.

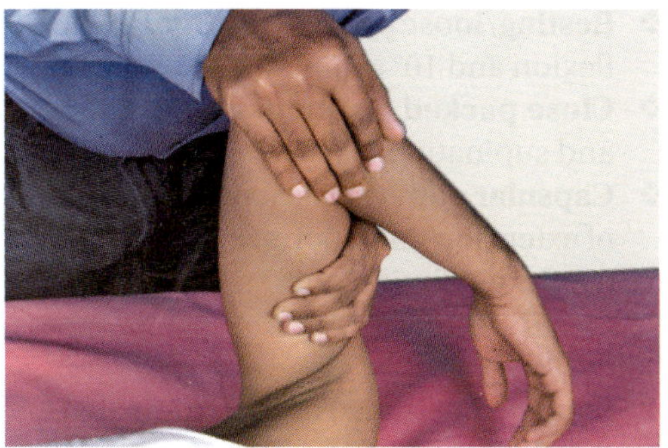

**Fig. 10.30:** Shoulder joint dorsal gliding progression.

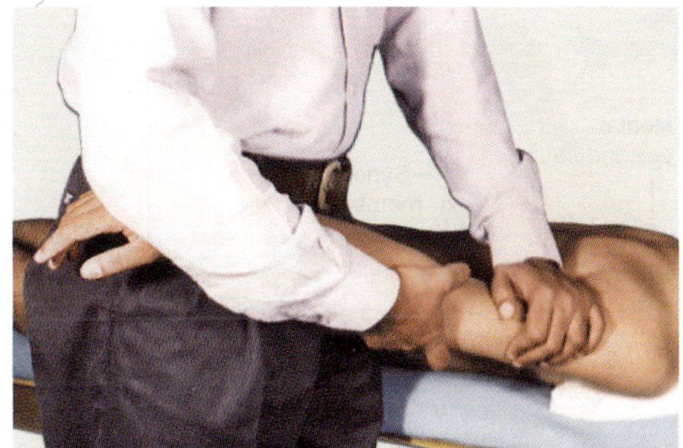

**Fig. 10.31:** Shoulder joint ventral gliding.

- To increase the flexion and internal rotation from the available range.

*Position of the Patient*

Supine lying with the glenohumeral joint in available flexed position.

*Fixation*

Scapular movements are restricted by body weight.

*Support*

Patient's hand is positioned on the chest wall of his own.

*Therapist's Position*

- Therapist stands beside the patient by facing the glenohumeral joint.
- Therapist's right hand is positioned over the olecranon process of the ulna.
- Therapist's left hand is positioned in the middle of the humerus.

*Procedure*

- Distraction is given by the therapist's left hand towards the lateral side.
- Therapist's right hand glides the humerus in the posterior direction.

**Ventral Gliding (Fig. 10.31)**

*Goal*

- To improve joint play movements of the glenohumeral joint.
- To increase the extension and external rotation of the shoulder joint.

*Position of the Patient*

Prone lying with the glenohumeral joint in slightly abducted position and placed in the end of the couch. A fold of towel supports the coracoid process and anterior chest wall.

*Fixation*

Scapular movements are restricted by the body weight.

*Support*

Forearm and the hand of the patient is supported by therapist's forearm and hand.

*Position of the Therapist*

- Standing beside the patient by facing the glenohumeral joint.
- Therapist's right hand is positioned in the middle part of the humerus.
- Therapist's left hand holds the upper part of the arm.

*Mobilizing Force*

- Traction applied by the therapist's right hand.
- Therapist's left hand glides the humerus in the ventral direction.

## *Elbow Joint (Figs. 10.32A and B)*

**Type**

Synovial joint of hinge variety.

**Articular surfaces**

1. Lower end of the humerus (convex)
2. Head of the radius (concave)
3. Upper end of the ulnar (concave).

**Ligaments**

- Ulnar collateral ligament
- Radial collateral ligament.

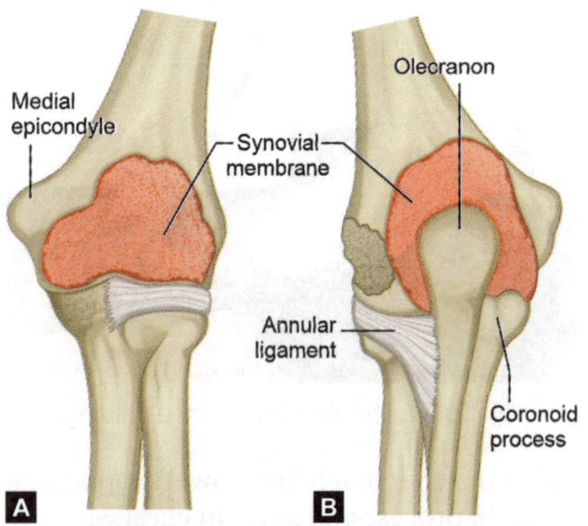


**Figs. 10.32A and B:** (A) Anterior view; (B) Posterior view of elbow joint.

### Movements

*Osteokinematics*

- Flexion—muscles: Biceps brachii, brachialis, brachioradialis.
- Extension—muscles: Triceps, anconeus.

### Arthrokinematics

Arthrokinematics relations with the osteokinematics are:

- **Flexion:** Medial gliding, lateral gliding of ulnohumeral joint and the ventral gliding of the radiohumeral joint.
- **Extension:** Medial gliding, lateral gliding of the ulnohumeral joint and the dorsal gliding of the radiohumeral joint.

### Range of Motion of Elbow Joint

Refer **Table 10.12**.

## *Position*

### Ulnohumeral Joint

- **Starting position:** Forearm supinated and the elbow extended.

**Table 10.12:** ROM of elbow joint.

| *Movement* | *Range of motion* |
|---|---|
| Flexion | 0°–120° to 150° |
| Extension | 0° |

- **Resting/loose packed position:** Elbow 70° flexion and 10° supination.
- **Close packed position:** Elbow extension and supination.
- **Capsular pattern:** Flexion—extension. 10° of extension limitation seen only when the 90° flexion limitation.

### Radiohumeral Joint

- **Starting position:** Forearm supinated and the elbow extended.
- **Resting/loose packed position:** Full extension and supination.
- **Close packed position:** 90° flexion and 5° supination.
- **Capsular pattern:** Flexion and extension. 10° of extension limitation seen when the 90° flexion limitation.

## *Ulnohumeral Joint (Fig. 10.33)*

### Joint Distraction

*Goal*

- To increase the joint play movement of the elbow joint.
- To reduce the pain around the elbow joint.

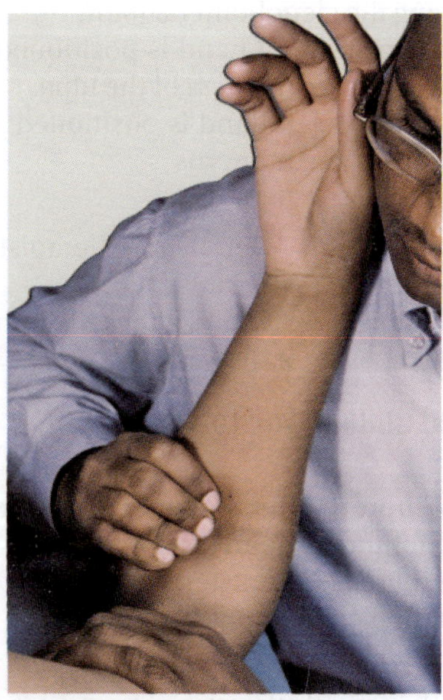

**Fig. 10.33:** Ulnohumeral distraction.

*Position of the Patient*
Supine lying or long sitting and the elbow is positioned in actual resting position.

*Fixation*
Arm of the patient is fixed by the assistant or it may be fixed by the therapist's left hand.

*Support*
Patient's forearm and hand are supported by the therapists shoulder.

*Position of the Therapist and Grasping*
- ❖ Therapist is standing at the side of the bed, stabilizing the arm with the left hand.
- ❖ Therapist's right hand fingers grasp the proximal end of the ulna.

*Procedure*
Therapist's right hand applies long axis distraction force over the patient's elbow in 45° flexion.

**Medial Gliding (Fig. 10.34)**

*Goal*
- ❖ To increase the joint play movement of the ulnohumeral joint.
- ❖ To reduce the pain around the ulnohumeral joint.
- ❖ To increase the elbow extension and flexion of ulnohumeral joint.

*Position of the Patient*
Supine lying'

*Fixation*
Therapist's left hand grasping the distal humerus and restricting the movement over the shoulder joint.

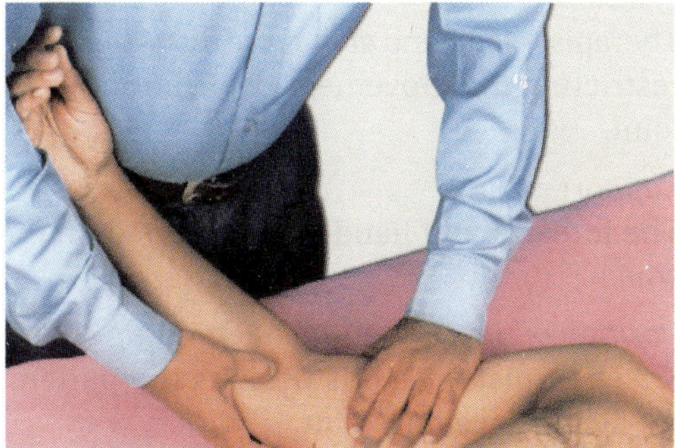

**Fig. 10.34:** Ulnohumeral medial gliding.

*Support*
Patient's forearm and hand are supported by the therapist's forearm.

*Position of the Therapist and Grasping*
- ❖ Therapist is standing besides the patient and facing the elbow joint.
- ❖ Therapist's left hand grasping the distal humerus and restricting the proximal joint motion.
- ❖ Therapist's right hand fingers are placed posteriorly and grasping the olecranon process of ulna and the thumb is placed on proximal part of anterior aspect of the ulna.

*Procedure*
Therapist's right thumb applies distraction force and the fingers grip the olecranon and glides the ulna medially.

**Lateral Gliding (Fig. 10.35)**

*Goal*
- ❖ To increase the joint play movement of the ulnohumeral joint.
- ❖ To reduce the pain around the ulnohumeral joint.
- ❖ To increase the elbow extension and flexion.

*Position of the Patient*
Supine lying.

*Fixation*
Therapist's left hand grasps the distal humerus and restricts the movement over the shoulder joint.

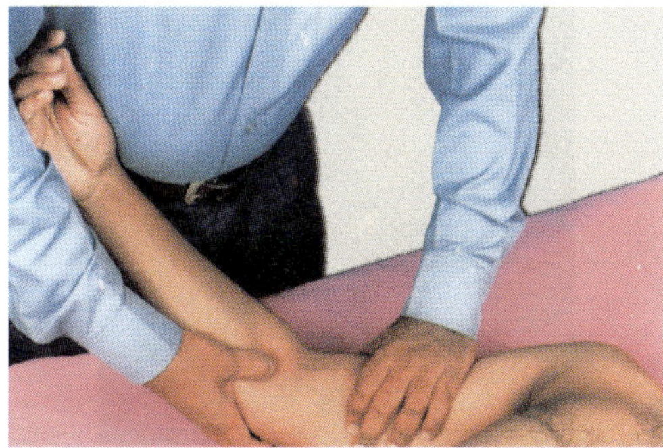

**Fig. 10.35:** Ulnohumeral lateral gliding.

*Support*

Patient's forearm and hand are supported on the therapist's forearm.

*Position of the Therapist and Grasping*

- ❖ Therapist stands besides the patient and faces the elbow joint.
- ❖ Therapist's left hand grasps the distal humerus, restricting the proximal joint motion.
- ❖ Therapist's right hand fingers placed posteriorly and grasping the olecranon process of ulna and the thumb is placed on the proximal part of anterior aspect of the ulna.

*Procedure*

Therapist's right thumb applies the distraction force and the thumb web and fingers perform the lateral gliding of the ulna.

## *Humeroradial Joint (Fig. 10.36)*

### Distraction

*Goal*

- ❖ To increase the joint play movement of the humeroradial joint.
- ❖ To reduce the pain around the humeroradial joint.
- ❖ To increase the elbow extension and flexion.

*Position of the Patient*

Supine lying.

*Fixation*

Therapist's left hand grasps the distal humerus, restricting the movement over the shoulder joint.

*Support*

No need of support for this mobilization.

*Position of the Therapist and Grasping*

- ❖ Therapist is standing besides the patient and facing the elbow joint.
- ❖ Therapist's left hand grasps the distal humerus, restricting the proximal joint motion.
- ❖ Therapist's right hand grasps the lower end of radius.

*Procedure*

Therapist's right hand pulls the radius downwards, applying the distraction force.

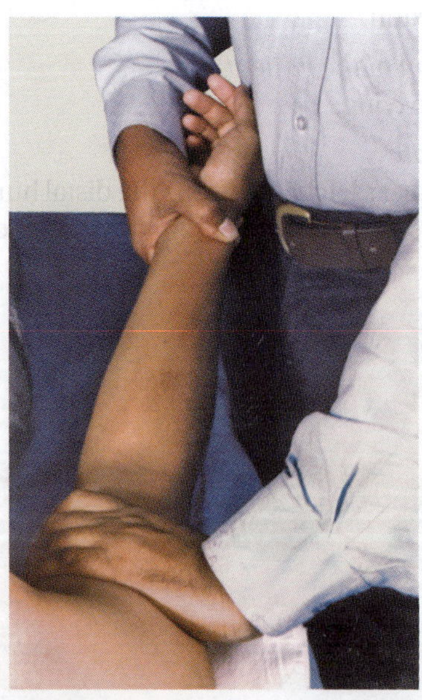

**Fig. 10.36:** Radiohumeral distraction

### Dorsal Gliding (Fig. 10.37A)

*Goal*

- ❖ To increase the joint play movement of the radiohumeral joint.
- ❖ To reduce the pain around the radiohumeral joint.
- ❖ To increase elbow extension ROM.

*Position of the Patient*

Supine lying.

*Fixation*

Therapist's left hand grasps the distal humerus restricting the movement over the shoulder joint.

*Support*

The forearm and hand are supported on the couch.

*Position of the Therapist and Grasping*

- ❖ Therapist is stands besides the patient, facing the elbow joint.

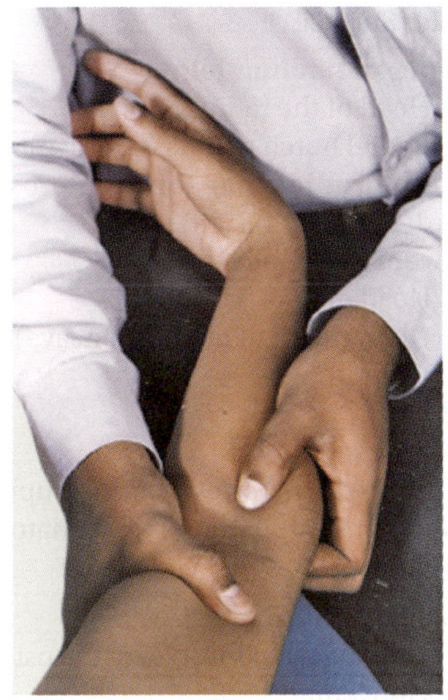

**Fig. 10.37A:** Radiohumeral dorsal gliding.

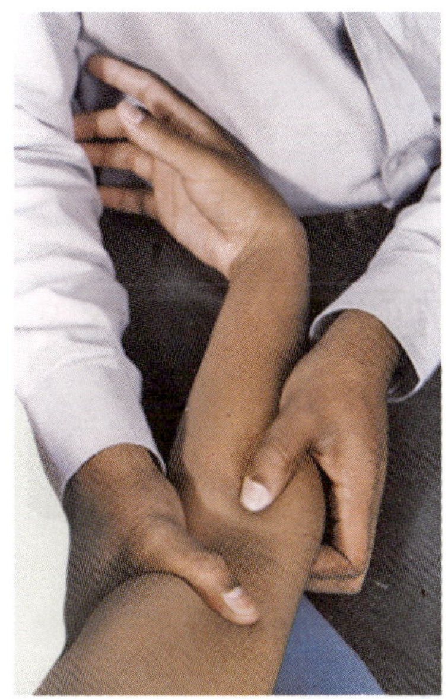

**Fig. 10.37B:** Radiohumeral ventral gliding.

- Therapist's right hand grasps the distal humerus, restricting the proximal joint motion.
- Therapist's left hand grasps the proximal radius with the thumb anteriorly and fingers posteriorly.

*Procedure*

Therapist's left hand glides the radius posteriorly.

**Ventral Gliding (Fig. 10.37B)**

*Goal*

- To increase the joint play movement of the radiohumeral joint.
- To reduce the pain around the radiohumeral joint.
- To increase the elbow flexion ROM.

*Position of the Patient*

Supine lying.

*Fixation*

Therapist's right hand grasps the distal humerus, restricting the movement over the shoulder joint.

*Support*

Patient's forearm and are supported on the couch.

*Position of the Therapist and Grasping*

- Therapist stands besides the patient, facing the elbow joint.
- Therapist's right hand grasps the distal humerus, restricting the proximal joint motion.
- Therapist's left hand grasps the proximal radius with the thumb anteriorly and fingers posteriorly.

*Procedure*

Therapist's left hand glides the radius anteriorly.

**Compression (Fig. 10.38)**

*Goal*

To reduce the positional fault of the radius.

*Position of the Patient*

Supine lying with elbow in 70–90° flexion.

*Fixation*

Therapist's left hand grasps the distal humerus, restricting the movement over the shoulder joint.

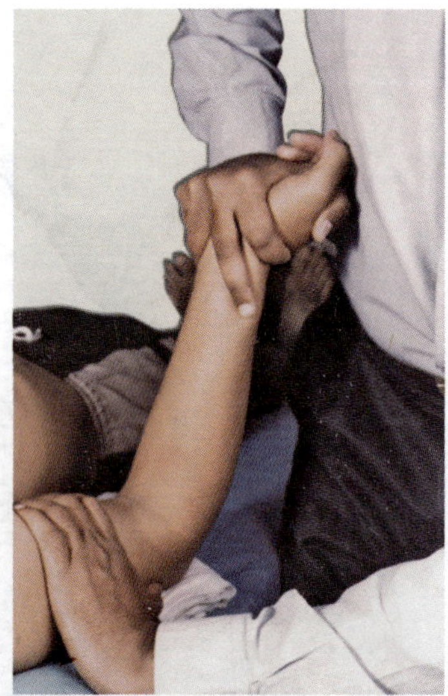

**Fig. 10.38:** Radiohumeral compression.

*Support*

Therapist's right hand grasps the patient's hand and supporting the distal parts.

*Position of the Therapist and Grasping*

- Therapist stands besides the patient, facing the elbow joint.
- Therapist's left hand grasps the distal humerus, restricting the proximal joint motion.
- Therapist's right hand grasps the patient's hand.

*Procedure*

Therapist's right hand applies downward force and compresses the radiohumeral joint through wrist joint.

## *Radioulnar Joint (Fig. 10.39)*

### Types

- Upper radioulnar joint—synovial
- Middle radioulnar joint—fibrous
- Lower radioulnar joint—synovial

### Variety

- Upper radioulnar joint—pivot
- Middle radioulnar joint—syndesmosis
- Lower radioulnar joint—pivot

### Articular Surface

- **Upper radioulnar joint**:
  - Head of the radius (convex)
  - Radial notch of ulna (concave)
- **Middle radioulnar joint:** Interosseous border of the ulna and radius.
- **Lower radioulnar joint:**
  - Head of ulna (convex)
  - Ulnar notch of radius (concave).

### Movements

*Osteokinematics*

- Supination—muscles—biceps, supinator.
- Pronation—pronator teres, pronator quadratus.

*Arthrokinematics*

Arthrokinematics relations with the osteokinematics movements are:

- **Upper radioulnar joint:**
  - Supination—ventral gliding
  - Pronation—dorsal gliding
- **Lower radioulnar joint**
  - Supination—dorsal gliding
  - Pronation—ventral gliding.

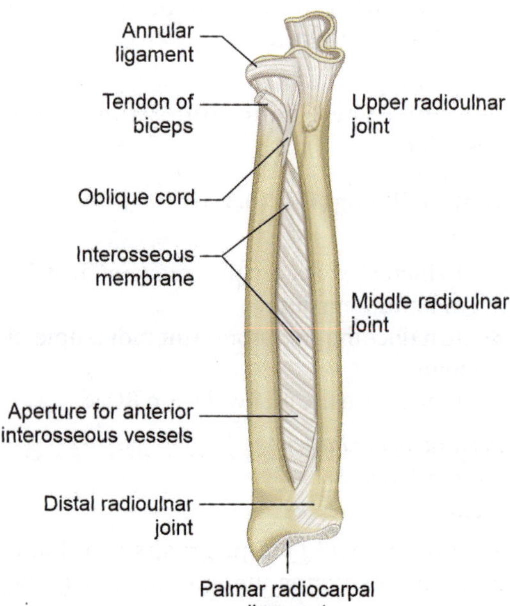


**Fig. 10.39:** Proximal and distal radioulnar joint.

- **Range of motion**
  - Supination—90°
  - Pronation—90°

**Positions**

*Starting Position*

Arm is parallel to the trunk with the elbow at right angle.

*Resting Position*

- Proximal radioulnar joint supination 35°, elbow flexion 70°.
- Distal radioulnar joint supination 10°.

*Close Packed Position*

Proximal radioulnar joint 5° supination.

*Capsular Pattern*

Supination—pronation, equally limited.

## Proximal Radioulnar Joint

### Dorsal Gliding (Fig. 10.40)

*Goal*

- To increase the joint play movement of the proximal radioulnar joint.
- To reduce the pain around the proximal radioulnar joint.
- To increase the pronation of the proximal radioulnar joint.

*Position of the Patient*

Supine lying.

*Fixation*

Proximal ulna is fixed with the right hand of the therapist.

*Support*

Distal part is stabilized by the couch itself.

*Position of the Therapist and Grasping*

- Therapist is stands beside the patient, facing the proximal radioulnar joint.
- Therapist's right hand fixes the proximal ulna of the patient.
- Therapist's left hand grasps the proximal radius of the patient.

*Procedure*

Therapist's left hand glides the radius in the dorsal and ventral direction.

### Ventral Gliding (Fig. 10.41)

*Goal*

- To increase the joint play movement of the proximal radioulnar joint.
- To reduce the pain around the proximal radioulnar joint.
- To increase the supination of the proximal radioulnar joint.

(Dorsal gliding increases pronation and ventral gliding increases the supination.)

*Position of the Patient*

Supine lying or long sitting.

*Fixation*

Proximal ulna is fixed with the left hand of the therapist.

*Support*

Distal part is stabilized by the couch itself.

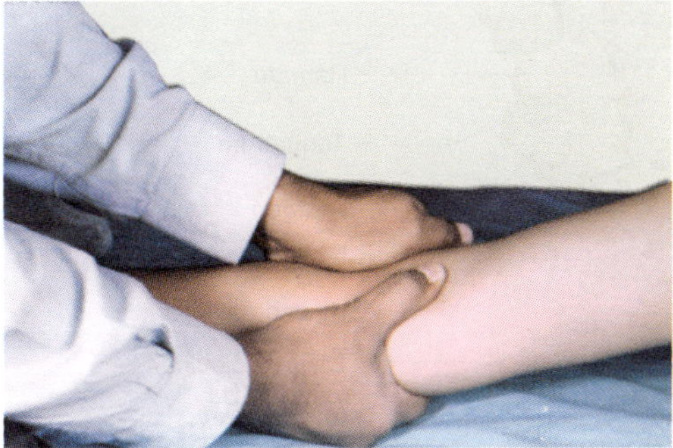

**Fig. 10.40:** Proximal radioulnar joint dorsal gliding.

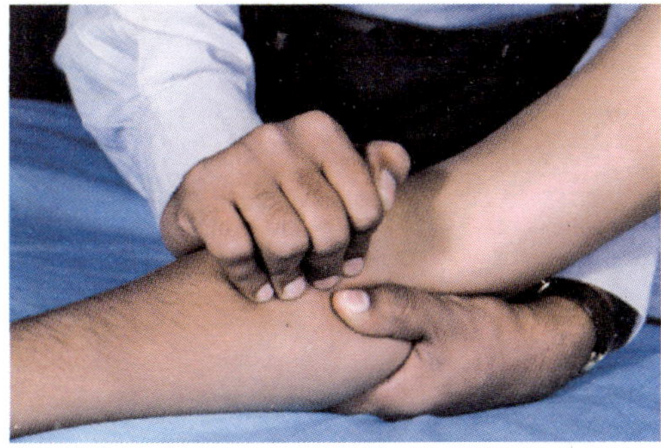

**Fig. 10.41:** Proximal radioulnar joint ventral gliding.

*Position of the Therapist and Grasping*

- ❖ Therapist stands beside the patient, facing the proximal radioulnar joint.
- ❖ Therapist's left hand fixes the proximal ulna of the patient.
- ❖ Therapist's right hand grasps the proximal radius of the patient.

*Procedure*

Therapist's right hand glides the radius in the dorsal and ventral direction.

## *Distal Radioulnar Joint*

### Dorsal and Ventral Gliding (Fig. 10.42)

*Goal*

- ❖ To increase the joint play movement of the distal radioulnar joint.

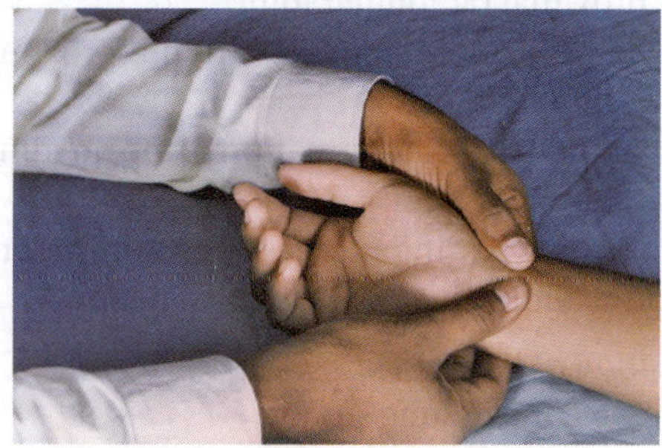

**Fig. 10.42:** Distal radioulnar joint dorsal and ventral gliding.

- ❖ To reduce the pain around the distal radioulnar joint.
- ❖ To increase the supination and pronation of the distal radioulnar joint.

*Position of the Patient*

Supine lying or long sitting.

*Fixation*

Distal ulna is fixed with the right hand of the therapist.

*Support*

The hand is supported on the couch.

*Position of the Therapist and Grasping*

- ❖ Therapist stands besides the patient, facing the proximal radioulnar joint.
- ❖ Therapist's right hand fixes the distal ulna of the patient.
- ❖ Therapist's left hand grasps the distal radius of the patient.

*Procedure*

Therapist's left hand glides the radius in the dorsal and ventral direction.

### Wrist Joint (Fig. 10.43)

*Type*

Synovial joint of ellipsoid/condyloid type.

*Articular Surfaces*

- ❖ Lower end of radius—Proximally (concave)

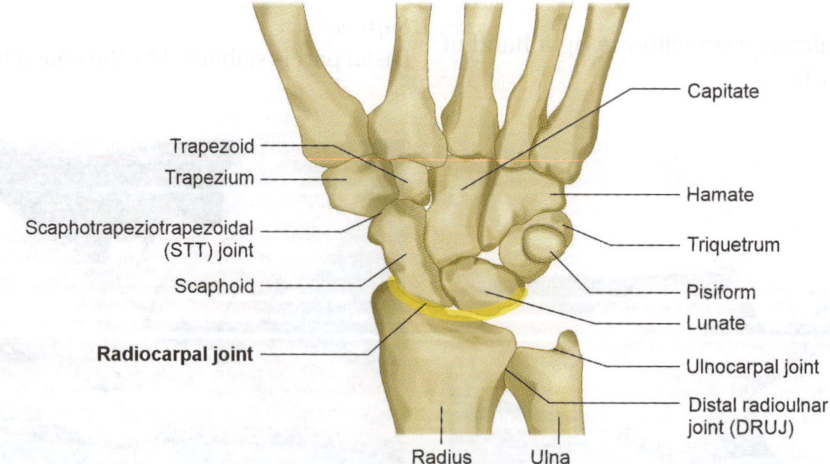


**Fig. 10.43:** Wrist and hand.

- Scaphoid, lunate and triquetral—distally (convex).

**Ligaments**

- Ulnar collateral ligaments
- Radial collateral ligaments
- Palmar ulnocarpal ligaments
- Dorsal radiocarpal ligaments
- Palmar radiocarpal ligaments.

**Movements**

*Osteokinematics*

**Flexion:** Muscles include:

- Flexor carpi radialis
- Flexor carpi ulnaris
- Palmaris longus
- Flexor digitorum profundus
- Flexor digitorum sublimis.
- Flexor pollicis longus.

**Extension:** Muscles include:

- Extensor carpi radialis longus
- Extensor carpi radialis brevis.
- Extensor carpi ulnaris
- Extensor digitorum
- Extensor indicis
- Extensor digiti minimi.
- Extensor pollicis longus.

**Ulnar deviation:** Muscles include:

- Flexion carpi ulnaris
- Extension carpi ulnaris.

**Radial deviation:** Muscles include:

- Flexor carpi radialis
- Extension carpi radialis longus
- Extensor carpi radialis brevis.

**Arthrokinematics**

Arthrokinematics relations with the osteokinematics movements are:

- Flexion—dorsal gliding
- Extension—ventral gliding
- Ulnar deviation—radial gliding
- Radial deviation—ulnar gliding.

**Range of Motion of Wrist Joint**

Refer **Table 10.13**.

**Table 10.13:** ROM of wrist joint.

| *Type of movement* | *Range of motion* |
|---|---|
| Flexion | 70–90° |
| Extension | 60–70° |
| Ulnar deviation | 30–45° |
| Radial deviation | 15–20° |

## *Position for Mobilization*

**Starting position**

Wrist in neutral.

**Resting/loose packed position**

Neutral with slight ulnar deviation.

**Close packed position**

Maximum extension and radial deviation.

**Capsular pattern**

Flexion and extension are equally limited.

**Distraction (Fig. 10.44)**

*Goal*

- To increase the joint play movement of the radiocarpal, ulnocarpal and intercarpal joint.
- To reduce the pain around the radiocarpal, ulnocarpal intercarpal joint.
- To increase the ROM of the radiocarpal, ulnocarpal and intercarpal joints.

*Position of the Patient*

Supine lying/long sitting and the wrist is placed at the side of the couch.

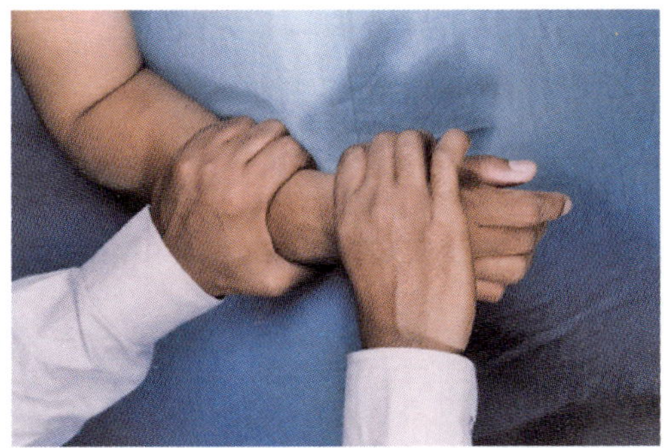

**Fig. 10.44:** Wrist distraction.

*Fixation*

Distal ulna and radius of the patient is fixed with the therapist's left hand.

*Support*

Therapist's right hand grasps the hand region of the patient.

*Position of the Therapist and Grasping*

- Therapist is stands beside the patient, facing the wrist of the patient.
- Therapist's left hand grasp the distal ulna and radius of the patient.
- Therapist's right hand grasps the metacarpal region of the patient.

*Procedure*

Therapist's right hand applies the distraction.

**Ventral Gliding (Fig. 10.45)**

*Goal*

- To increase the joint play movement of the radiocarpal, ulnocarpal and intercarpal joints.
- To reduce the pain around the radiocarpal, ulnocarpal and intercarpal joints.
- To increase wrist extension ROM.

*Position of the Patient*

Supine lying/long sitting and the wrist is placed at the side of the couch.

*Fixation*

Distal ulna and radius of the patient are fixed with the therapist's left hand.

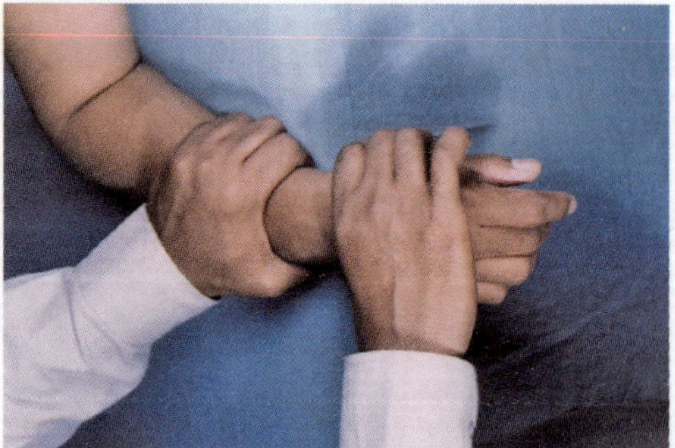

**Fig. 10.45:** Wrist ventral gliding.

*Support*

Therapist's right hand grasps the hand region of the patient.

*Position of the Therapist and Grasping*

- Therapist is stand beside the patient, facing the wrist of the patient.
- Therapist's left hand grasp the distal ulna and radius of the patient.
- Therapist's right hand grasps the metacarpal region of the patient.

*Procedure*

Therapist's right hand performing the ventral gliding of the radiocarpal, ulnocarpal and intercarpal joints.

**Dorsal Gliding (Fig. 10.46)**

*Goal*

- To increase the joint play movement of the radiocarpal, ulnocarpal and intercarpal joints.
- To reduce the pain around the radiocarpal, ulnocarpal and intercarpal joints.
- To increase the wrist flexion ROM.

*Position of the Patient*

Long sitting/supine lying and the wrist is placed at the side end of the couch and the forearm in supinated position.

*Fixation*

Distal ulna and radius of the patient are fixed with the therapist's left hand.

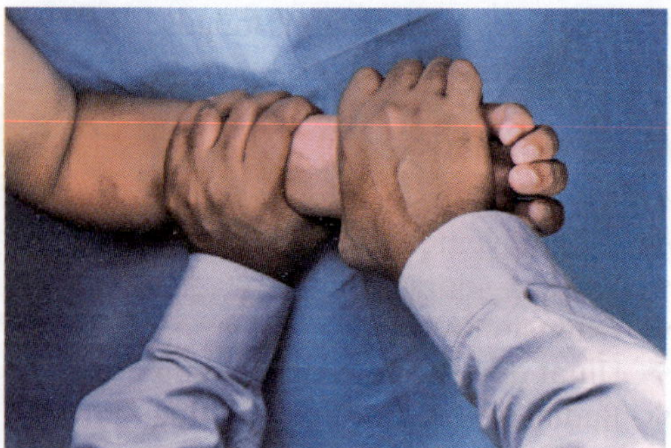

**Fig. 10.46:** Wrist joint dorsal gliding.
(*Note:* The same position as described for ventral gliding, can also be used for dorsal gliding maneuver)

*Support*

Therapist's right hand grasps the hand region of the patient.

*Position of the Therapist and Grasping*

- Therapist is standing beside the patient and facing the wrist of the patient.
- Therapist's left hand grasps the distal ulna and radius of the patient.
- Therapist's right hand grasps the metacarpal region of the patient.

*Procedure*

Therapist's right hand performing the dorsal gliding of the radiocarpal, ulnocarpal and intercarpal joints.

### *Ulnar Gliding (Fig. 10.47)*

*Goal*

- To increase the joint play of the wrist joint.
- To reduce the pain over the wrist.
- To increase the radial deviation of the wrist.

*Position of the Patient*

Long sitting/supine lying and the wrist is placed at the side end of the couch. Patient's forearm in mid-prone position.

*Fixation*

Distal ulna and radius of the patient are fixed with the therapist's left hand.

*Support*

Therapist's right hand grasps the hand region of the patient.

*Position of the Therapist and Grasping*

- Therapist is standing beside the patient and facing the wrist of the patient
- Therapist's left hand grasps the distal ulna and radius of the patient
- Therapist's right hand grasps the metacarpal region of the patient.

*Procedure*

Therapist's right hand glides the wrist in ulnar direction.

### Radial Gliding (Fig. 10.48)

*Goal*

- To increase the joint play of the wrist joint.
- To reduce the pain over the wrist.
- To increase the ulnar deviation of the wrist

*Position of the Patient*

Long sitting/supine lying and the wrist is placed at the side end of the couch. Patient's forearm in mid prone position.

*Fixation*

Distal ulna and radius of the patient are fixed with the therapist's left hand.

*Support*

Therapist's right hand grasps the hand region of the patient.

*Position of the Therapist and Grasping*

- Therapist is standing beside the patient and facing the wrist of the patient.
- Therapist's left hand grasps the distal ulna and radius of the patient.

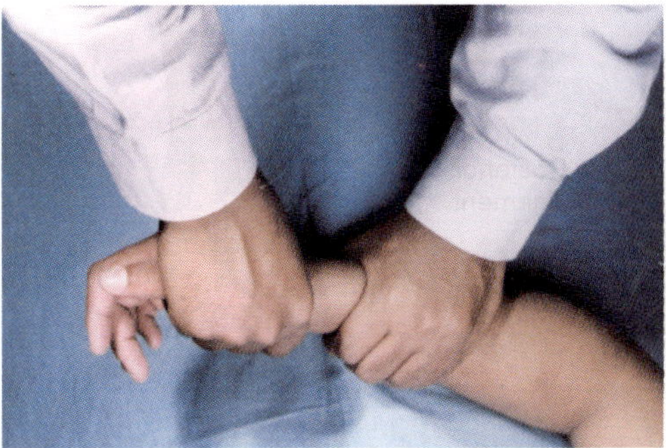

**Fig. 10.47:** Wrist ulnar gliding.

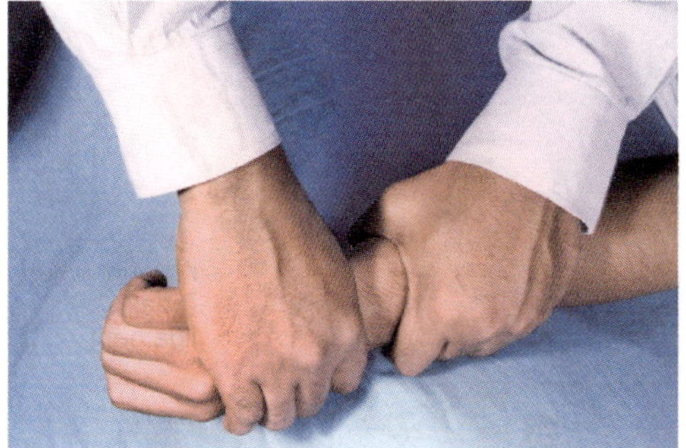

**Fig. 10.48:** Wrist joint radial gliding.

- Therapist's right hand grasps the metacarpal region of the patient.

*Procedure*

Therapist's right hand glides the wrist in the radial direction.

### *Thumb (1st Carpometacarpal Joint)*

**Type**

Synovial joint—saddle type.

**Articular surfaces**

- Trapezium (concavoconvex)
- Proximal part of 1st metacarpal (concavoconvex)

**Ligaments (Figs. 10.49A and B)**

- Capsular ligament
- Posterior oblique ligament.
- Dorsoradial ligament.
- Posterior intermetacarpal ligament.
- Anterior volar (break) ligament.
- Anterior intermetacarpal ligament.

**Movements**

*Osteokinematics*

**Flexion:** Muscles include:

- Flexion pollicis longus and brevis
- Opponens pollicis.

**Extension:** Muscles include:
Extensor pollicis longus and brevis

**Abduction:** Abductor pollicis longus and brevis.

**Adduction:** Adductor pollicis.

**Opposition:** Opponens pollicis.

*Arthrokinematic*

Arthrokinematics relations with the osteokinematics movement are:

- Flexion—ulnar gliding
- Extension—radial gliding
- Abduction—dorsal gliding
- Adduction—ventral gliding.

*Positions*

**Starting position:** Midway between flexion extension and abduction and adduction.

**Resting/loose packed position:** Midway between flexion extension and abduction and adduction.

**Close packed position:** Full opposition.

**Capsular pattern:** Movement is restricted in abduction and extension.

**Distraction (Fig. 10.50)**

*Goal*

- To increase the joint play in 1st carpometacarpal joint.
- To increase the ROM of thumb.

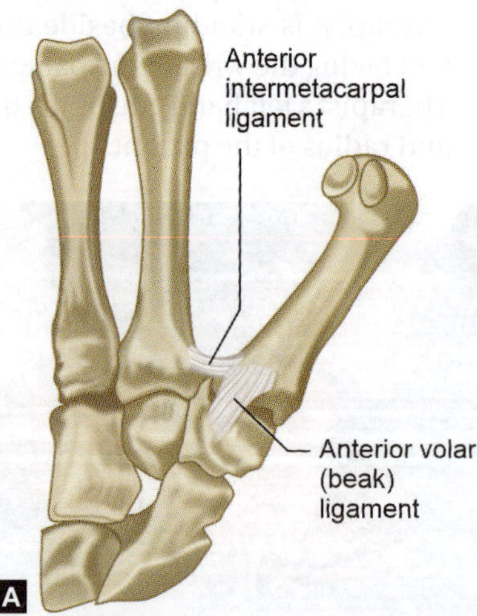


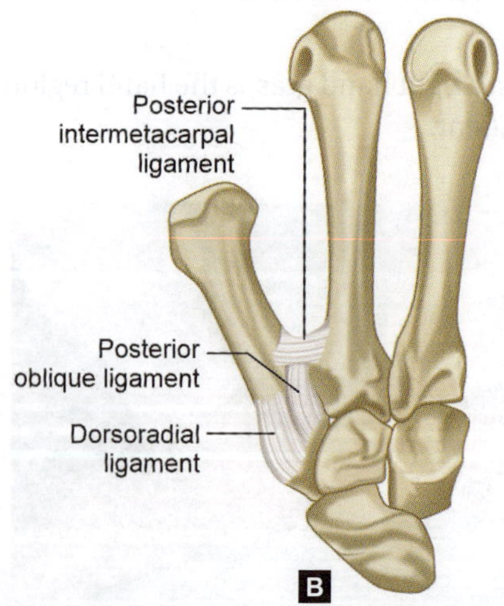


**Figs. 10.49A and B:** Ligaments of carpometacarpal joint of right thumb: (A) Palmar view; (B) Dorsal view.

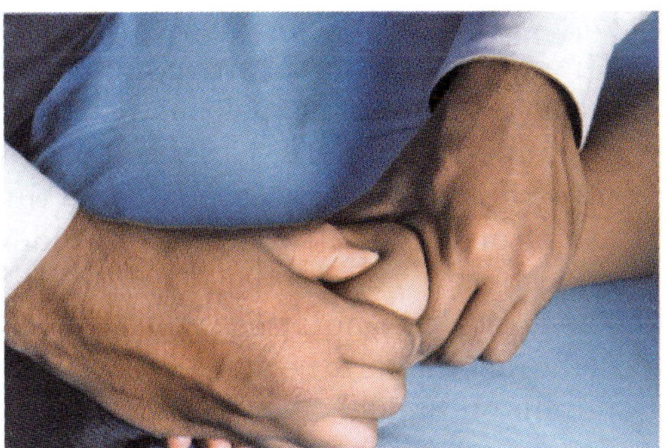

**Fig. 10.50:** Thumb joint—joint distraction.

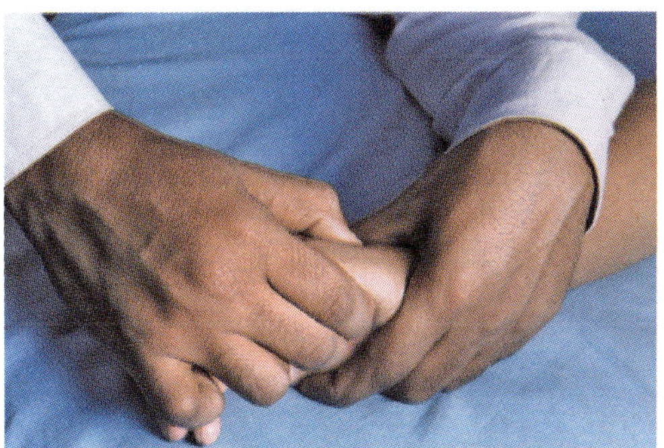

**Fig. 10.51:** Carpometacarpal joint of thumb, dorsal and ventral gliding.

- ❖ To reduce pain in 1st carpometacarpal joint.

*Patient's Position*

Supine lying/sitting.

*Fixation*

Carpal bones are fixed by therapist's left hand with the thumb on the dorsal surface and the finger on ventral surface.

*Support*

Distal part is supported on the table/bed.

*Therapist's Position and Grasping*

- ❖ Therapist stands near the patient, facing the carpometacarpal joint.
- ❖ Therapist's right hand grasps the base of the 1st metacarpal with the thumb on the dorsal surface and the fingers on the ventral surface.
- ❖ Therapist's left hand grasps the distal row of the carpal bones with the thumb on the dorsal surface and the fingers on the ventral surface.

*Procedure*

Therapist's right hand pulls 1st the metacarpal distally from the trapezium for mobilization of carpometacarpal joint of thumb.

*Note:* For mobilization of the carpometacarpal joints of fingers the metacarpal bones are pulled from the relevant carpal bones (i.e., 2nd metacarpal on trapezoid, 3rd on capitate, 4th on hamate, 5th on hamate).

**Dorsal and Ventral Gliding (Carpometacarpal Joints of Fingers and Thumb) (Figs. 10.51 and 10.52)**

*Goal*

- ❖ To increase the joint play around the, 1st, 2nd to 5th carpometacarpal joints.
- ❖ To increase the flexion and extension of the 2nd to 5th fingers (dorsal gliding increases flexion and ventral gliding increases extension of carpometacarpal joints) and abduction and adduction of thumb.
- ❖ To reduce the pain around the carpometacarpal joints.

*Patient's Position*

As said in distraction.

*Fixation*

As said in distraction.

*Support/Stabilization*

As said in distraction.

*Therapist's Position*

As said in distraction.

*Procedure*

Therapist's right hand glides the metacarpals on the relevant carpal bones in the volar and dorsal direction (i.e., 1st metacarpal on trapezium, 2nd metacarpal on trapezoid, 3rd metacarpal on capitate, 4th metacarpal on capitate and hamate, 5th metacarpal on hamate).

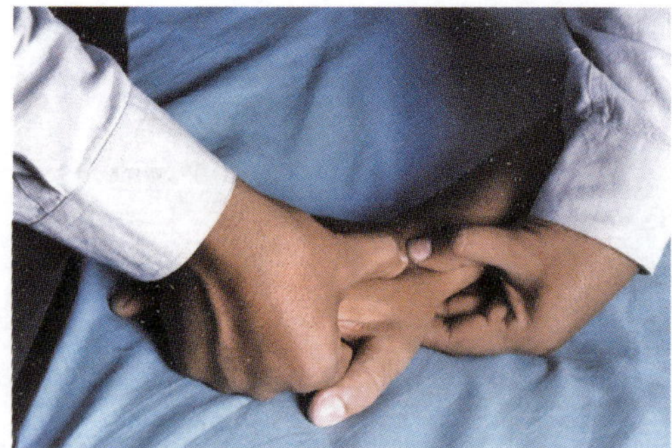

**Fig. 10.52:** Carpometacarpal joint (2nd–5th) dorsal and ventral gliding.

### *Intermetacarpal Joints*

**Dorsal and Ventral Gliding (Fig. 10.53)**

*Goal*

- ❖ To increase the joint play around the intermetacarpal joint.
- ❖ To reduce the pain around the intermetacarpal joint.

*Patient's Position*

As said in the distraction of the carpometacarpal joint of thumb.

*Fixation*

Therpist's right hand fixes the adjacent mid shaft of the metacarpals with the thumb on the dorsal surface and the index finger on the ventral surface.

*Support*

The hand is supported on the bed.

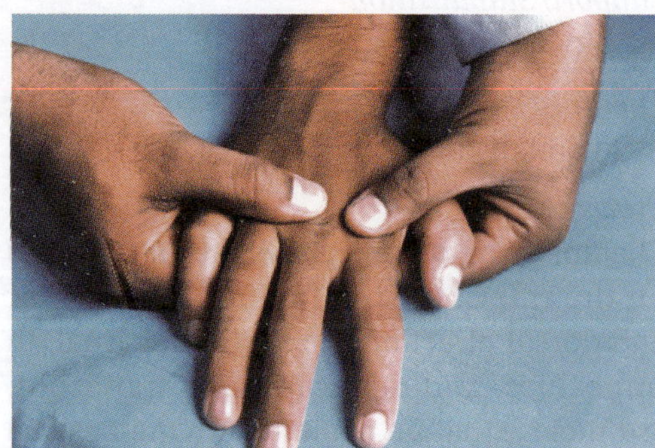

**Fig. 10.53:** Intermetacarpal joint dorsal and ventral gliding.

*Therapist's Position*

- ❖ Therapist stands near the patient and facing the intermetacarpal joint.
- ❖ Therapist's right hand fixes the adjacent mid-shaft of the metacarpal with the thumb on the dorsal surface and the index finger on the ventral surface.
- ❖ Therapist's left hand is grasps the mid-shaft of the metacarpal to be mobilized with the thumb on the dorsal surface and index finger on the ventral surface.

*Procedure*

Therapist's left hand glides each metacarpal on the adjacent metacarpal in the dorsal and ventral direction (1st metacarpal on 2nd metacarpal, 2nd metacarpal on the 3rd metacarpal, 4th metacarpal on the 3rd metacarpal, 5th metacarpal on the 4th metacarpal).

### *Metacarpophalangeal Joints*

**Metacarpophalangeal Joint of Thumb**

**Type:** Synovial joint—hinged type.

*Articular Surface*

- ❖ Head of the metacarpal (convex)
- ❖ Proximal end of proximal phalanx (concave).

*Ligaments*

- ❖ Palmar ligament
- ❖ Collateral ligaments—medial, lateral.

*Movements*

**Osteokinematics:** The movements produced in the joint are flexion and extension. Abduction and adduction are insignificant in this joint, which are mostly produced at the CMC joint.

**Flexion:** Muscles include:
1st MCP—flexor pollicis longus and brevis.

**Extension**

1st MCP—extensor pollicis longus and brevis.

**Range of motion:**

- ❖ **Flexion:** 10–60°.
- ❖ **Extension:** 10–0°.

*Note:* At rest MCP joint of thumb remains at about 10° of flexion.

**Arthrokinematics**

Arthrokinematic relations with the osteokinematics.

- ❖ Flexion—ventral gliding
- ❖ Extension—dorsal gliding

*Positions*

**Starting position**

Metacarpals and phalanx are in straight line.

**Resting/loose packed position**

Slight flexion.

**Close packed position**

1st MCP—maximum extension

**Capsular pattern**

Flexion limited more than extension.

**Distraction of MCP Joint of Thumb**

*Goal*

- ❖ To increase the joint play in 1st MCP joint.
- ❖ To increase the ROM of thumb.
- ❖ To reduce pain in 1st MCP joint.

*Patient's Position*

Supine lying/sitting.

*Fixation*

The MCP joint of thumb is held by the therapist's left hand.

*Support*

Distal part is supported on the table/bed.

**Therapist's position and grasping:**

- ❖ Therapist stands near the patient, facing the 1st MCP joint.
- ❖ Therapist's right hand grasps the base of the proximal phalanx of thumb.
- ❖ Therapist's left hand grasps 1st metacarpal.

**Procedure:** Therapist's right hand pulls proximal phalanx distally from the 1st metacarpal for mobilization of the 1st MCP joint of thumb, as done for distraction of carpometacarpal joint.

**Metacarpophalangeal Joint of Fingers (2–5)**

**Type:** Synovial joint—condyloid type.

**Articular surface**

- ❖ Head of the metacarpal (convex)
- ❖ Proximal end of proximal phalanx (concave).

**Ligaments**

- ❖ Palmar ligament
- ❖ Collateral ligaments—medial, lateral.
- ❖ Deep transverse metacarpal ligament.

**Movements**

**Osteokinematics:** The movements produced in the joint are flexion and extension, abduction, adduction and circumduction.

**Flexion:** Muscles include:
2nd–5th MCP—lumbricals, flexion digitorum superficialis, flexor digitorum profundus.

**Extension:** 2nd–5th MCP—extensor digitorum, extensor digiti minimi (little finger extension), extensor indicis (index finger extension).

**Abduction:**

- ❖ 2nd–4th MCP—dorsal interossei.
- ❖ 5th MCP—abductor digiti minimi.

**Adduction:** The 1st palmar interosseous also called as pollical palmar interosseous, is often found rudimentary, which produces thumb adduction along with adductor pollicis.

- ❖ 2nd MCP—2nd palmar interosseous
- ❖ 4th MCP—3rd palmar interosseous
- ❖ 5th MCP—4th palmar interosseous.

## Arthrokinematics

### *Arthrokinematic Relations with the Osteokinematics*

- ❖ Flexion—ventral gliding
- ❖ Extension—dorsal gliding
- ❖ Abduction—2nd–3rd MCP radial gliding

- Abduction—4th-5th MCP medial gliding.
- Adduction—2nd MCP medial gliding.
- Adduction—4th-5th MCP radial gliding.

## *Range of Motion*

- Flexion—80-90°.
- Extension—10-30° (nearly 10° in index finger and 30° in little finger).
- Abduction—25-30°
- Adduction—0°

### Positions

**Starting position:** Metacarpals and phalanx are in straight line.

**Resting/loose packed position:** Slight flexion in all joints.

**Close packed position:** 2nd-5th MCP—maximum flexion.

**Capsular pattern:** Restricted in all directions.

### Distraction (Fig. 10.54)

*Goal*

- To increase the joint play around the metacarpophalangeal joint.
- To reduce the pain around the metacarpophalangeal joint.
- To increase the ROM of the metacarpophalangeal joint.

*Patient's Position*

As said in the distraction of the metacarpophalangeal joint of thumb.

*Fixation*

Therapist's left hand fixes the head of the metacarpals with the thumb on the dorsal surface and the index finger on the ventral surface.

*Support*

Not necessary.

*Therapist's Position*

- Therapist is standing near to the patient and facing the metacarpophalangeal joint.
- Therapist's right hand grasps the proximal end of the proximal phalanx with the thumb on the dorsal surface and the index finger on the ventral surface.
- Therapist's left hand fixes the head of the metacarpal with the thumb on the dorsal surface and the index finger on the ventral surface.

*Procedure*

Therapist's right hand pulls the proximal phalanx distally.

### Dorsal Gliding and Ventral Gliding (Fig. 10.55)

*Goal*

- To increase the joint play around the metacarpophalangeal joint.
- To increase the flexion and extension of the metacarpophalangeal joint (dorsal gliding increases the extraction, ventral gliding increases the flexion).
- To reduce the pain around the metacarpophalangeal joint.

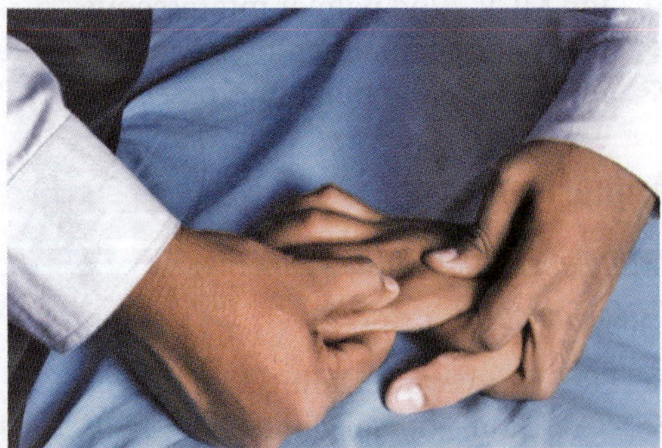

**Fig. 10.54:** Metacarpophalangeal joint distraction.

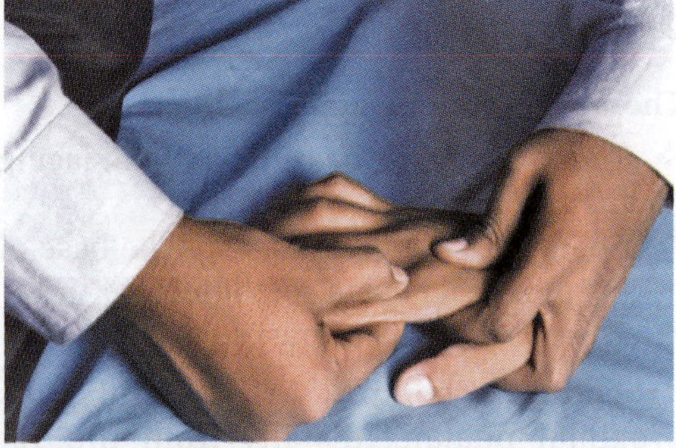

**Fig. 10.55:** Metacarpophalangeal joint dorsal, ventral, medial and lateral gliding.

*Patient's Position*
As said in the distraction.

*Fixation*
As said in the distraction.

*Support*
As said in the distraction.

*Therapist's Position*
As said in the distraction.

*Procedure*
Therapist's right hand glides the proximal phalanx on the metacarpal in the dorsal and ventral directions.

### Medial and Lateral Gliding

*Goal*
- ❖ To increase the joint play around the metacarpophalangeal joint of fingers.
- ❖ To increase the ROM around the metacarpophalangeal joint (Medial gliding increases the adduction of index finger, ulnar abduction of middle finger and abduction of ring and little finger. Lateral gliding increases the abduction of index finger radial abduction of middle finger, and adduction of ring and little fingers).
- ❖ Reduce the pain around the metacarpophalangeal joint.

*Patient's Position*
As said in distraction.

*Fixation*
As said in distraction.

*Support*
As said in distraction.

*Therapist's Position*
As said in distraction.

*Procedure*
Therapist grasps the respective metacarpals with the left hand. The right hand glides the proximal phalanx in the medial and lateral direction.

## *Interphalangeal Joints of Thumb and Fingers*

**Type:** Synovial joint of hinge variety.

### Articular Surfaces

- ❖ Distal end of the proximal phalanx (convex)
- ❖ Proximal end of the distal phalanx (concave).

### Ligaments

- ❖ Medial collateral ligament
- ❖ Lateral collateral ligament
- ❖ Palmar collateral ligament.

### Movements

*Osteokinematic*

**Flexion:** Muscles include:
- ❖ 1st IP—flexor pollicis longus
- ❖ 2nd-5th IP—flexor digitorum sublimis and flexor digitorum profundus.

**Extension**
- ❖ 1st IP—extensor pollicis brevis and longus.
- ❖ 2nd-5th IP—extension digitorum.
- ❖ 2nd IP—extensor indicis.
- ❖ 5th IP—extensor digiti minimi.

## *Range of Motion*

### Thumb

- ❖ Flexion—0-80°-90°
- ❖ Extension—0°-10° (hyperextension in IP joint occurs in forceful movements of thumb).

## *Fingers*

### Flexion

- ❖ PIP flexion: 0° to 100-110°.
- ❖ DIP flexion: 0° to 70-80° [digit 3 has highest range of flexion (80°), and digit 5 has lowest range of flexion (70°)].

**Extension:** Active extensions at PIP joints of digits 2-5 are limited to 2° and for DIP joints the active extensions are limited to 5°.

*Positions*

**Starting position:** Both the phalanges are in straight line.

**Resting/loose packed position:** Slight flexion.

**Close packed position:** Maximum extension.

**Capsular pattern:** Restricted in all directions: Flexion is more limited than extension.

**Distraction (Fig. 10.56)**

*Goal*

- ❖ To increase the joint play in the interphalangeal joint.
- ❖ To reduce the pain in the interphalangeal joint.
- ❖ To increase the ROM in the interphalangeal joint.

**Patient's position:** Sitting/supine lying.

*Fixation*

Therapist's left hand fixes the distal end of the proximal phalanx with the thumb on the dorsal surface and the index finger on the ventral surface.

**Support:** Not necessary.

**Therapist's position**

- ❖ Therapist stands/sits at the side facing the interphalangeal joint.
- ❖ Therapist's right hand grasps the proximal end of the distal phalanx with the thumb on the dorsal surface and the index finger on the ventral surface.
- ❖ Therapist's left hand grasps the distal end of phalanx with the thumb on the dorsal surface and the index finger on the ventral surface.

*Procedure*

Therapist's right hand pulls the distal phalanx distally.

**Dorsal and Ventral Gliding (Fig. 10.57)**

*Goal*

- ❖ To increase the joint play around the interphalangeal joint.
- ❖ To increase the flexion and extension of the interphalangeal joint (dorsal gliding increases the extension, ventral gliding increases the flexion).
- ❖ To reduce the pain.

*Patient's Position*

As said in distraction.

*Fixation*

As said in distraction.

*Support*

As said in distraction.

*Therapist's Position*

As said in distraction.

*Procedure*

Therapist's right hand glides the distal phalanx on the proximal phalanx in the ventral and dorsal direction.

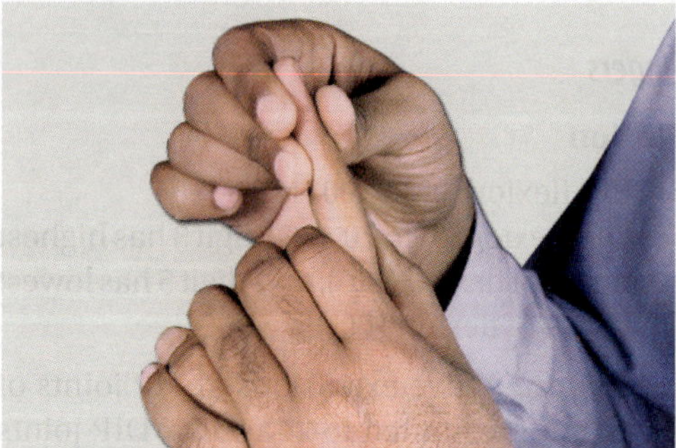

**Fig. 10.56:** Interphalangeal joint distraction.

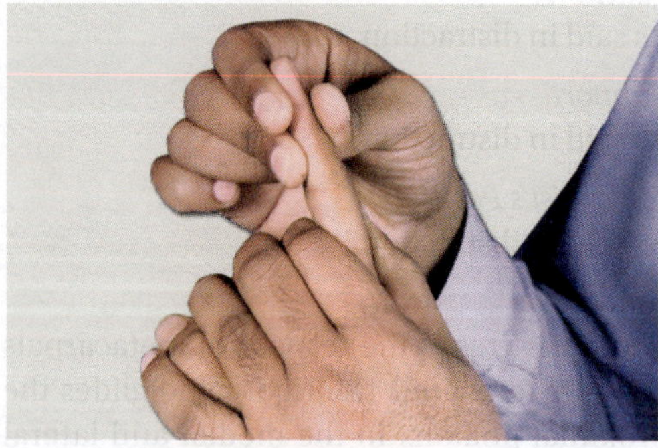

**Fig. 10.57:** Interphalangeal joint dorsal and ventral gliding.

## *Hip Joint*

**Type:** Synovial joint of ball and socket variety.

### Articular Surfaces

- Acetabulum of the pelvis (concave)
- Head of the femur (convex).

### Ligaments (Figs. 10.58A and B)

- Iliofemoral ligament
- Pubofemoral ligament
- Ischiofemoral ligament
- Transverse ligament
- Round ligament.

### Movements

*Osteokinematics*

The muscles responsible for hip movements are shown in **Figures 10.59A to C**.

*Flexion*

Iliacus, psoas major, sartorius, rectus femoris, lateral part of pectineus.

*Extension*

Gluteus maximum, hamstrings.

*Abduction*

- Gluteus medius, gluteus minimus
- Sartorius, tensor fascia lata.
- Gluteus maximus, piriformis.

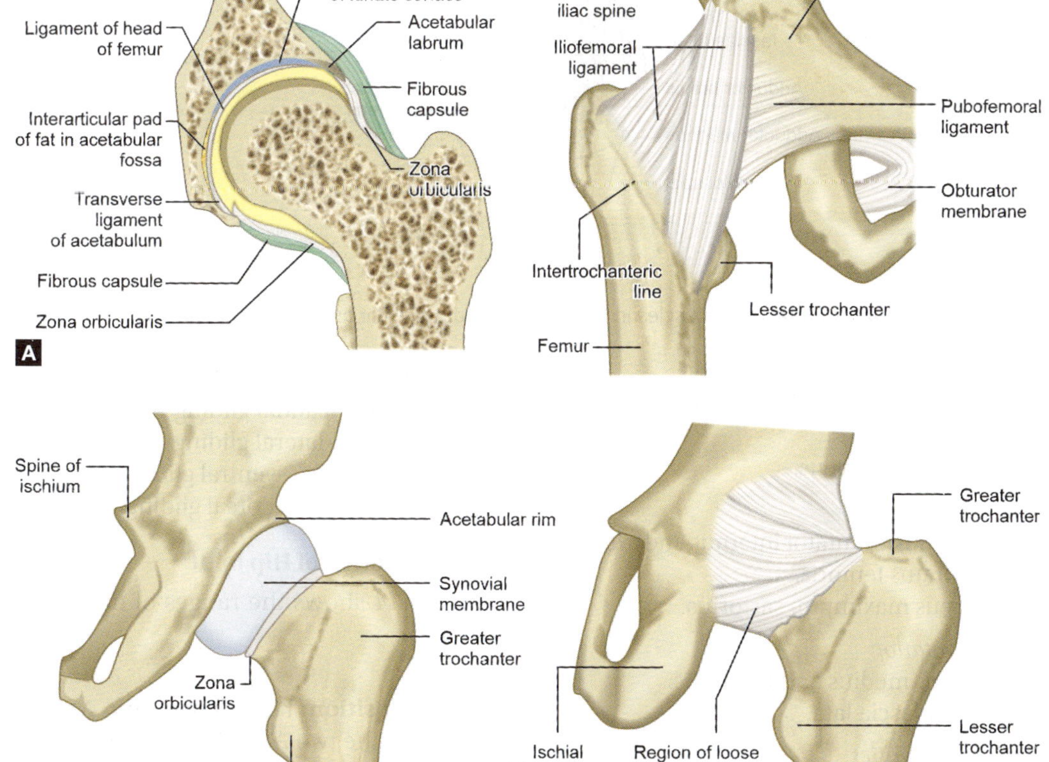


**Figs. 10.58A and B:** Hip joints.

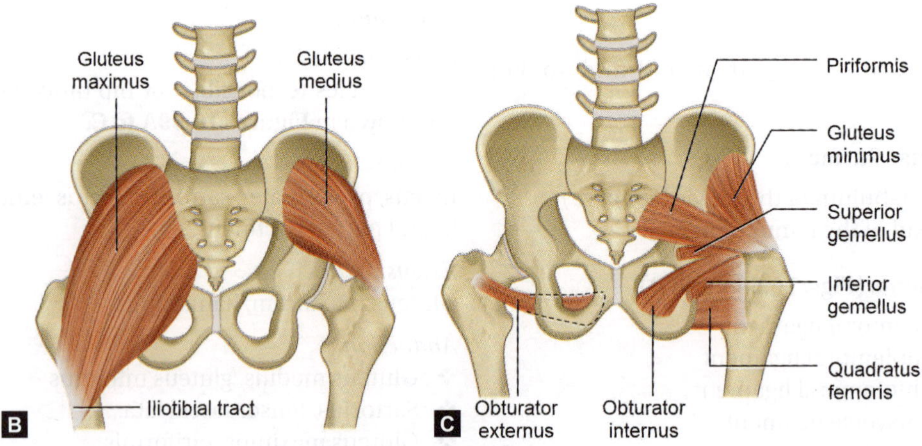


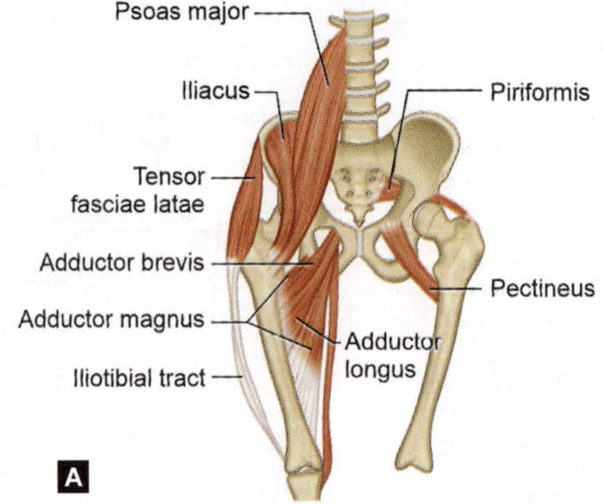


**Figs. 10.59A to C:** Muscles in the anterior and posterior aspects of hip joints.

*Adduction*

- ❖ Adductor longus, adductor brevis, adductor magnus
- ❖ Gracilis, pectineus.

*Lateral rotation*

- ❖ Piriformis, obturator internus and externus, quadratus femoris.
- ❖ Gluteus maximum, sartorius.

*Medial rotation*

- ❖ Gluteus medius and minimus.
- ❖ Tensor fascia lata.

*Arthrokinematics*

Arthrokinematics relations with the osteokinematics movements are:

- ❖ Flexion—dorsal gliding
- ❖ Extension—ventral gliding
- ❖ Abduction—caudal gliding
- ❖ Adduction —lateral gliding
- ❖ Lateral rotation—ventral gliding
- ❖ Medial rotation—dorsal gliding.

**Range of Motion of Hip Joint**

**Table 10.14** shows the ranges of motion of hip joint.

*Position*

**Starting position:** Line drawn from ASIS to patella and the two ASIS lies at right angle to each other.

**Resting position:** 30° hip flexion, 30° abduction, slight external rotation.

**Table 10.14:** Ranges of motion of hip joint.

| | |
|---|---|
| Flexion | 0–120° (with knees flexed)<br>0–90° to 100° (with the knee extended) |
| Extension | 0–30° |
| Abduction | 0–45° |
| Adduction | 0–20° |
| Medial rotation | 0–40° |
| Lateral rotation | 0–50° |

**Close packed position:** Maximum extension, medial rotation, abduction.

**Capsular Pattern**

- Restriction of the movements in this order
- Medial rotation > flexion > abduction.

### Distraction (Fig. 10.60)

*Goal*

- To increase the ROM around the hip joint.
- To increase the joint play around the hip.
- To reduce the pain around the hip.

*Patient's Position*

Supine lying.

*Fixation*

Patient's pelvis is fixed by the assistance of another person/body weight/by the belt.

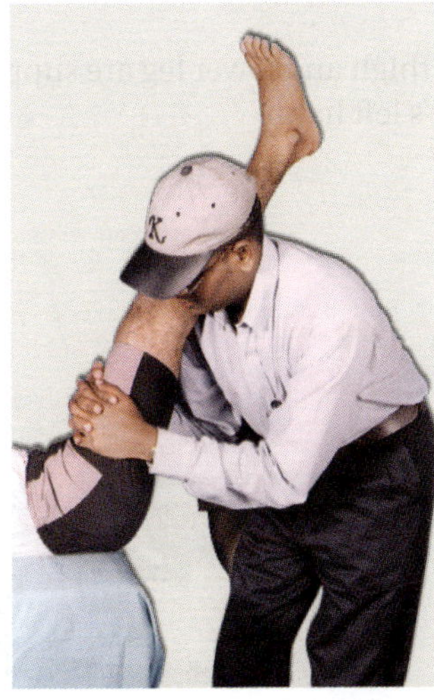

**Fig. 10.60:** Hip joint distraction.

*Support*

Patient leg is kept on the therapist's shoulder.

*Therapist's Position and Holding*

- Therapist stands at the foot end of the patient, facing the patient's hip.
- Therapist's both the hands grasp the upper thigh of the patient.
- Patient's hips and knees are flexed and the patient's leg is kept on the therapist's shoulder.

*Procedure*

Therapist's both the hands apply the distraction force on the hip joint.

### Caudal Gliding (Fig. 10.61)

*Goal*

- To increase the hip abduction movement.
- To increase the joint play around the hip.
- To reduce pain around hip.

*Patient's Position*

Supine lying.

*Fixation*

Patient's pelvis is fixed and the movement is restricted by the assistance of another person/body weight or by the belt.

*Support*

The entire lower limb is supported on bed.

*Therapist's Position*

- Therapist stands at the foot end of the patient, facing the hip joint of the patient.
- Therapist's both the hands grasp the lower leg of the patient above the ankle joint.

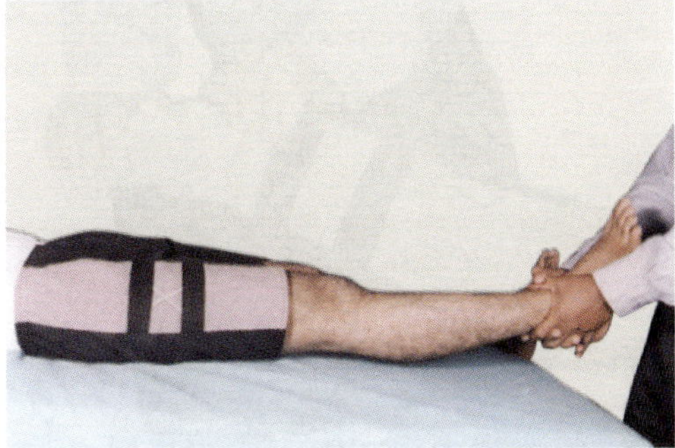

**Fig. 10.61:** Hip joint caudal gliding.

*Procedure*

Therapist's both the hands pull the leg down to achieve caudal gliding with mild distraction.

### Ventral Gliding (Figs. 10.62A and B)

*Goal*

- ❖ To increase the extension and external rotation of the hip.
- ❖ To increase the joint play around the hip.
- ❖ To reduce the pain around the hip.

*Patient's Position*

Trunk prone lying, with the hip at the end of the bed. The affected thigh supported on the therapist's hand. Alternatively, side lying with the affected side hip facing upwards may also be considered.

*Fixation*

Patient's pelvic is fixed by the assistant/belt/ weight of body.

*Support*

In trunk prone lying, the lower leg of the patient is supported by the therapist's right hand. In side lying the lower limb is supported on the lower leg or on pillows.

*Therapist's Position*

- ❖ Therapist stands at the foot end of the patient facing the posterior aspect of the hip of the patient, or at the posterior aspect of the patient, who is in side lying.
- ❖ Therapist's left hand is placed over the posterior aspect of the upper thigh of the patient placed in trunk prone lying and the right hand supports the leg of the patient.
- ❖ If mobilization is given in side lying, the left hand stabilizes the pelvis and right hand is placed at the back of upper thigh.

*Procedure*

Therapist's left hand applies anterior force and performing the anterior gliding around the hip joint of the patient with mild distraction, when mobilization is done in trunk prone lying. When placed in side lying, the gliding force is given by the right hand of the therapist.

### Dorsal Gliding (Fig. 10.63)

*Goal*

- ❖ To increase the hip flexion and medial rotation.
- ❖ To increase the hip joint play movement.
- ❖ To reduce the hip pain.

*Patient's Position*

Supine lying, with the patient's hip placed at the bed end.

*Fixation*

Patient's pelvis is fixed to the couch by body weight/belt.

*Support*

Patient's thigh and lower leg are supported by therapist's left hand.

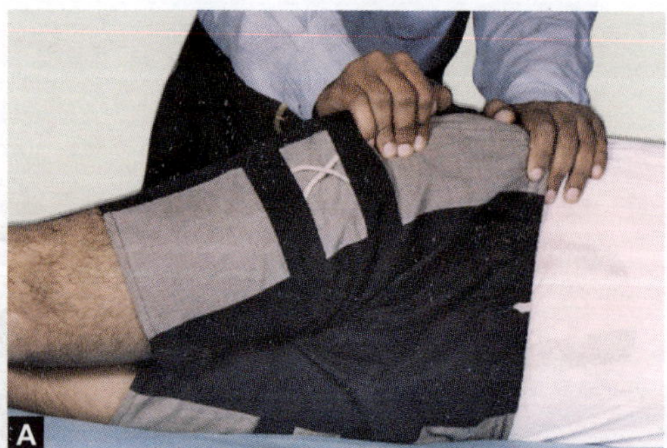


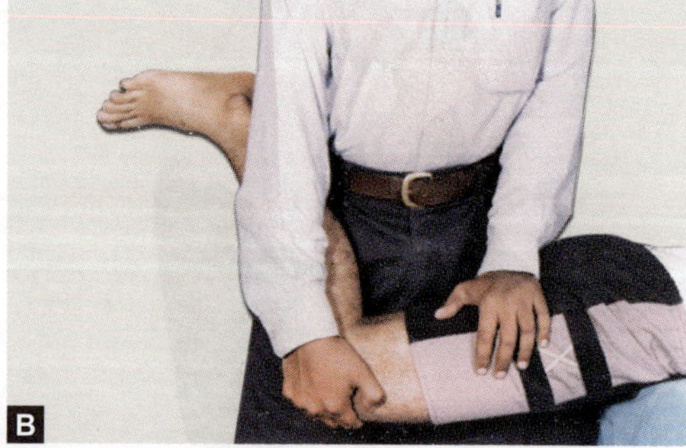


**Figs. 10.62A and B:** Hip joint ventral gliding.

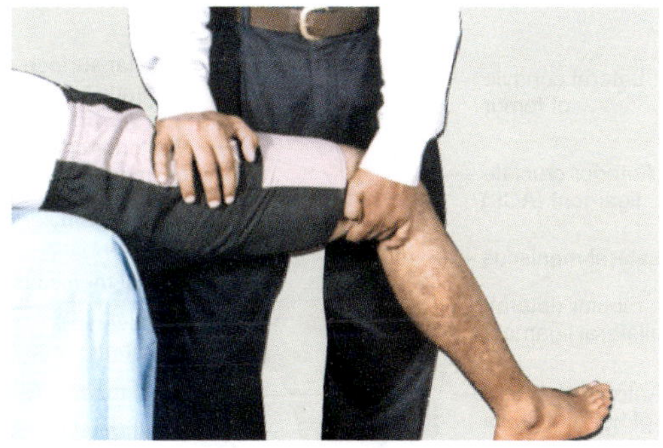

**Fig. 10.63:** Hip joint dorsal gliding.

*Therapist's Position and Holding*

- Therapist stands at the foot end of the patient and faces the hip joint of the patient.
- Therapist's right hand is placed on the anterior aspect of the upper thigh of the patient.
- Therapist's left hand grasps around the knee and the supports the lower leg of the patient.

*Procedure*

Therapist's right hand applies posterior force and hand performs the dorsal gliding of the hip of the patient with mild distraction.

**Lateral Gliding (Fig. 10.64)**

*Goal*

- To increase the internal rotation and adduction.
- To reduce the pain around the hip joint.
- To increase the joint play movement around the hip.

*Position of the Patient*

Supine position.

*Fixation*

Pelvic is already fixed by the positioning itself.

*Support*

The patient's flexed leg is supported on the therapist's shoulder.

*Therapist's Position*

- Therapist is standing near the patient's lower extremity.

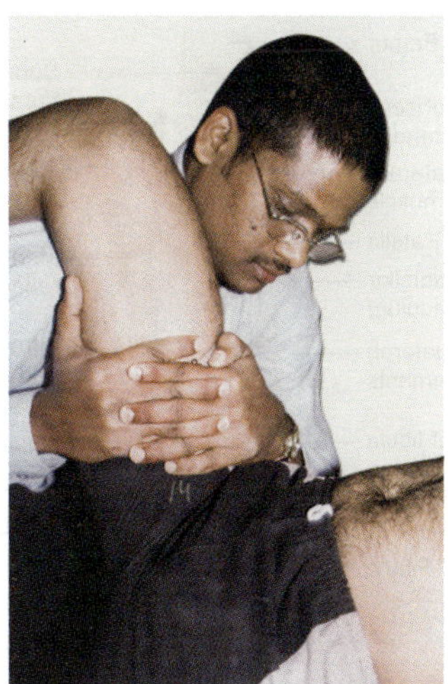

**Fig. 10.64:** Hip joint lateral gliding.

- Therapist's left and right hands grasp the upper thigh of the patient.

*Procedure*

Therapist's both the hands are gliding the femur in lateral direction. A belt tied to the upper thigh of patient and pelvis of therapist can also be used to give lateral gliding.

## Knee Joint

**Type:** Synovial joint of condyloid/modified hinged variety. It is often termed a compound joint having tibiofemoral and patellofemoral components. It is the largest joint in the human body.

**Tibiofemoral Joint**

**Articular surfaces:**

Lower end of femur (convex) and upper end of tibia (concave).

*Ligaments* ***(Figs. 10.65A to C)***

- Medial collateral ligament
- Lateral collateral ligament.
- Transverse ligament.
- Anterior and posterior meniscofemoral ligament.
- Meniscotibial ligaments.
- Medial and lateral patellar retinacular ligament.

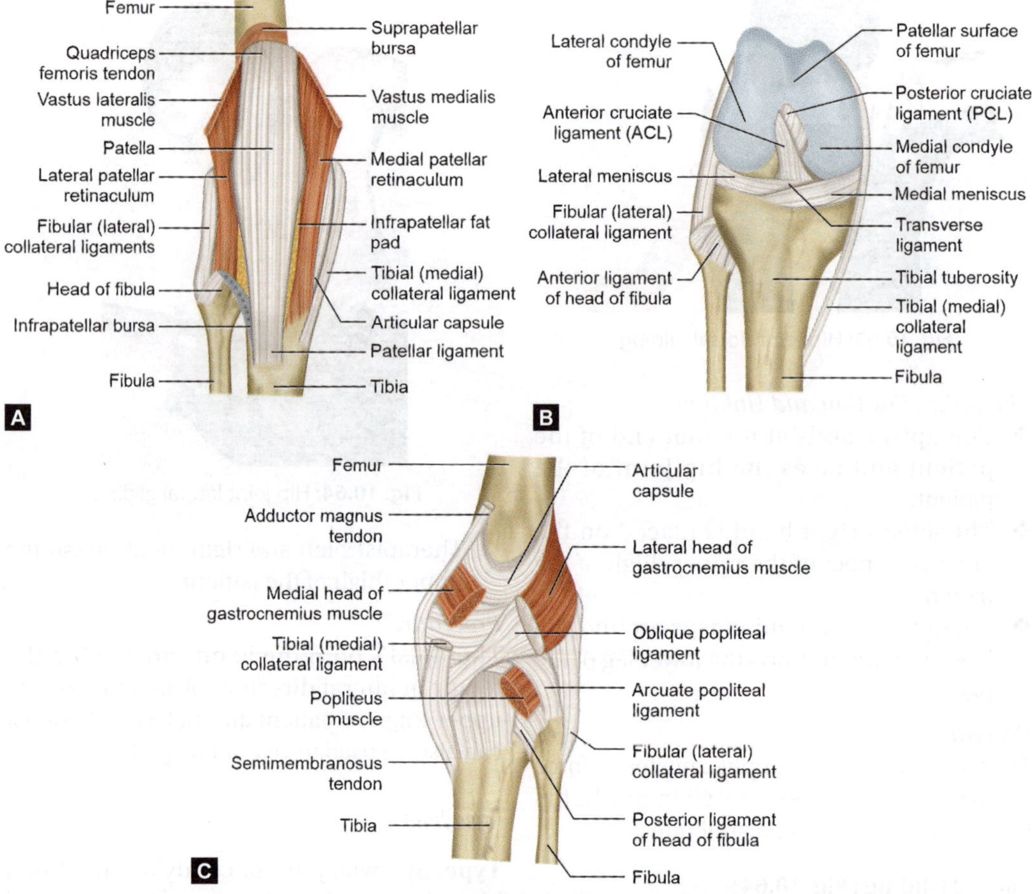


**Figs. 10.65A to C:** Anterior and posterior view of knee joint showing the ligaments: (A) Anterior view (superficial); (B) Anterior view (deep); (C) Posterior view (deep).

- Arcuate popliteal ligament.
- Oblique popliteal ligament.
- Ligamentum patellae
- Cruciate ligaments (anterior, posterior).

**Menisci:** There are two menisci in the knee, the medial (inner) and the lateral (outer). The menisci act as shock absorbers and separate the two ends of bone in the knee joint. The blood flow of the meniscus is from the periphery (outside) to the central meniscus. Blood flow decreases with age and the central meniscus is avascular by adulthood, which slows healing.

**Movements**

*Osteokinematics*

Muscles include:

- Flexion—hamstrings, popliteus, gracilis, sartorius, gastrocnemius, plantaris.
- Extension—quadriceps
- Medial rotators—semimembranosus, semitendinosus.
- Lateral rotators—biceps femoris

**Arthrokinematic**

Arthrokinematic relations with the osteokinematic movements are:

- Flexion—posterior gliding
- Extension—anterior gliding

- Medial rotators—posterior gliding
- Lateral rotators—anterior gliding.

### Range of Motion

Flexion and extension are the movements of the knee joint, which are the voluntary physiological movements. Rotations in the knee do not occur isolately, they are combined with flexion and extension, i.e., extension is associated with lateral rotation of tibia and flexion is associated with medial rotation. Ranges of motion of knee are as per the **Table 10.15**.

*Positions*

**Starting position:** Knee in neutral position.

**Resting/loose packed position:** 25° of flexion.

**Close packed position:** Maximum extension and lateral rotation.

**Capsular pattern:** Restriction of the movement: Flexion > extension.

## *Tibiofibular Joint (Fig. 10.66)*

### Type

- Superior tibiofibular joint—synovial joint—plane variety.
- Middle tibiofibular joint—fibrous joint
- Inferior tibiofibular joint—fibrous joint.

### Articular Ends

**Superior tibiofibular joint:**

- Articular facet on the lateral condyle of the tibia (concave)
- Articular facet of the head of fibula (convex).

**Inferior tibiofibular joint:**

- Lateral surface of the lower end of the tibia (concave)
- Medial surface of the lower end of the fibula (convex)

**Table 10.15:** Shows ROM of knee joint.

| *Movement* | *ROM* |
|---|---|
| Knee flexion | 0 –120 ° to 150° |
| Knee extension | 0° |

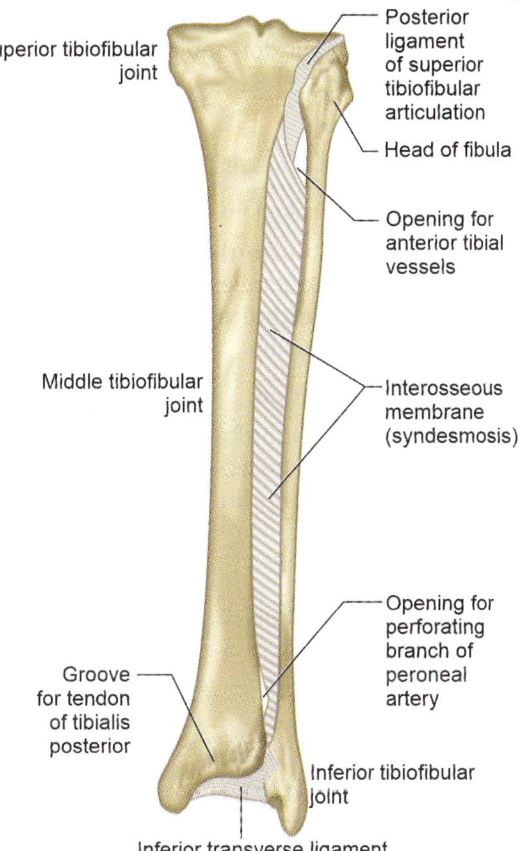


**Fig. 10.66:** Proximal and distal tibiofibular joint.

**Middle tibiofibular joint:** Shafts of tibia and fibula

### Ligaments

Ligaments of superior tibiofibular joint is are:

- Anterior tibiofibular ligament.
- Posterior tibiofibular ligament.

Ligaments of the inferior tibiofibular joint are:

- Interosseous tibiofibular ligament.
- Anterior—inferior tibiofibular ligament.
- Posterior—inferior tibiofibular ligament.
- Transverse tibiofibular ligament.

### Movements

*Osteokinematics*

- **Superior tibiofibular joint:** Gliding helps in knee flexion and extension.

- **Inferior tibiofibular joint:** Gliding helps in ankle dorsiflexion and plantar flexion.

*Positions*

**Starting position:**

Neutral position of ankle.

**Resting/loose packed position:**

- **Superior tibiofibular joint:** 25° knee flexion, 10° plantar flexion
- **Inferior tibiofibular joint:** 10° plantar flexion, 5° inversion.

**Close packed position:**

- Superior tibiofibular joint—maximum dorsiflexion of ankle.
- Inferior tibiofibular joint—maximum dorsiflexion of ankle

**Capsular pattern:**

- Superior tibiofibular—pain over the joint, when stressed
- Inferior tibiofibular—none.

### *Tibiofemoral Joint Mobilization*

**Distraction (Fig. 10.67)**

*Goal*

- To increase the joint play around knee joint.
- To increase the ROM around knee joint.
- To reduce the pain around the knee joint.

*Patient's Position*

Sitting on bed, with affected knee hanging at the edge.

*Fixation*

The lower thigh is fixed on the bed, with the help of the assistance.

*Support*

Therapist's both the hands grasp the leg of the patient.

*Therapist's Position*

- Therapist is sitting opposite to the patient on the stool and facing the patient's knee joint.

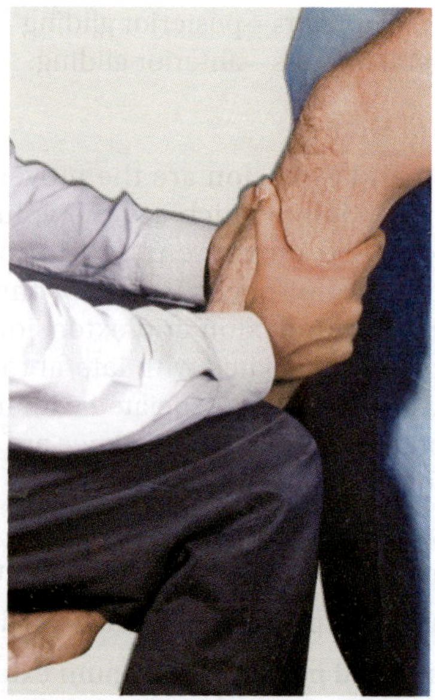

**Fig. 10.67:** Tibiofemoral distraction.

- Therapist's both hands grasp the upper leg of the patient.
- Therapist's both legs support the lower leg of the patient.

*Procedure*

Therapist perform the distraction over the knee by pulling the tibia downwards

**Dorsal/Posterior Gliding (Fig. 10.68)**

*Goal*

- To increase the joint play of the knee joint
- To increase the flexion ROM of the knee joint.

*Patient's Position*

Sitting on the bed with the leg hanging at the end of bed, with the knee in available range of knee flexion (almost extended).

*Fixation*

The thigh is fixed on the bed by an assistant/ with sand bag.

*Support*

Distal part of the leg is grasped by the therapist right hand.

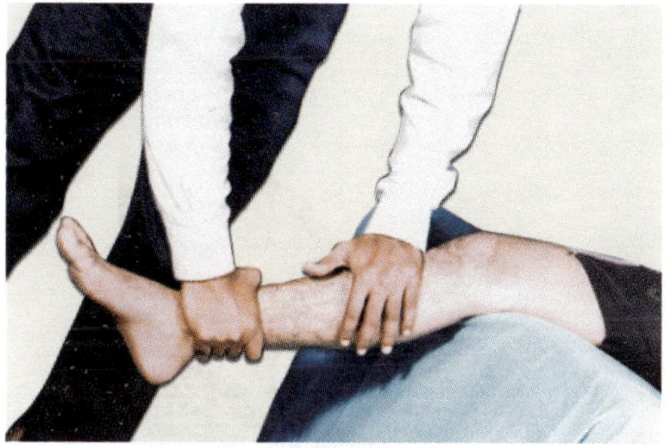

**Fig. 10. 68:** Tibiofemoral dorsal/posterior gliding.

*Therapist's Position and Grasp*

- Therapist stands opposite to the patient, facing the patient's knee joint.
- Therapist's left hand grasps the proximal tibia of the patient.
- Therapist's right hand is grasps the distal tibia of the patient.

*Procedure*

- Therapist's right hand applies mild-distraction of the knee joint.
- Therapist's left hand glides the tibia dorsally/posteriorly.

**Dorsal/Posterior Gliding (Progression) (Fig. 10.69)**

*Goal*

- To increase the maximum ROM of the knee joint.
- To increase the maximum flexion of the knee joint.
- To reduce the pain of the knee joint.

*Patient's Position*

Patient is sitting on bed. Knee is kept in maximum available flexed position.

*Fixation*

The thigh is fixed on the bed by an assistant/ with sand bag.

*Support*

Lower leg is supported by therapist's both the knee joints.

*Therapist's Position and Grasp*

- Therapist is sitting opposite to the patient.

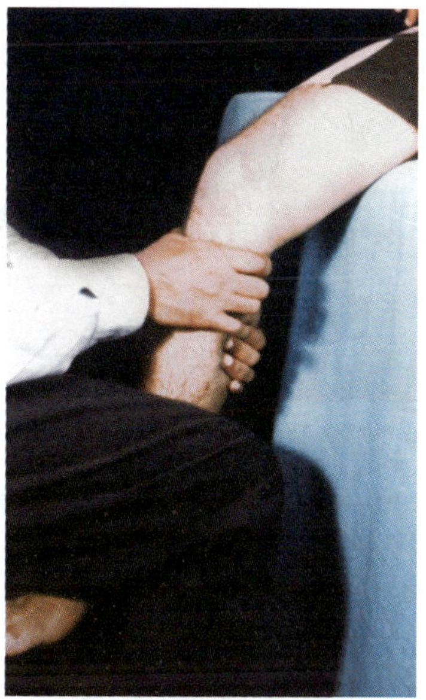

**Fig. 10.69:** Tibiofemoral dorsal/posterior gliding progression.

- Therapist's right hand grasps the anterior part of the proximal part of the tibia of the patient.
- Therapist's left hand grasps the posterior part of the proximal part of the tibia of the patient.
- Therapist's knee and leg provide support to the lower leg of the patient.

*Procedure*

- Therapist's leg and the left hand apply minimal traction around the knee of the patient.
- Therapist's right hand performs dorsal/ posterior gliding around the knee joint of the patient.

**Ventral/Anterior Gliding (Fig. 10.70)**

*Goal*

- To increase the ROM of the knee joint.
- To increase the joint play around the knee joint.
- To increase the extension of the knee joint.

*Patient's Position*

Prone lying and the knee is in available extension position. A pad of towel may be

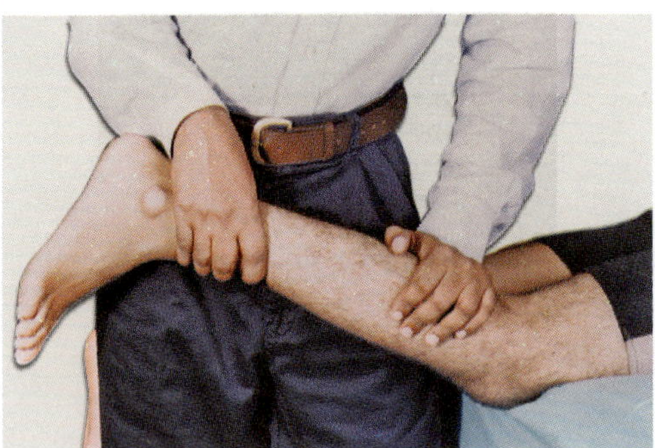

**Fig. 10.70:** Tibiofemoral ventral gliding.

placed under the lower thigh to prevent compression over the patella.

*Fixation*

The thigh is fixed by sand bag/assistant.

*Support*

Therapist's right hand holds/supports the lower leg.

*Therapist's Position and Grasp*

- ❖ Therapist stands at the foot end of the bed, facing the knee joint.
- ❖ Therapist's left hand is placed over the posterior aspect of the upper part of the tibia.
- ❖ Therapist's right hand grasps the lower end of the tibia and fibula.

*Procedure*

- ❖ Therapist's left hand performs the ventral/anterior gliding.
- ❖ Therapist's right hand applies minimal distraction force.

**Ventral Gliding—Second Technique (Fig. 10.71)**

*Goal*

- ❖ To increase the joint play around the knee joint.
- ❖ To increase the ROM of the knee joint.
- ❖ To increase the extension range around the knee joint.

*Patient's Position*

Sitting and the legs are kept hanging at the end of the couch.

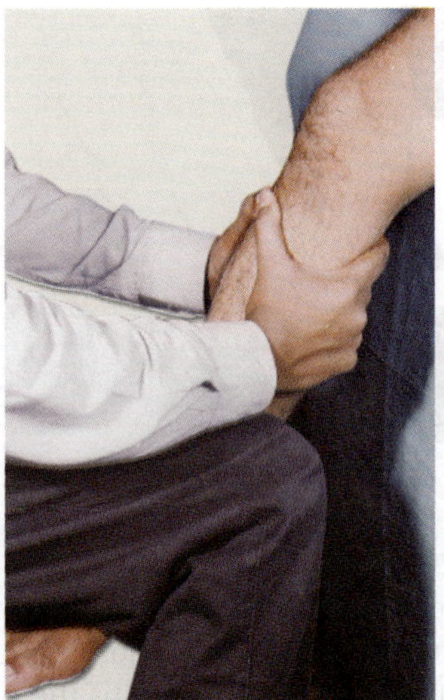

**Fig. 10.71:** Tibiofemoral joint ventral/anterior gliding.

*Fixation*

Thigh is fixed by sand bag/assistant.

*Support*

The patient's leg is supported by both the knees of therapist.

*Therapist's Position and Grasp*

- ❖ Therapist sit's in front of the patient and supports the patient's lower leg with both of his knees.
- ❖ Therapist's both the hands grasp the upper part of the tibia.

*Procedure*

Therapist's both the hands perform ventral/anterior gliding with the minimal traction. Therapist's legs also maintain the traction.

## *Patellofemoral Joint*

The patellofemoral joint is a diarthrodial plane joint that consists of the posterior surface of the patella and the trochlear surface of the distal anterior femur.

**Close packed position:** 60-90 degrees of knee flexion.

**Loose packed position:** Full knee extension.

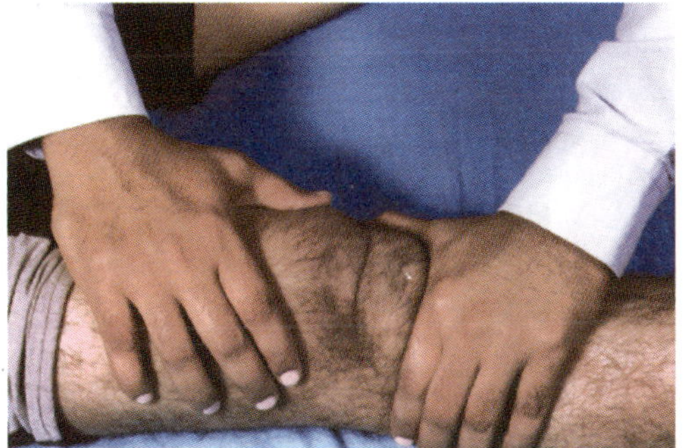

**Fig. 10.72:** Patellofemoral cranial/superior gliding.

### Cranial/Superior Gliding (Fig. 10.72)

*Goal*

- ❖ To increase the joint play in the patellofemoral joint.
- ❖ To increase the knee extension ROM.

*Patient's Position*

Supine lying.

*Fixation*

Weight of the lower limb provides fixation.

*Support*

Entire lower limb is supported on the bed.

*Therapist's Position and Grasp*

- ❖ Therapist stands at the side of the bed, facing the knee joint.
- ❖ Therapist's left hand thumb web space is placed over apex of the patella.
- ❖ Therapist's right hand is placed over the base of the patella.

*Procedure*

Therapist's left hand performs the cranial/superior gliding of the patella.

### Caudal/Inferior Gliding (Fig. 10.73)

*Goal*

- ❖ To increase the joint play around the patellofemoral joint.
- ❖ To increase the knee flexion ROM.

*Patient's Position*

Supine lying.

*Fixation*

As said in cranial gliding.

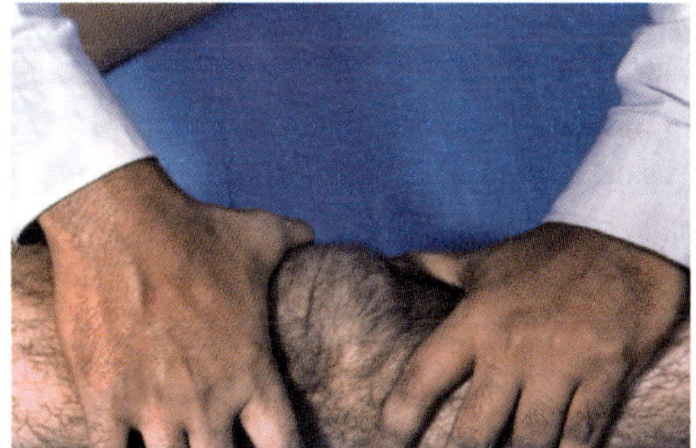

**Fig. 10.73:** Patellofemoral caudal gliding.

*Support*

As said in cranial gliding.

*Therapist's Position and Grasp*

- ❖ Therapist stands near to the patients lower extremity, facing the knee joint of the patient.
- ❖ Therapist's right hand is placed over the base of the patella patient.
- ❖ Therapist left hand is placed over the apex of patella.

*Procedure*

Therapist's right hand performs the caudal gliding of the patella.

### Medial Gliding (Fig. 10.74)

*Goal*

- ❖ To increase the joint play in patellofemoral joint.
- ❖ To increase the knee flexion ROM.

*Patient's Position*

Supine lying.

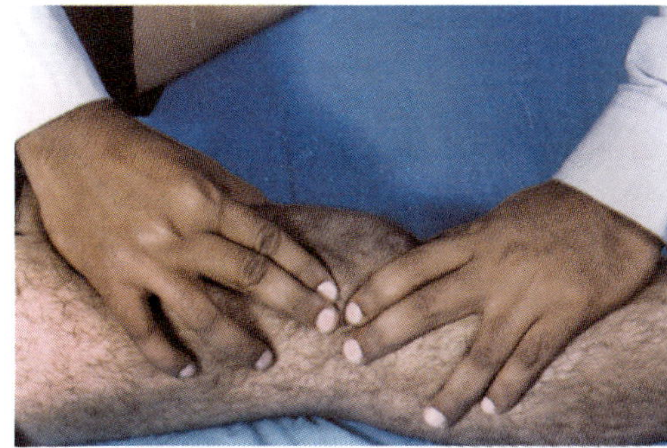

**Fig. 10.74:** Patellofemoral medial gliding.

*Fixation*
As said in cranial gliding.

*Support*
As said in cranial gliding.

*Therapist's Position and Grasp*
- ❖ Therapist stands near to the patient's lower extremity.
- ❖ Therapist's both hands index and middle fingers are placed over the lateral margin of the patella of the patient, and both the thumbs are placed over the medial aspect of the patella.

*Procedure*
Therapist's both hands, index and middle fingers perform the medial gliding over the patellofemoral joint.

**Lateral Gliding (Fig. 10.75)**

Positioning and grasp are same like the medial gliding of the patella, described above. With the thumbs of therapist placed over the medial margin of patella, the therapist produces gliding of patella, laterally.

## Tibiofibular Joint

### *Upper Tibiofibular*

**Dorsal/Posterior Gliding (Fig. 10.76)**

*Goal*
- ❖ To increase the joint play around the upper tibiofibular joint.
- ❖ To reduce the pain over the upper tibiofibular joint.

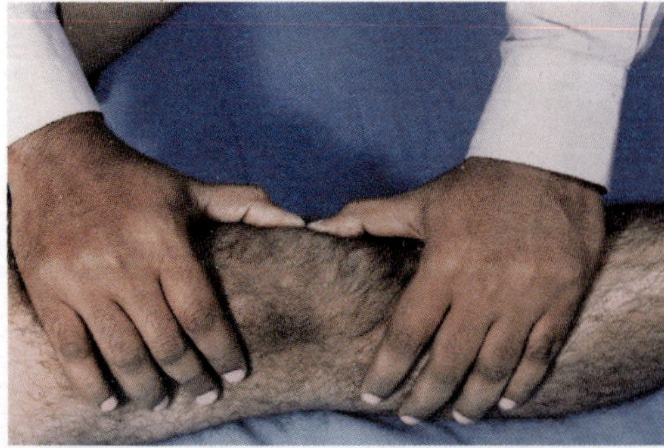

**Fig. 10.75:** Patellofemoral—lateral gliding.

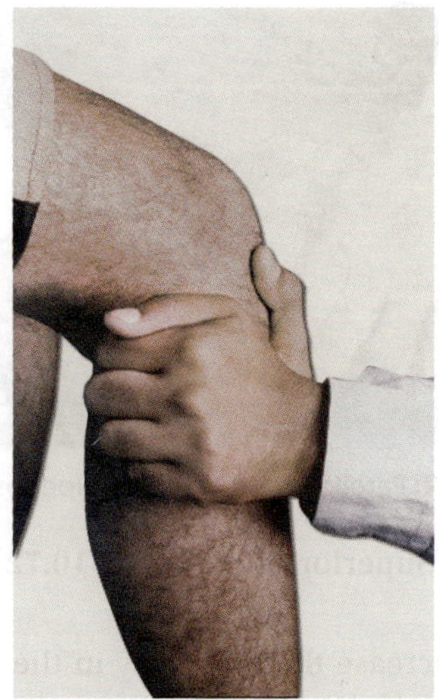

**Fig. 10.76:** Upper tibiofibular joint dorsal/posterior gliding.

*Patient's Position*
Supine lying or sitting in the bed end.

*Fixation*
Therapists—right hand fixes the upper end of tibia.

*Support*
Not required.

*Therapist's Position and Grasp*
- ❖ Therapist stands near the lower extremity of the patient, facing the upper tibiofibular joint.
- ❖ Therapist's right hand fixes the upper end of tibia of the patient.
- ❖ Therapist's left hand grasps the head of the fibula.

*Procedure*
Therapist's left hand performs the dorsal/posterior gliding of the fibular head over the tibia.

**Ventral Gliding (Fig. 10.77)**

*Goal*
- ❖ To increase the joint play around the upper tibiofibular joint.
- ❖ To reduce the pain around the upper tibiofibular joint.

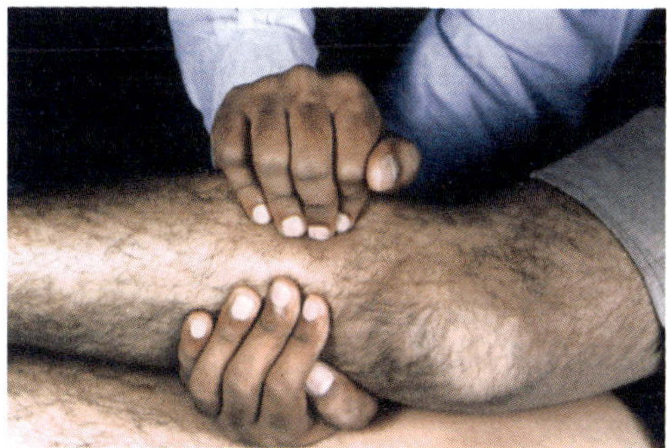

**Fig. 10.77:** Upper tibiofibular joint ventral gliding.

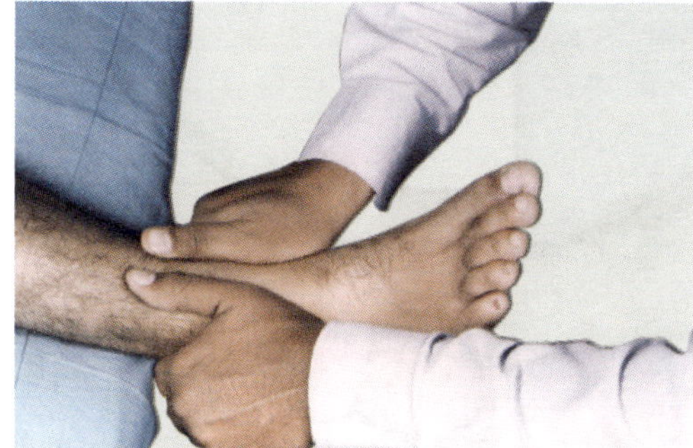

**Fig. 10.78:** Lower tibiofibular joint distraction.

*Patient's Position*

Prone lying or side lying.

*Fixation*

Therapist's left hand fixes the upper end of the tibia by grasping it in posteromedial aspect.

*Support*

The distal leg is supported by the couch/bed.

*Therapist's Position and Grasp*

- Therapist stands at the side of bed, facing the legs.
- Therapist's left hand grasps the fibular head.
- Therapist's right hand grasps the upper end of the posteromedial aspect of tibia.

*Procedure*

Therapist's right hand glides the fibula in ventral/anterior direction on the tibia.

### *Lower Tibiofibular Joint*

**Distraction (Fig. 10.78)**

*Goal*

- To increase the joint play around the lower tibiofibular joint.
- To increase the dorsiflexion ROM of the ankle.
- To reduce the pain around the lower tibiofibular joint.

*Patient's Position*

Supine lying. Ankle and foot at the foot end of the bed.

*Fixation*

No need of proximal joint fixation already it is done by the positioning itself.

*Support*

No need of distal support.

*Therapist's Position and Grasp*

- Therapist stands near to the lower extremity of the patient, facing the lower tibiofibular joint.
- Therapist's right hand is grasps the medial malleolus of the patient.
- Therapist's left hand grasps the lateral malleolus of the patient.

*Procedure*

Therapist's both the hands move the tibia and fibula away from each other.

**Dorsal Gliding (Fig. 10.79)**

*Goal*

- To increase the joint play in the distal tibiofibular joint.
- To increase the plantar flexion ROM of the ankle.
- To reduce the pain around the lower tibiofibular joint.

*Patient's Position*

Supine lying.

*Fixation*

Therapist's right hand fixes the medial malleolus of the patient.

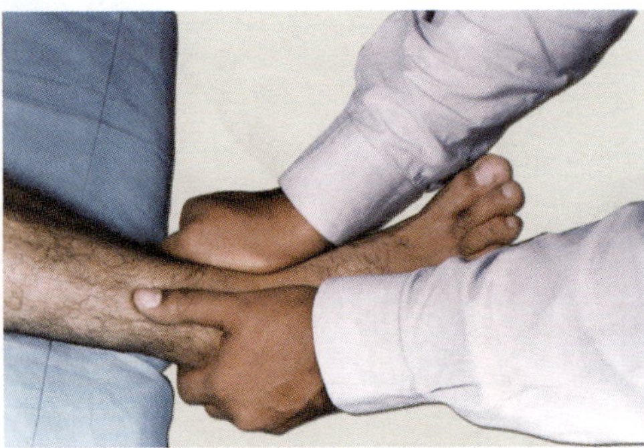

**Fig. 10.79:** Lower tibiofibular joint dorsal gliding.

*Support*

As said in distraction of lower tibiofibular joint.

*Therapist's Position and Grasp*

- Therapist stands near the foot end of the patient, facing the lower tibiofibular joint.
- Therapist's right hand fixes the medial malleolus.
- Therapist's left hand grasps the lateral malleolus of the patient.

*Procedure*

Therapist's left hand glides the lateral malleolus in dorsal direction.

### Ventral Gliding (Fig. 10.80)

*Goal*

- To increase the joint play around lower tibiofibular joint.
- To increase the dorsiflexion ROM of the ankle.
- To reduce the pain over the lower tibiofibular joint.

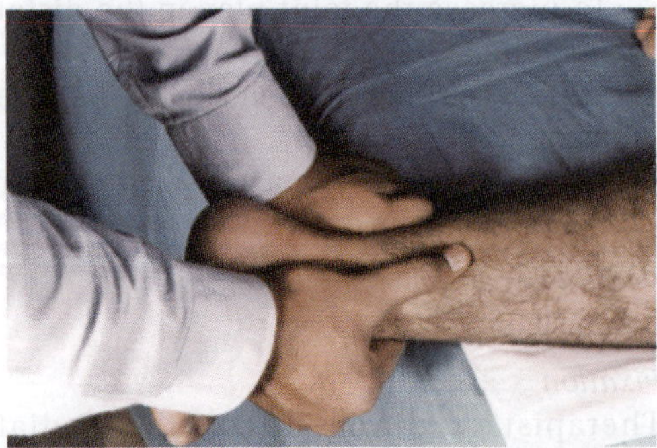

**Fig. 10.80:** Lower tibiofibular joint ventral gliding.

*Patient's Position*

Prone lying. Ankle and foot at the edge of the bed.

*Fixation*

Therapist's right hand fixes the medial malleolus of the patient.

*Support*

No support of distal part is required.

*Therapist's Position*

- Therapist is standing near the foot of the patient and facing the lower tibiofibular joint.
- Therapist's right hand fixes the medial malleolus of the patient.
- Therapist's left hand gasps the lateral malleolus of the patient.

*Procedure*

Therapist's left hand glides the lateral malleolus in ventral/anterior direction.

### Caudal Gliding (Fig. 10.81)

*Goal*

- To decrease the pain over the lower tibiofibular joint.
- To increase the plantar flexion of the ankle.

*Patient's Position*

Supine lying. Foot at the edge of foot end of bed.

*Fixation*

Therapist's left hand fixes the lateral malleolus.

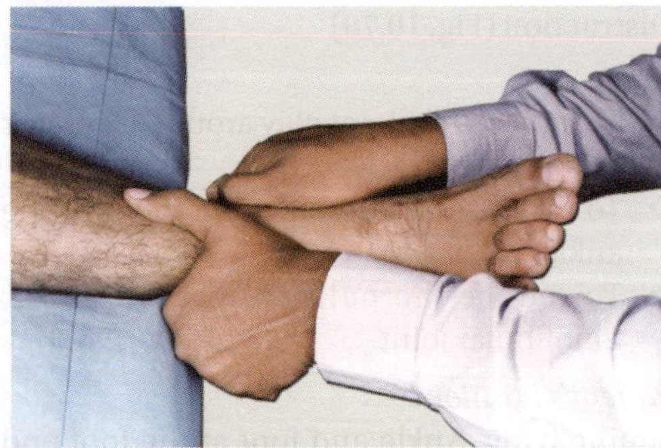

**Fig. 10.81:** Lower tibiofibular joint caudal gliding.

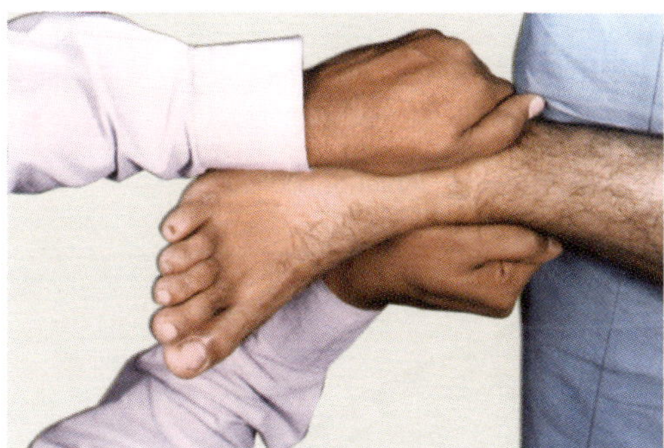

**Fig. 10.82:** Lower tibiofibular joint cranial gliding.

*Support*

Support to distal part is not required.

*Therapist's Position and Grasp*

- ❖ Therapist stands at the foot end of the patient, facing the lower tibiofibular joint.
- ❖ Therapist's left hand fixes the lateral malleolus of the patient.
- ❖ Therapist's right hand grasps the medial malleolus of the patient.

*Procedure*

Therapist's right hand glides the medial malleolus in the caudal direction.

### Cranial Gliding (Fig. 10.82)

*Goal*

- ❖ To increase the joint play around the lower tibiofibular joint.
- ❖ To reduce the pain over the lower tibio-fibular joint
- ❖ To increase the dorsiflexion ROM of the ankle.

*Patient's Position*

Side lying. The foot is kept at the end of the bed.

*Fixation*

Therapist's left hand fixes the lateral malleolus.

*Support*

Support to distal part is not required.

*Therapist's Position and Grasp*

Therapist stands facing the lower tibiofibular joint, grasping the medial malleolus.

*Procedure*

Therapist's right hand glides the medial malleolus in cranial direction.

## *Ankle Joint/Talocrural Joint (Figs. 10.83A and B)*

**Type:** Synovial joint—hinge variety.

### Articular Ends

*Proximally*

- ❖ Distal articular surface of tibia (concave)
- ❖ Lateral surface of medial malleolus (flat)
- ❖ Medial surface of lateral malleolus (flat).

*Distally*

- ❖ Trochlear surface of talus (convex)
- ❖ Coma-shaped facet of talus (flat)

### Ligaments

- ❖ Medial ligament: Deltoid ligament.
- ❖ Lateral ligament:
  - ▪ Anterior talofibular ligament.
  - ▪ Posterior talofibular ligament.
  - ▪ Calcaneofibular ligament.

### Movements

**Osteokinematics:** Muscles include:

- ❖ Dorsiflexion: Tibialis anterior, extensor hallucis longus, extensor digitorum longus.
- ❖ Plantar flexion: Soleus, gastrocnemius, flexor hallucis longus, flexor digitorum longus.

**Arthrokinematics**

- ❖ Dorsiflexion—posterior gliding
- ❖ Plantar flexion—anterior gliding.

### Range of Motion

- ❖ Plantar flexion: 0 to 40–50°
- ❖ Dorsiflexion: 0 to 20°

### Positions

**Starting position:** Neutral position of the ankle.

**Resting/loose packed position:** 10° plantar flexion and midway between the inversion and eversion.

**Close packed position:** Maximum dorsiflexion.

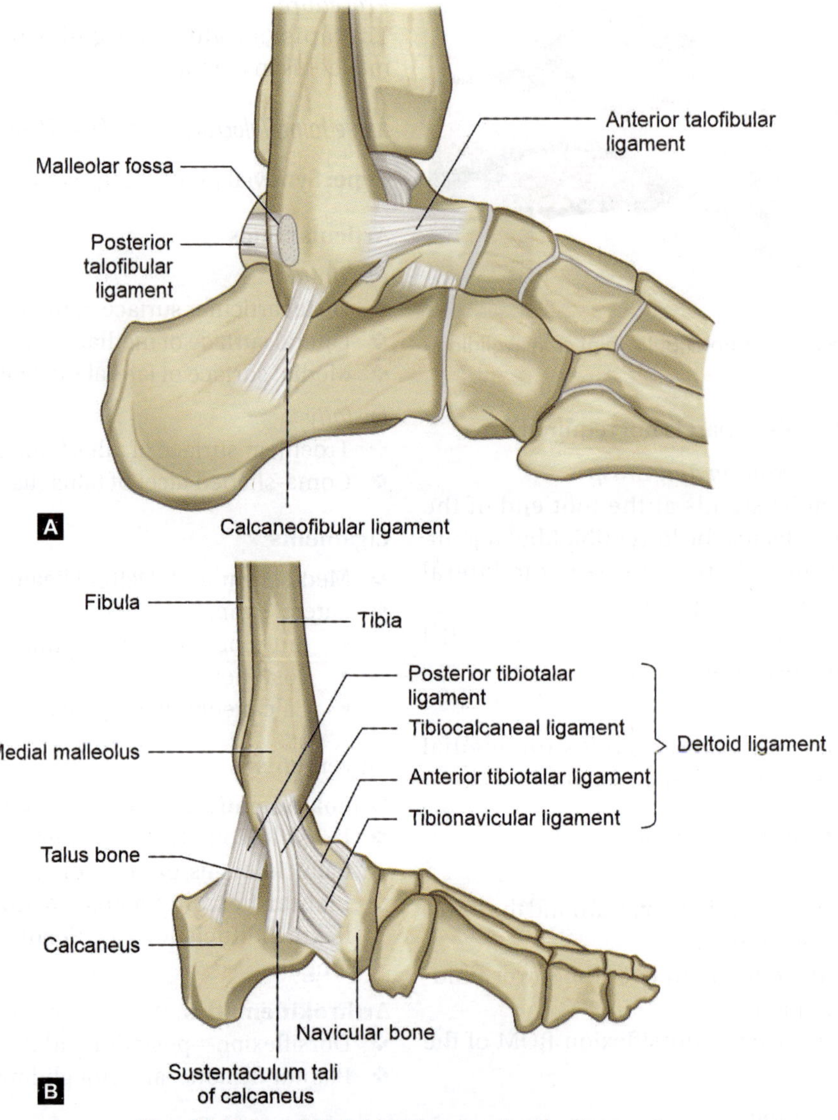


**Figs. 10.83A and B:** Ankle joint showing the ligaments.

**Capsular pattern:** Movements restricted: Plantar flexion > dorsiflexion.

**Distraction (Fig. 10.84)**

*Goal*

- ❖ To increase the joint play over the ankle.
- ❖ To increase the ROM of the ankle joint.
- ❖ To decrease the pain around the ankle.

*Patient's Position*

Supine lying, ankle and foot at the edge of foot end of bed.

*Fixation*

Proximal part is already fixed by the position itself.

*Support*

No support to distal part is needed.

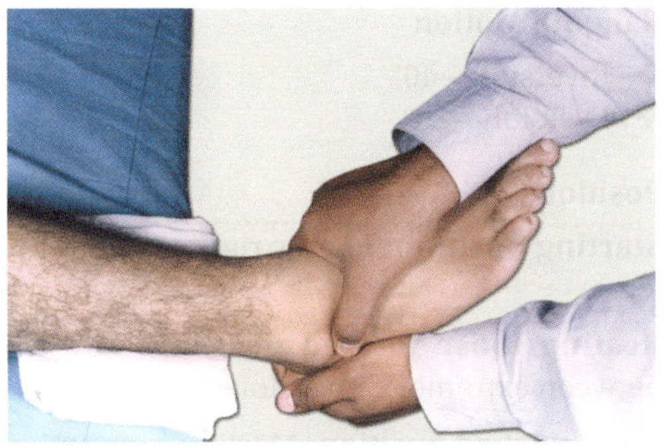

**Fig. 10.84:** Ankle distraction.

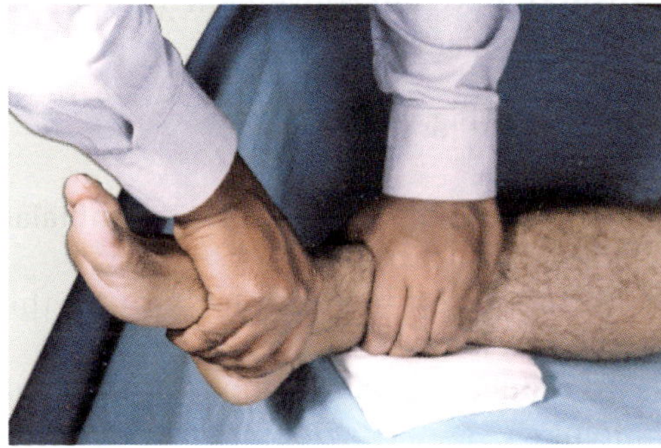

**Fig. 10.85:** Ankle posterior gliding.

*Therapist's Position and Grasp*

❖ Therapist stands at the foot end of patient and facing the ankle joint.
❖ Therapist's right hand grasps the proximal talus anteriorly.
❖ Therapist's left hand grasps the calcaneus of the patient.

*Procedure*

Therapist's both the hands apply downward pull separating the joints.

**Posterior Gliding (Fig. 10.85)**

*Goal*

❖ To increase the joint play in the ankle.
❖ To increase dorsi flexion ROM of ankle.
❖ To reduce the pain around the ankle.

*Patient's Position*

Supine lying, foot at the edge of foot end of bed.

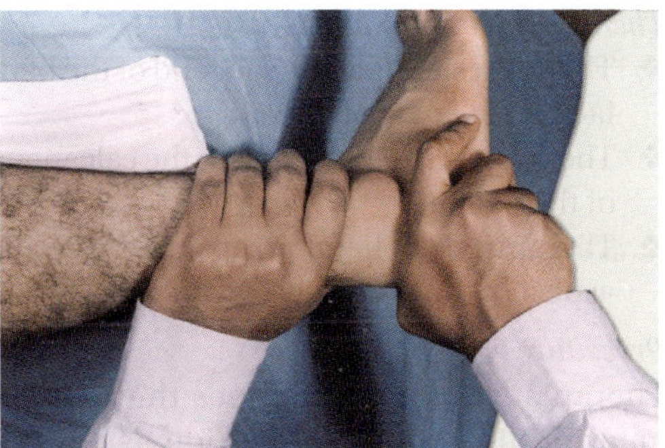

**Fig. 10.86:** Ankle anterior gliding.

*Fixation*

Therapist's left hand fixes the distal part of lower leg of the patient.

*Support*

No support is necessary for distal part.

*Therapist's Position and Grasp*

❖ Therapist stands at the foot end of the patient.
❖ Therapist's right hand grasps the dorsal talus and the foot with the web space.
❖ Therapist's left hand fixes the dorsal surface of the distal lower leg.

*Procedure*

Therapist's right hand glides the talus in the dorsal direction with the traction as per the grading.

**Anterior Gliding (Fig. 10.86)**

*Goal*

❖ To increase the joint play in the ankle.
❖ To increase the plantar flexion in the ankle.
❖ To reduce the pain over the ankle.

*Patient's Position*

Prone lying.

*Fixation*

Therapist's left hand fixes the posterior aspect of the distal leg.

*Support*

No support is needed for the distal part.

*Therapist's Position and Grasp*

- ❖ Therapist stands at the foot end of the bed, facing the ankle of patient.
- ❖ Therapist's right hand grasps the calcaneus of the patient.
- ❖ Therapist's left hand grasps the posterior aspect of the distal leg.

*Procedure*

Therapist's right hand glides the talus in anterior direction with traction as per the gliding.

## *Talocalcaneal/Subtalar Joint*

**Type:** Synovial joint of plane variety, with 3° of freedom.

### Articular surfaces

This joint is formed by the posterior articular surfaces of talus and calcaneus.

- ❖ Calcaneus: Convex area of upper surface of the middle third of the calcaneus.
- ❖ Talus: Concave area of the lower surface of the body of talus.

### Ligaments

- ❖ Fibrous capsule.
- ❖ Medial and lateral talocalcaneal ligament
- ❖ Interosseous talocalcaneal ligament.
- ❖ Cervical ligament.

### Movements

Supination (inversion of hind foot, adduction of forefoot and plantar flexion) and pronation (eversion of hind foot, abduction of forefoot and dorsiflexion).

**Osteokinematics:** Muscles include:

**Inversion:** Tibialis anterior and tibialis posterior.

**Eversion:** Peroneus longus and brevis, peroneus tertius.

**Arthrokinematics:**

- ❖ Inversion—medial gliding
- ❖ Eversion—lateral gliding.

### Range of Motion

- ❖ Inversion—40°
- ❖ Eversion—20°

### Positions

**Starting position:** Foot is right angle to the leg.

**Resting/loose packed position:** Midway between extreme of inversion and eversion.

**Close packed position:** Maximum inversion (supination).

**Capsular pattern:** Movement limitation: Inversion > eversion.

### Distraction (Fig. 10.87)

*Goal*

- ❖ To increase the ROM around the subtalar joint.
- ❖ To increase the joint play around the subtalar joint.
- ❖ To reduce the pain around the subtalar joint.

*Patient's Position*

Prone lying/side lying and the ankle is kept at the foot end of bed.

*Fixation*

Talus is fixed with the therapist's right hand in the posterior aspect.

*Support*

No need of the distal joint support.

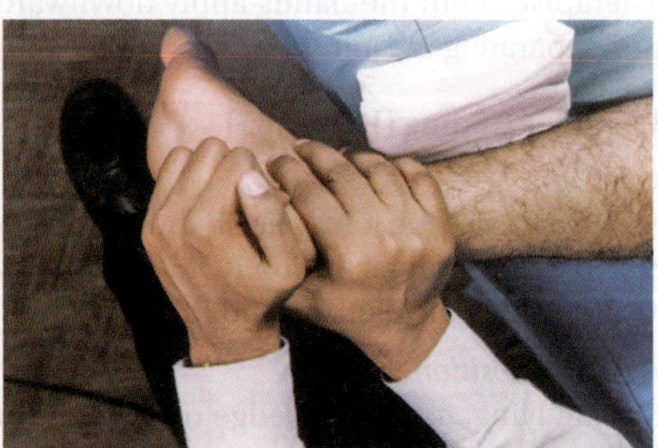

**Fig. 10.87:** Subtalar joint distraction.

*Therapist's Position and Grasp*

- Therapist is standing at the foot of the patient.
- Therapist's left hand grasps the calcaneus of the patient.
- Therapist's right hand grasps the ventral aspect of the talus.

*Procedure*

Therapist's left hand moves the calcaneus distally.

**Medial Gliding (Fig. 10. 88)**

*Goal*

- To increase the joint play around the subtalar joint.
- To increase the eversion movement of foot.
- To reduce the pain round the subtalar joint.

*Patient's Position*

Prone lying/side lying.

*Fixation*

Therapist's right hand fixes the talus of the patient.

*Support*

No support is necessary for the distal joint.

*Therapist's Position and Grasp*

- Therapist stands at the foot end of the patient and facing the talocalcaneal joint.
- Therapist's right hand fixes the talus.
- Therapist's left hand grasps the calcaneus at the posterolateral aspect.

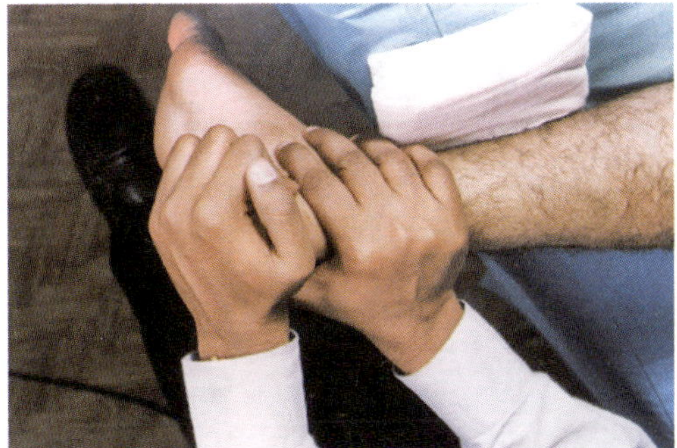

**Fig. 10.88:** Talocalcaneal joint/subtalar joint—medial gliding.

*Procedure*

Therapist's left hand is glides the calcaneus in the medial direction.

**Lateral Gliding (Fig. 10.89)**

*Goal*

- To increase the joint play around the talocalcaneal joint.
- To increase the inversion movement
- To reduce the pain around the talocalcaneal joint.

*Patient's Position*

Prone lying/side lying.

*Fixation*

Therapist's left hand grasps the talus of the patient.

*Support*

No need of the support for distal joints.

*Therapist's Position and Grasp*

- Therapist stands at the foot end of the bed, facing the talocalcaneal joint.
- Therapist's left hand fixes the talus of the patient.
- Therapist's right hand grasps the postero-medial aspect of the calcaneus.

*Procedure*

Therapist's right hand performs the lateral gliding the calcaneus.

### *Talonavicular Joint/Talocalcaneonavicular Joint*

**Type**

- Talonavicular joint: Synovial joint of saddle variety.

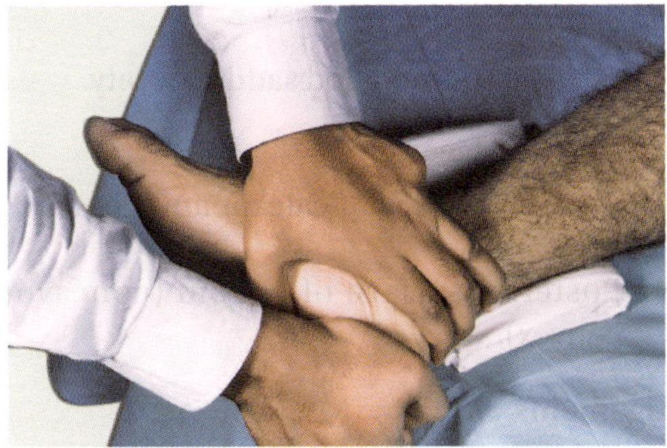

**Fig. 10.89:** Talocalcaneal lateral gliding.

- Talocalcaneonavicular joint: Synovial joint of ball and socket variety.

**Articular Surfaces (Talonavicular Joint)**

- Head of the talus (convex)
- Proximal end of the navicular (concave)

**Articular Surfaces (Talocalcaneonavicular Joint)**

- Head and plantar surface of neck of talus (convex).
- Calcaneus and navicular articulating surface (socket-concave).

**Ligaments**

- Dorsal talonavicular ligament.
- Plantar calcaneonavicular ligament/spring ligament
- Calcaneonavicular part of bifurcate ligament

**Osteokinematics of Talonavicular/Talocalcaneonavicular Joint**

The joints allow motion with 3° of freedom.

- Inversion/eversion
- Abduction/adduction.
- Plantar flexion/dorsiflexion.

*Talonavicular*

- Inversion—dorsal/anterior gliding
- Eversion—ventral/posterior gliding

The muscles involved are:

- Inversion: Tibialis posterior/tibialis anterior.
- Eversion: Peroneus longus/peroneus brevis/peroneus tertius.

### *Calcaneocuboid Joint*

Synovial joint—modified saddle variety.

**Articular surfaces**

- Anterior surface of calcaneum (concavo-convex)
- Posterior surface of cuboid (concavo-convex).

**Ligaments**

- Dorsal calcaneocuboid ligament.
- Plantar calcaneocuboid ligament.
- Part of bifurcated ligament.
- Long plantar ligament.

**Movements**

**Osteokinematics:** The joint is described as one of the least mobile joint of the human foot. Movements are limited to single rotation and some translation. The cuboid rotates to about 25° around an oblique axis, during inversion/eversion, called as involution.

- Inversion—tibialis anterior and posterior
- Eversion—peroneus longus and brevis, peroneus tertius.

**Arthrokinematics:** Calcaneocuboid joint:

- Inversion—ventral/posterior gliding
- Eversion—dorsal/anterior gliding.

**Position**

**Starting position:** Foot and leg are perpendicular to each other.

**Resting/loose packed position:** Midway between supination and pronation with 10° plantar flexion.

**Close packed position:** Full supination.

**Capsular pattern:** Movement restrictions: Supination > pronation.

**Talonavicular Joint: Dorsal Gliding (Fig. 10.90)**

*Goal*

- To increase the joint play around the talonavicular joint.

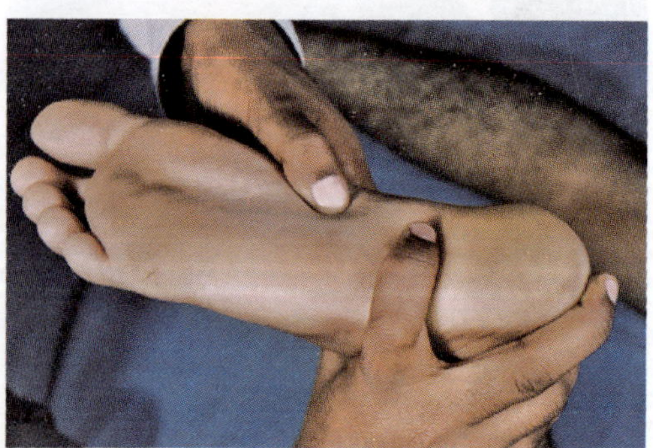

**Fig. 10.90:** Talonavicular dorsal gliding.

- To increase the inversion movement.
- To increase the dorsiflexion movement.
- To reduce the pain around the talonavicular joint.

*Patient's Position*

Prone lying with the knee in flexed position and the sole of the foot facing up.

*Fixation*

Therapist right hand fixes the talus of the patient.

*Support*

No need of the support for distal joints.

*Therapist's Position and Grasp*

- Therapist stands at the foot end of the patient, facing the talonavicular joint.
- Therapist's right hand fixes the talus of the patient.
- Therapist's left hand index finger down thumb up holds the navicular.

*Procedure*

Therapist's left hand glides the navicular bone in dorsal direction.

**Plantar Gliding (Fig. 10.91)**

*Goal*

- To increase the joint play around the talonavicular joint.
- To increase the midtarsal eversion movement.
- To increase the midtarsal plantar flexion.
- To reduce the pain around the talonavicular joint.

*Patient's Position*

Supine lying.

*Fixation*

Therapist's left hand fixes the talus of the patient.

*Support*

As said in dorsal gliding.

*Therapist's Position and Grasp*

- Therapist stands at the foot end of the patient.
- Therapist's left hand fixes the talus in the plantar aspect of the patient.
- Therapist's right thumb is in dorsal aspect and the index finger is in plantar surface of navicular bone.

*Procedure*

Therapist's right hand glides the navicular in plantar direction.

**Calcaneocuboidal Joint Dorsal Gliding (Fig. 10.92)**

*Goal*

- To increase the joint play over the calcaneocuboidal joint.
- To increase the midtarsal eversion.
- To increase the midtarsal plantar flexion.
- To reduce the pain around the calcaneocuboidal joint.

*Patient's Position*

Prone lying with the knee in flexed position and the sole of the foot facing up.

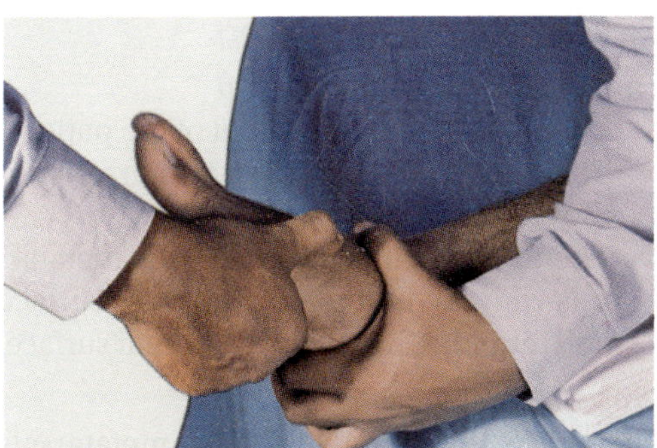

**Fig. 10.91:** Talonavicular plantar gliding.

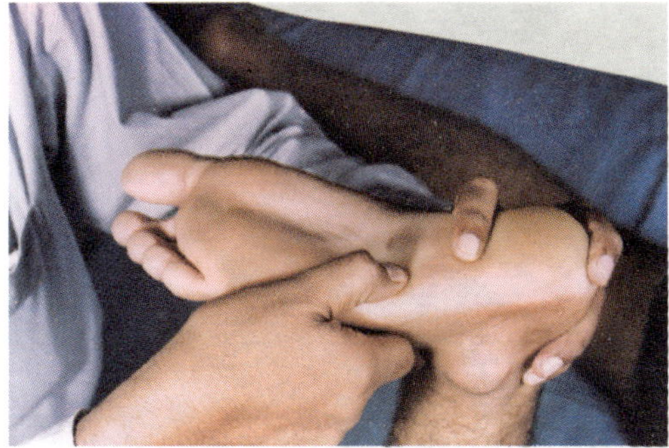

**Fig. 10.92:** Calcaneocuboidal dorsal gliding.

*Fixation*

Therapist's left hand fixes the calcaneus in the dorsal aspect along with ankle joint.

*Support*

No support of distal part is required.

*Therapist's Position and Grasp*

- ❖ Therapist stands at the foot of the patient.
- ❖ Therapist's right hand grasps the cuboid with the thumb on plantar surface and the index finger on the dorsal surface.
- ❖ Therapist's left hand fixes the calcaneus.

*Procedure*

Therapist's left hand performs the dorsal gliding of the cuboid.

**Calcaneocuboid: Plantar Gliding (Fig. 10.93)**

*Goal*

- ❖ To increase the joint play around the calcaneocuboidal joint.
- ❖ To increase the midtarsal inversion.
- ❖ To increase the midtarsal dorsiflexion.
- ❖ To reduce the pain over the calcaneocuboidal joint.

*Patient's Position*

Supine lying, ankle and foot at the foot end of bed.

*Fixation*

Therapist's right hand fixes the calcaneus with finger in dorsal and plantar aspect.

*Support*

No support to distal part is required.

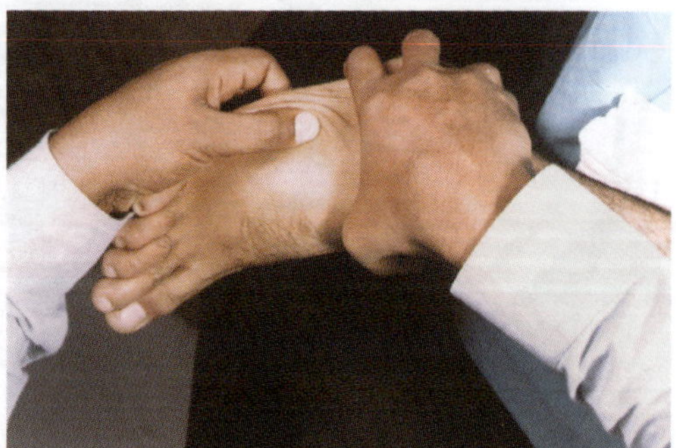

**Fig. 10.93:** Calcaneocuboidal plantar gliding.

*Therapist's Position and Grasp*

- ❖ Therapist stands at the foot end of the patient.
- ❖ Therapist's right hand fixes the calcaneus with the finger in dorsal and plantar surface.
- ❖ Therapist's left hand grasps the cuboid with the thumb in dorsal surface and the index finger in plantar surface.

*Procedure*

Therapist's left hand glides the cuboid in plantar direction.

**Tarsometatarsal Joint: Plantar/Dorsal Gliding**

The tarsometatarsal joint (Lisfranc's joint) is an articulation, where 3 cuneiforms and the cuboid articulate with 5 metatarsals. The articulations formed between the distally located tarsal bones (cuboid and cuneiforms) and the metatarsals are plane type synovial joints that allow some gliding movements.

*Goal*

- ❖ To increase the joint play around the tarsometatarsal joint.
- ❖ To increase the plantar flexion/dorsiflexion (plantar gliding increases the plantar flexion, dorsal gliding increases dorsiflexion).
- ❖ To reduce the pain around the tarsometatarsal joint.

*Patient's Position*

Supine lying.

*Fixation*

Therapist's left hand fixes the tarsal joints.

*Support*

No need of distal joint support.

*Therapist's Position and Grasp*

- ❖ Therapist stands at the foot of the patient.
- ❖ Therapist's left hand fixes the tarsal joint movements.
- ❖ Therapist's right hand grasps the metatarsals with the thumb on the dorsal surface and the index finger is in the plantar surface.

*Procedure*

Therapist's right hand glides the metatarsals in the plantar/dorsal direction.

### *Intermetatarsal Joint*

These joints located at the base of metatarsals are very strong plane type of synovial joints in the foot.

#### Dorsal and Plantar Gliding

*Goal*

- ❖ To increase the joint play around the intermetatarsal joint.
- ❖ To reduce pain around the intermetatarsal joint.

*Patient's position*

Supine lying.

*Fixation*

Therapist's left hand grasps the mid-shaft of the first metatarsal with the thumb in dorsal surface and the finger in the plantar surface of the patient.

*Support*

No need of support for the distal joint.

*Therapist's Position and Grasp*

- ❖ Therapist stands at the foot of the patient.
- ❖ Therapist's left hand grasps the mid-shaft of the first to 5th metatarsal one after other with the thumb on the dorsal surface and the finger in the plantar surface.
- ❖ Therapist's right hand grasps the mid-shaft of the adjoining metatarsals one after other, with the thumb on the dorsal surface and the finger on the plantar surface.

*Procedure*

Therapist's right hand performs the dorsal and plantar gliding of the intertarsal joints one after other.

#### Metatarsophalangeal Joint Distraction (Fig. 10.94)

They are condyloid joints, meaning that an elliptical or rounded surface (of the metatarsal bones) comes close to a shallow cavity (of the proximal phalanges). The movements permitted in the metatarsophalangeal joints are flexion, extension, abduction, adduction and circumduction.

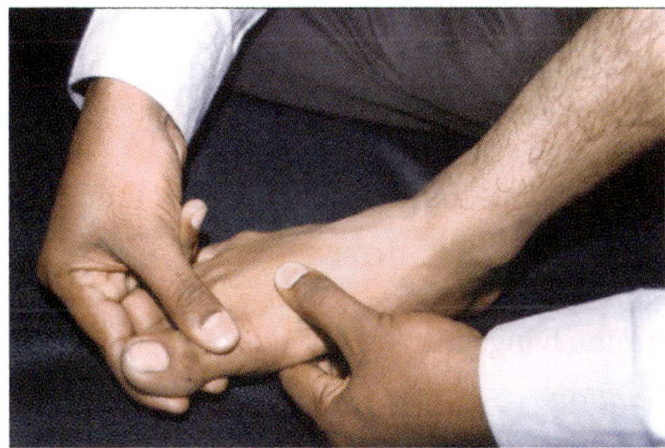

**Fig. 10.94:** Metatarsophalangeal joint distraction, medial, lateral, dorsal and plantar glidings.

*Goal*

- ❖ To increase the joint play around the metatarsophalangeal joint.
- ❖ To increase the ROM of the metatarsophalangeal joint.
- ❖ To reduce the pain around the metatarsophalangeal joint.

*Patient's Position*

Supine lying.

*Fixation*

Therapist's left hand grasps the mid-shaft of the metatarsals, restricting the movement.

*Support*

Distal joints are supported with the therapist's right hand.

*Therapist's Position*

- ❖ Therapist stands near the foot of the patient.
- ❖ Therapist's left hand grasps the mid-shaft of the metatarsals and restricting the movement.
- ❖ Therapist's right hand grasps the mid-shaft of the proximal phalanx of the patient.

*Procedure*

Therapist's right hand pulls the proximal phalanx distally.

#### Dorsal and Plantar Gliding

*Goal*

- ❖ To increase the joint play at the metatarsophalangeal joint.

- ❖ To increase the flexion and extension of the metatarsophalangeal joint (dorsal gliding increase the extension, plantar gliding increases the flexion).
- ❖ To reduce the pain over the metatarsophalangeal joint.

*Patient's Position*
Supine lying.

*Fixation*
As said in distraction.

*Support*
As said in distraction.

*Therapist's Position*
As said in distraction.

*Procedure*
Therapist's right hand glides the phalanx in dorsal and plantar direction.

**Medial Lateral Gliding**

*Goal*

- ❖ To increase the joint play and the metatarsophalangeal joint.
- ❖ To increase the abduction and adduction movements of the metatarsophalangeal joints (medial gliding increases the abduction of the digit 1 and 2, tibial abduction of digit 3 and adduction of digit 4 and 5. Lateral gliding increases the adduction of the digit 1 and 2, fibular abduction of the digit 3 and abduction of digits 4 and 5).

*Patient's Position*
As said in distraction.

*Fixation*
As said in distraction.

*Support*
As said in distraction.

*Therapist's Position*
As said in distraction.

*Procedure*
Therapist's right hand glides the phalanx in the medial and lateral directions.

### *Interphalangeal Joint*

These are synovial joints of hinge variety, permitting flexion and extension of the interphalangeal joints.

**Proximal Interphalangeal Joints Toes (2–5)**

Formed between the convex trochlear surface on the head of a proximal phalanx and the corresponding concave articular surface on the adjacent base of a middle phalanx.

**Distal Interphalangeal Joints of Toes (2–5)**

Formed between the trochlear surfaces on the heads of a middle phalanx and the corresponding concave articular surface on the adjacent bases of a distal phalanx.

**Interphalangeal Joint of Big Toe**

Formed between the trochlear surface on the head of the proximal phalanx and the concave articular surface of the base of the distal phalanx.

Plantar gliding of middle and distal phalanges increases toes flexion and dorsal gliding improves toes extension. Plantar gliding of the distal phalanx improves flexion of IP joint and dorsal gliding improves extension of IP joint of great toe.

# 11 CHAPTER

# Spinal Mobilization

## INTRODUCTION

Spinal mobilization is a type of passive movement of a spinal segment or region, which could be accessory and physiological. It is usually performed with the aim of achieving a therapeutic effect. It is the application of gentle/high velocity, graded oscillatory, passive physiological movements applied to a spinal region or segment to increase the passive range of motion of that segment or region, so that pain and movement limitations are reduced. The purpose of spinal mobilization is to provide short term pain relief and to restore pain-free, functional movements by achieving full range at the particular segment/region.

Research reveals mobilization of the spine used as therapy produces significant mechanical and neurophysiological effects, causing pain relief and movement restoration.

### Effects of Mobilization of Spine

#### *Pain Relief*

The pain gate mechanism, where stimulation of mechanoreceptors due to mobilization produce short term pain relief through the mechanism of pain gating, explains pain relief by mobilization. Spinal soft tissues are highly innervated and may provide a large degree of afferent input into the central nervous system. This input can come from multiple sources such as type I and II mechanoreceptors and free nerve endings found in facet joints and muscle spindles of the spine. Mobilization of the spine also leads to activation of descending pain inhibitory pathways that originate in the midbrain and travel down the spinal cord, through the release of enkephalins and beta endorphin at the posterior horn cell. Mobilization also causes adaptation to pain, by increasing the pain threshold, a phenomenon called relative hypoalgesia.

The breaking of pain spasm cycle and the psychological benefits (placebo effects) may also contribute for pain relief.

#### *Increase of ROM of Spine*

Mobilizations of the spine stretches the shortened fibrous tissue, producing "creep" (ability of the soft tissue to change shape/undergo deformation, when a constant load is applied), thereby increasing the ROM of the stiff segment and region of the spine. Once the length of the shortened tissue is increased, through mobilization (which is temporary), permanent gain in flexibility of spine is achieved, by functional integration and through regular active exercises. The mechanical effects, besides increasing the tensile strength of tight soft tissues, breaks intra-articular adhesions and releases the facet joints from meniscoid entrapment.

#### *Effect on Autonomic Nervous System*

Mobilization has been found to influence sympathetic activity, affecting heart rate, blood pressure, and respiratory rate. Teodorczyk-Injeyan et al. (2006) found that mobilization effected the levels of blood components, with a reduction in inflammatory proteins, suggesting mobilization as a potential therapeutic modality to reduce inflammatory response in spine.

### *Nutritional Effects*

Distraction or small gliding movements, causes movement of synovial fluid, which improves nutrient exchange, to the joints, which were impaired due to joint immobilization and swelling.

## Types of Spinal Mobilization

### *Accessory Mobilization*

Pressure (oscillatory movements) to the vertebral segment affected is applied by the therapist through the thumb or pisiform bone, to produce required amount of movement, as per the selected grade.

### *Physiological Movements*

These are movements like flexion/extension/side flexions/rotations, which are done either passively or actively, in a slow and smooth manner, without causing much discomfort. If treatment is for dysfunction (stiffness), physiological movements are given in the direction of dysfunction, whereas for active derangements like prolapsed intervertebral disc (PIVD), movements are given in the opposite direction that, causes derangement (disc bulge). For example: In flexion dysfunction of lumbar spine, causing flexion limitation, mobilization exercises in the direction of flexion are recommended, where as in flexion derangements, causing disc bulge, physiological movements in the opposite direction (towards extension), is recommended.

## Techniques of Mobilization

There are different techniques of mobilization which are briefly discussed below. However, for detailed knowledge of the manual therapy techniques, the reader is advised to read specific manual therapy literature. The techniques of mobilization are:

### *Maitland Mobilization (Fig. 11.1)*

The Maitland concept uses passive and accessory mobilizations of the spine to treat mechanical pain and stiffness. There are 5 grades of mobilization in the Maitland concept **(Fig. 10.11B)**, shown in Chapter 10.

**Grade I:** Small movements of the spine performed within the spines resistance (at the initial range of pathology).

**Grade II:** Larger movements of the spine but still performed within the spines resistance (the range of oscillation/movement is grater than grade-I, but without touching the pathological limit).

**Grade III:** Large movements of the spine performed into the spines resistance (oscillations/movements are given up to the pathological limit).

**Grade IV:** A small movement of the spine performed into the spines resistance (oscillations are given at the pathological limit).

**Grade V:** A high velocity movement performed into the spines resistance (between the pathological and anatomical limits).

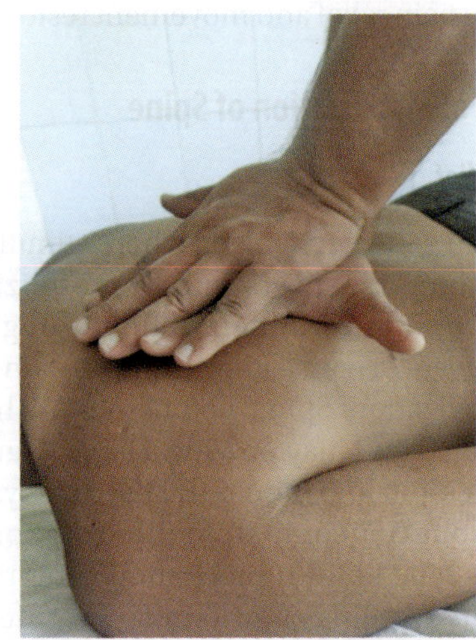

**Fig. 11.1:** Maitland central postero-anterior mobilization of thoracic spine.

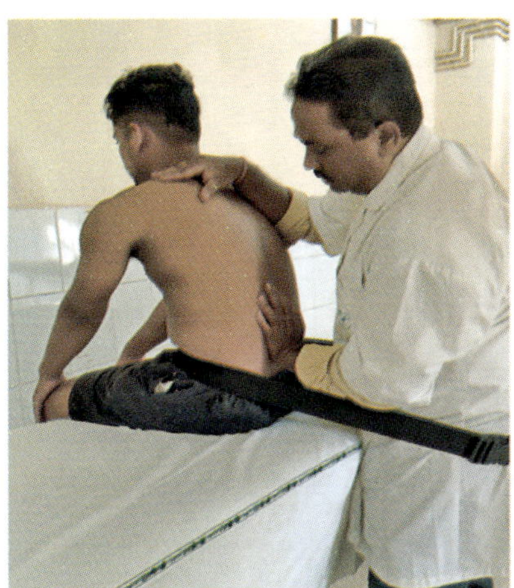

**Fig. 11.2:** Mulligan's mobilization using belt to increase lumbosacral flexion.

### *Mulligan's Mobilization*

This technique of mobilization, called mobilization with movement (MWM), is a manual therapy treatment approach developed by Brian Mulligan in New Zealand, used for treatment of joint dysfunction involving spinal and peripheral joints. The technique involves application of mobilization force by therapist (distraction/glide) during active movement to reduce pain and increase mobility. A belt is used by the therapist to apply glides during mobilization. **Figure 11.2** shows mobilization of lumbar spine using the technique.

### *McKenzie Method*

The McKenzie method or mechanical diagnosis and therapy (MDT) is a system of diagnosis and treatment for spinal and extremity musculoskeletal disorders. It was introduced in 1981 by Robin McKenzie (1931–2013), a physical therapist from New Zealand. The technique involves 4 steps, such as:

**1. Assessment**

Besides the history of symptoms, the clinician makes the patient perform repeated or sustained movements to determine its effect on symptoms.

**2. Diagnosis**

Based on the outcome of repeated or sustained movement tests, the clinician classifies patient's symptoms arising from three syndromes such as:

- ❖ Postural syndrome (performing movements in a direction opposite to the painful posture/movement reduces patient's symptoms).
- ❖ Dysfunction syndrome (movement limitation with pain).
- ❖ Derangement syndrome (production of movement in the opposite direction of pain/movement limitation, reduces radicular pain).

**3. Treatment**

It consists of first finding a repeated or sustained movement or posture that reduces the symptoms and making the patient practice the tested movement repeatedly to cause centralization of symptoms (reduction of leg pain in patients with lumbar PIVD with leg pain) **(Fig. 11.3)** or gain of pain free movements in lumbar dysfunction **(Fig. 11.4)** or achieve maintenance of pain free posture. Next, the goal is to maintain this improvement for several days, gradually integrating the gain of the symptom free movements/posture into function.

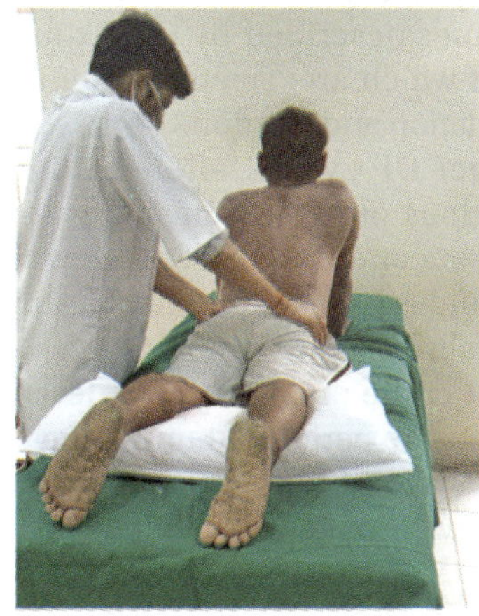

**Fig. 11.3:** Repeated extension of L-S spine to cause centralization of symptoms in lumbar PIVD.

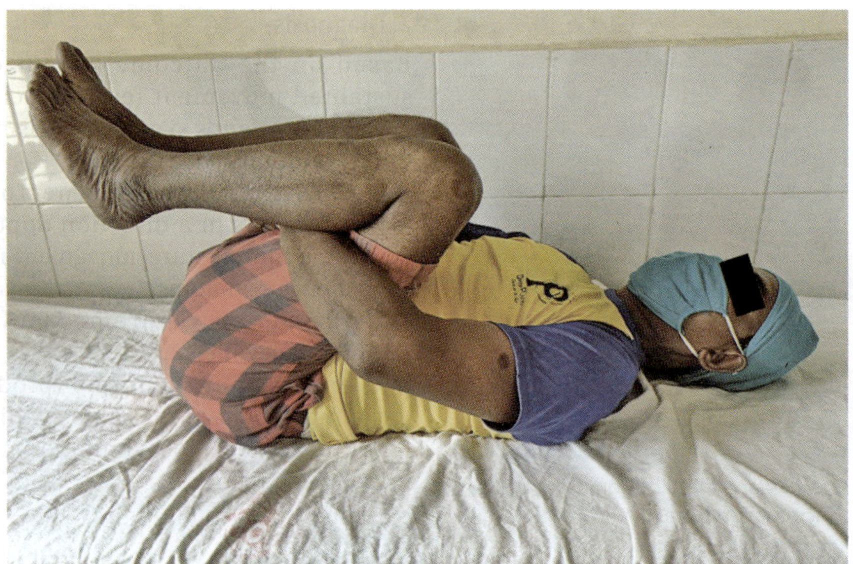

**Fig. 11.4:** McKenzie flexion exercise for lumbosacral dysfunction syndrome.

**4. Prevention**

The final step consists of educating and encouraging the patient to exercise regularly and prevent recurrence.

### *Cyriax Method*

This manual therapy technique, was invented by Dr James Cyriax who also coined the term "orthopedic medicine", and regarded as father of orthopedic medicine. There are various techniques described by Cyriax under the concept which are: Deep friction massage, manipulation and traction.

As per Dr Cyriax, after the age of 60, the nucleus pulposus, becomes hard and disappears and the disc becomes uniform (i.e., annulus fibrosus and nucleus pulposus structurally become same).

Most of the manipulations described by Dr Cyriax, are performed under traction. For the cervical and thoracic spines, traction is applied by the therapist/manipulator with the help of a fixing belt, or by an assistant, whereas for the lumbar spine traction is already built into the maneuver. The techniques involve:

- Application of manual traction.
- Moving the joint into extreme range (to take the slack).
- Application of overpressure.

Three grades of mobilization/manipulation are used, such as:

**Grade-A:** Mobilizations within pain free range.

**Grade-B:** Sustained stretch at the end of range.

**Grade-C:** High velocity low amplitude manipulation at the end of the range.

Grade "A" and "B" mobilizations are movements of low velocity with varying amplitude, remaining within the physiological limit and within the patients tolerance and control, where as a grade "C" mobilization/manipulation usually consists of a single thrust of high velocity and low amplitude, performed at the end of the passive movement, after the slack has been taken up.

Besides mobilization and manipulations described by Dr Cyriax, techniques for correction of listing (lateral deviation of spine), has also been described.

## Indications of Spinal Mobilization

Spinal manipulation exercises are indicated for treating a variety of spinal disorders, listed below. However, the therapist should have enough hands on practice and skill to apply the techniques. A thorough checking for contraindications and precautions discussed below, should be made before the techniques are selected for application. The indications include:

- **Prolapsed intervertebral disc (PIVD) with/without peripheral symptoms:** The McKenzie method of positioning and repeated movements, in the opposite direction of movements that caused the derangement is selected.
- Degenerative spinal diseases (spondylosis), Inflammatory spinal diseases (spondylitis), etc., where Maitland mobilization, McKenzie's method of mobilization for dysfunction syndrome are selected.
- Postural syndrome, causing back pain, neck pain are treated using McKenzie's technique for postural syndrome.
- Hard disk lesion, Locked facets causing spinal movement limitation and pain are treated using either Cyriax or Maitland techniques.

## Contraindications and Precautions to Spinal Mobilizations/Manipulations

### *Neurological Conditions*

- Bladder and bowel dysfunction.
- Saddle (perianal anesthesia).
- Cord signs (spasticity, extensor plantar response).

### *Radiological Changes*

- Severe osteoporosis.
- Hemangiomas in vertebral body/bone tumors (both benign and malignant).
- Severe joint dysfunction in rheumatoid arthritis/psoriatic arthritis/osteoarthritis, where forceful mobilizations are contra-indicated.
- Osteoporosis due to prolong steroid therapy.
- Vertigo, due to vertebra basilar insufficiency in cervical disorders, where careful monitoring should be done while mobilization exercises are performed.
- **Hypermobility.**
- **Vascular: Haemophilia.**
- **Pregnancy.**
- **Spinal disorders such as:** Spondylolysis, Spondylolisthesis, Koch's spine.

# 12 CHAPTER Stretching

## DEFINITION

Stretching is a physical exercise, that involves elongation of the pathologically shortened or tightened soft tissues with the help of some therapeutic techniques, that involve putting a body part in a certain position or application of a constant load/force for considerable duration, that helps in lengthening of the soft tissues and thus enhancing its flexibility and elasticity.

These are forceful movements, where sustained stretching force is applied to tight soft tissues either manually or mechanically by therapists using weight and pulley, weight cuffs, or devices like dynamometers, etc., to elongate tight structures to correct deformities, improve joint range of motion and to restore function. Before stretching is performed, the differentiation between tightness (a state of shortening of soft tissues, which can be elongated by passive force) and contracture (a state of shortening of soft tissues, which can not be elongated by passive force) should be made.

## Types of Stretching Exercises

Stretching exercises are classified into the following types, depending upon the mode of their performance, such as passive or active, manual or mechanical.

### *I. Passive Stretching*

The act of passive stretching entails the use of an external force on a tight muscle/soft tissue to produce a stretch. This external force could be multiple things such as: own body weight, a strap, spring, weight cuff, another person, some form of leverage, gravity etc. The types of passive stretching are:

#### Static Stretching

This is the most commonly performed stretching exercise, where the tight soft tissues are lengthened past the point of tissue resistance and held in the lengthened position for an extended period of time preferably 30 seconds or more with a maintained stretch force. It is done manually by therapists or mechanically.

The slow and prolonged stretch applied avoids reflex contraction of the muscle by inhibition of muscle spindle, due to lengthening of the spindle along with the extrafusal muscle fibers, hence the muscle relaxes. The Golgi tendon organ protects the muscle from the stretch by firing the impulse through type Ib fibers. This type Ib fiber stimulation relaxes the muscle by autogenic inhibition.

#### Static Progressive Stretching

In this type of stretching exercise, the tight soft tissues are held in the lengthened position, until a degree of relaxation is achieved. Then the shortened structured are further lengthened and held in the new lengthened position for some time.

#### Cyclic Stretching/Intermittent Stretching

In this type of stretching, a relatively short duration stretch force is applied repeatedly and gradually with intermittent release to cause elongation of tight tissues. This can be done manually or mechanically.

In cyclic mechanical stretching, the stretching program can be given in cyclic manner with the help of mechanical devices. The intensity and duration of stretch and number of stretch cycle per minute can be set in the mechanical device itself. Thus, manual and mechanical stretching have different effect. The mechanical stretching (long duration, cyclic) gives more flexibility in a short period than the manual method of applying stretching.

**Mechanical Stretching**

The stretch is given by low intensity external force for longer duration with the help of mechanical instrument. In this type of stretching, devices like orthotics, serial casts, weights (weight cuffs/sand bags), theraband, weight and pulley circuits, traction devices, automated devices such as CPM, Dynamometers, etc. are used to apply a sustained stretch to elongate tight soft tissues. The low intensity and long duration stretch gives more flexibility in the muscle and connective tissue than the less duration stretch. The stretch, which is given from 20 minutes to several hours, gives good effect than the stretch applied for less than 20 minutes.

## *II. Active Stretching*

Active stretching (also referred as static-active stretching), involves assumption of a position of joint by contraction of the agonists, so that the tension in the agonist in the active stretch relaxes the muscle being stretched (antagonist) through reciprocal inhibition. Active stretches are usually difficult to be maintained for more than 10 seconds, and rarely needed to be held longer than 15 seconds. The various forms of active stretching are:

**Dynamic Stretching**

Dynamic stretching, according to Kurz, involves moving parts of the own body and gradually increasing reach, speed of movement or both. It consists of controlled leg and arm swings, that moves the joint to the limits of range of motion. In this stretching, there are no bounces or jerky movements. Examples of dynamic stretching include, slow and controlled leg/arm swings and torso twists etc. to increase dynamic flexibility. These exercises are performed in the sets of 8–12 repetitions. These are basically used as home exercise program.

**Ballistic Stretching**

This is a rapid, forceful, high velocity, high intensity intermittent stretch, performed by the patient as per instruction of the therapist to increase flexibility of soft tissues and increase joint range of motion. The Codman's exercise used to mobilize shoulder joint, uses ballistic stretching **(Fig. 12.1)**.

For athletes, a ballistic type of stretching called "progressive velocity flexibility program", based on velocity (slow, fast), and ROM (end range, full) is used. The athletes performing the stretch, undergo a series of stretching program. First the athletes are given static stretching. After sometime it is changed to slow and controlled stretching with mild oscillation in the end range. Then the athlete is progressed to perform the full-length muscle stretch. Once he is mastered in it, he is progressed to fast

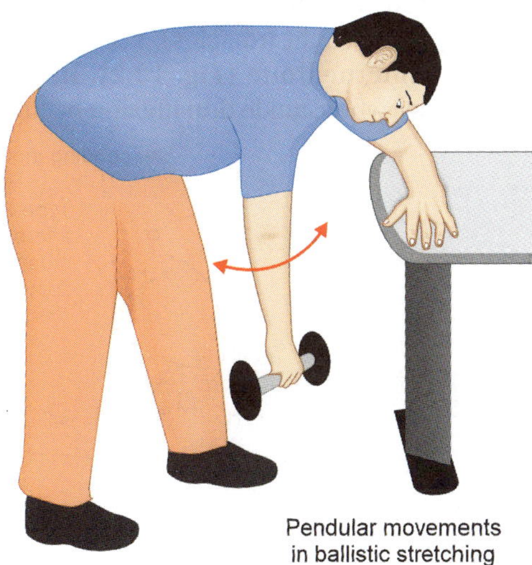


**Fig. 12.1:** Ballistic stretching to shoulder.

stretching in shortened range called as fast short end range (FSER) stretch. Finally, he is made to perform the fast full range stretch.

**PNF Stretching**

This stretching is based on the ideas of autogenic inhibition and reciprocal inhibition.

Autogenic inhibition is what occurs in a contracted or stretched muscle in the form of a decrease in the excitability because of inhibitory signals sent from the GTOs of the same muscle (Sharman et al., 2006). This tension causes activation of Ib afferent fibers within the GTOs.

The GTO senses increased tension when the muscle contracts or stretches, and it responds by inhibiting this contraction and contracting the opposing muscle group. Autogenic inhibition plays an important role in flexibility. When the GTO inhibits the agonist muscle's contraction and allows the antagonist muscle to contract more readily, the muscle can be stretched further.

Reciprocal inhibition, refers to relaxation of the muscles on one aspect of the joint (antagonists), to accommodate contraction of the muscle on the other aspect of the joint (agonists). When the agonists (muscles opposite to the tight muscles) contract, the type Ia, afferent of the muscle spindle is stimulated, which triggers relaxation of the antagonists (tight muscles), via type-Ia, inhibitory interneurone **(Fig. 12.2)**. In the figure, below, when, ankle dorsiflexion occurs actively, the ankle plantar flexors relax by reciprocal inhibition.

The different types of PNF stretching are:

- **Hold and relax:** The tight muscle is kept in a comfortably lengthened position and the patient is asked to isometrically contract the muscle against the resistance given by the therapist. This contraction activates the GTO, which stimulates type-Ib afferents and, subsequently inhibits (relaxes) the muscle through autogenic inhibition. As the patient relaxes, the therapist moves the extremity through the gained range to a new position. After reaching the new position, the above said process may be repeated again.
- **Contract-relax:** This is a stretching technique, that utilizes the natural reflexes and synergies to enhance the stretch response. The steps include:
  - Moving the joint to a position (actively by patient/passively by therapist), where the tight muscle is maximally lengthened.
  - Producing isometric contraction of the opposite muscle/muscle groups, followed by relaxation.
  - After the tight muscle is elongated by reciprocal inhibition, the joint is actively moved to a new position, where the tight muscle is maximally lengthened and again isometric

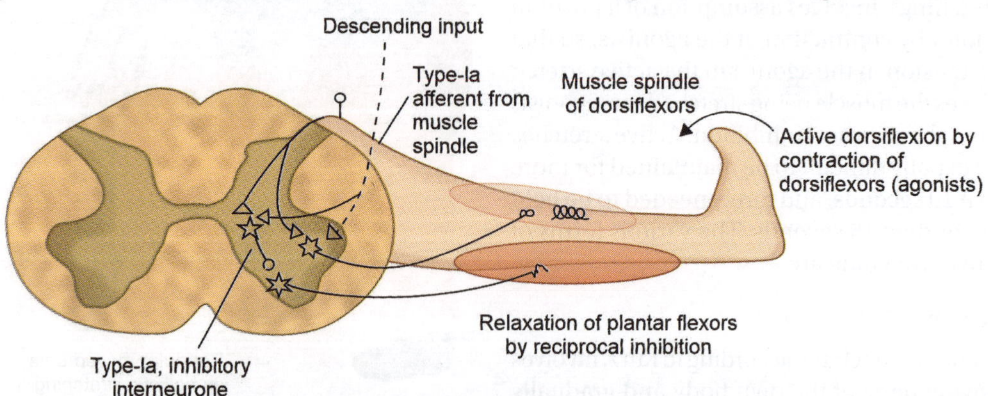


**Fig. 12.2:** Shows mechanism of reciprocal inhibition.

contraction of the opposite muscles are performed.

- The above events are repeated several times to achieve elongation of the tight muscle(s).

For example, in hamstring stretching, the knee is extended, and hip is flexed with the patient in supine lying. After attaining the end range, the patient is asked to contract the opposite muscles to the muscle being stretched, i.e., the hip flexor and quadriceps are made to contract isometrically, which results in maximum stretching of the hamstrings. Normally, in any synergic group, contraction of agonist results in reflexive relaxation of the antagonist, i.e., hip flexors and quadriceps contraction causes the hamstring relaxation. After the consecutive contraction of the hip flexors and quadriceps, the therapist/patient moves the limb still more forward, i.e., more hip flexion with knee extension and a new position is attained. The same procedure is repeated several times without lowering legs.

❖ **Hold-relax with agonist contraction:** The technique is similar to hold relax technique, but differs in the final stretch. The technique involves:
  - Moving the joint to a position, where the tight muscle is maximally lengthened.
  - Isometric contraction of the tight muscle against the resistance offered by therapist, followed by relaxation of the tight muscle(s).
  - Concentric contraction of the opposite muscle groups of the target muscle group that is being stretched and holding the contraction for 30 seconds to relax the tight muscle and increase ROM.

❖ **Agonist contraction:** The tight muscle is passively lengthened to a comfortable position, and subsequently the patient is asked to contract the agonist muscle (opposite of tight muscle) concentrically. The therapist applies mild resistance to the contracting muscle. The tight muscle will relax and lengthen as a result of reciprocal inhibition.

❖ **Slow reversal:** This technique of PNF, involves alternating contraction of the agonist and antagonist muscle groups, without pause/relaxation. It is based on the principles of successive induction, which means that the excitability of one reflex is increased, after another reflex is elicited.

The technique involved for stretching include, moving the patient's limb through a complete ROM, against maximum resistance to both the agonist and antagonist muscle groups alternatively. When the antagonist muscle groups of the tight muscles, contract, the tight agonists relax through reciprocal inhibition. When the tight muscle groups contract against resistance, the muscles relax through autogenic inhibition.

### Self-stretching

The patient himself/herself does this stretching exercise as per the advice of the therapist, as a home exercise program. This type of exercise is valuable in the early stage, of recovery, as the patient applies the stretching force himself/herself using own hand/towels/straps under the guidance of the therapist within the limit of pain (tolerance) **(Figs. 12.3A and B)**.

## *III. Hyperbolic Stretching*

Hyperbolic stretching is an online program that focuses on increase of flexibility, improve posture and relieve back and hip pain, regardless of age or body type. It is a rising star in the world of "next best thing" in fitness programming. The gender-specific program is based on the idea that full-body flexibility can be transformed in four weeks (eight minutes per day) and that men and women need different stretching techniques to achieve their fitness goals. It mostly targets the hips, back, and legs, as well as increases the range of motions in a safe way **(Figs. 12.4A and B)**.

This is the stretching program designed by Alex Larsson. The program combines several methods of stretching, including PNF stretching as well as dynamic and

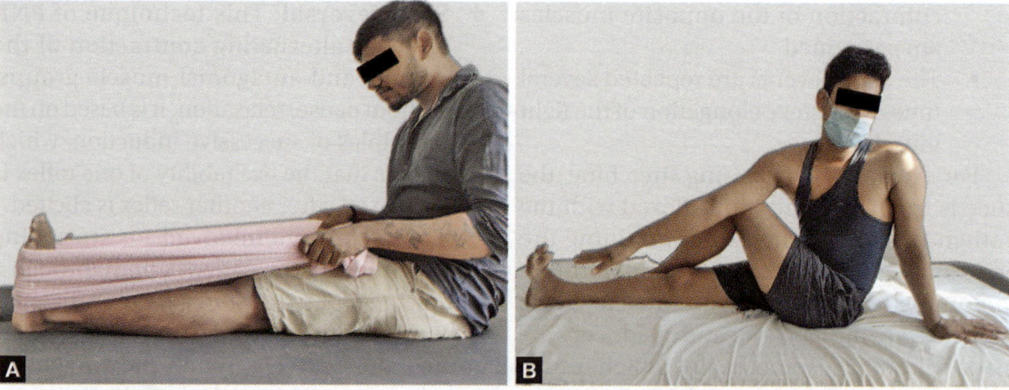

**Figs. 12.3A and B:** (A) Self-stretching of tendo-Achilles using towel; (B) Self-stretching of piriformis muscle in sitting.

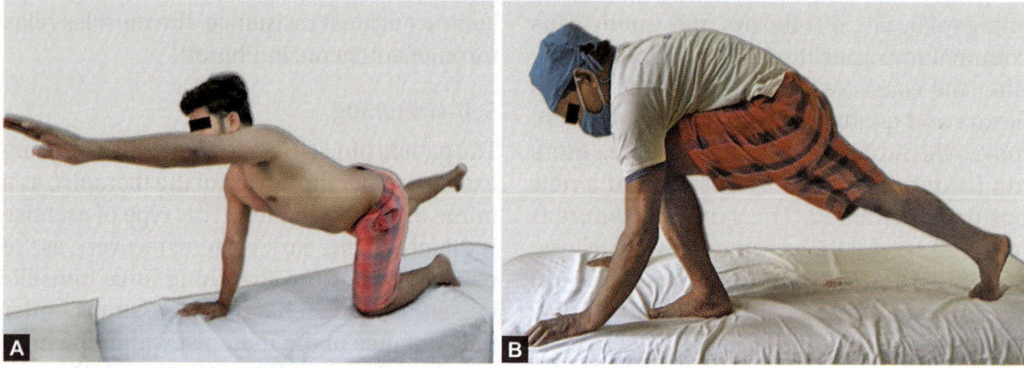

**Figs. 12.4A and B:** Hyperbolic stretching exercises.

static stretches. The program relies on three principles discussed below to help improve flexibility.

- The inverse survival reflex-based on PNF concepts of hold and relax. The muscles are kept in a stretched position and made to contract isometrically, which triggers a reflex that allows one to move deeper into the stretch.
- The second principle is "S.A.I.D." or Specific Adaptation to Imposed Demands. Basically, this means if someone wants to do the splits (routines to focus on different muscle groups on different days), one actually needs to practice stretches that mimic this motion.
- The third principle is using strengthening exercises to get the muscles primed for stretching. The program claims this not only to make the muscles stronger but also "pre-exhausts" the muscles for optimal stretching.

## Mechanism of Stretching

While stretching the tightened joint or muscle the therapist may feel the restriction by the surrounding structures. Limitations may be due to capsule, ligaments, muscle, skin, fascia, cartilages tightness or adhesions. The stretching of a muscle fiber begins with stretching of the sarcomere, resulting in decreasing overlap between actin and myosin filaments, allowing the muscle fibers to elongate. Once the muscle fiber is at its maximum resting length (where all the sarcomeres are fully stretched), additional stretching using a constant load, applied for sufficient duration, places force on the surrounding connective tissues elongating the same by the mechanism of creep (permanent deformation of soft tissues due to a constant load). As the tension in the soft tissues stretched, increases, the collagen fibers in the connective tissue align themselves along the same line of force as the tension.

The proprioceptors related to stretching are located in the tendons and in the muscle fibers. The muscle spindles (intrafusal fibers), that lie parallel to the extrafusal fibers, are also stretched, resulting in reduction of the bias of the spindle to contract and increase tension in the muscles, leaving the muscles in the state of relaxation. The Golgi tendon organ, located in the tendon, near the end of the muscle fibers, help in relaxation of the muscles stretched, due to autogenic inhibition.

The role of the extensibility of the soft tissue, the stress-strain curve gives the perfect knowledge about the load deformation of the soft tissue. Whenever the external force is applied to a soft tissue, it goes for more stress and strain. The first phase is "elastic phase", the stretched tissue will go for normal position after removing the external force. The second is "plastic phase", the stretched tissue may remain in the elongated state when the external force is removed. Third phase is "failure point", the stretched tissue may be teared or separated. Normally, stretch techniques are done up to the limit of the plastic range and sometimes about to reaching the breaking point but without causing any tissue damage. If the breaking point is felt, the treatment should be terminated **(Figs. 12.5A and B)**.

The limitations or restrictions to stretch is felt by the therapist is called as first tissue stop. Normally, the passive movement can cross the first tissue stop. If the therapists add more force after the first tissue stop, he may feel again the restriction to stretch by some structures, which is called as second tissue stop. If a force more than the first tissue stop is applied the

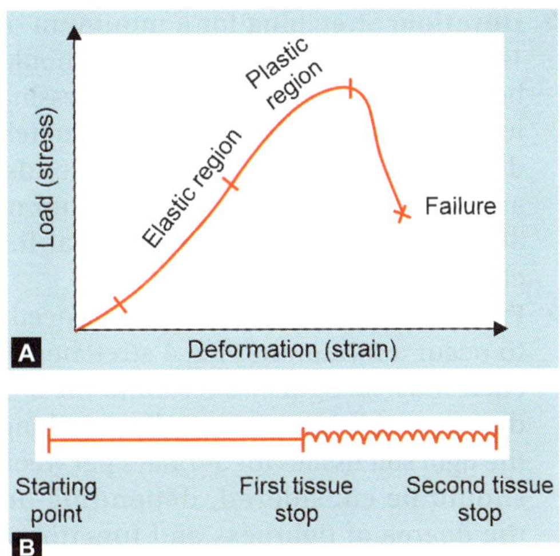


**Figs. 12.5A and B:** (A) Stress-strain curve; (B) Tissue restriction with the stretch.

tissue will be attaining the plastic range. But if the therapist crosses the second tissue stop, the tissue may be separated or teared. So, the stretching technique should be performed within the second tissue stop.

### *Determinants of Stretching Exercises*

- **Intensity:** The lower the intensity, the longer the time the patient will tolerate stretching and soft tissues can be held in a lengthened position. The higher the intensity, the less frequently the stretching intervention can be applied. However, the intensity should be strong to produce creep (discussed below), but care should be taken for prevention of rupture, due to a very high intensity. The soft tissues should be stretched to the point of tightness or mild discomfort.

  Creep is a phenomenon that occurs in viscoelastic materials when a constant stress is applied over an extended period. Over time, the material deforms slowly under the stress, which leads to a permanent change in its shape. In soft tissue, this can occur when the tissue is under a constant load or is exposed to repetitive loading.

- **Duration:** Stretching for a minimum of 10 seconds for very tight muscles should be given with an emphasis on progressing to 30–90 seconds. However, most stretch durations are maintained at 30 seconds, as research reveals that a minimum of 30 seconds of stretch is beneficial for elongating tight soft tissues.
- **Frequency:** Frequency of stretching needs to occur a minimum of 2–4 stretches of each muscle/tight tissue, done for 2–3 days per week. However, ideally stretching the tight soft tissues for 5–7 days per week should be considered, depending on the degree of tightness and functional integration of the affected segment.
- **Speed of stretching:** To cause the elongation of tight soft tissues, the speed of stretch should be slow, as compared to fast speed, as faster speed, elicits the stretch reflex, producing muscle contraction, instead of elongation.
- **Mode:** Mode of stretch is the manner in which the stretch force is applied (static, ballistic, cyclic); degree of patient participation (passive, assisted, active); or the source of the stretch force (manual, mechanical, self).

**Effect and uses of stretching exercises:** The effect and uses of stretching exercises include the followings:

- Stretching improves flexibility and maintains fitness of body.
- It corrects deformities, that result from soft tissue tightness and increases the joint range of motion.
- It reduces the risk of injuries, hence used in sports personnel regularly and before starting outdoor sports.
- It improves blood circulation, reduces muscle soreness and time for recovery. Hence used before and after high intensity exercises.
- It maintains normal neuromuscular balance between muscle groups, hence help in correcting postural deviations and restoration of balance.

## Indications of Stretching Exercises

- Post-traumatic stiffness.
- Post-immobilization stiffness/restrictive mobility.
- Congenital or acquired deformity.
- Joint pathology resulting in soft tissue stiffness.
- Soft tissue pathology leading to relative soft tissue stiffness.
- Healed burn scars.
- To break the pain-spasm cycle, where movement is permissible.
- Adhesion formation over soft tissue.
- Spasticity of muscles.

## Contraindications for Stretching Exercises

Stretching exercises are contraindicated in the following conditions:

- Acute inflammation/acute soft tissue injuries.
- Loose bodies/bony blocks in joints, limiting movement.
- Myositis ossificans/heterotrophic ossification.
- Acute fracture/nonunion of fracture.
- Early tendon transfer/tendon repair.
- Prolonged steroid therapy.
- Hypermobile joints.
- Charcot's (insensitive) joints.
- Chronic rheumatoid arthritis.
- Malignancy.
- In conditions, where, tightness/spasticity is used to hold a posture/perform functional movements.

## Methods for Effective Stretching

Some of the physical modalities are helpful to increase the effect of stretching. The assistive modality that increases the quality of stretch can be given before/during the stretching regime. Some of them are:

- Heat.
- Cold (Cryo-stretch): Given during the performance of stretching exercises.

- Massage.
- Oscillation.
- Joint mobilization.
- Active exercise (warm-up exercises).

**Heat**

Heat increases the relaxation and lengthens the muscle fastly. Normally, heat increases relaxation, circulation, and nutrition, to tissue and decreases spasm and tightness. Stretching performed after applying heating modality requires less force to stretch, as the extensibility of collagen fibers increases with application of heat. The physiotherapy modalities like hot water fomentation, IRR, wax bath, ultrasound, SWD/MWD etc., produces heat in the tissue. So, they can be applied before performing the stretching. The heat stimulates Aβ fibers, resulting in pain inhibition and helps reduction of muscle spasm.

**Cold**

If pain induced by stretch, increases muscle spasm, preventing muscle elongation to stretch, cold application is combined with stretching, to reduce pain and muscle spasm, and achieve muscle lengthening, called cryo-stretch. Though prolonged application of cold, is beneficial for spastic muscles, it has the disadvantage of increasing the viscosity of muscle cells, hence, should be considered carefully, while stretching soft tissues, that undergoes tightness, due to lower motor neuron pathology.

**Massage**

Massage can be applied after application of heat therapy, improving its effect, thereby helpful in stretching.

Effective maneuver of massage produces the followings:

- It increases blood circulation.
- It increases tissue nutrition.
- It enhances local relaxation.
- It decreases spasm.

**Active exercise/warm-up exercises**

Active exercises produces heat inside the body. Warm tissue can be stretched easily. Active exercise like walking, jogging, cycling increases local blood circulation thereby increases the intramuscular temperature. Stretching which is performed after an active exercise will be more effective.

**Joint mobilization**

Before doing the joint stretching, joint mobilization is done; which reduces the stiffness of the joint by breaking the adhesion formed and makes the joint free. Joint traction breaks the adhesion and stretches the tightened structures. The pendular and oscillatory movements relaxes and reduces the tightness of the soft tissue in the joint. Once the joint is made mobile, it will be easier to elongate the tight muscles, that produce joint deformity.

*Note:* The stretching can be given up to the second tissue stop without causing the microtrauma. If the microtrauma occurs during stretching, then icing can be done to constrict the blood vessels, thereby reducing the local blood circulation which prevents further damage. Icing also reduces the post-stretching muscular soreness.

Normally, three varieties of stretching can be performed in body. They are:

a. Muscular stretching.
b. Joint stretching.
c. Skin stretching.

## *a. Muscular Stretching*

To stretch one particular muscle, the opposite action of that muscle should be performed. Some of the muscles that commonly become tight in injuries and diseases and their method of stretching are discussed below:

**Tendo-Achilles Stretching**

Action—Flexion of knee, plantar flexion of ankle.

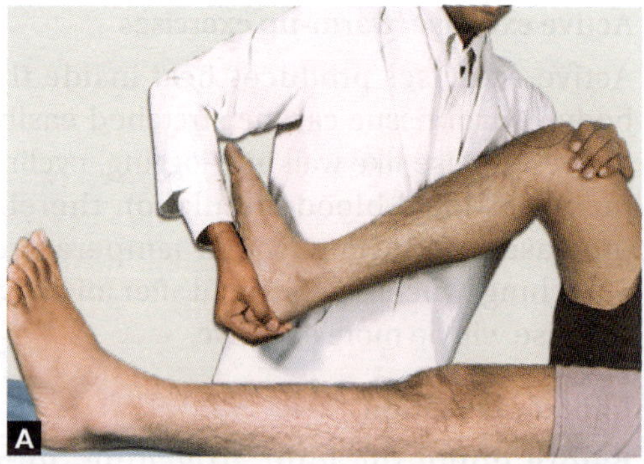
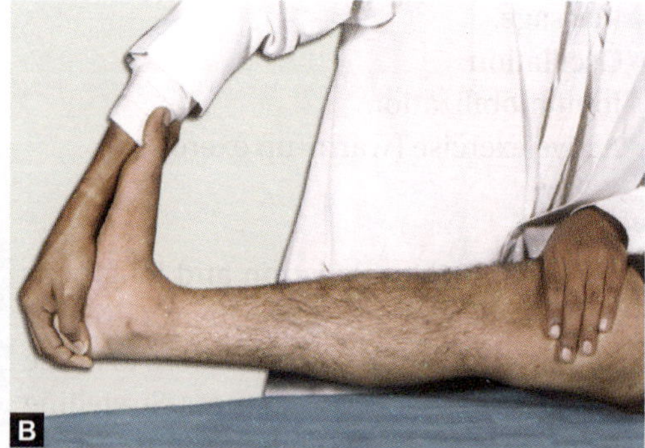

**Figs. 12.6A and B:** (A) Starting stage of tendo-Achilles stretching; (B) End stage of tendo-Achilles stretching.

**Passive Stretching (Figs. 12.6A and B)**

**Position of patient:** Supine lying.

**Position of therapist:** Standing beside the patient.

**Procedure (for right TA tightness):**

- The therapist holds the lower thigh region with his left hand and flexes the affected knee.
- The therapist's right hand holds the heel and pushes the ankle into dorsiflexion.
- Maintaining the ankle in maximum dorsiflexion with the right hand, the therapist slowly extends the knee and holds the stretch for 30 seconds, followed by rest.

While extending the knee, it is advisable to place the hand at the posterior aspect of the knee, unless the patient has associated knee flexion deformity.

**Self-stretching:**

- Standing on slopping surface and leaning forwards for stretching of soleus **(Fig. 12.7A)**.
- Standing on the steps with the ball of the toes for stretching of gastrocnemius **(Fig. 12.7B)**.
- Doing towel stretch **(Fig. 12.3A)**.

*Note:* For soleus stretching knee extension should be avoided. Gastrocnemius flexes the

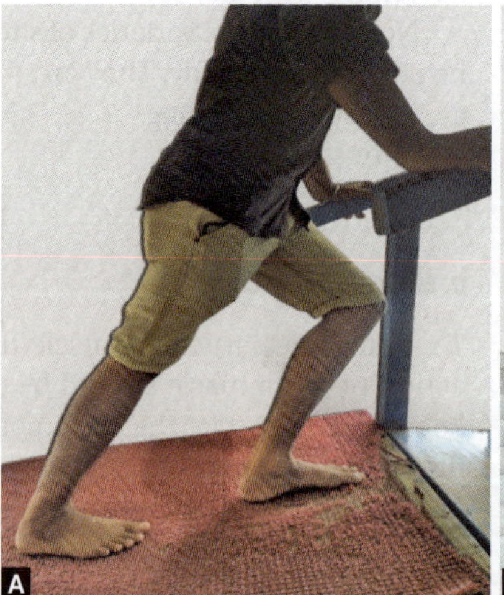
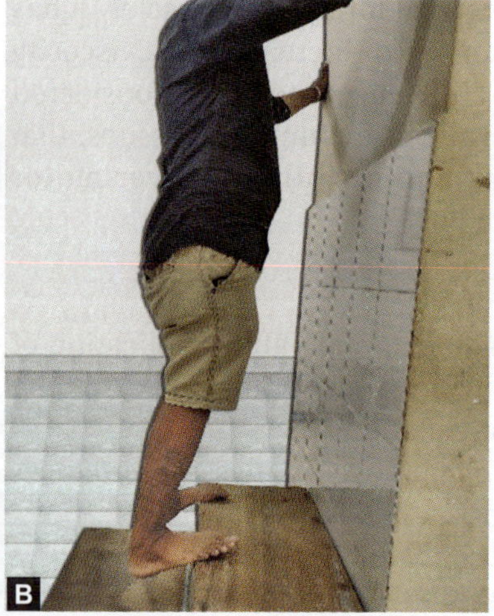

**Figs. 12.7A and B:** (A) Stretching of right gastrocnemius and left soleus; (B) Stretching of bilateral gastrocnemius on a step.

knee and plantar flexes the ankle but soleus is purely for ankle plantar flexion.

### Ankle Dorsiflexor Stretching (Left Side)

*Passive stretching*

**Position of patient:** Supine lying.

**Position of therapist:** Standing beside the patient.

**Procedure:** Therapist's right hand holds the leg region and left hand holds the foot, plantar flexing the ankle (pulling the ankle downwards) **(Fig. 12.8A)**.

**Self-stretching:**

Sitting on the stool/bed by leg hanging, right foot is placed on the dorsum of left foot and pushes the left foot down for stretching the dorsiflexors **(Fig. 12.8B)**.

### Quadriceps Stretching

**Action:** Hip flexion and knee extension (rectus femoris—hip flexion and knee extension, vastus medialis, vastus lateralis, vastus intermedius—knee extension).

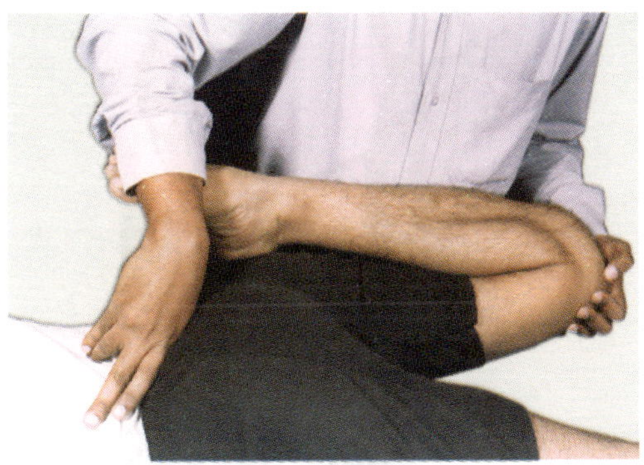

**Fig. 12.9:** Quadriceps stretching in prone lying.

*Passive stretching*

**Method—I (Fig. 12.9)**

**Position of the patient:** Prone lying.

**Position of the therapist:** Standing beside the patient and looking the stretched part.

**Procedure:** For right quadricep, patient's knee is flexed and the therapist's left hand holds the anterior portion of the knee, lifting the thigh upwards to cause hip extension, right hand holds the ankle of the patient in plantar flexion, while forearm and elbow stabilizes

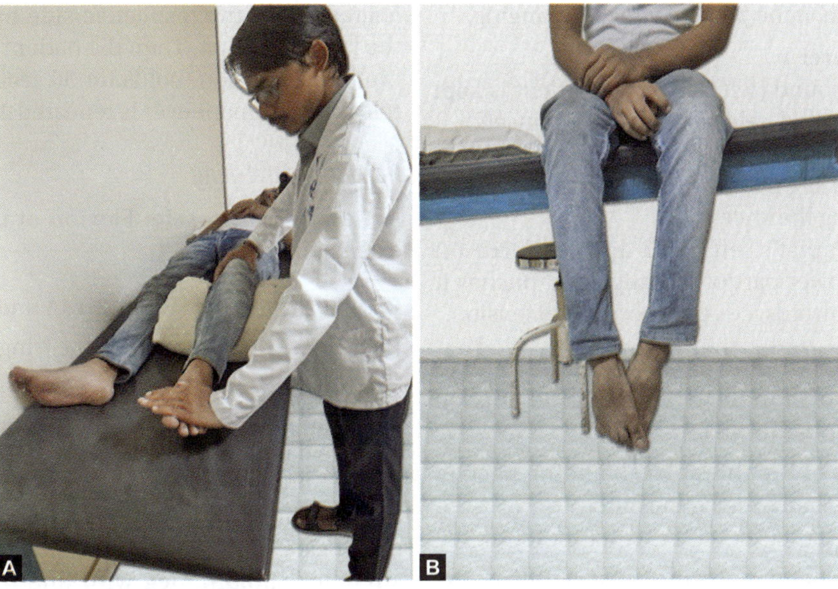

**Figs. 12.8A and B:** (A) Passive stretching of left ankle dorsiflexors; (B) Self-stretching of dorsiflexors.

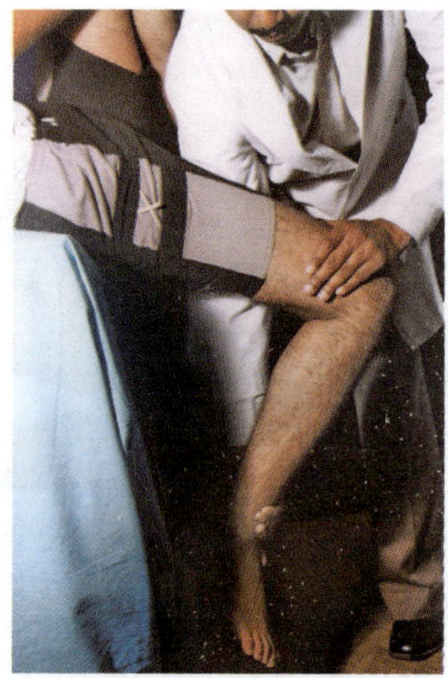

Fig. 12.10: Quadriceps stretching in supine lying in bed end.

the patient's pelvis. The position is held for 30 seconds and then released. 2–4 stretches are given in a session.

**Method—II (Fig. 12.10)**

**Position of the patient:** Supine lying with the lower limb kept hanging at the end of the couch (from the hip region).

**Position of the therapist:** Standing beside the leg region of the patient, which is hanging.

**Procedure:**

- The sound (left) leg of the patient is kept flexed and held by the patient himself.
- Therapist's right hand holds the affected lower leg pushing it towards inside, i.e., flexing the knee.
- Therapist's left hand applies force on the lower part of the thigh and pushes it downwards, i.e., produces hip extension.

**Method—III (Fig. 12.11)**

**Position of the patient:** Side lying (description is for left quadriceps).

**Position of the therapist:** Standing back to the patient and seeing the limb.

**Procedure:**

- Right hand of the therapist stabilizes the affected pelvis and restrict the movement.

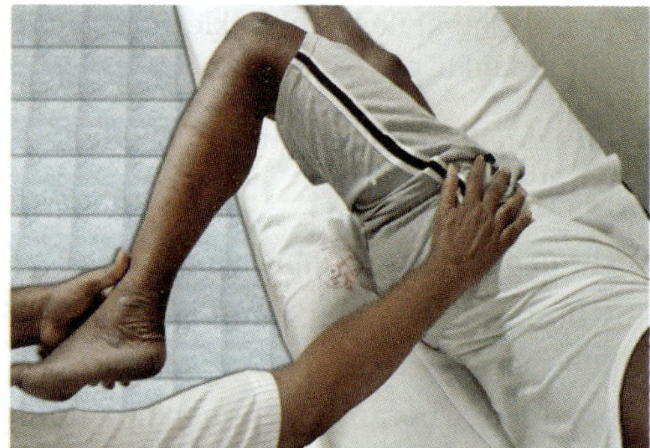

Fig. 12.11: Quadriceps stretching in side lying.

- Left hand of the therapist holds the left knee in flexed position and forearm supporting the leg.

  After maximum flexion of the knee, hip extension is made by pulling the leg backwards.

*Self-stretching* ***(Fig. 12.12)***

Patient standing on one leg and stretching right quadriceps **(Fig. 12.12A)**/side lying, stretching left quadriceps **(Fig. 12.12B)**/prone lying, stretching left quadriceps **(Fig. 12.12C)**/ half kneeling, stretching right quadriceps **(Fig. 12.12D)**/supine lying, stretching left quadriceps **(Fig. 12.12E)**. The affected foot is grasped by the respective side hand with the knee in flexion. Then the patient pulls the hip into extension, holds for 30 seconds and releases. The maneuver is repeated 2–4 times.

## *Hamstring Stretching*

**Action of the muscle:** Flexion of the knee, extension of the hip.

**Passive Stretching (Figs. 12.13A and B)**

**Position of the patient:** Supine lying.

**Position of the therapist:** Therapist is kneeling near the leg region of the patient and the patient's leg is kept over his shoulder and the other hand of therapist stabilizes the opposite hip in extension/therapist standing at the side of the bed close to the leg to be stretched, holding leg with one hand and thigh with the other hand.

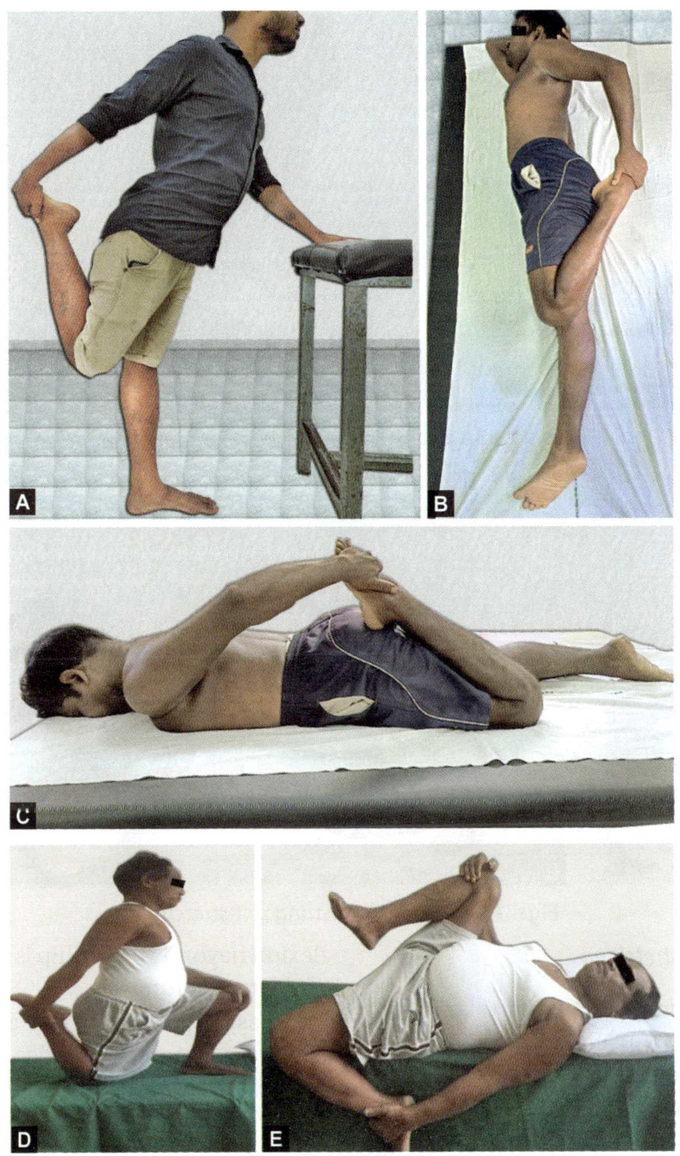

**Figs. 12.12A to E:** Self-stretching of the quadriceps.

**Procedure:** With the knee extension therapist flexes the hip of the patient.

**Self-stretching:**

❖ Patient standing on one leg and other leg over an elevated platform with the knee in extension. Stretching of the hamstrings is done by bending the hip and trunk **(Fig. 12.14A)**. Alternatively, patient lying in supine, is advised to raise the affected leg off the bed, maintaining knee extension by a towel **(Fig. 12.14B)**/Long sitting on the floor—grasping the toes by the corresponding hand and bending the trunk forwards, can also be advised to some patients **(Fig. 12.14C)**.

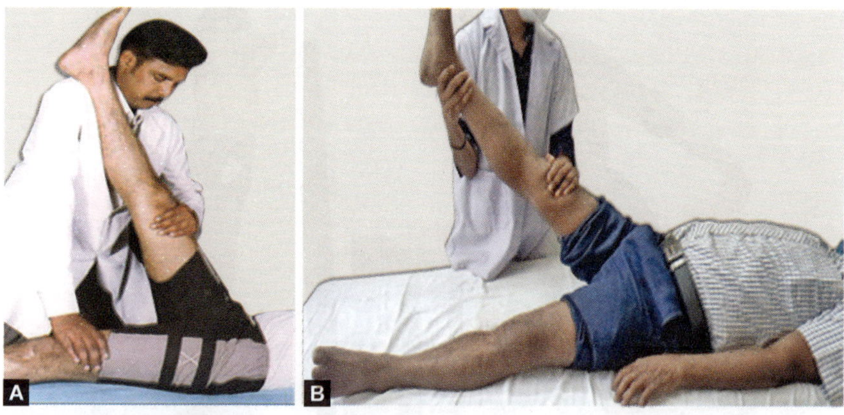

**Figs. 12.13A and B:** Hamstring passive stretching.

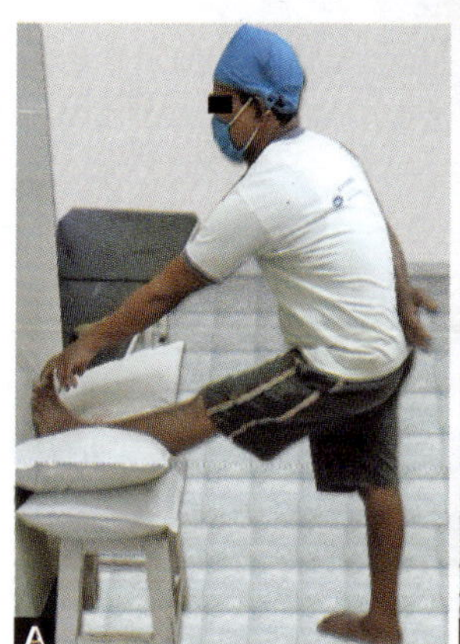

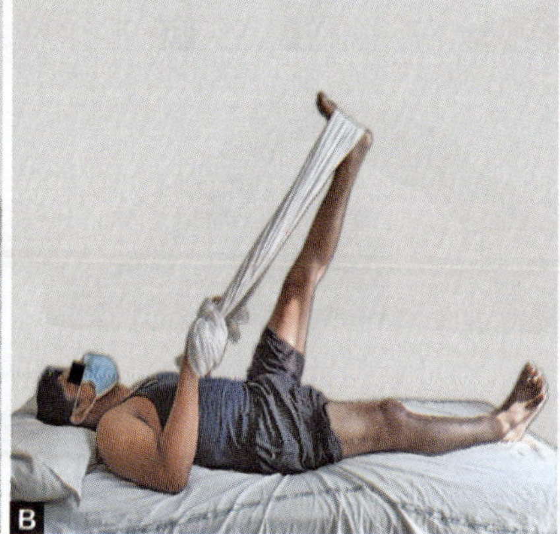

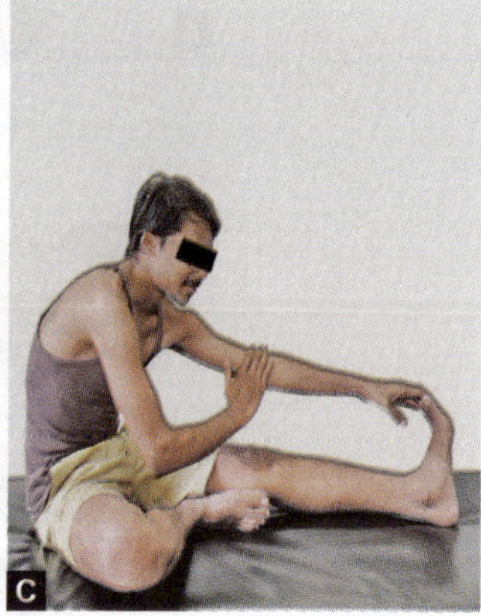

**Figs. 12.14A to C:** Hamstring self-stretching.

### *Piriformis Muscle Stretching*

This is a small muscle, which takes origin from the ventral surface of sacrum and is inserted over the greater trochanter of femur. The muscle laterally rotates the femur with hip extension and abducts the femur with hip flexion. When the hip is flexed to 90°, piriformis abducts the femur at the hip and reverses primary function, internally rotating the hip when the hip is flexed at 90° or more. Tightness of this muscle very often compresses the sciatic nerve on the same side producing pain along the course of sciatic nerve (sciatica). When the muscle is stretched with the hip flexion limited to 90°, the hip is flexed, adducted and medially rotated, whereas if stretching is done with hip flexion beyond 90°, the hip is flexed, adducted and laterally rotated.

Passive stretching of right piriformis is shown in **Figure 12.15**. Please note, with the hip flexed >90 degrees, the affected side hip is adducted and laterally rotated.

**Self-stretching:** It can be stretched in lying **(Fig. 12.16A)**, sitting **(Figs. 12.16B, 12.3B)**—Please note, in **Figure 12.3B**, as the hip flexion is <90 degrees, the affected hip is rotated medially while stretching the muscle.

### *Hip Flexor (Iliacus and Psoas Major) Stretching*

**Action of muscle:** Hip flexion.

**Passive stretching:**
**Method—**I **(Fig. 12.17)**.

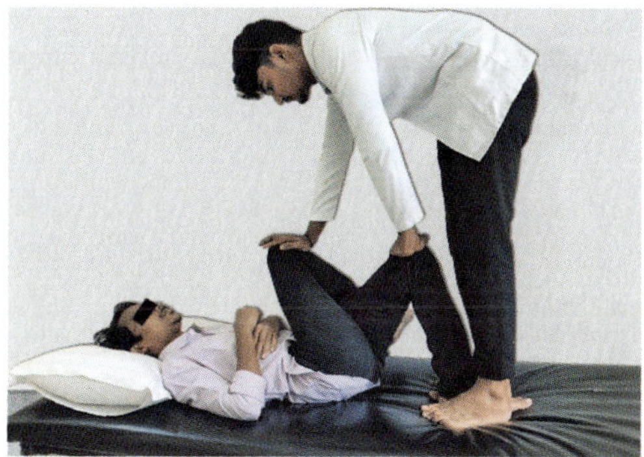

**Fig. 12.15:** Passive stretching of piriformis.

**Position of the patient:** Supine lying with the lower part of the body hanging at the end of the couch.

**Position of the therapist:** Therapist is standing near to the leg region of the patient.

**Procedure:**
- ❖ Normal side hip and knee are kept flexed and held by the patient himself.
- ❖ Therapist grasps the other leg and performs hip extension by pushing the leg down.

**Method—II (Fig. 12.18)**

**Position of patient:** Side lying.

**Position of therapist:** Standing back to the patient.

**Procedure:**
- ❖ Therapist's left hand stabilizes the pelvis and right hand grasps the lower thigh and

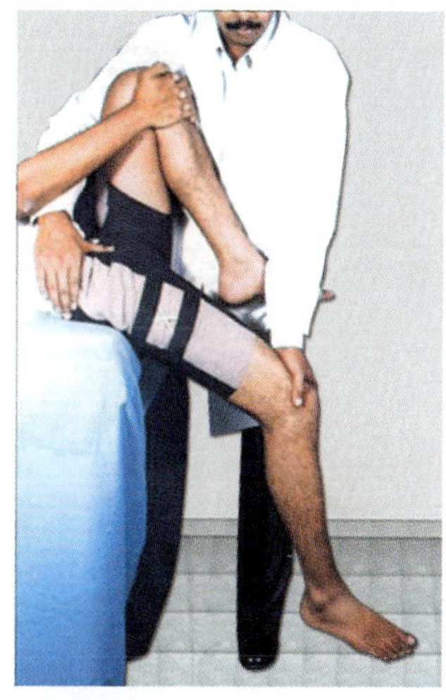

**Fig. 12.17:** Iliopsoas passive stretching in supine position.

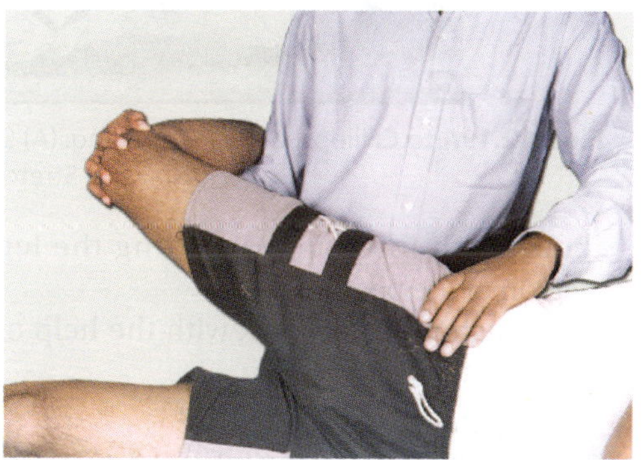

**Fig. 12.18:** Iliopsoas passive stretching in side lying position.

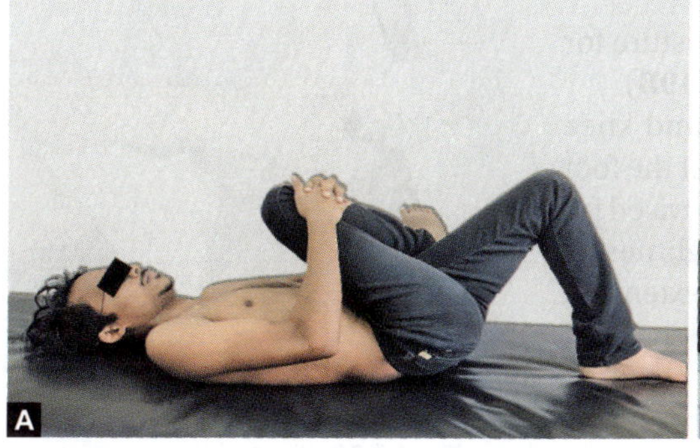



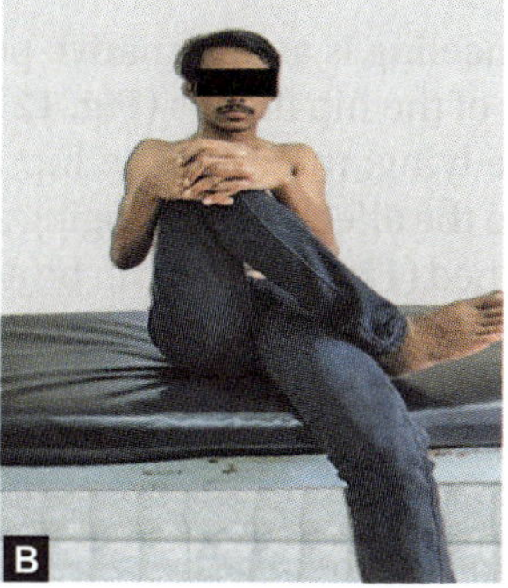



**Figs. 12.16A and B:** Self-stretching of piriformis: (A) In supine lying; (B) Sitting.

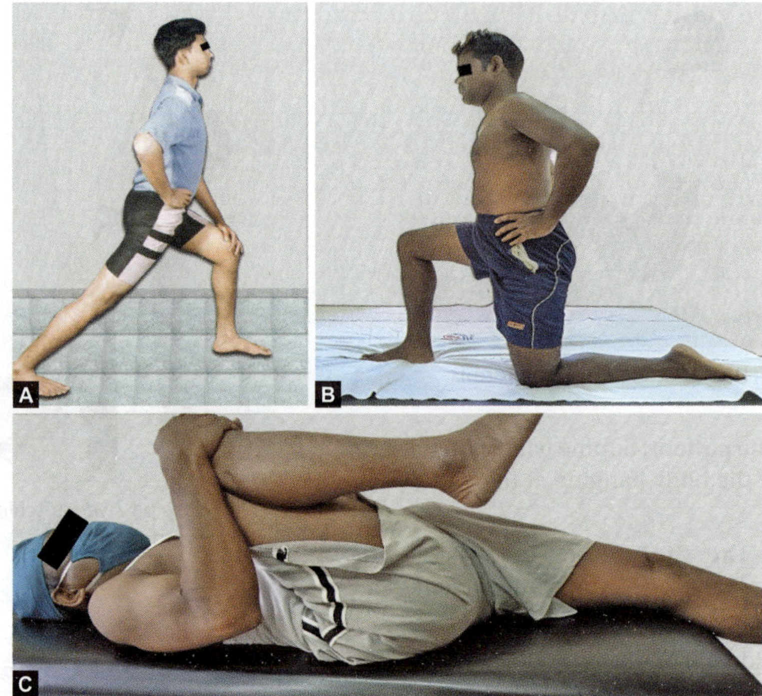

**Figs. 12.19A to C:** Iliopsoas self-stretching: (A) Stretching of right hip flexor; (B) Stretching of left hip flexors; (C) Stretching of left hip flexor.

knee, with forearm supporting the leg region of the patient.

- The thigh is pulled back with the help of right hand.

**Self-stretching:**

Fall out standing posture stretches the iliopsoas **(Fig. 12.19A)**. Stretched side hip and knee are extended and kept backwards, the opposite side hip and knee are partially flexed and kept forwards.

Half kneeling is an alternative posture for stretching of the hip flexors **(Fig. 12.19B)**.

Supine lying, the opposite hip and knee flexed, and the affected leg hanging at the foot end of the bed **(Fig. 12.19C)** can be advised for stretching of hip flexors, where the tightness is very less and the thigh is pushed into extension by gravity.

### *Gluteus Maximus Stretching*

**Action:** Hip extension.

**Passive Stretching (Fig. 12.20)**

**Position of patient:** Patient is lying supine.

**Position of therapist:** Therapist is standing beside the patient and facing the limb.

**Procedure:**

- Therapist's right hand grasps the ankle while his left hand holds the knee posteriorly.

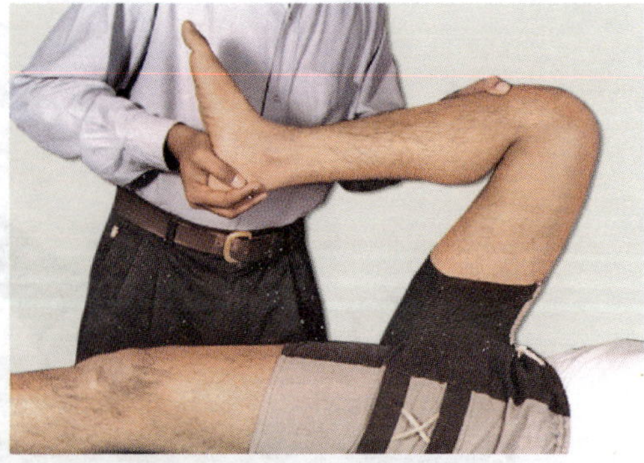

**Fig. 12.20:** Right gluteus maximus passive stretching.

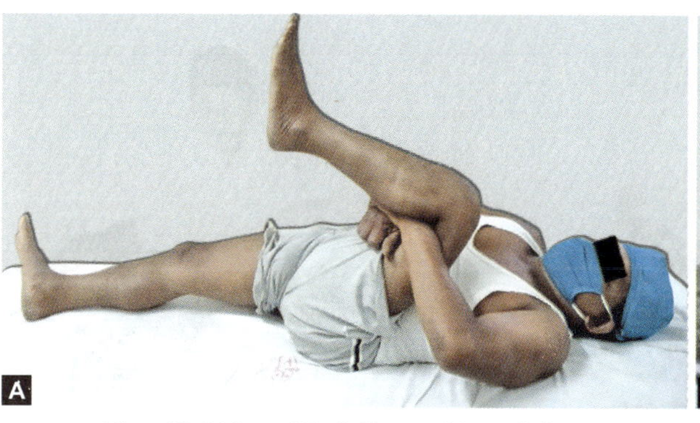


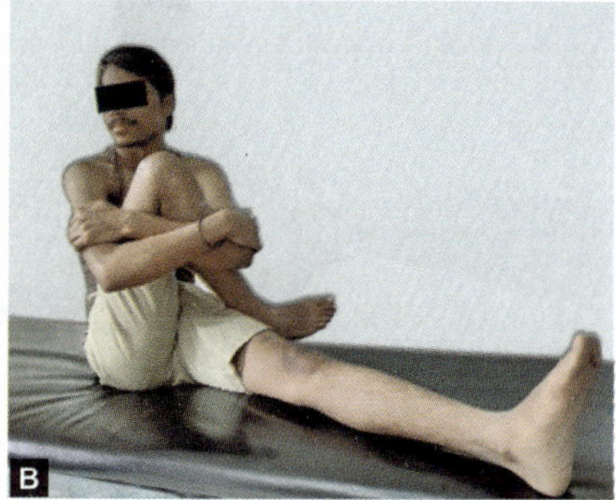


**Figs. 12.21A and B:** Self-stretching of gluteus maximus: (A) In supine; (B) In long sitting.

- The affected leg is lifted with hip and knee flexed, towards the cranial side of the patient.

**Self-stretching:**

- Kneel sitting is one way of stretching the gluteus maximum.
- Patient flexing the hip and knee himself, with his/her hands in supine **(Fig. 12.21A)**/ long sitting **(Fig. 12.21B)** maintains a good stretch.

### *Hip Adductor Stretching*

Passive stretching of short hip adductors (Adductor longus, Adductor brevis, Adductor magnus) **(Fig. 12.22).**

**Position of patient:** Crook lying.

**Position of therapist:** Standing or sitting beside the patient, facing the limb.

**Procedure:** Both the heels are kept together and the knees are drawn apart.

**Self-stretching:**

- Ride sitting stretches the short hip adductor.
- Circle sitting, both the sole of feet touching together. Pressure is applied on the medial aspect of the knees towards the floor **(Fig. 12.23)**.

**Passive stretching** of long hip adductors (gracilis and medial hamstrings) **(Fig. 12.24)**.

**Position of patient:** Supine lying with the knees extended.

**Position of therapist:** Standing at the foot end of the bed, facing the patient.

**Procedure:** The therapist passively abducts both hips simultaneously, holds the position for 30 seconds and then relaxes.

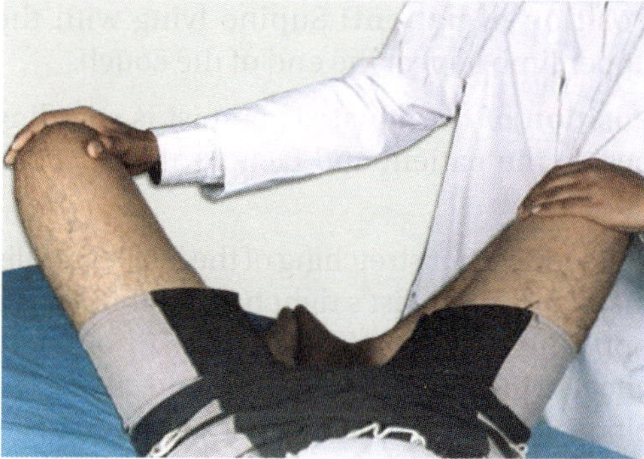

**Fig. 12.22:** Hip adductor passive stretching (Short adductors).

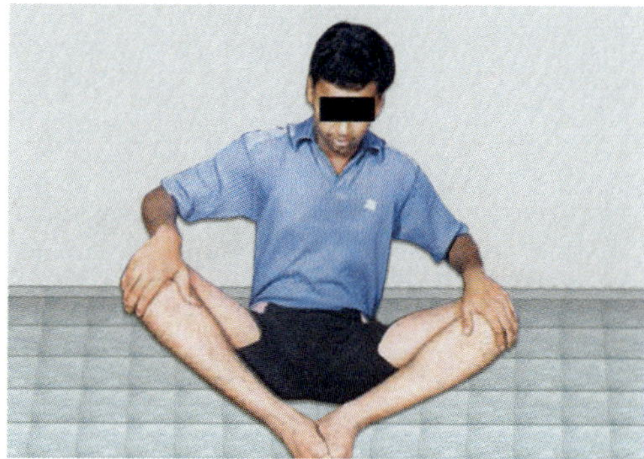

**Fig. 12.23:** Self-stretching of short adductors of hips.

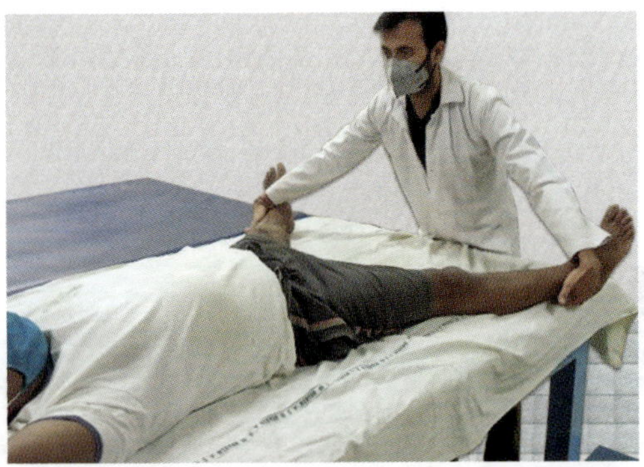

**Fig. 12.24:** Passive stretching of long adductors of hips.

**Self-stretching:** Stride sitting, touching both feet with hands **(Fig. 12.25)**.

### *Iliotibial Tract*

**Passive Stretching (Fig. 12.26)**

**Action of IT band:** Flexion, abduction, external rotation of hip, flexion/extension of knee.

**Position of patient:** Side lying.

**Position of therapist:** Standing back to the patient and facing the limb.

**Procedure:**

- Therapist's left hand stabilizes the pelvic and right hand grasps the patient knee with the leg placed over the forearm. The lower side hip and knees should be flexed, to prevent movement of the pelvis (stabilize pelvis).

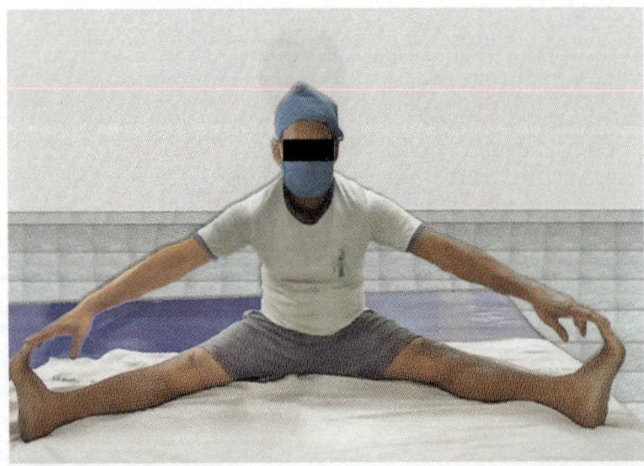

**Fig. 12.25:** Self-stretching of long adductors of hips.

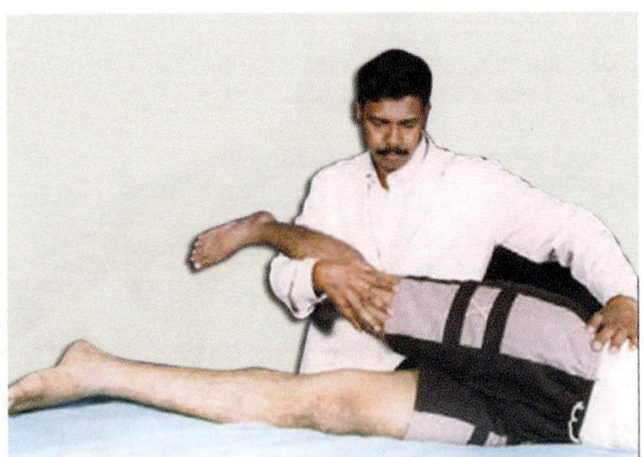

**Fig. 12.26:** Iliotibial tract passive stretching.

- Hip is extended, adducted and medially rotated, finally the knee is flexed to stretch the iliotibial tract.

**Self-stretching:**

- Patient is standing and feet away from the wall and leaning forward with one leg placed in front and the other internally rotated, adducted and extended **(Fig. 12.27A)**.
- In side lying the patient's upper most hip is extended, adducted and medially rotated, with the knee held in flexion by the patient's hand. The hip is pushed into adduction by the lower side foot **(Fig. 12.27B)**.

### *Pectoralis Major Stretching*

**Passive Stretching (Figs. 12.28A and B)**

**Action of the muscle:** Flexion, horizontal adduction, and medial rotation of the shoulder.

**Position of patient:** Supine lying with the upper limb kept at the end of the couch.

**Position of therapist:** Therapist is standing beside the patient and facing the respective upper limb.

**Procedure:** For stretching of the left pectoralis major, the therapist's right hand stabilizes the opposite shoulder. The therapist holds the affected arm with his/her left hand, above the elbow (the patient may grasp the therapist's elbow keeping his/her elbow flexed). Then the left hand performs the reverse action

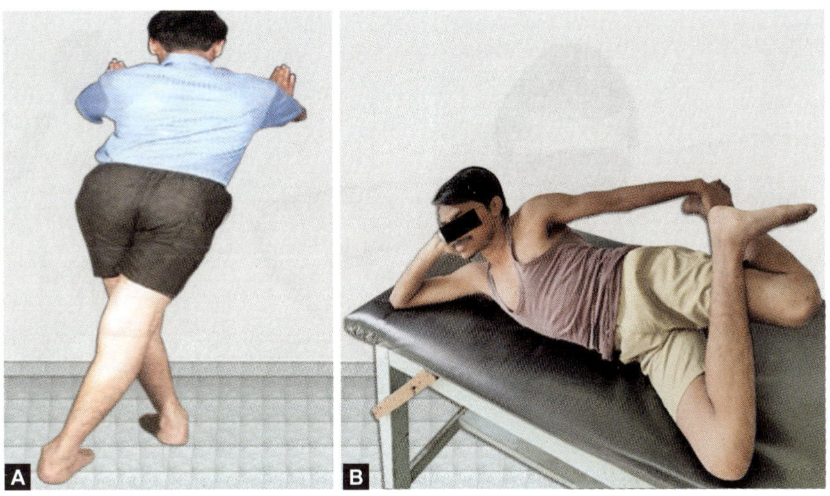


**Figs. 12.27A and B:** Iliotibial tract self-stretching: (A) Standing; (B) Side lying.

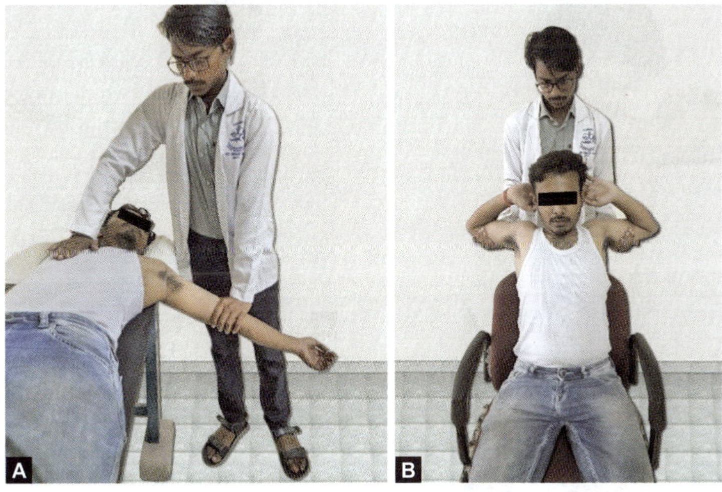


**Figs. 12.28A and B:** Pectoralis major passive stretching: (A) Supine lying; (B) Sitting.

of pectoralis major, i.e., lateral rotation, abduction and extension of shoulder **(Fig. 12.28A)** Alternatively, the patient is made to sit on the chair with both hands at the back of head. The therapist stands at the back of patient, holds the patients arm and pulls the shoulders towards, extension, abduction and external rotation **(Fig. 12.28B)**.

**Self-stretching:**

- Both the hands grasped behind the head in supine lying and the patient is asked to relax and drop the elbows down to touch the support surface **(Fig. 12.29A)**.
- The patient stands, facing the corner of the room, with both shoulders abducted and laterally rotated, and hands over the side walls. Then, he/she pushes the body towards the corner, holds for 30 seconds and then relaxes **(Fig. 12.29B)**.

### *Biceps Brachii Stretching*

**Action:** Flexion of shoulder and elbow, supination of forearm.

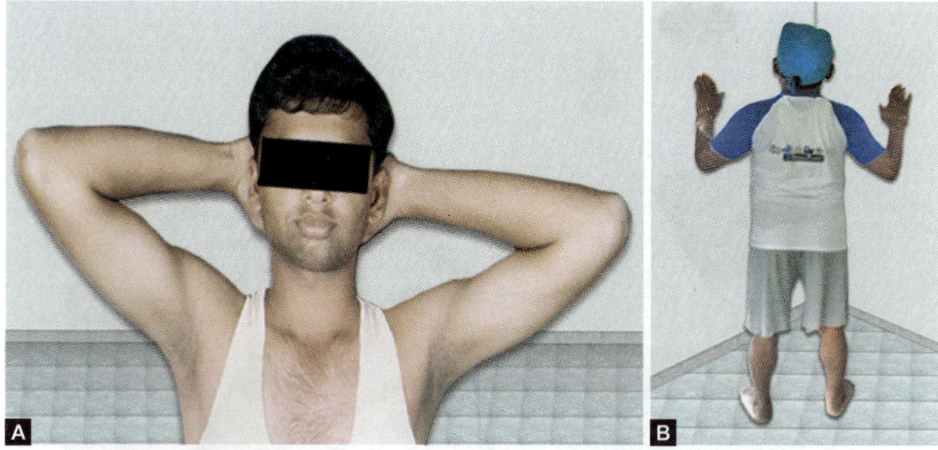

**Figs. 12.29A and B:** Pectoralis major self-stretching: (A) On bed; (B) Corner stretch.

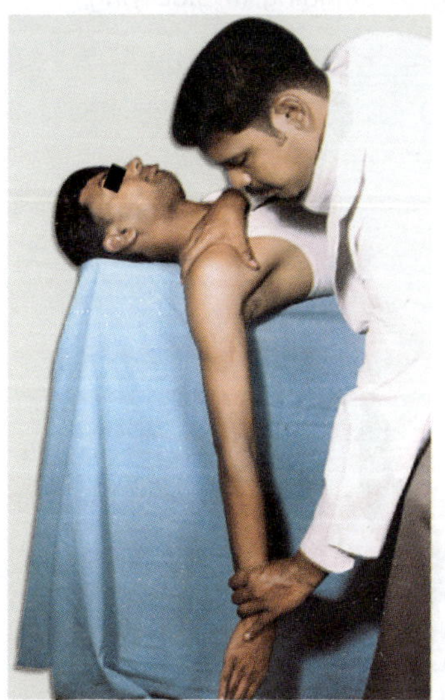

**Fig. 12.30:** Biceps brachii passive stretching.

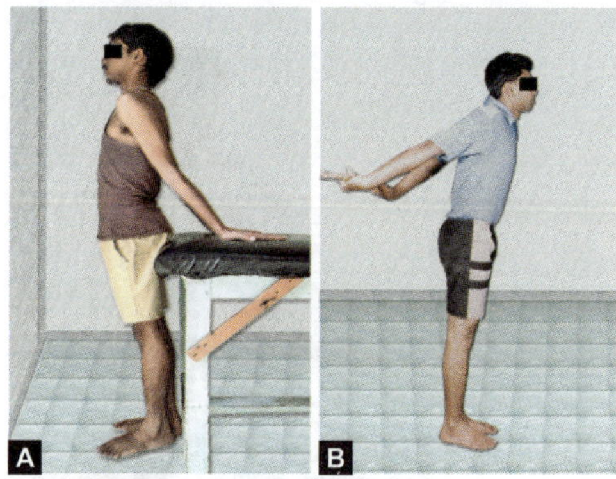

**Figs. 12.31A and B:** Biceps self-stretching: (A) Placing the hands on table; (B) Stretching the arms backwards holding a stick.

**Passive Stretching (Fig. 12.30)**

**Position of patient:** Supine lying.

**Position of therapist:** Therapist is standing at the side of the bed, facing the affected limb.

**Procedure:**

For stretching of right side biceps brachii, therapist's left hand grasps the wrist and hand of the patient, maintaining elbow extension and forearm pronation, while right hand stabilizes the scapula.

Left hand performs the shoulder extension, and medial rotation, with elbow in extension and forearm in pronation.

**Self-stretching (Figs. 12.31A and B)**

- In high sitting/standing, the patient places the hands at the back of the body on the surface and stretches the biceps **(Fig. 12.31A)**.
- In standing, the patient stretches the arms backwards, holding the stick **(Fig. 12.31B)**.

## *Triceps Brachii Stretching*

**Action of muscle:** Shoulder extension and elbow extension.

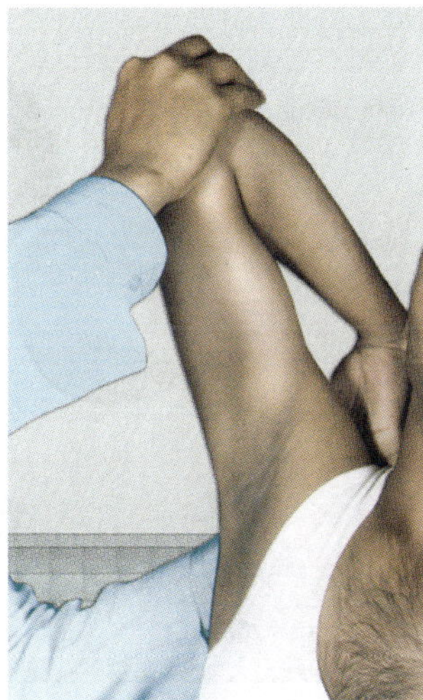

**Fig. 12.32:** Triceps brachii passive stretching.

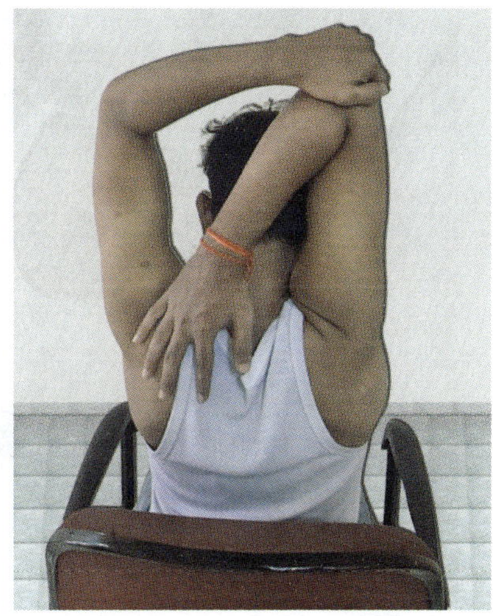

**Fig. 12.33:** Triceps brachii-self-stretching.

**Passive Stretching (Fig. 12.32)**

**Position of patient:** Supine lying or sitting.

**Position of therapist:** Therapist is stands beside the patient, and holds the affected elbow in flexion.

**Procedure:**

- For right triceps brachii, the left hand of the therapist stabilizes the scapula, whereas the right hand flexes the affected shoulder with the elbow maintained in flexion.

**Self-stretching (Fig. 12.33)**

In sitting or standing, the opposite side hand, pulls the shoulder into flexion with the elbow in flexion.

### *Extensor Compartment Muscles of Forearm Stretching*

**Passive stretching:** The muscles are commonly affected in tennis elbow. The stretching is started with the elbow in a bent position. The wrist is fully flexed and ulnar deviated. Then the elbow is extended and the position is maintained for 30 seconds. 3–4 stretches are given which are shown in **Figures 12.34A and B**.

**Self-stretching (Fig. 12.35)**

### *Flexor Compartment Muscles of Forearm Stretching*

These muscles are commonly inflamed in golfer's elbow.

**Action of the muscles:** Wrist flexion, elbow flexion, finger flexion (MCP, PIP, DIP).

**Passive stretching (Fig. 12.36)**

**Position of the patient:** Sitting or supine lying, side lying.

**Position of the therapist:** Standing beside the patient.

**Procedure:**

- For muscles of right side, the therapist's left hand grasps the lower arm preventing the shoulder movement.
- Therapist's right hand grasps the hand and the fingers.
- Therapist extends the fingers and wrist after the elbow extension. Here the whole flexor compartment muscles undergo stretching.

**Self-stretching (Figs. 12.37A and B)**

Place the hand on the couch with wrist, fingers and elbow extended for stretching the flexor compartment of the forearm **(Fig. 12.37A)**. Alternatively, the patient is sits with the affected side elbow extended. He/she extends

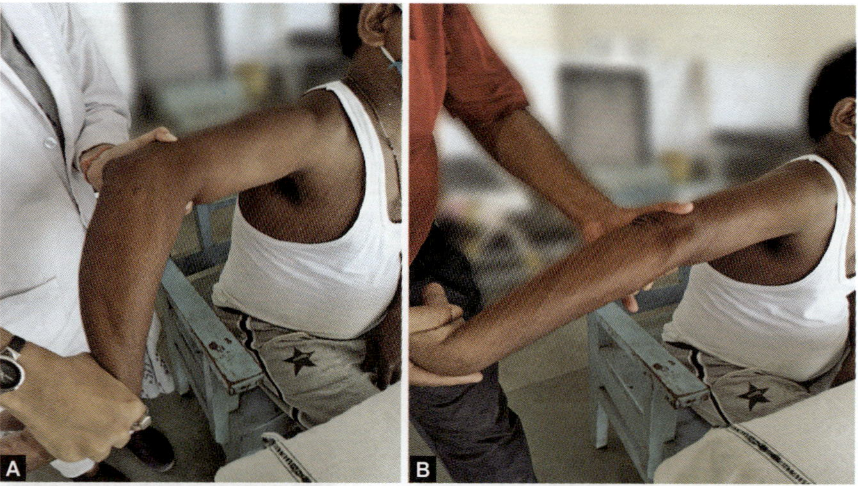

**Figs. 12.34A and B:** Passive stretching of extensor muscles of forearm: (A) Beginning; (B) Ending.

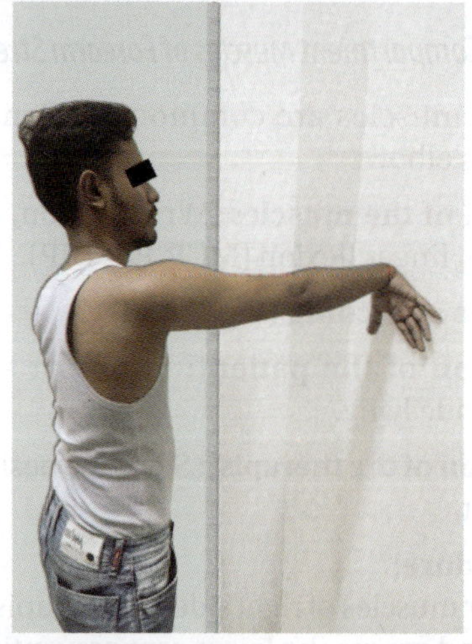

**Fig. 12.35:** Self-stretching of extensor muscles of forearm.

the wrist and fingers with the opposite hand, maintains extension for 30 seconds and repeat the same for 3–4 times **(Fig. 12.37B)**.

### *Sternocleidomastoid Stretching*

**Passive stretching:**

**Action:** Same side flexion and opposite side rotation of the neck and also forward flexion of the neck.

**Position of the patient:** Sitting or supine lying with the neck placed at the end of the couch.

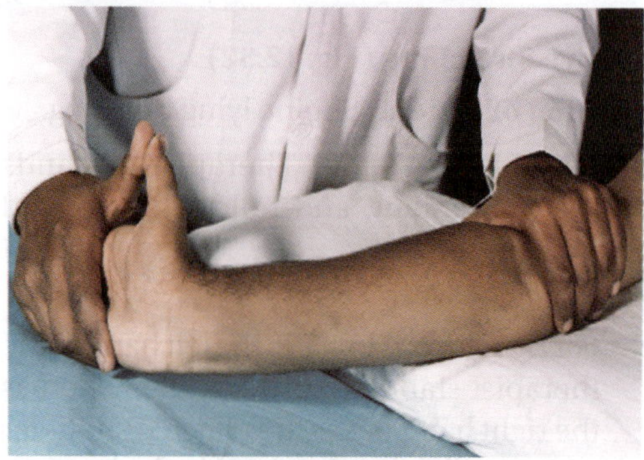

**Fig. 12.36:** Flexor compartment of the forearm passive stretching.

**Position of the therapist:** Therapist is standing behind the patient's head.

**Procedure:** The therapist holds the patient head with both the hand (one below the occiput other below the chin) and performs the opposite action of the sternomastoid, i.e., opposite side flexion and same side rotation and extension of the neck **(Fig. 12.38)**.

**Self-stretching (Fig. 12.39):** The patient sitting on chair/bed, and performs the followings:

- ❖ Tuck the chin inward and downward.
- ❖ Bends the neck to opposite side by placing the hand on the tight side of the head, so that ear is between middle and ring fingers.

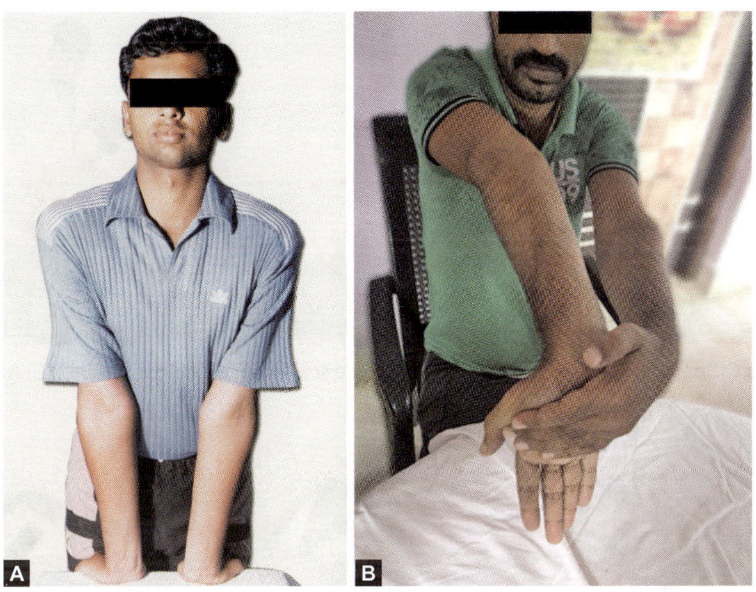

**Figs. 12.37A and B:** Flexor compartment of the forearm self-stretching.

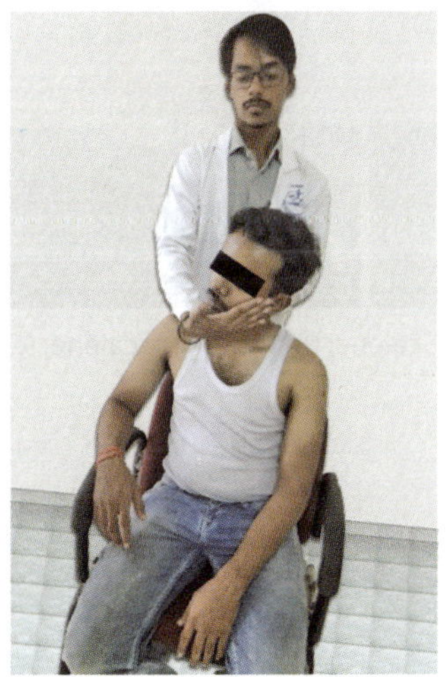

**Fig. 12.38:** Sternocleidomastoid stretching (right side)..

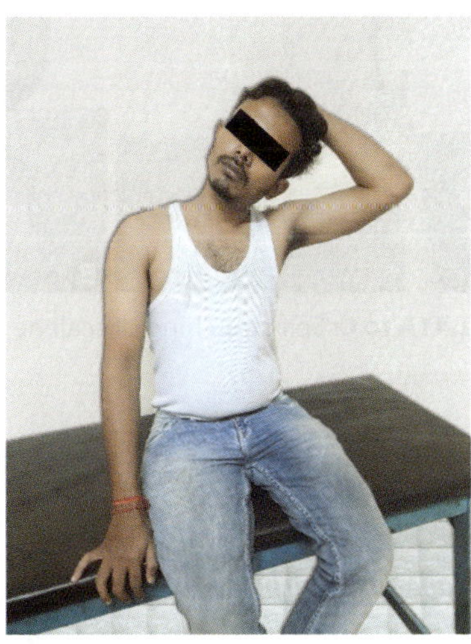

**Fig. 12.39:** Self-stretching of sternocleidomastoid.

- Bends the head backward.
- Gently turns the head to the opposite side.

### *Scalene Muscle Stretching*

#### Action of Muscle

**Anterior scalene muscle:** Bilateral contraction produces neck flexion. Unilateral contraction: Same side neck lateral flexion, and elevation of 1st rib.

**Middle scalene muscle:** Produces same side neck lateral flexion and elevation of 1st rib.

**Posterior scalene muscle:** Produces same side neck lateral flexion and elevation of 2nd rib.

**Passive stretching:** (left side) **(Figs. 12.40A to C)**

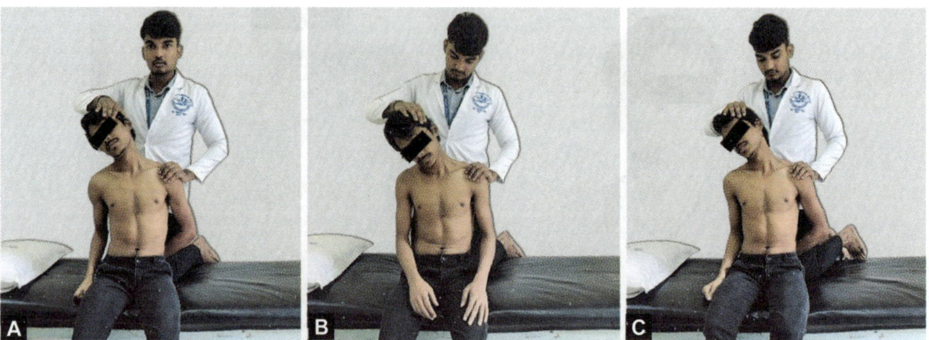

**Figs. 12.40A to C:** Stretching of scalene muscles: (A) Middle scalene; (B) Posterior scalene; (C) Anterior scalene.

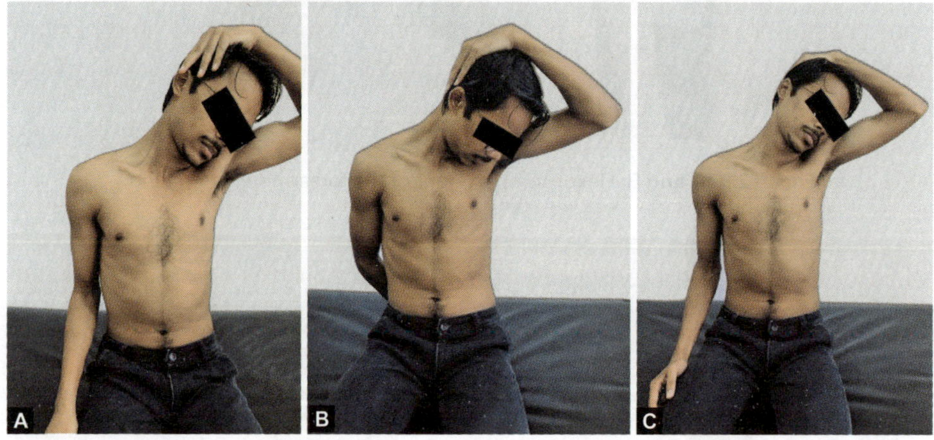

**Figs. 12.41A to C:** Self-stretching of scalene muscles: (A) Middle Scalene; (B) Posterior scalene; (C) Anterior scalene.

**Self-stretching:** (Right side) **(Figs. 12.41A to C).**

### *Upper Trapezius Stretching*

**Passive stretching:** (left side) **(Fig. 12.42)**

**Self-stretching:** (Right side) **(Fig. 12.43)**.

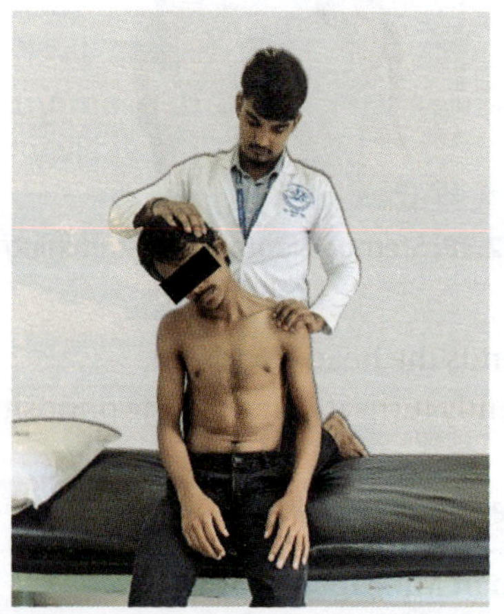

**Fig. 12.42:** Passive stretching of left upper trapezius.

### *Levator Scapulae Stretching*

**Passive stretching (Fig. 12.44)**.

**Self-stretching** of levator scapulae **(Figs. 12.45A and B)**.

### *Rhomboids Stretching*

**Passive stretching (Fig. 12.46)**

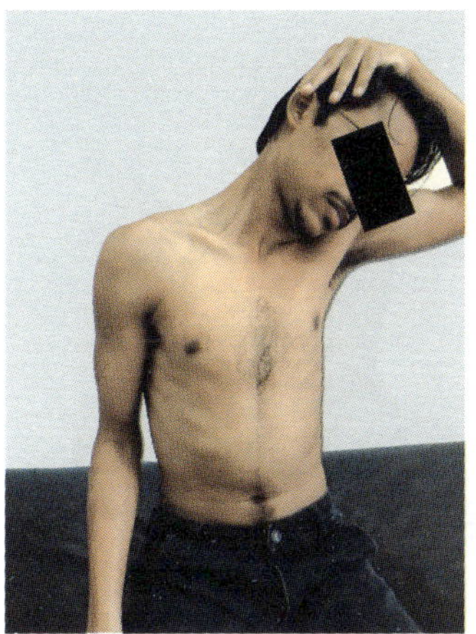

**Fig. 12.43:** Self-stretching of right upper trapezius.

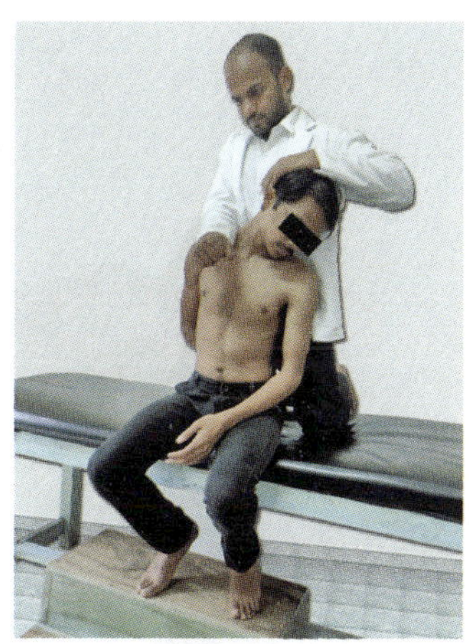

**Fig. 12.44:** Passive stretching of right levator scapulae.

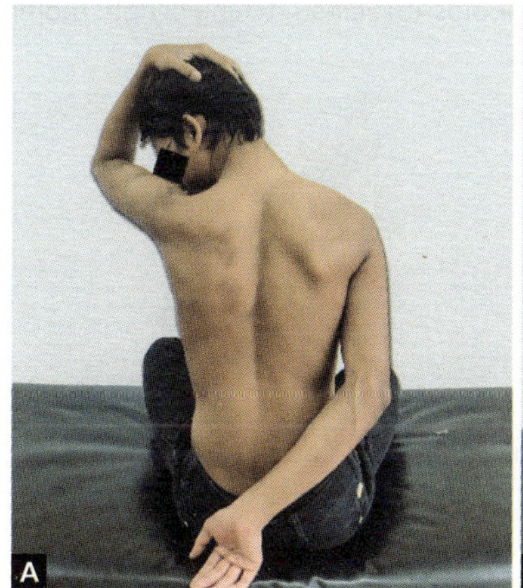

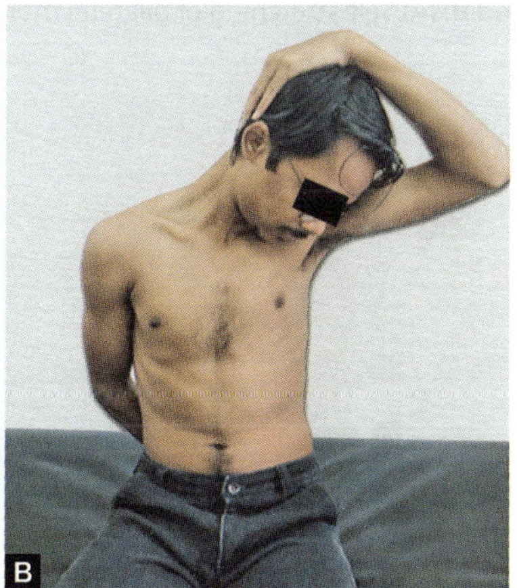

**Figs. 12.45A and B:** Self-stretching of levator scapulae: (A) Posterior view; (B) Anterior view.

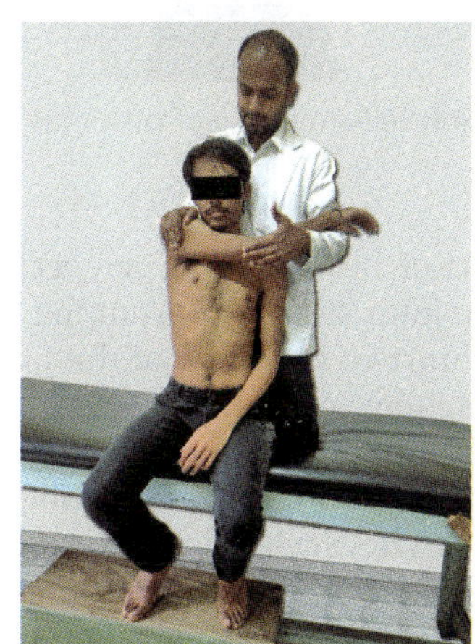

**Fig. 12.46:** Passive stretching of right rhomboids.

**Self-stretching** of rhomboids **(Figs. 12.47A and B)**.

### *Latissimus Dorsi Stretching*

**Passive stretching** can be done in sitting/ standing **(Fig. 12.48)**.

**Self-stretching** of latissimus dorsi **(Fig. 12.49)**.

### *Stretching of Trunk Lateral Flexors*

The lateral flexor stretching is commonly performed for correction of lateral bending deformity of spine (scoliosis). It can be done in

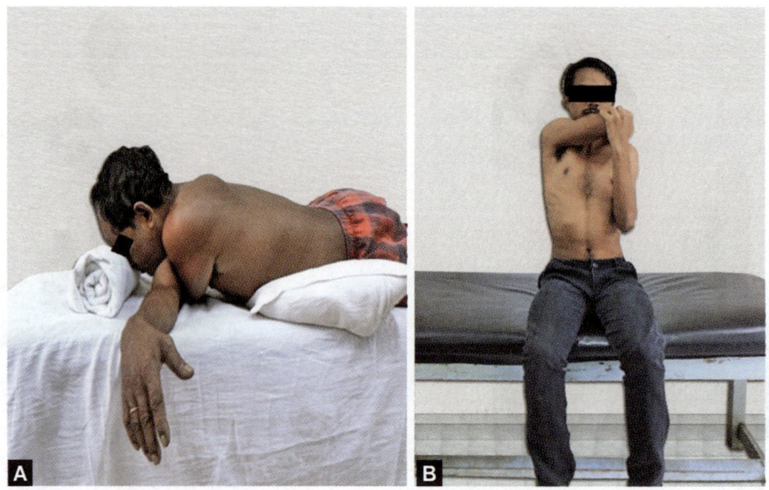

**Figs. 12.47A and B:** (A) Self-stretching of bilateral rhomboids; (B) Self-stretching of right rhomboids in sitting.

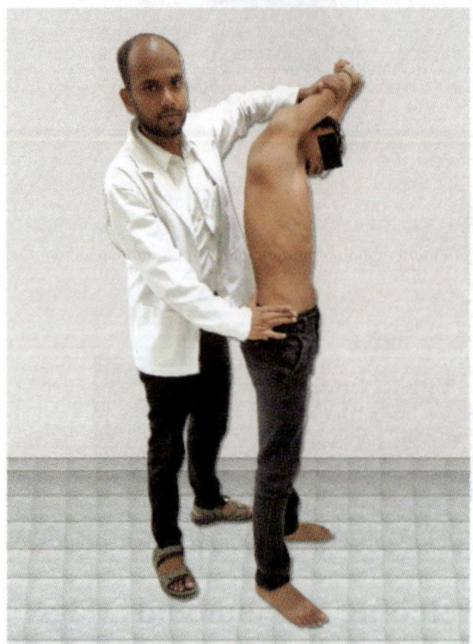

**Fig. 12.48:** Passive stretching of latissimus dorsi in standing.

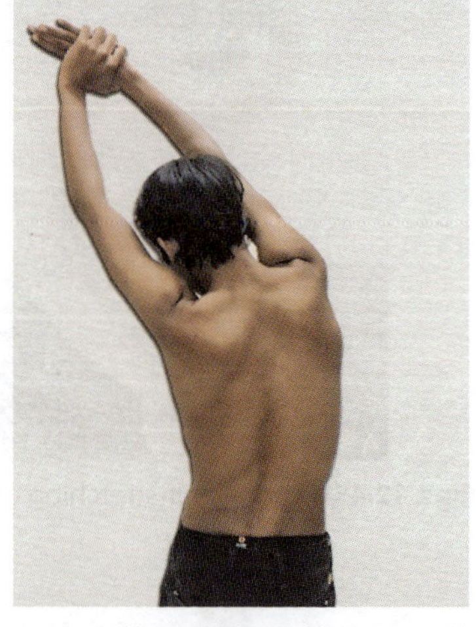

**Fig. 12.49:** Self-stretching of latissimus dorsi in standing.

various ways, and two simple methods of self-stretching are shown in **Figures 12.50A and B.**

### *b. Joint Stretching*

Joint stretching means the stretching of the soft tissue around the joint including the muscles. The individual muscles can be stretched as mentioned earlier but we need to stretch the ligaments, bursae, capsule, cartilage and other soft tissues of the joint which may get tight and make the joint stiff. To prevent the stiffness and to improve the ROM of the joint, this joint stretching will be helpful. To stretch one particular muscle, the opposite action of the muscle has to be done. To stretch one joint we have to analyze which action or movement has been restricted and same action or movement has to be performed to stretch the structures, which is stiff.

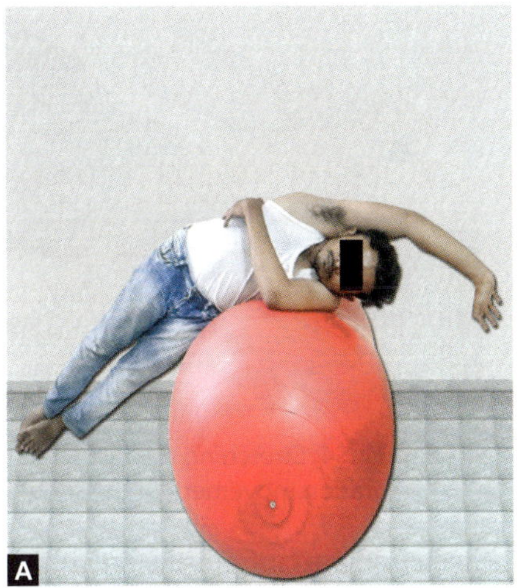
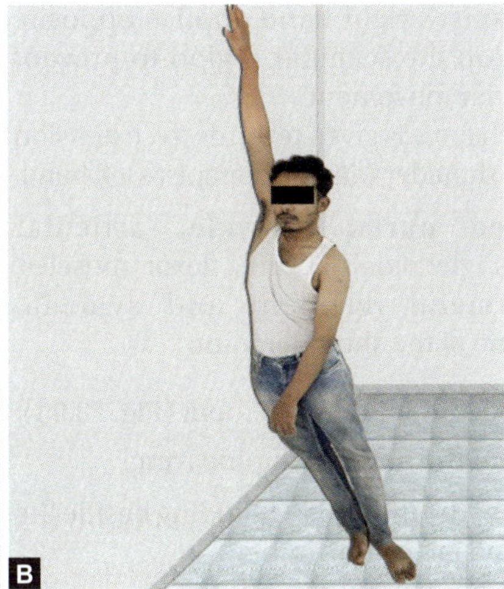

**Figs. 12.50A and B:** (A) Self-stretching of right flexors on Swiss ball; (B) Self-stretching of right trunk lateral flexors against the wall'.

## *Shoulder Joint*

### For Restricted Flexion Movement (Fig. 12.51).

**Position of the patient:** Supine lying.

**Position of the therapist:** Therapist is standing beside the patient and facing the limb.

**Procedure (for right shoulder):**

- Therapist's left hand grasps the lower arm region and the patient's forearm resting over the therapist's forearm.
- Therapist's right hand apply opposite force on the scapular region to prevent excessive scapular movement and to allow proportionate scapular movement.
- Stretch force is given towards the flexion of the shoulder with the therapist's left hand.

**Stretched parts:** Capsule, articular cartilages, glenoidal labrum, extensor muscles and synovial membrane of the shoulder joint.

### Restricted Extension Movement (Fig. 12.52)

**Position of the patient:** Prone lying.

**Position of the therapist:** Therapist is standing beside the patient and facing the limb.

**Procedure (for right shoulder):**

- Therapist's left hand grasps the lower arm region and the patient's forearm resting over the therapist's forearm.

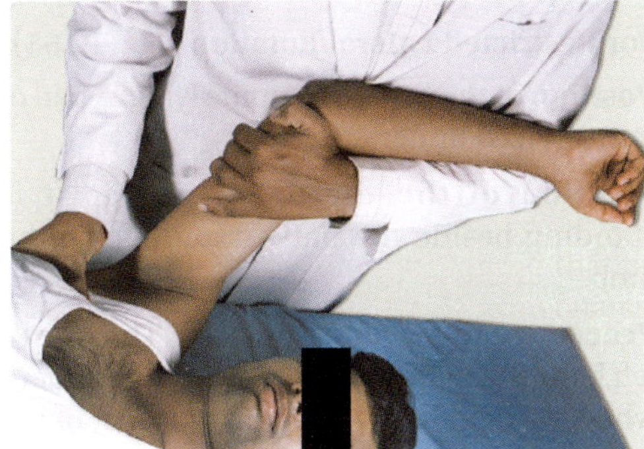

**Fig. 12.51:** Stretching the restricted flexion movement of the shoulder.

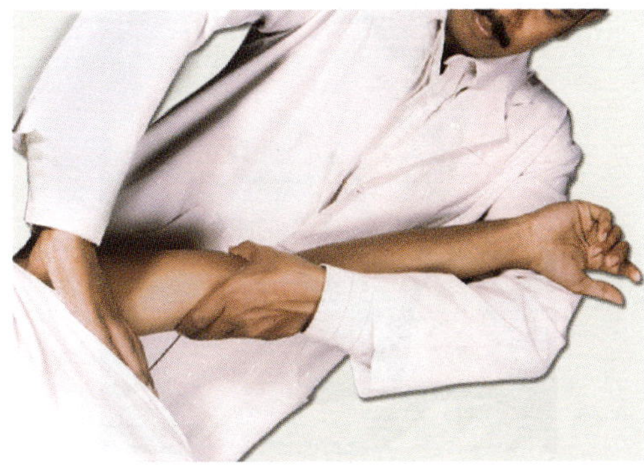

**Fig. 12.52:** Stretching the restricted extension movement of the shoulder.

- Therapist's right hand applies opposite force on the scapular region to prevent scapular movement.
- Stretch force is given towards the extension of the shoulder with the therapist's left hand.

**Stretched parts:** Capsule, articular cartilages, glenoidal labrum, flexor muscles, glenohumeral ligament and synovial membrane of the shoulder joint.

**Restricted Abduction Movement (Fig. 12.53):**

**Position of the patient:** Supine lying.

**Position of the therapist:** Standing beside the patient and facing the limb.

**Procedure (for right shoulder):**

- Therapist's left hand grasps the lower arm region and the patient's forearm resting over the therapist's forearm.
- Therapist's right hand applies opposite force on the scapular region to prevent scapular movement.
- Stretch force is given towards the abduction of the shoulder with the therapist's left hand.

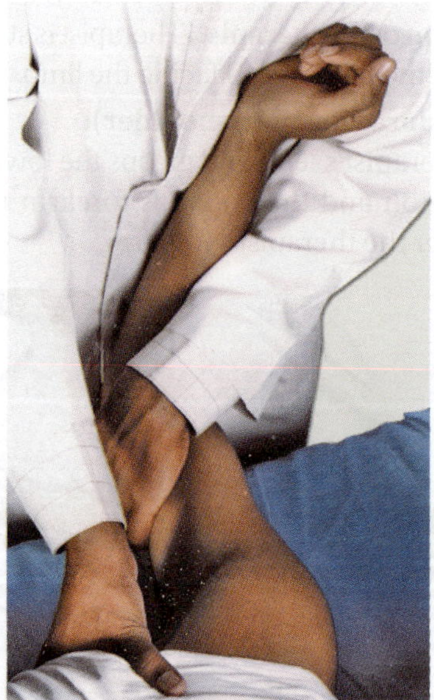

**Fig. 12.53:** Stretching the restricted abduction movement of the shoulder.

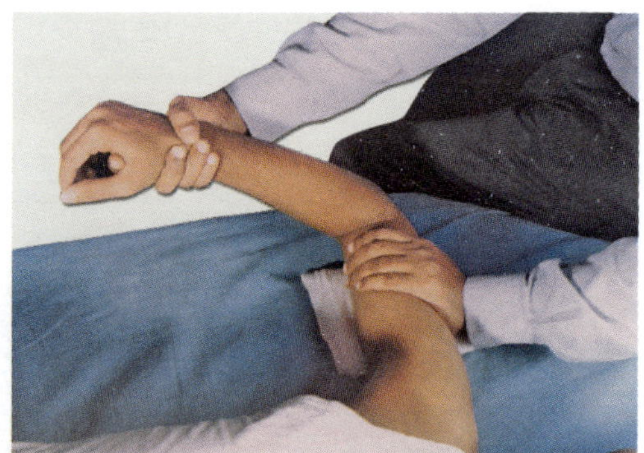

**Fig. 12.54:** Stretching the restricted medial rotation movement of the shoulder.

**Stretched parts:** Capsule, articular cartilages, glenoidal labrum, adductor muscles and synovial membrane of the shoulder joint.

**For Restricted Medial Rotation (Fig. 12.54):**

**Position of the patient:** Supine lying. Arm supported on a pad of towel.

**Position of the therapist:** Therapist is standing beside the patient and facing the limb.

**Procedure (for right shoulder):** Therapist's left hand grasping the lower arm of the patient while his right hand grasping the wrist and applying the stretch force towards the medial rotation.

**Stretched parts:** Capsule, articular cartilages, glenoidal labrum, lateral rotator muscles and synovial membrane of the shoulder joint.

**For Restricted Lateral Rotation (Fig. 12.55):**

**Position of the patient:** Supine lying. A pad of towel placed under the arm.

**Position of the therapist:** Therapist is standing beside the patient and facing the limb.

**Procedure (for right shoulder):** Therapist's left hand grasping the lower arm of the patient while his right hand grasping the wrist of the patient and applying the stretch force towards the lateral rotation.

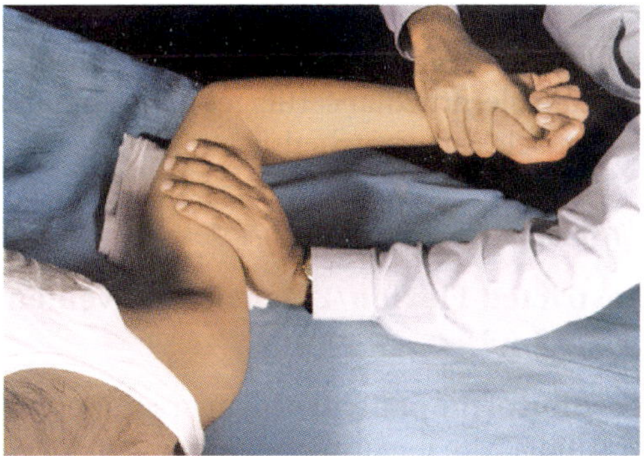

**Fig. 12.55:** Stretching the restricted lateral rotation movement of the shoulder.

**Stretched parts:** Capsule, articular cartilages, glenoidal labrum, medial rotator muscles and synovial membrane of the shoulder joint.

### *Elbow Joint*

**For Restricted Flexion Movement (Fig. 12.56):**

**Position of the patient:** Supine lying. A pad of towel is placed under the arm.

**Position of the therapist:** Therapist is standing beside the patient and facing the limb.

**Procedure (for right elbow):**

- ❖ Therapist's left hand grasping the lower arm of the patient and stabilizing the proximal joint.
- ❖ Therapist's right hand grasping the lower forearm and wrist of the patient.

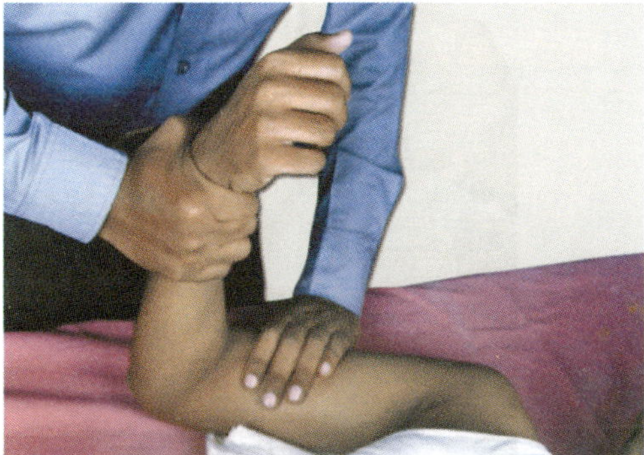

**Fig. 12.56:** Stretching the restricted flexion movement of the elbow.

- ❖ Stretch force is applied with the right hand of the therapist towards the flexion of the elbow.

**Stretched parts:** Capsule, articular cartilages, elbow extensor muscles, radial and ulnar collateral ligament.

**For Restricted Extension Movement (Fig. 12.57):**

**Position of the patient:** Supine lying. A pad of towel placed under the arm.

**Position of the therapist:** Therapist is standing beside the patient and facing the limb.

**Procedure (for right elbow):**

- ❖ Therapist's left hand grasping the lower arm of the patient and stabilizing the proximal joint.
- ❖ Therapist's right hand grasping the lower forearm and wrist of the patient.
- ❖ Stretch force is applied with the right hand of the therapist towards the extension of the elbow.

**Stretched parts:** Capsule, articular cartilages, elbow flexor muscles, radial and ulnar collateral ligament.

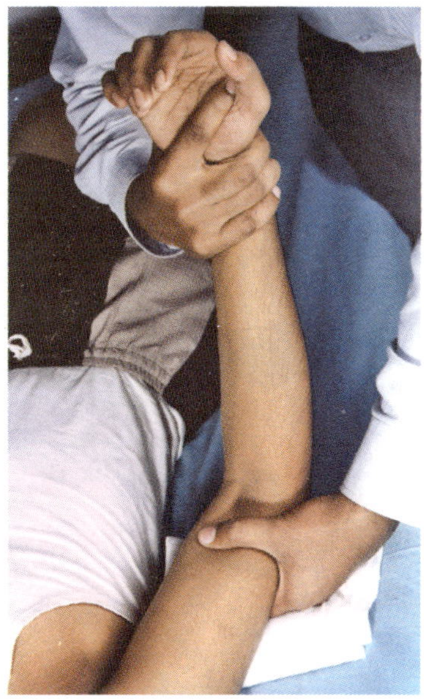

**Fig. 12.57:** Stretching the restricted extension movement of the elbow.

## Forearm

**For Restricted Supination and Pronation Movement (Fig. 12.58):**

**Position of the patient:** Supine lying. A pad of towel is placed under the arm.

**Position of the therapist:** Therapist is standing beside the patient and facing the limb.

**Procedure (for right side):**
- Therapist's left hand stabilizing the anterior aspect of proximal humerus of the patient.
- Therapist's right hand grasping the lower forearm, wrist and hand of the patient with elbow is in 90° flexed position.
- Therapist's right hand supinates and pronates the forearm and stretches the structures.

**Stretched parts:**
- While performing supination: Annular ligament, ulnar collateral ligament, capsule, articular cartilages and pronator muscles are stretched.
- While performing pronation: Annular ligament, radial collateral ligament, capsule, articular cartilages and supinator muscles are stretched.

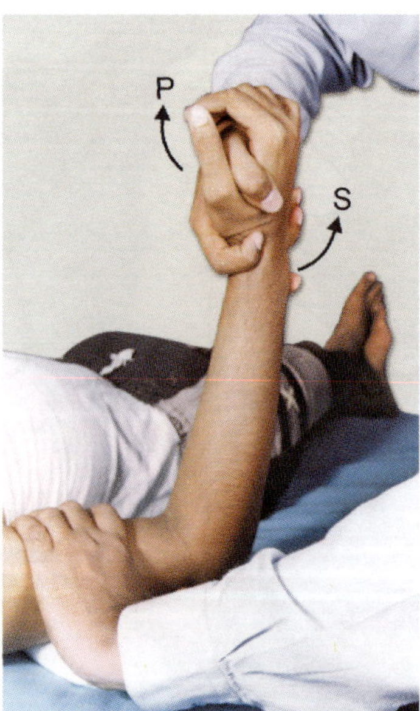


**Fig. 12.58:** Stretching the restricted supination and pronation movement of the forearm.

## Wrist Joint

**Restricted Flexion/Extension Movement (Fig. 12.59):**

**Position of the patient:** Patient in supine lying or sitting, with forearm supported on pillow.

**Position of the therapist:** Therapist is standing beside the patient and facing his wrist.

**Procedure (for right side):**
- Therapist's left hand grasping the lower forearm of the patient while his right hand grasps the palm and fingers.
- The therapist flexes/extends the wrist of the patient with his right hand.

**Stretched parts for flexion:** Articular disc, capsule, extensor muscles of the wrist, ulnar and radial ligament, extensor retinaculum.

**Stretched parts for extension:** Articular disc, capsule, flexor muscles of the wrist, ulnar and radial ligament, flexor retinaculum.

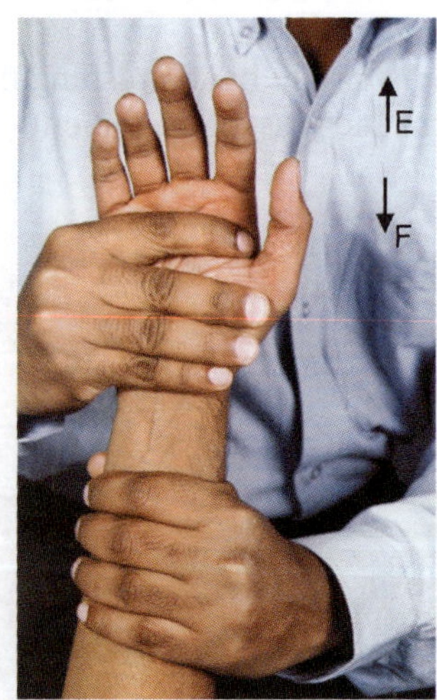


**Fig. 12.59:** Stretching the restricted flexion and extension movement of the wrist.

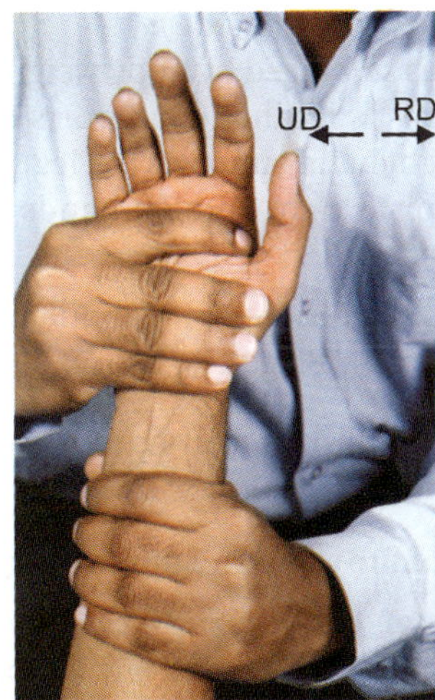


**Fig. 12.60:** Stretching the restricted ulnar and radial deviation movement of the wrist.

**Restricted Ulnar/Radial Deviation Movement (Fig. 12.60):**

**Position of the patient:** Patient is sitting with forearm supported on pillow or supine lying.

**Position of the therapist:** Therapist is standing beside the patient and facing his wrist.

**Procedure (for right side):**

- Therapist's left hand grasping the lower forearm of the patient while his right hand grasp the palm and fingers.
- The therapist performs the ulnar/radial deviation of the wrist of the patient with his right hand.

**Stretched parts for ulnar deviation:** Articular disc, capsule, radial deviation muscles of the wrist, radial ligament, radial part of extensor and flexor retinaculum.

**Stretched parts for radial deviation:** Articular disc, capsule, ulnar deviation muscles of the wrist, ulnar ligament, ulnar part of extensor and flexor retinaculum.

## *Hip Joint*

**Restricted Flexion Movement (Fig. 12.61):**

**Position of the patient:** Supine lying.

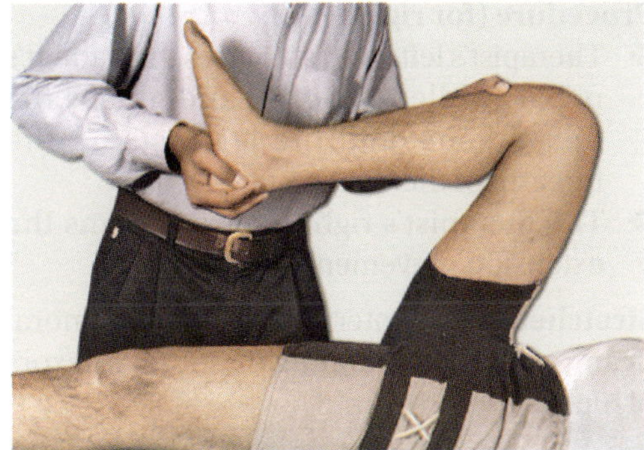

**Fig. 12.61:** Stretching the restricted flexion movement of the hip.

**Position of the therapist:** Therapist is standing beside the patient and facing the hip joint.

**Procedure (For right side):**

- Right hand of the therapist is grasping the heel of the patient while left hand grasping the patient's upper leg.
- Therapist's both the hands flexes hip and knee of the patient.

**Stretched parts:** Posterior capsule, ischiofemoral ligament, extensors of hip, articular cartilages.

**Restricted Extension Movement (Fig. 12.62):**

**Position of the patient:** Side lying.

**Position of the therapist:** Therapist is standing beside the patient and facing the hip joint.

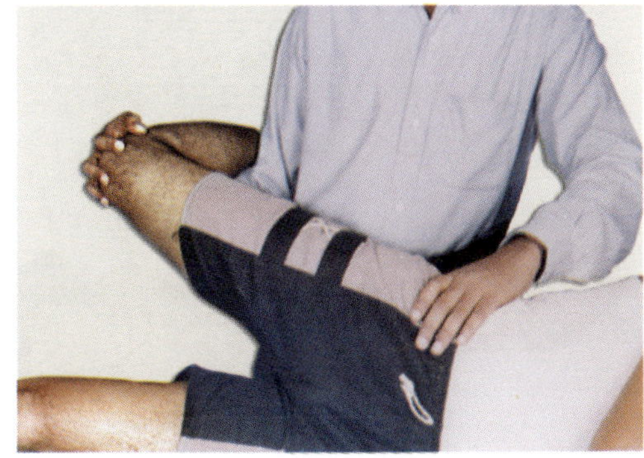

**Fig. 12.62:** Stretching the restricted extension movement of the hip.

**Procedure (for right side):**

- Therapist's left hand stabilizes the patient's pelvis, while his right hand grasps the flexed knee, and the leg rests on the forearm of the therapist.
- The therapist's right hand performs the extension movement of the hip.

**Stretched parts:** Anterior capsule, iliofemoral ligament, pubofemoral ligament and flexors of hip.

**Restricted Abduction Movement (Fig. 12.63):**

**Position of the patient:** Supine lying.

**Position of the therapist:** Therapist is standing beside the patient and facing the hip joint.

**Procedure (for right side):**

- Therapist's left hand stabilizes the opposite thigh, while his right hand grasps the lower thigh and the leg is placed on the therapist's forearm.
- Leg is pulled apart by the therapist's right hand.

**Stretched parts:** Capsule, transverse ligaments, articular cartilage, adductor muscles.

**Restricted Adduction Movement:**

**Position of the patient:** Supine lying.

**Position of the therapist:** Therapist is standing beside the patient and facing the hip joint.

**Procedure (for right side):**

- Pelvis is stabilized by body weight.
- Therapist's left hand supports the thigh and right hand supports the leg.
- Therapist's right and left hands push the leg inside.

**Stretched parts:** Capsule, abductors of the hip, articular cartilages.

**Restricted Medial and Lateral Rotation Movement (Fig. 12.64):**

**Position of the patient:** Supine lying.

**Position of the therapist:** Therapist is standing beside the patient and facing the hip joint.

**Procedure (for right side):**

- Therapist's left hand stabilizes the thigh of the patient, while his right hand grasps the heel and lower leg.
- Hip and knee are kept in 90° flexed position.
- Therapist performs stretching in both the medial and lateral rotation directions.

**Stretched parts:**

- During medial rotation: Capsule, ischiofemoral ligament, articular cartilage, lateral rotators.
- During lateral rotation: Capsule, pubofemoral ligament, iliofemoral ligament, transverse ligament, round ligament, articular cartilages, medial rotators.

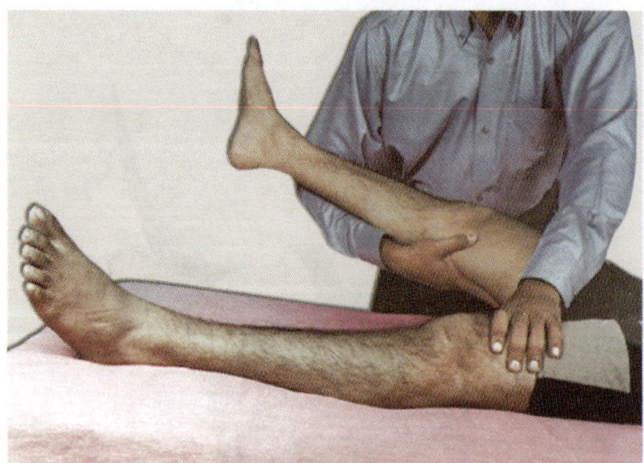

**Fig. 12.63:** Stretching the restricted abduction movement of the hip.

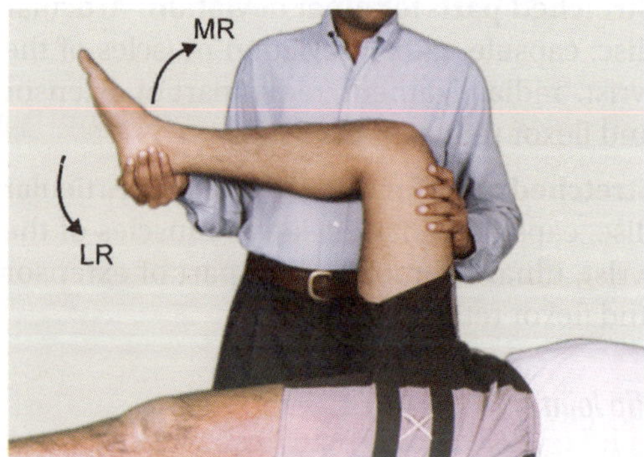


**Fig. 12.64:** Stretching the restricted medial and lateral rotation movements of the hip.

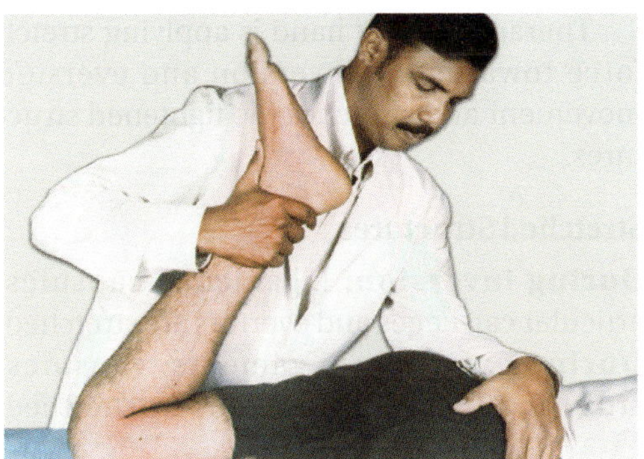

**Fig. 12.65:** Stretching the restricted flexion movement of the knee.

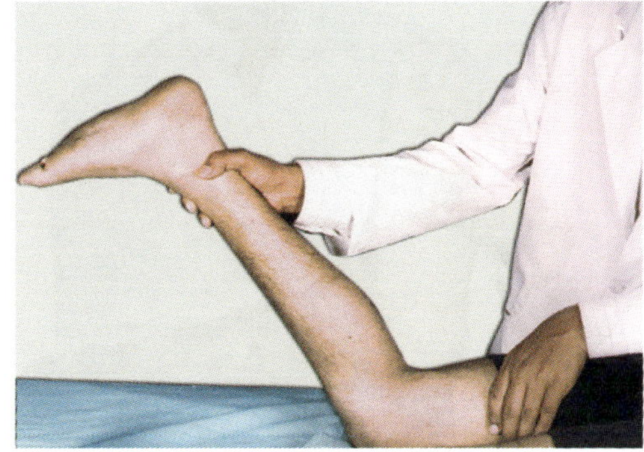

**Fig. 12.66:** Stretching the restricted extension movement of the knee.

### *Knee Joint*

**Restricted Flexion Movement (Fig. 12.65):**

**Position of the patient:** Prone lying.

**Position of the therapist:** Therapist is standing beside the patient and facing the knee joint.

**Procedure (for left side):**

- Therapist's left hand stabilizes the pelvis and upper thigh of the patient while his right hand grasps the lower leg region.
- Therapist's right hand flexes the knee and stretches the tightened structures.

**Stretched parts:** Ligaments, medial and lateral meniscus, capsule, bursae and extensor muscles (quadriceps femoris).

**Restricted Extension Movement (Fig. 12.66):**

**Position of the patient:** Prone lying.

**Position of the therapist:** Therapist is standing beside the patient and facing the knee joint.

**Procedure (for left side):**

- Therapist's left hand stabilizing the thigh of the patient while his right hand grasps the lower leg region, with the knee in maximum extension.
- Therapist's right hand extends the knee and stretches the tightened structures.

**Stretched parts:** Ligaments, medial and lateral meniscus, capsule, bursae and flexor muscles.

### *Ankle Joint*

**Restricted Plantar Flexion/Dorsiflexion Movement (Fig. 12.67):**

**Position of the patient:** Supine lying, with the hips and knees flexed and leg supported on therapist's forearm.

**Position of the therapist:** Therapist is standing beside the patient and facing the ankle joint.

**Procedure (for right side):**

- Therapist's left hand supports the lower leg region and his right hand holds the heel of the patient in such a way that, the thumb encircles the dorsal aspect of hind foot.
- Therapist's right hand plantar flexes/dorsiflexes the ankle and stretches the tightened structures.

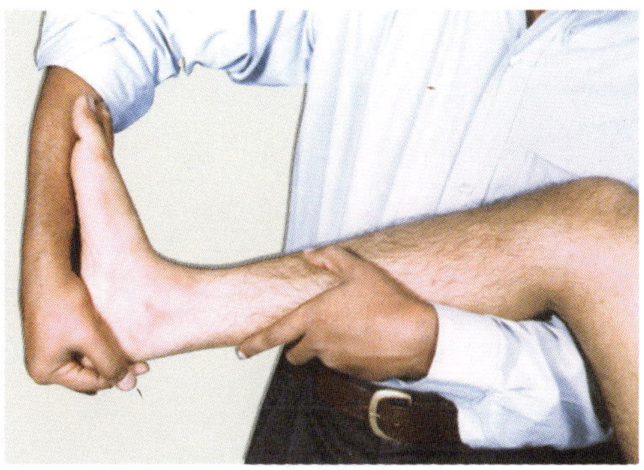

**Fig. 12.67:** Stretching the restricted plantar and dorsiflexion movement of the ankle.

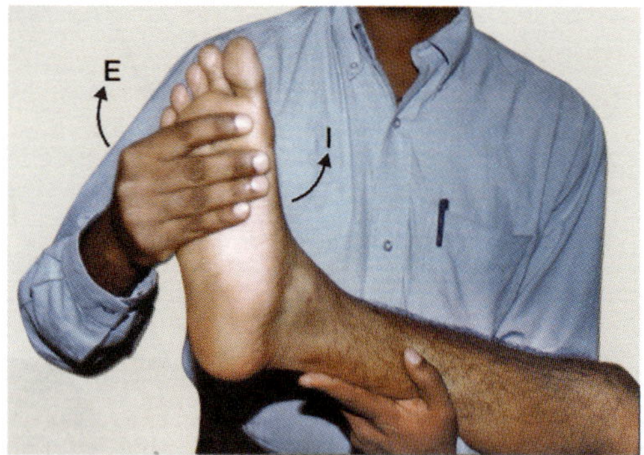


**Fig. 12.68:** Stretching the restricted inversion and eversion movement of the subtalar joint.

**Stretched parts for plantar flexion:** Ligaments, capsule and dorsi-flexors.

**Stretched parts for dorsiflexion:** Ligaments, capsule and plantar flexors.

### *Subtalar Joints*

**Restricted Inversion Eversion Movement (Fig. 12.68):**

**Position of the patient:** Supine lying.

**Position of the therapist:** Therapist stands beside the patient facing the ankle joint.

**Procedure (for right side):**
Therapist's left hand grasp the ankle joint of the patient while his right hand grasping the foot region.

Therapist's right hand is applying stretch force towards the inversion and eversion movement and stretches the tightened structures.

**Stretched Structures**

**During inversion:** Ligaments, capsules, articular cartilages and evertors are stretched.
**During eversion:** Ligaments, capsules, articular cartilages and invertors are stretched.

### *c. Skin Stretching*

It is also like the joint stretching, the stretching has to be performed in the opposite direction to the aspect of the tightened skin/fascia. This type of stretching mainly performed for the burns contracture, prolonged immobilization contracture and traumatic contractures. For example, if the skin is tight in the necks that restrict the extension movement (the skin/fascia over the flexor aspect is tight), stretching in the direction of neck extension should be performed. The same procedure as said in the joint stretching has to be followed.

# 13 CHAPTER

# Functional Re-education Training

## INTRODUCTION

Functional re-education is a phase of the rehabilitation process, that includes a series of exercises, aimed at re-educating the body or part of it for normal motor and postural activities.

Re-education means educating something, which was already known by an individual in the past, but due to some injury or disease, the person is not able to perform the activities currently. Here the patient knows the activities or movements that has, to be performed but due to his impairment or diseased pathology he is not able to perform it properly. The functional re-education program designed by therapists, helps the patient to make him independent. "Making the person independent" is the main goal for the functional re-education program.

In the functional re-education training, sequence of progressions of the position like the development of the milestone of the child from the lying to the walking is followed, though not very rigidly. Soon after childbirth, the baby can adopt the supine position, and later, as stability improves, it achieves the side lying. From the side lying it progresses to the prone. After achieving the prone it tries to lift its head and the trunk with help of the elbow and the forearm, thus it attains the prone on elbow position. As the child achieves this position, it begins to creep and achieve its first mobility. Subsequently the child sit and tries to achieve prone-on-hand position. In the prone-on-hand position the child pulls its lower limb upwards and adopt the quadruped position, with which the child crawls. From quadruped the child holds the furniture, wall or some objects and achieve the kneeling position, with that it starts kneel walking with the support. After development of the stability it attains the standing position with help of the support from the kneeling.

Depending on the condition and the level of the independence the program can be designed for a patient. Depending on the condition, the sequence can be planned and the multiple postures may be overlapped during that program. The sequence activities, techniques also can be varying from one patient to another. The functional re-education program is helpful for all patients with orthopedics, neurology and cardio-respiratory conditions to overcome their impairment/ disability and improve function.

It helps to:

- Increase the dynamic and static stability.
- Improve the coordination and balance.
- Increase the strength and endurance (both muscular/cardiorespiratory).
- Increase the pelvic stability.
- Enhance the proprioception function.
- Correct the postural instability.
- Improve the ambulatory skill and function.

## POSTURES

The functional re-education training consists of preambulatory mat exercise and ambulatory training in various postures.

- Supine lying.
- Rolling
- Supine to side lying

- Side lying to prone lying
- Prone to side lying
- Side lying to supine
- Prone lying
- Prone lying on elbows.
- Sitting
- Quadruped position
- Kneeling
- Half-kneeling
- Standing
- Walking.

In each and every posture many of the exercises can be practiced for the progression and to improve the stability as well as mobility. This progressive exercise program in each position makes the patient master skill in that particular posture and also gives more confidence for the next progressive posture.

## Supine

### *Progressive Activities in Supine*

Most of the exercises can be performed in the supine lying posture.

- Neck stability and strengthening exercises.
- Upper and lower limb coordination as well as strengthening programs.
- Trunk exercises.
- Postural drainage techniques.

And also supine position is the very much convenient posture to adopt for long period. All the strengthening exercises starts with assisted exercise progressing to active free and active assisted resisted exercise, and ends with resisted exercises.

Assisted → Active free → Assisted resisted → Resisted.

The activities performed in supine are:

**Bridging (Fig. 13.1)**

In the supine lying both the knees are flexed and the feet are placed on the couch. Patient is asked to raise his lower trunk from the floor or couch. The hip knee trunk aligns in straight line. In hemiplegic's condition early weight bearing is facilitated through bridging and practice of the activity improves the independency. This activity when mastered, helps to insert the bed pan for toileting. Some salient points regarding bridging include the followings:

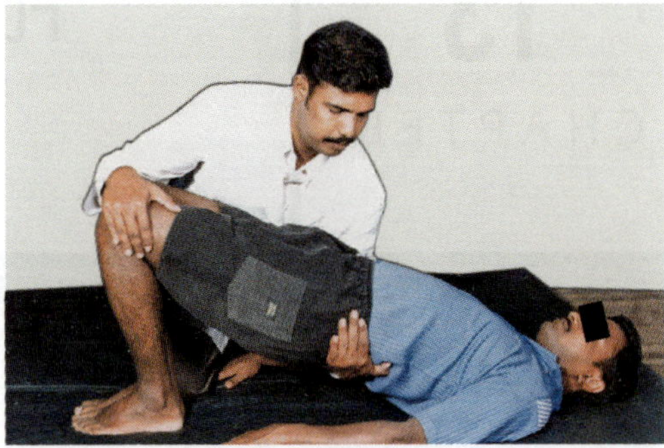

**Fig. 13.1:** Bridging with assistance of the therapist.

1. This is the important exercise to be practiced to improve the trunk stability. It improves the pelvic and trunk stability as well as facilitates hip abductors and adductors.
2. Earlier it started with the assisted type by decreasing leverage (heels close to buttocks, to reduce weight arm), and movements practiced with the assistance/support, which prevents knees from falling apart.
3. Once skill developed, the patient is made to practice independently without any support or assistance to improve the ability to hold the trunk for some time after rising from the floor.
4. Modification can be made to improve the stability and endurance. Performing the bridging exercise with feet away from the buttocks, and unilateral bridging (bridging with one lower extremity support and another lower extremity off the bed with hip flexed and knee extended) are the progressions.
5. Once the skill improved, practice is made with the manual resistance by the therapist and later with mechanical resistance.

This exercise program can be altered for the hemiplegia and paraplegic patients.

**Supine to Side Lying (Fig. 13.2)**

Rolling can be practiced with the assistance. While rolling towards left side, below mentioned sequences are performed.

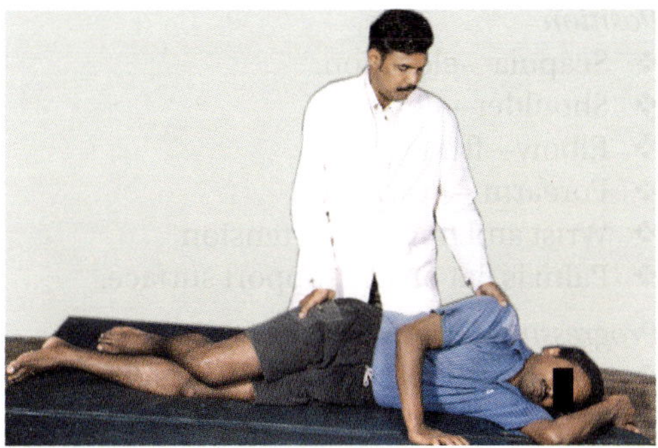

**Fig. 13.2:** Rolling from supine to side lying with assistance of the therapist.

- Right hand pulls the upper body, i.e., upper trunk and pelvic towards left side by holding the bed end or bedside bars in the left side.
- Right knee is flexed and with the foot, the pelvis and lower trunk pushed towards left side. In paraplegic patients, who cannot move the lower limbs, the patient is taught to pull the lower limbs forward with the help of his/her hands.
- Left leg can be hooked over the bed end for rotation of the lower trunk.
- Left hand also may assist to turn the upper trunk by grasping the bed end.

Though, rolling should be performed on both sides, in hemiplegic patients, emphasis should be given on rolling first towards the sound side, using the affected side trunk, upper and lower limbs. The pattern of rolling varies from hemiplegic patients to paraplegic patients.

*Uses of Rolling*

- Useful in bed making activities.
- Useful in preventing the bedsore.
- Easy to progress to next posture, i.e., sitting.

*Uses of Side Lying*

- Some of exercises like upper and lower extremities facilitation/strengthening exercises can be performed.
- Coordination exercises can be performed.
- Postural drainage techniques can be performed.
- Position of choice for stroke/head injury patients to inhibit spasticity.
- Assistive movements can be performed in the early stage.
- Independent activities can be practiced.
- If the stability and strength is more the patient can practice the resisted exercises.
- Depending on the muscle power, exercise programs are selected in side lying.

### Side Lying to Prone

*For Left Side Lying to Prone*

- Left shoulder adducted and elbow extended and placed under the body.
- Right hand grasping the head end bedside bars or bed end the patient is assisted to rotate the upper trunk.
- Left upper extremity extended throughout.
- Right knees flexed and the foot pushes the mat to rotate the lower trunk.

*Progressive Activities in Prone Lying*

- Neck stability exercises can be performed mainly extension and side flexion movement.
- Spinal extensor exercises can be practiced.
- Some of the upper and lower extremity exercises can be practiced.
- Starts with the assisted exercise and ends in the resisted exercises to improve the strength of the muscles.

*Uses*

- Useful for bed activities.
- Useful for postural drainage techniques.
- Prevent bedsore.
- Useful to perform above said exercises.
- Useful to expand the lungs and enhance breathing.

### Prone to Side Lying

*For Prone to Left Side Lying*

- Right hand placed sideways and the pressure applied over the mat by which the upper trunk and the head can be raised up.
- Right knee flexed and the pressure applied on the mat to rotate the lower trunk.

- Left hand holds the bedside bars or right side bed end and pushes the body towards left side.

Here the total body rotates 90° and the left hand goes down and right hand comes up.

### Side Lying to Supine

*Left Side Lying to Supine Lying*

- Right hand holds the bed end or the side bars and pulls the upper trunk towards back side.
- Left lower limb hooks the bed end and pushes the lower trunk towards the right side.
- Left hand applies pressure over the bed or the bedside bars and pushes body back side.

Above mentioned all the rolling techniques done with assistance in the early stage and it is progressed into independent rolling.

Assisted → Independent → Resisted

### Prone Lying on Elbows (Fig. 13.3)

The elbow and the forearm supports patient's upper trunk and the weight is transmitted through the elbow. This position is achieved from the prone lying.

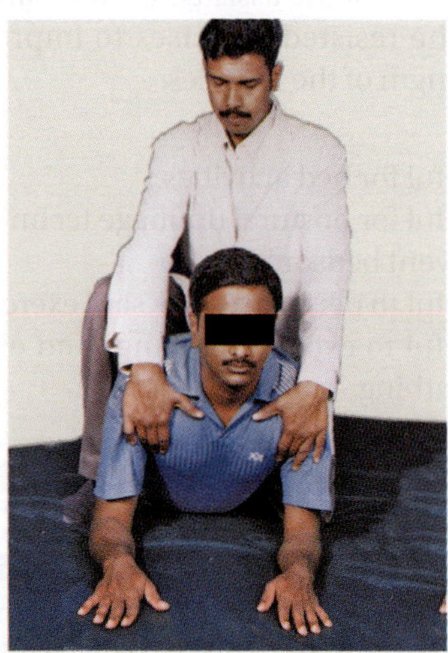

**Fig. 13.3:** Achieving the prone on elbow positioning with assistance of the therapist.

*Position*

- Scapula—elevation.
- Shoulder—flexion.
- Elbow—flexion
- Forearm—pronation
- Wrist and fingers—extension
- Palm is flat on the support surface.

*Progressive Activities*

- This position can be adopted with help of the assistance from the prone lying. Progression can be made to maintain the posture independently.
- Manual approximation force can be applied from one side to another to improve the dynamic stability of shoulder girdle and the upper extremities.
- Elbow walking/creeping can be practiced.
- Shifting the weight from side to side also improves the proprioception of the shoulder joints.
- The resistance can also be applied manually to improve the strength.

*Uses*

- Bed making.
- Dressing activities.
- Patient can hold the magazine and read in this position.
- These activities are more helpful for the paraplegic patients to improve their upper limb stability.
- The posture helps to reduce spasticity of hand muscles, in stroke/head injury patients.
- Stimulates neck control and creeping in cerebral palsy.

### Hand Prone Lying (Fig. 13.4)

This position is same like the prone lying on elbows. In this position the BOS decreases slightly and COG is raised comparatively with the prone lying on elbows. Here instead of weight bearing on the elbow, the weight is transmitted through the hand and wrist. This is intermediate position between the prone lying on elbows and the quadruped position.

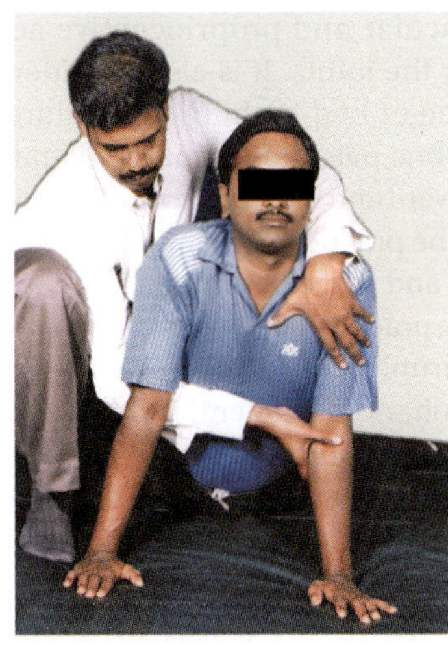

**Fig. 13.4:** Achieving the hand prone lying position from prone on elbow position with assistance of the therapist.

Hyperextension of spine as well as hip joint occurs more, which is useful for postural alignment during ambulation. In beginning this position can be achieved by the assistance of the therapist.

Like prone on elbow position, many of the progressive activities can be performed.

*Position*

- Shoulder—elevation, flexion, and abduction
- Elbow—extension
- Wrist—hyperextension
- Fingers—extension
- Forearm—pronation.

*Progressive Activities*

- Position may be achieved by the assistants and the support given to maintain the posture during the early stage.
- Preparing the patient to maintain the posture independently without any assistants.
- Approximation can be applied in sideways, anteroposterior direction by which we can achieve the proximal muscle stability as well as coordination.
- Weight shifting from one side to another can be practiced to increase the muscle power as well as proprioception activities over the shoulder joint.
- Hand walking can be practiced to improve the dynamic stability over the upper limb.
- Push-up exercise may helpful to improve the static as well as dynamic stability of the upper limb.
- Pegboards can be used to improve the hand coordination.

*Uses*

- This position is helpful for the paraplegic patient to improve the upper limb muscle power and strength.
- It is used for spastic patients to reduce tone in the flexor muscles of upper limbs.
- Bed mobility can be improved.

### Quadruped Position (Fig. 13.5)

It is otherwise called as four-footed position or animal position or prone kneeling position. In this position the BOS decreases while compared with the hand prone lying and the COG increases. It is the first position in which the weight bearing through the hip joint takes

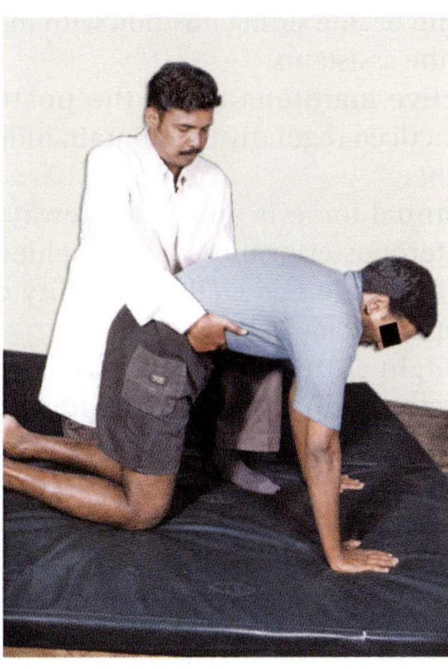

**Fig. 13.5:** Achieving the quadruped from hand prone lying position with assistance of the therapist.

place in the re-education training. It can be achieved from: (1) hand prone lying, (2) side sitting.

*From Hand Prone Lying*

From the hand prone lying hip and knee are flexed and the pelvis is taken up to the knee level and the body is raised with the help of therapist's support.

*From Side Sitting*

From the side sitting the trunk is rotated and raised up. Both the upper limbs are placed in front, allowing weight bearing on the knees and the hands.

*Position*

- Trunk—forward flexion (placed horizontal to the floor)
- Hip—flexed 90°
- Knee—flexed 90°
- Elbow—extension
- Wrist—extension
- Shoulder—flexion
- Forearm—pronation
- Palm—flat and placed on the floor.

*Progressive Activities*

- This position is achieved from the prone on hand or side sitting position with the help of the assistants.
- Active maintenance of the posture is practiced regularly to maintain independence.
- Manual force is applied sideways and anteroposterior direction to achieve the coordination as well as stability of the upper and lower limbs.
- Weight shifting sideways and anteroposterior direction can be practiced to improve the dynamic stability of the trunk and limbs.
- Weight bearing on the contralateral upper and lower extremities are practiced, which is helpful during the upper limb swinging walking.
- Crawling movement can be practiced to improve the dynamic stability of the neck, trunk and limbs. It improves the neuromuscular and proprioceptive activities over the joints. It is also considered as a mode of bed mobility for children with cerebral palsy and spinal cord injured.
- Forward and backward crawling movement can be practiced.
- 'Cat and camel' exercise for the trunk has to be practiced, i.e., raising and lowering of the trunk in the quadruped position.
- 'Elephant movement', i.e., forward, backward and sideways oscillatory movement of the body can be done in the quadruped position, which increases the static and dynamic stability of the limbs.
- During the above-mentioned activities manual resistance can be applied to improve the muscle strength.

*Uses*

- Floor level activities like playing with the kids, seeding, weeding and gardening, floor cleaning activities.
- It is useful for the patients who cannot walk to ambulate inside the house.

**Elbow Side Lying**

This can be achieved from the side lying. The BOS is less and the COG is high while compared with the elbow prone lying. It is the very much unstable and inconvenient for an individual to maintain for the longer period. This posture can be supported with the opposite side hand placing over the mat in front.

*Position*

Same like the side lying but the elbow is flexed and placed on the mat and the upper trunk weight is transmitted through the weight-bearing elbow.

- Elbow — flexion
- Shoulder—extension, elevation and internal rotation.

*Progressive Activities*

- This position is achieved from the elbow prone lying with the help of the assistant.

- ❖ Independently maintaining the position also can be practiced.
- ❖ Creeping with the help of the elbow on the mat is taught to improve the dynamic and static stability as well as proprioception activities.
- ❖ Manual approximation force is applied to increase the static stability over the upper limb.
- ❖ Resisted activities can be performed to improve the muscle power.

*Uses*

- ❖ Mat mobility activities.
- ❖ Relaxed position for reading books and watching television.
- ❖ This is the enroute for achieving sitting position.

**Side Sitting (Fig. 13.6)**

This position can be achieved from the elbow side lying as well as from kneel sitting. Here the BOS still reduces and the COG rises while comparing with elbow side lying and it is more stable than kneel sitting posture.

Both thc upper extremities will be supporting this posture.

*From Elbow Side Lying*

This can be achieved from elbow side lying. The hip and knee are flexed, elbow extended, palm is flat and placed on the floor and the trunk is raised.

We can achieve from the elbow side lying hip and knee is flexed, elbow extended, palm is flat and placed on the floor and the trunk raised.

*From Kneel Sitting*

From kneel sitting, the pelvis is made to move further posterior and one side of the hip is placed on the floor with the same side upper limb support.

*Position*

- ❖ Hip and knees are flexed and kept in the side.
- ❖ Weight is transmitted through one upper limb and the pelvis of the one side.

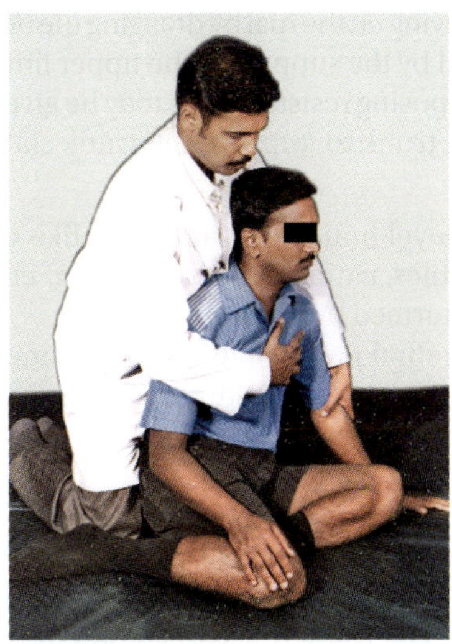

**Fig. 13.6:** Achieving the side sitting position from elbow side lying position with assistance of the therapist

- ❖ Shoulder is abducted and elevated.
- ❖ Elbow is extended.
- ❖ Lower hip is flexed, abducted and laterally rotated.
- ❖ Upper hip is medially rotated and flexed.

*Progressive Activities*

- ❖ Earlier this position is adopted from the elbow side lying and kneel sitting with the help of assistance of the therapist. Therapist will be sitting side to the patient and assist for flexing both the hip and knees, and extending the elbow.
- ❖ The patient is made to practice to maintain the posture without any support.
- ❖ Side sitting will be practiced for the both sides.
- ❖ Manual approximation force is given in anterior and posterior as well as lateral direction also to improve the static stability of the trunk as well as the weight-bearing limb.
- ❖ Weight shifting over the upper limb will be practiced to activate the proprioceptors over the shoulder and elbow joint.
- ❖ Balancing exercise will be practiced by removing the upper limb support.

- Moving on the mat by dragging the buttocks and by the support of the upper limb.
- Opposing resisted force may be given over the trunk to improve the trunk stability.

*Uses*

Floor level household activities like cutting vegetables, eating, garland making, etc., can be performed by using this posture.

Cerebral palsy children, sometimes drag the buttock in this posture (bottom shuffling) for ambulation inside home.

### Long Sitting

This is very stable position to maintain for longer period. This can be achieved from side sitting. The trunk muscles should have good power and strength to maintain the trunk in erect posture independently. Patients with trunk muscles weakness are made to sit by placing both upper limbs by sides. Sometime the upper limbs may be placed posteriorly to avoid back falling **(Fig. 13.7)**.

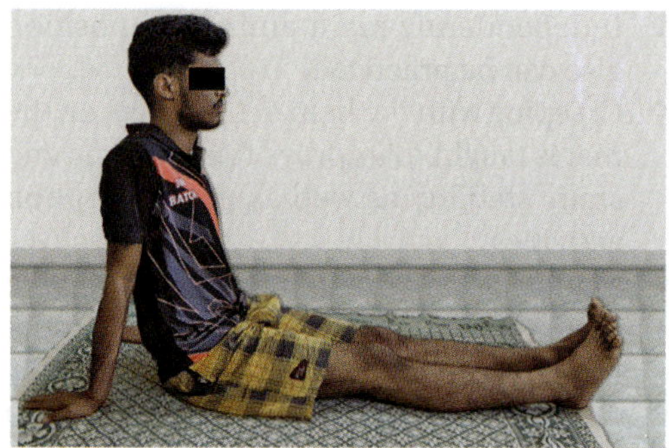

**Fig. 13.7:** Long sitting with hands placed behind for support.

*Position*

- Spine—erect
- Shoulder—abduction and elevation
- Elbow—extension
- Wrist—extension
- Hip—flexion and lateral rotation
- Knee—extension.

*Progressive Activities*

- Posture is achieved with the help of the therapist. Therapist grasping the trunk and making it straight.
- Patient is made to maintain this posture with the help of the upper limb support without any external support.
- Balancing forces can be applied from the sides as well as in anteroposterior direction.
- The patient should be taught balancing exercises, in long sitting, first with wide base, gradually decreasing the base of support and with both shoulders abducted to side-using the high guard posture **(Fig. 13.8A)**, gradually progressing to mid-guard and low-guard postures.
- Weight shifting from one upper extremity to another will improve the proprioceptor activity over the shoulder region.
- Some of the trunk, upper extremity, lower extremity strengthening exercise can be performed in this posture.
- Mat crutch exercise can be practiced with the help of the crutches.
- **Hitching and hiking**: Both the hips when lifted with the help of the upper limb support is called as hitching. Forward backward and sideways movements can be practiced in this position. Sandbags, wooden blocks or small size crutches can be used for performing hitching. Lifting one side of the pelvic up is called as hiking. Hiking is the most important movement to be practiced because during the swing phase hip hiking is must to clear the foot from the floor.
- Patient is made to practice sitting without the support of the upper extremity.
- Walking on the buttocks can be practiced to improve the dynamic stability.
- Sitting push-ups can be performed in chair sitting/wheel chair sitting which gives more stability and strength to the upper extremity **(Fig. 13.8B)**.
- Sitting with leg crossed can be performed.

### Kneel Standing (Fig. 13.10)

Standing on both the knees are called as kneel standing. This can be achieved from the quadruped position and side sitting. In

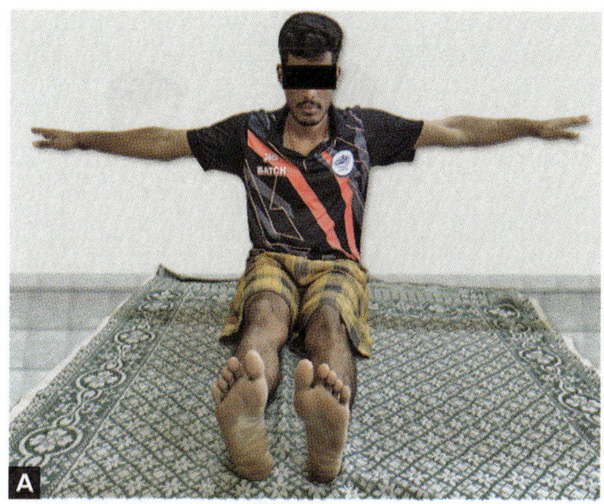

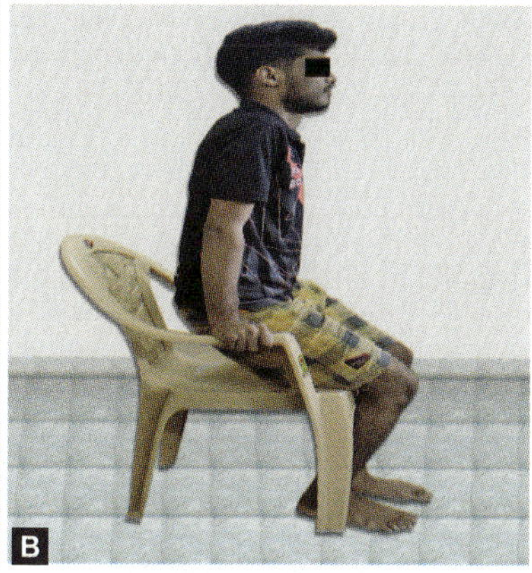

**Figs. 13.8A and B:** (A) Long sitting in high guard posture; (B) Sitting push-ups.

this position BOS is decreased and the COG is raised. This is very much inconvenient posture to maintain for long-time. Stability in this posture also very less.

*From Quadruped Position*

Therapist, standing back of the patient grasping the upper trunk and lifting the trunk and upper extremity up. The posture is maintained by the help of the back support by the therapist.

*From Side Sitting*

Same like quadruped position the therapist grasping the upper trunk by standing back to the patient and lifting him. In the middle sometime the kneel sitting **(Fig. 13.9)** also may be attained before achieving kneel standing posture **(Fig. 13.10)**.

*Progressive Activities*

- Patient is assisted to maintain the posture in the beginning stage.
- Independent maintenance the posture can be practiced.
- Manual approximation force is applied in the anteroposterior as well as lateral directions to improve the static and dynamic stability of the patient.
- Hip hiking can be practiced in this posture as said in the long sitting.
- Kneel walking may be encouraged to increase the dynamic stability of the patient.

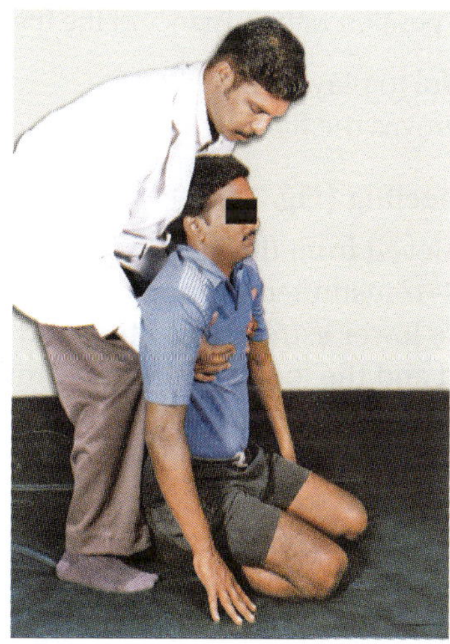

**Fig. 13.9:** Achieving the kneel sitting from side sitting position with assistance of the therapist.

- Mat crutch activities can be practiced, by swinging the upper extremity by holding the crutches. Lifting the body by holding the furniture/stable support can be practiced.
- Progression can be made to walk in side-ways.

*Uses*

- For dressing activities.
- Useful for mobility in small tunnels, as well in patients who have knee flexion deformity.

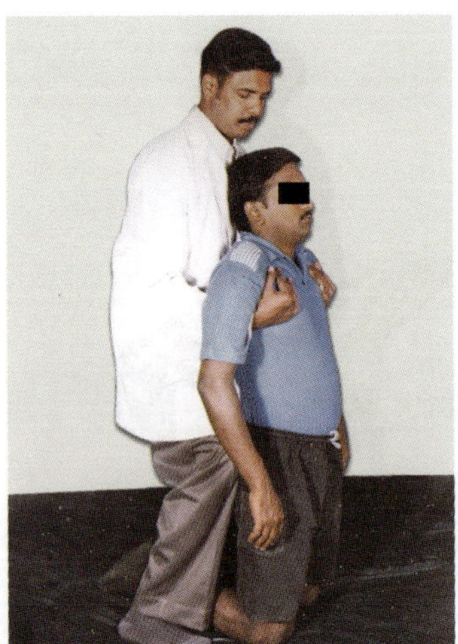

**Fig. 13.10:** Achieving the kneel standing from kneel sitting position with assistance of the therapist.

- ❖ Useful to play with the kids.
- ❖ Improves the floor level activities.

### Half-Kneeling (Fig. 13.11)

It is achieved from the kneel standing, where weight is transmitted to one side knee and the opposite lower extremity is lifted and the hip is flexed and the foot is placed in front on the mat. In this posture the BOS is more the COG is little low while comparative to the kneeling posture and it is stable than the kneel standing. It is the intermediate posture between the kneel standing and the standing.

*Position*

Weight bearing over one side knee, and another side hip and knees are flexed and the foot is kept on the floor.

*Progressive Activities*

- ❖ Weight shifting activities can be performed with/without assistance.
- ❖ Push-ups can be practiced to come out of this posture and go for the standing posture with the help of the furniture or wall/therapist.

*Uses*

- ❖ Sometimes used by weak/aged individuals while moving from floor sitting to standing.

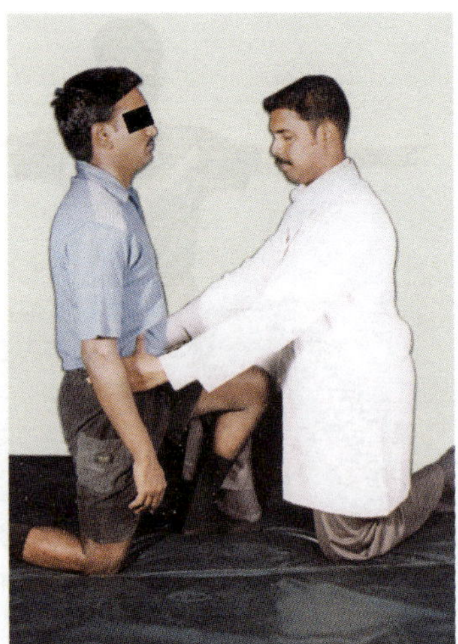

**Fig. 13.11:** Half-kneeling with the support of the therapist

- ❖ Can be used in therapy to reduce lower limb spasticity and to promote standing.

*Standing*

Here the BOS is less and the COG is high. So, this is the unstable posture to maintain for prolonged time. This is the intermediate position between the half-kneeling and the walking. It can be achieved from the half kneeling and chair sitting. This is the starting position for walking.

*Standing from Half-Kneeling*

Therapist is standing back to the patient and grasping the upper trunk with both the hands and lifting the patient up. The kneeling leg moves forwards and the foot is placed on the mat or floor. The patient can also hold the furniture or the wall, and lift his body up, to reach standing with the help of the assistance.

*From Sitting to Standing*

From the sitting the therapist has to sit in front of the patient on the stool and has to lock the patient's knee with his knee, while he is made to stand **(Fig. 13.12A)**. The therapist has to hold the pelvis of the patient and lift him. The patient should hold the shoulder region of the therapist to avoid falling. However, for patients of hemiplegia, while making a patient stand, instead of locking the patient's knee in

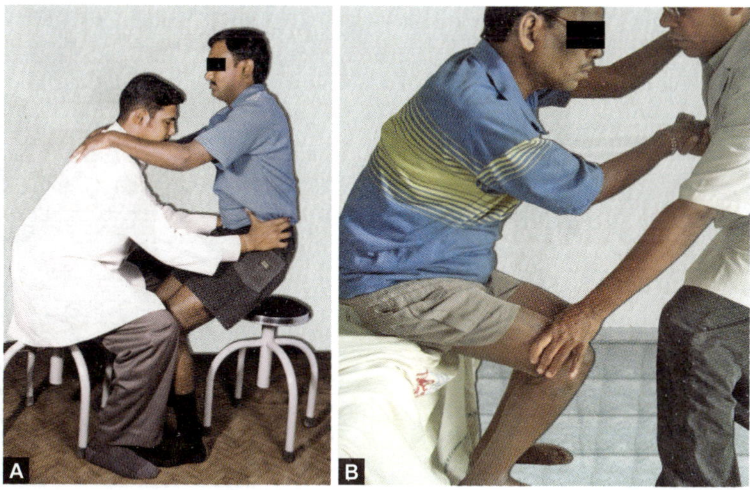


**Figs. 13.12A and B:** Achieving the standing position from sitting position with assistance of the therapist: (A) With the knees locked in a paraplegic patient; (B) Pushing at the lower thigh in a right hemiplegic patient.

extension, the therapist should push the lower thigh of the affected side, as locking the knees prevents displacement of COG forward and upwards, which is required in standing from sitting **(Fig. 13.12B)**.

Whenever the patient is allowed standing for first time, the therapist should be alert to complaint of nausea, light-headedness due to the sudden drop of the BP. The patient should be supported as per need, while made to stand **(Fig. 13.13)**.

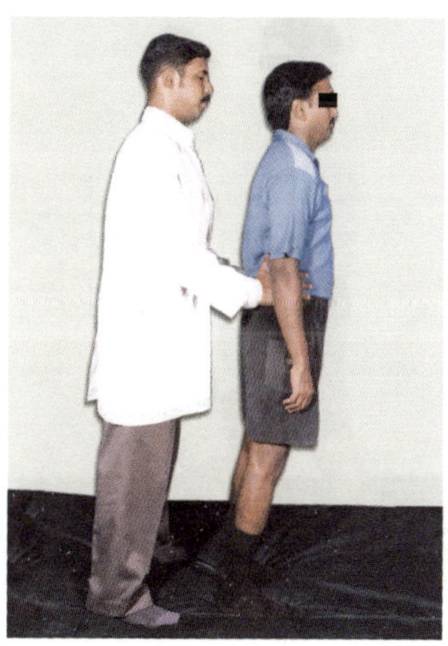

**Fig. 13.13:** Standing with support of therapist.

*Progressive Activities*

- At the beginning the patient is made to stand in the corner of the wall with the therapist's support in front, so that the patient cannot fall front, back, and sideways.
- Independent maintaining the standing posture can be performed to improve the static stability.
- Approximation force is applied in front, back, and lateral direction to improve the lateral stability.
- Weight shifting from one side to another will be carried out to increase the proprioceptor and the balancing activity. It may be started with the support of an object or the therapist.
- Crutch exercises may be performed in this posture to improve the crutch activities **(Fig. 13.14)**. Many of the upper and lower extremities exercises can be performed.
- Forward, backward, and sideways stepping can be practiced to improve the dynamic stability and to attain earlier walking.
- Walking training should be given with support of therapist **(Fig. 13.15)**, followed by walker/crutches, if independent walking is not possible.

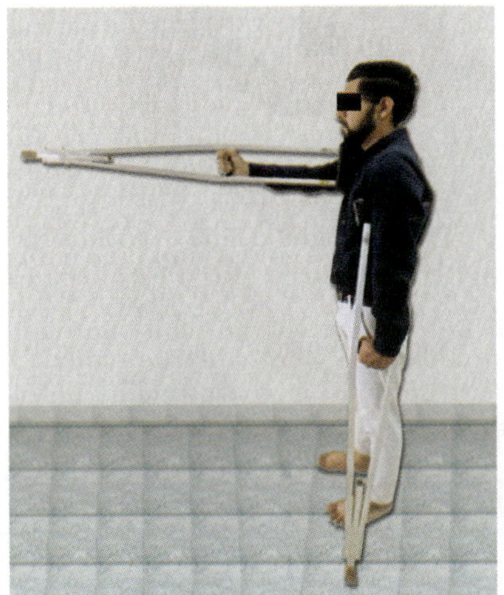

**Fig. 13.14:** Crutch balance training.

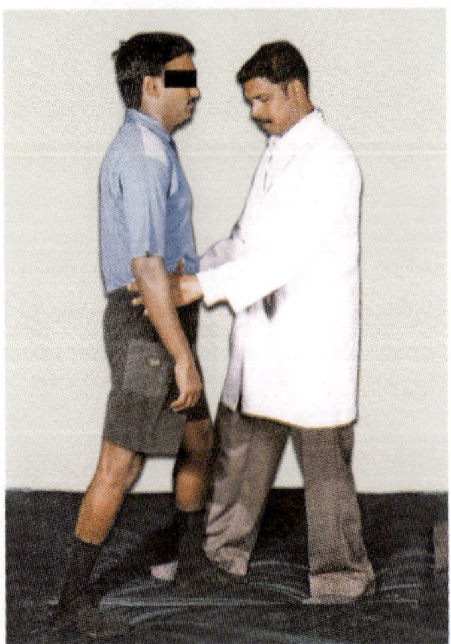

**Fig. 13.15:** Walking training with the support of therapist.

**Uses**

- Many of the functional activities at home and industries are done in standing.
- Standing in a parallel bar and stepping limbs forwards and backwards alternatively will have carryover into walking.

**Parallel Bar Walking**

As soon as the motor control is achieved in the standing posture, the parallel bar activities can be introduced. Before going for the parallel bar activities the parallel bar should be adjusted depending on the patient's height. Normally, the height of the parallel bar should be up to the level of the patient's greater trochanter **(Fig. 13.16)**.

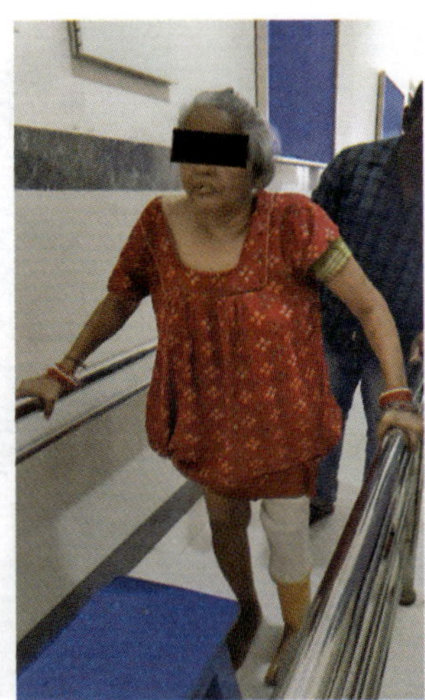

**Fig. 13.16:** Below-knee amputee fitted with artificial limb (prosthesis), receiving gait re-education training in parallel bar.

*General Instructions*

Proper instructions in parallel bar activities should be given throughout the walking training. It includes walking pattern, progressive activities, turning techniques, stability, balance and coordination. Generally, the verbal command improves or facilitates the activities more. The support or assistance of the therapist will be given in the weaker side limb to increase more stability. In some conditions like unstable knee, the therapist should lock the knee of the patient and body weight is transmitted through the locked knee joint.

During the initial range of the parallel bar activities the therapist should give support to the patient preventing from falling. Normally, the therapist has to stand towards the weaker side to give the stability. Guarding belt or the towel tied over the waist is used to guard the patient from falling. During the initial standing the therapist should be careful about the

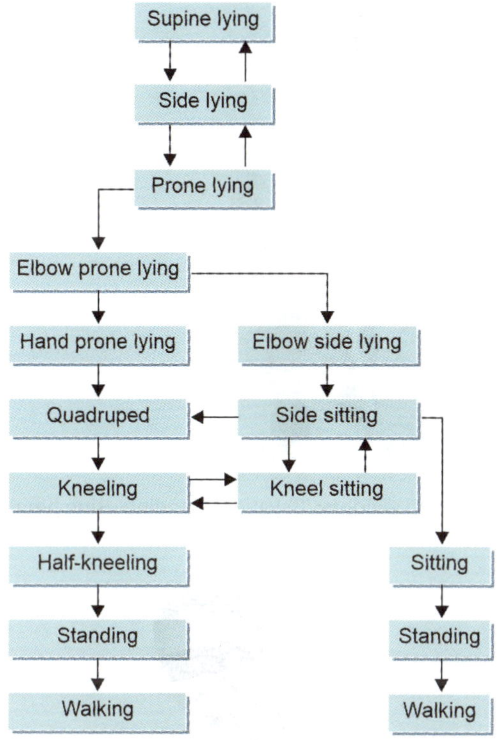


**Fig. 13.17:** Progressive positions in the functional re-educational training.

complaints of the light headedness, nausea due to postural hypotension.

*Progressive Activities In Functional Re-educational Training (Fig. 13.17)*

The progressive activities to improve posture and movement in patients with functional limitations are given in **Figure 13.17**.

During functional re-education training, patients should be made to practice the below mentioned progressive exercises to improve walking.

- Patient is made to stand with the support of the parallel bar without the therapist's support in the early stage.
- **Weight shifting:** Shifting the weight lateral, anterior, posterior sides are performed without altering the hand position in the parallel bar.
- **One leg standing**: Patient is recommended to stand with one leg support and transmitting whole weight over the supported leg.
- **One hand support standing**: Patient's one hand is removed from the parallel bar and make him to stand with the one hand support.
- **Hip hiking**: Patient is asked to practice the hip hiking movements, which is helpful to clear the foot from the ground and the forward propulsion of the body during ambulation.
- **Stepping forward and backward**: Patient is practiced to keep one leg forward, bring back to the normal position and the one step backward movement, and bring back to the neutral position by standing in same place.
- **Parallel bar push-ups:** Patient lifting his body with the upper limb support on parallel bar, is called as parallel bar push up. This is to be practiced, to improve upper extremity strength and power.
- **Turning technique**: The turning in the parallel bar is important and useful like turning in the normal floor walking. Generally, the patient is made to turn towards the normal side by avoiding turning towards the affected side. Avoiding pivot is also most helpful to show easy mastering in the turning technique. For example, while turning towards right side, right leg is raised and placed on the floor 90° to the previous position and the same was followed by the left foot, which is kept parallel to the right foot. Next to that the left hand is removed from the left side and placed, on the right side parallel bar to attain perfect support. The therapist may help the patient supporting him by standing back to him.
- **Resisted forward progression**: Resistance force is applied over the chest region of the patient while walking in the parallel bar.
- **Backward walking:** Backward walking can be practiced by the patient to get good standing.

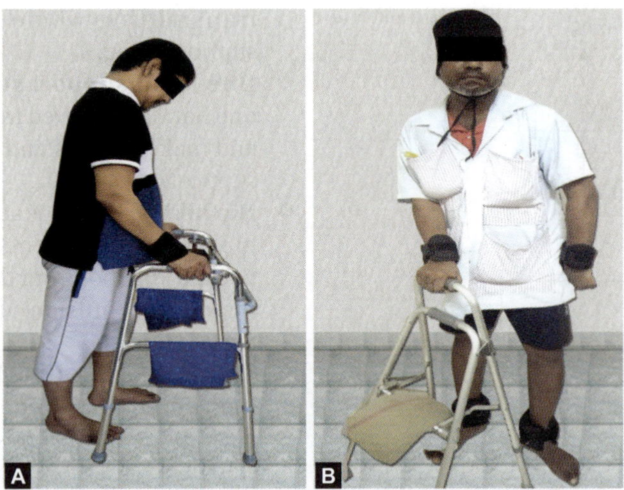

**Figs. 13.18A and B:** (A) Ataxic patient walking using walker with weights; (B) Patient standing using hemi-walker and weight jackets/weight cap/weight cuffs.

- **Side walking**: Side walking can also be practiced to improve the stability and balance.
- **Air cycling:** Parallel bar push-ups have to be done first followed by the cycling activity with the lower extremity in the air.
- **Step-up**: Inside the parallel bar the step is placed and the patient is instructed to practice the step-up activity. Standing on one leg and swing the opposite side unsupported lower extremity, will also carry over into stepping.

**Use of assistive technologies for improvement of function**: As per the need of the patient, assistive technologies, such as a hemi walker/walker **(Fig. 13.18A)**/crutches/walking sticks, for walking, and universal cuffs with attachments for spoon/comb, etc., should be selected and used for the patient during functional re-education. Involuntary movements, like tremor/jerky movements (chorea), etc., should be controlled by selecting appropriate strategies, such as weight cuffs/ weight jackets/weight cap, etc. **Figure 13.18B**, shows a patient with basal ganglia disorder, with severe involuntary jerky movements, made to stand with weight jacket, weight cap, weight cuffs in the limbs and a hemi walker on right side, as his left hand function is severely impaired.

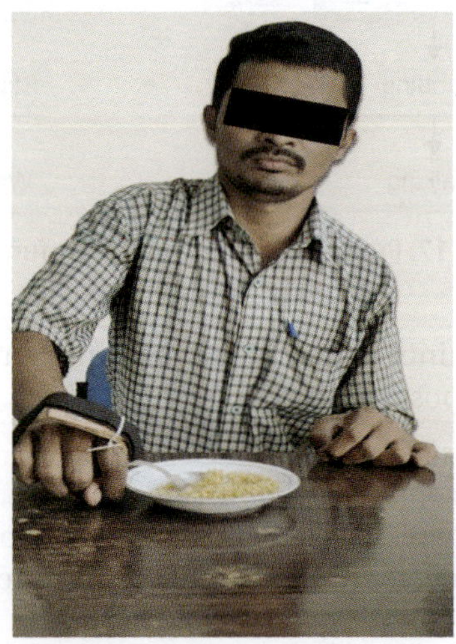

**Fig. 13.19:** Use of universal cuff with spoon for eating.

**Re-education of hand function:** Besides re-education for bed mobility, sitting, standing and walking (gait re-education), the therapist should re-educate hand function with or without adaptive devices such as universal cuff for taking food to mouth **(Fig. 13.19)**.

# 14 CHAPTER Coordination and Balance

## DEFINITION FOR COORDINATION

Coordination is the ability to execute smooth, rhythmical, accurate, controlled motor responses, performed in correct sequence of the group actions of muscles, to maintain posture and balance, and perform purposeful movements.

The cerebellum is the primary center in the brain for coordination of movement and the ability to execute smooth accurate motor response. It enable the person to select the right muscle at the right time with proper intensity to achieve proper action.

### Factors Affecting Coordinated Movements

#### *Volition*

It is the ability to initiate, maintain or stop an activity or motion at own will.

#### *Perception*

Movement production is the interaction, between cognition, perception and action. Intact proprioception and subcortical centers integrate motor impulses and the sensory feedback to recognize the task and movement parameters to accomplish the task. When proprioception is affected, movement becomes uncoordinated, which is compensated with visual feedback.

#### *Engram*

It is the abstract representation that stores the memory of rules of performance of various purposeful movements. This is a physical or biochemical change in neural tissue, which stores the memory of movement. A high repetitions of precise performance is required in order to develop an engram. Coordination is developed in proportion to the number of repetitions of movement to strengthen the engram.

Motor coordination to complete a task is a collaboration of three skills.

### Skills for Motor Coordination

#### *Fine Motor Skills*

Require coordinated movement of small muscles of hands, face etc., e.g., writing, drawing, buttoning a shirt, blowing bubbles.

#### *Gross Motor Skills*

Require coordinated movement of large muscles or groups of muscles of trunk and extremities, e.g., walking, running, lifting activities.

#### *Eye-Hand Skills*

The ability of the visual system to coordinate visual information and then direct the hands for the accomplishment of a task, e.g., catching a ball, sewing, operation of computer mouse, etc.

### Ataxia

Ataxia/asynergia is a condition that affects the coordination of movement. Coordinated movement requires a functioning cerebellum, spinal cord and peripheral nervous system. Diseases and injuries that damage or destroy any of these structures can lead to ataxia.

There are different types of ataxia, depending on the cause and the affected part of the body. Some of the main types of ataxia are:

### *Cerebellar Ataxia*

It caused by a problem in the cerebellum, a part of the brain that controls coordination and balance. The patient walks with a wide based, unsteady gait, with hypotonia, tremor, loss of balance, dysmetria (undershooting/overshooting), dysdiadokokinesia (inability to perform rapid, alternating movements), slurred/dysarthric speech, nystagmus, poor eye hand coordination, etc.

### *Sensory Ataxia*

It is caused by a problem in the sensory nerves that relay information about the position of the body parts to the brain. It affects patients with significant proprioceptive loss. The dorsal column of the spinal cord fails to carry proprioceptive information from the body to the brain. Characteristically, the patient looks down and walks as if throwing his feet, which tend to slap on the ground. Sensory ataxia is distinguished from cerebellar ataxia by the presence of near-normal coordination when the movement is visually observed by the patient, but marked worsening of coordination when the eyes are shut, indicating a positive Romberg's sign. This type of ataxia is found in patients of syringomyelia, tabes dorsalis, leprosy, diabetic neuropathy, etc., who develop insensitive (charcot's joints).

### *Vestibular Ataxia*

The term vestibular ataxia is used to indicate ataxia due to dysfunction of the vestibular system (made up of the inner ear and the semicircular canals that contain the semicircular fluid, which senses the position of head in space, helping in balance and spatial orientations). It results in vertigo, nausea and vomiting.

### *Genetic Ataxia*

These inherited ataxias develop from mutations in specific genes that are inherited from the parents. Some examples are ataxia telangiectasia, Friedreich's ataxia, and spinocerebellar ataxia (please refer some neurology books to know in detail about the ataxias, particularly the genetic ataxias).

## Tests for Incoordination

### *Upper Limb*

**Finger-Nose Test (Refer Fig. 3.25 from Chapter 3)**

The finger-nose test is used to assess coordinated, target-driven movement of the upper limb. The shoulder of the seated patient is abducted to 90° with the elbow extended. The patient is then asked to bring the tip of the index finger to the tip of his/her nose. Alternatively, the test is performed by making the patient and the therapist sit opposite to each other. The therapist's index finger is held in front of the patient and the patient is asked to touch the tip of his index finger to the therapist's index finger and then touch his/her nose. A positive test in the form of intention tremor, dysmetria (undershooting/overshooting) indicates cerebellar pathology. In posterior column disease, the patient can touch the nose accurately with eye-opened but he cannot do with closed eyes.

**Finger-to-Finger Test (Refer Fig. 3.26 from Chapter 3)**

The patient is asked to abduct both the shoulders 90° with elbow in extension and bring both the index fingers towards midline and touch each other. Cerebellar diseased patient may touch each other by the wavering and oscillating fashion. But the posterior column diseased person can touch accurately with opened eyes, but not with closed eyes.

### Rapid Alternating Movement Test

The patient is asked to do the pronation and supination movement alternatively. In cerebellar lesion the patient feels difficulty in performing this movement, and this phenomena is called as dysdiadochokinesia.

## *Lower Limb*

### Finger-to-Toe Test (Refer Fig. 3.27 from Chapter 3)

The therapist's finger is pointed two feet above the patient's great toe and he/she is instructed to touch the finger with the great toe. The cerebellar disease patient can touch the finger with the oscillatory or light bouncing movements. But it can be done accurately with the eyes opened, but not with the eyes closed in patients with sensory ataxia (posterior column disease).

### Heel-to Shin Test (Refer Fig. 3.28 from Chapter 3)

The patient is in supine lying. He/she is asked to touch the knee with the opposite side heel and slide the heel on the shin towards the great toe. In cerebellar disease, when the heel is carried up, it overshoots the knee and if the heel is carried down, it begins to execute an action tremor. In posterior column disease the patient cannot perform it due to the inability to recognize the position of the joint.

### Romberg's Test (Refer Fig. 3.29 from Chapter 3)

The Romberg test is a test that measures a persons sense of balance. Specifically, the test assesses the function of the dorsal column of the spinal cord (the dorsal column is responsible for proprioception). The Romberg test is an appropriate tool to diagnose sensory ataxia.

Patient is made to stand straight with the eyes opened and feet close to each other. Then the patient is instructed to shut the eyes. Patient may begin to sway and may even fall, if he is not supported, when the eyes are closed. It occurs in patient's with posterior column disease. But cerebellar diseased patients can stand even their eyes are closed also.

### Walking Along a Straight Line, Foot Close to Foot

In case of cerebellar lesion, there is deviation of gait.

### Foot Tapping Test

The subject sits on a chair with adjustable height so that the bilateral soles made contact with the floor, and the hip and knee joints flexed at approximately 90°. He/she moves his/her toes up and down repeatedly to tap the floor as fast and as vigorously as possible for 10 sec with the heels planted on the floor. The test is performed for both sides separately. The examiner counts the number of taps for each side. This test is done for patients with cerebellar ataxia.

### Lower Extremity Motor Coordination Test (LEMOCOT)

The subject sits on a height adjustable chair with the feet resting flat on a thin rigid foam, heels on the proximal target, and knees at 90° of flexion. Then, after a familiarization trial, he/she is instructed to alternately touch the proximal and distal targets placed 30 cm apart with his/her big toe for 20 sec. The number of touched targets in 20 sec is recorded for the motor coordination of the lower limb.

# Correction of Incoordinated Movements/ Physiotherapy for Incoordination

## *Flaccidity/Weakness*

Muscle weakness and the muscular paralysis/ flaccidity can be analyzed with help of the muscle power grading techniques. Whenever the muscle is weak, the person should undergo strengthening and endurance exercises. Strengthening program is modified depending on the muscle power and has to be performed by the patient with the supervision of the therapist.

## *Spasticity*

It is a condition of velocity dependent increase in muscle tone, which also leads to incoordination. Soft tissue stretching, PNF techniques and spasticity relieving techniques, regular active movements, etc., are used to reduce the spasticity and make the movements coordinated and purposeful.

### *Loss of Kinesthetic Sensation/Sensory Ataxias*

Neuropathic joint patients are normally unaware of the joint movement and posture due to the loss of proprioceptor activity. Their walking patterns are like the "space walk". They raise their foot up in the air and stamp on the floor forcibly. Loss of joint sense leads to disuse of the limb, which leads to the hypotonia of the muscle. This lack of joint sense and the hypotonia of the muscle together results in the uncoordinated movement of the limb. To improve the joint sense and convey the kinesthetic sensation, the alternative nervous pathway has to be selected. Proprioceptive training in the form of weight bearing and weight shifting exercises, Frenkel's exercises, etc., are used to treat such disorders.

### *Cerebellar Ataxia*

The main aim of the treatment is to improve the stability and balance of the trunk and the proximal joints while treating the cerebellar ataxic cases. The stability as well as balancing training has to be practiced by the patients depending on the degree of the disability. Hypotonia is the main clinical feature in this disease. Isometric exercise program, strengthening and endurance exercises, PNF techniques of rhythmic stabilization, etc., have to be practiced by the patient to improve the coordinated movement production and balance. Some of the coordinated exercises can be followed from the Frenkel's exercise program (which is mostly used for the sensory ataxia).

## Frenkel Exercise

Frenkel exercises are a series of motions of increasing difficulty, performed by ataxic patients, to facilitate the restoration of rhythmic, smooth and coordinated movements, by the use of any part of the sensory mechanism, which are intact, such as vision, hearing, touch, etc., to compensate for the loss of kinesthetic sensation.

These exercises are a set of slow repetitive exercises developed by Professor Heinrich Sebastian Frenkel, Medical Superintendent of the Sanatorium Freihof, in Switzerland in 1889, to treat ataxic in patients of tabes dorsalis and sensory ataxias owing to loss of proprioception. These exercises are also applicable to cerebellar ataxic patients.

The exercises are designed to establish the voluntary control of movements by the use of any part of the sensory mechanism which is intact, such as vision, hearing, touch, etc., to compensate for the loss of kinesthetic sensation. The visual sense is the most important supporting factor in the treatment. The ultimate aim is to establish control of movements, so that the patient is confidently able in his ability to carry out activities, which are essential for independence in everyday life. While performing the exercises, the patient watches his hand or arm movements (for example, in training of upper limb) and corrects them as needed. Daily treatment sessions for at least 6 weeks are effective.

### *Indications of Frenkel's Exercise*

- Cerebellar ataxia.
- Sensory ataxia.
- Stroke.
- Cerebral palsy.
- Multiple sclerosis.
- Wilson's disease.
- Parkinson's disease.
- Other neurological disorders.

### *Principles of Frenkel's Exercises*

- Concentration
- Precision
- Speed and range
- Command
- Repetition
- Complication.

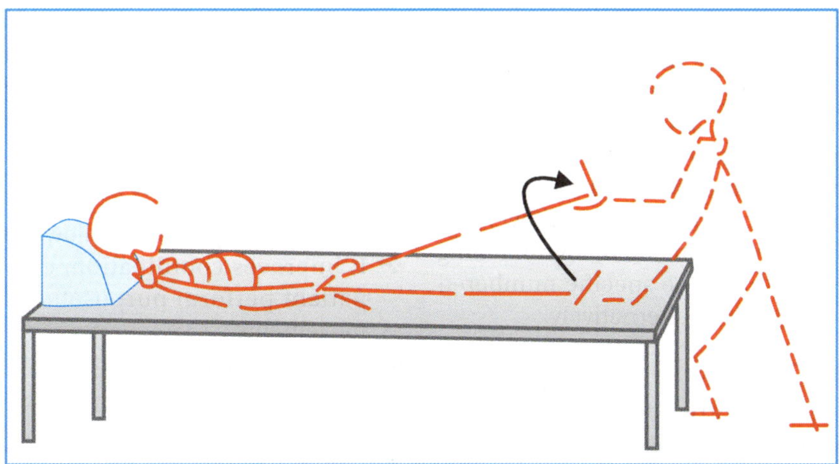

**Fig. 14.1:** Therapist directing movements to touch his/her hands placed in air.

The above principles are briefly discussed below:

### Concentration

The patient has to be positioned to watch every movement, which he performs. Normally, half-lying position is adopted during the treatment session. The patient must give full attention on the movement, which he performs. This attention of the movement may create the proprioceptor activities over the joint. The visually watching the movements are recorded in the brain and it may improve the kinesthetic sensation. Regular movements of the joint also may stimulate the proprioceptor activity.

### Precision

The movements should be accurate and rhythmical. There should not be any jerky, arrhythmic, and inaccurate movements, as the movement which the patient performs will be recorded in his brain through the visual pathways. The establishment of alternative sensory pathway will depend on the movements which the patient performs.

### Speed and Range

Quick movement needs less control than the slow movements. So, normally slow movements are recommended to be performed by the patient. The speed of movement should progress from high speed (which the patient usually performs) to low speed (which is required). Movements in large excursion/ROM involving big joints are selected first, subsequently, progressing to movements in small excursion/ROM and involving smaller joints. Selected range should be reached during each and every movement accurately and slowly. Selected range movements are indicated by marking the spot over the couch/floor or by the therapist placing the finger in the air **(Fig. 14.1)**.

### Command

Audition is another source of the sensory mechanism to compensate the proprioceptive activities and involuntary movements. Commanding is a very much necessary source to perform and progress the activity. With the command we can alter the speed, range of the movement, which the patient performs. All the instructions are mostly given in the form command through patient's own language, in this exercise regimen.

**Complexity**

Complexity (making the movement more and more difficult) introduced in the exercise regimen improves the coordination as well as proprioceptive activities. It may increase the concentration power and memorizing capacity of the brain on particular movement pattern. Complexity is made by commanding the patient to touch the specific numbered mark on the floor/bed alternatively.

**Repetition**

The movements are repeated until the accurate movements are performed by the patient (till the engram is developed). The repetition of the accurate movement improves the kinesthetic sense and the coordination. The exercises should be stopped whenever the patient feels tired. Frequent rest period must be allowed between repetitions. Repeating the movements are helpful for the cerebrum to record and memorize one particular movement perfectly.

### *Techniques of Frenkel's Exercise*

- The patient should be positioned comfortably, and suitably clothed, so that, he/she can see the movements, throughout the exercise program.
- The room should be well lighted, without distractions, for better learning and development of engram.
- The patient should be given a concise explanation and demonstration about the exercise program.
- The patient is requested to give attention to the movements, he/she is performing.
- ROM is indicated by drawing spot on floor/ bed or by placing hand in space, making the patient move the hand/foot to the spot/ or touch the hand of the therapist, held in space, as dictated by the therapist.
- Speed of movement is dictated by the therapist through rhythmic counting, which progresses from faster to slower movements/speed.
- Sufficient rest periods should be given between exercises to avoid fatigue.
- Exercises should be repeated, till it is easily and perfectly performed by the patient.

### *Benefits of Frenkel Exercises*

The exercises improve the followings:

- It improves coordination, enabling the patient perform purposeful functional movements.
- It improves postural control and balance, and prevents falls.
- It improves body awareness.
- It improves gait.
- It improves proprioception.

### *The Frenkel's Exercise Program*

For a patient with ataxia, the exercises should start in lying and gradually progress to sitting and standing. The exercises contain the followings:

**Exercises in Lying/Half Lying**

The movements in the form of flexion-extension, abduction-adduction, should be performed both unilaterally, starting from faster movements progressing to slower movements, as well as bilaterally. Bilateral movements, should occur simultaneously, progressing to alternate movements. The exercises for upper and lower limbs in lying are discussed below:

**Upper limb**

- Half-lying—abduction and adduction of shoulder.
- Half-lying—wrist flexion, extension, ulnar and radial deviation.
- Side lying—flexion and extension of elbow.
- Side lying—flexion and extension of shoulder.

**Lower limb**

- Half-lying—abduction and adduction of hip **(Fig. 14.2)**.
- Side lying—flexion and extension of hip.
- Side lying—flexion and extension of knee.

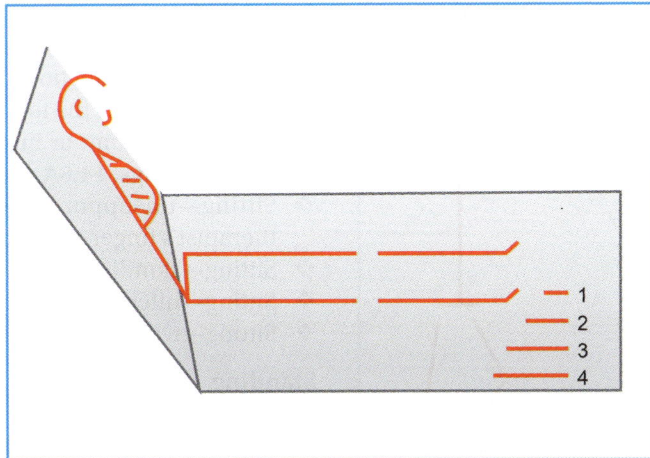


**Fig. 14.2:** Half lying, abduction/adduction of hips to the marks on bed/floor.

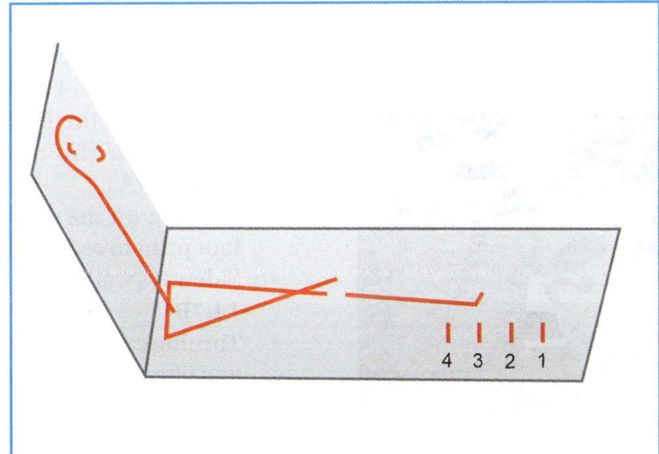


**Fig. 14.3:** Half lying, flexion/extension of hip and knees to reach at the marks on floor/bed.

- Half-lying—flexion and extension of hip and knee **(Fig. 14.3)**.

**Exercise in Sitting**

Sitting with support is started first, followed by sitting independently and performing the exercises.

Upper limb

- Sitting—alternating the movements like supination and pronation, flexion and extension, closing and opening the fist, touching the finger tips with the thumb.
- Sitting—reaching the therapist's hand/finger, which is placed in the air **(Fig. 14.4)**.
- Sitting—pegboard exercises **(Fig. 14.5)**.
- Sitting—separating the same colored blocks from the box.
- Sitting—constructing some objects like towers with help of the blocks
- Sitting—transferring the ball from one hand to another hand.
- Sitting—pushing and punching movements.
- Sitting—elbow flexing and touching the shoulder with the palm.
- Sitting—combing, drawing, tying the shoelace and normal household activities.

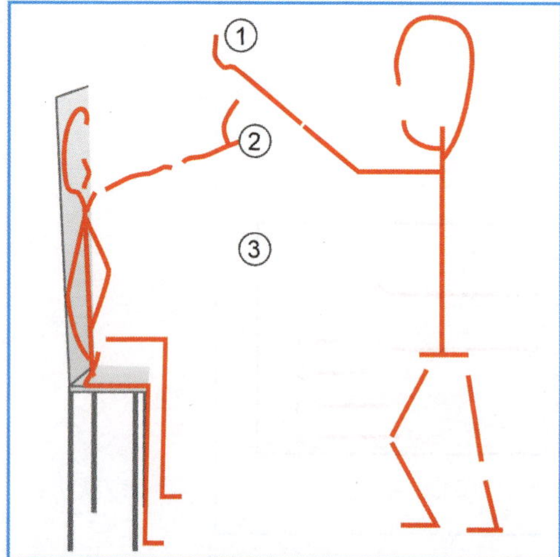


**Fig. 14.4:** Patient touching therapists hand/fingers placed in air.

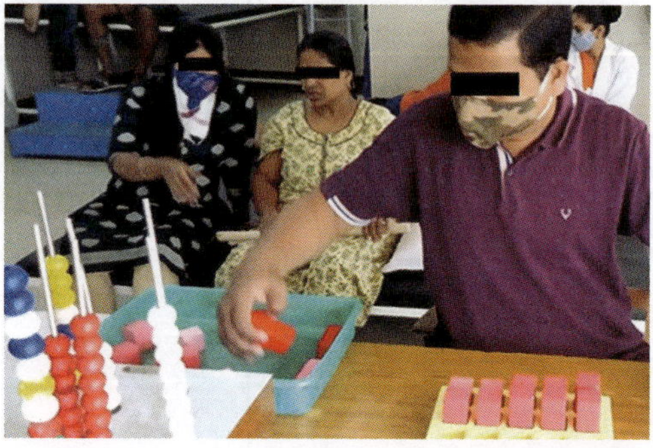

**Fig. 14.5:** Patient performing peg board exercises.

**Lower limbs**

- Sitting—knee flexion and extension.
- Sitting—hip abduction and adduction.
- Sitting—moving the foot and placing over the marked point or numbered board on the floor **(Figs. 14.6A and B)**.
- Sitting—unsupported foot touching the therapist's finger, which is placed in air.
- Sitting—standing and sitting down.
- Sitting—hitching, hiking movements.
- Sitting—walking on the buttocks.

**Standing**

- Standing with the support is practiced first.
- Walking training with help of the parallel bars.
- Walking training is given first with wider base later changing into narrow base.
- Frenkel's mat is used to improve the walking skill **(Figs. 14.7A and B)**
  - Walking on the both side footprints by leaving the middle footprints **(Fig. 14.7A)**.
  - Walking on the middle and one-side foot print to reduce the base.
  - Sideways walking on the foot mat **(Fig. 14.7B)**.
  - Turning can be practiced with pivoting and lifting and placing on the footmarks **(Fig. 14.8)**.
  - The turning/pivoting is done towards the weak side. The weak side will be

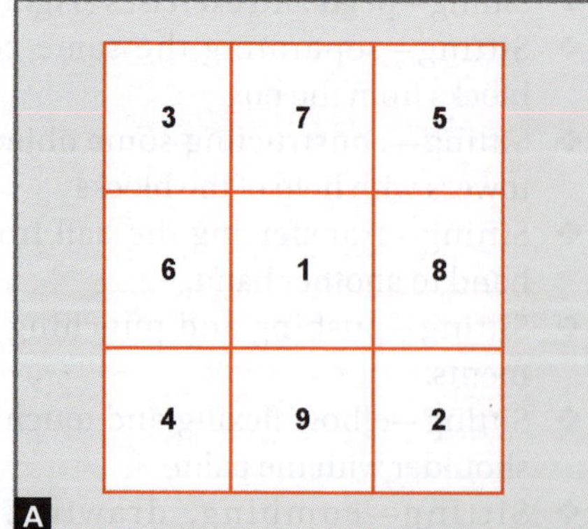


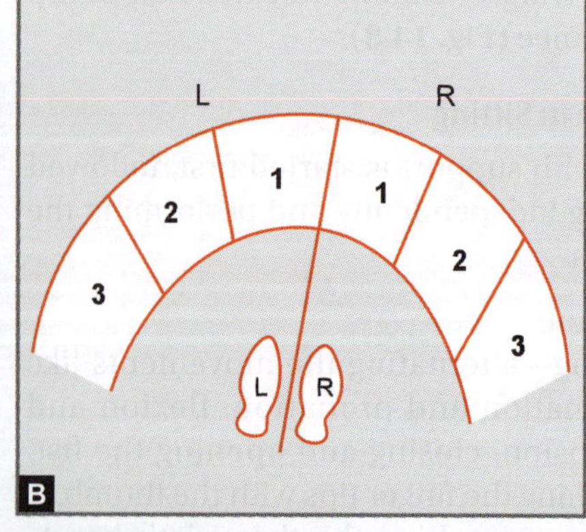


**Figs. 14.6A and B:** Lower limb movements in sitting.

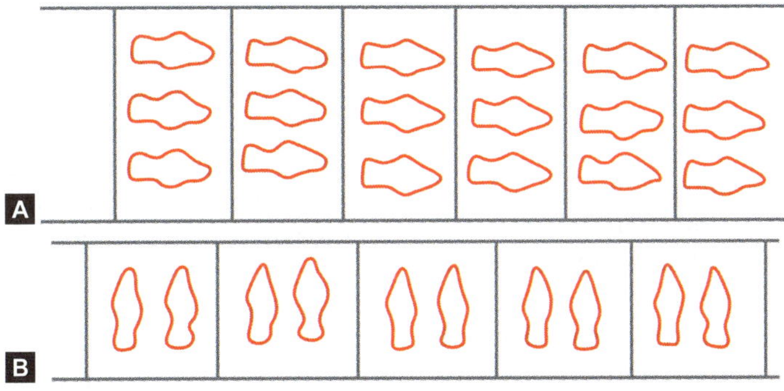


**Figs. 14.7A and B:** (A) Frenkel's foot mat; (B) Frenkel's mat for side walking training.

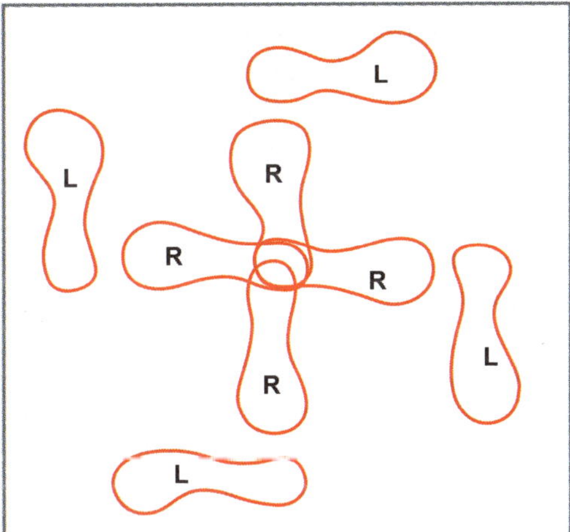


**Fig. 14.8:** Pivot turning

stable in one point and rotating with the fixed axis and another leg is lifted and kept on the marked place.

- While turning, the right foot is rotated or turned 90° and the left foot is raised and placed parallel to the right foot.

❖ Throwing and catching a ball in the hands and kicking balls forwards/backwards/sideways should be added as progression in standing. The therapist, should remain alert to prevent a fall from occurring.

### *Progression of Frenkel's Exercises*

❖ According to the impairment level, exercises should progress from lying to sitting and then standing.

❖ Movements can be made more difficult, by altering the speed (starting with high speed requiring less control and progressing to slow movements, that require high control.

❖ Gradually movements should be made more complex, like pivoting in one place, squatting, walking with arm swings, walking up and down steps/slopes, etc.

❖ Integrating the movement gain into functional activities.

## Balance

Balance refers to an individual's ability to maintain the line of gravity within the base of support (BOS). It can also be described as the ability to maintain equilibrium, where equilibrium can be defined as any condition in which all acting forces are cancelled by each other resulting in a stable balanced system.

Balance control is a complex body function that involves regulating posture and movement via the cerebellum by processing sensory inputs from the vestibular visual and proprioceptive systems in the cerebral cortex

The somatosensory system/proprioception, vestibular and visual systems, provide input to the CNS for the body's equilibrium and help in maintenance of balance.

### *Somatosensory System*

Activation leads to transmission of proprioceptive information in the spino-cerebellar pathways, for processing, unconsciously in the cerebellum, for the control of posture and balance.

### *The Vestibular System*

It generates compensatory responses to head motion via the postural, oculomotor and visceral responses, as discussed below, for maintenance of balance.

- Postural responses (vestibulospinal reflex), keep the body upright and prevent falls when the body is unexpectedly knocked off balance.
- Ocular-motor responses (vestibulo-ocular reflex) allows the eyes to remain steadily focused while the head is in motion.
- Visceral responses (vestibulocolic reflex), help keep the head and neck centered, steady, and upright on the shoulders.

### *The Visual System*

It helps maintain balance by interacting with the vestibular system via the vestibulo-ocular reflex. The eyes provide relevant information, about the body's position, relative to the environment and compensates for impairment of the visual and vestibular systems.

### *Classification of Balance*

**Static balance:** Static balance is the ability to maintain postural stability and orientation with center of mass over the base of support and body is at rest.

**Dynamic balance:** Dynamic balance is the ability to maintain postural stability and orientation with center of mass over the base of support while the body parts are in motion.

### *Causes of Loss of Balance*

Disorders that affect the somatosensory system/proprioception, visual and vestibular system are responsible for loss of balance. Such disorders are:

- **Benign paroxysmal positional vertigo (BPPV):** It is the most common inner ear condition that causes vertigo. It develops when calcium crystals in the ear (otoconia) move out of place. Symptoms come on suddenly with certain head movements. BPPV is diagnosed using a technique called the Dix-Hallpike maneuver. BPPV is treated using a technique called the Epley maneuver, performed by a healthcare provider, which helps relocate the crystals to their proper position in the inner ear.
- **Ménière's disease:** It is a condition that is caused by build up of fluid in the inner ear, which interferes with signals sent between the inner ear and the brain that help maintain balance.
- Peripheral neuropathies.
- **Labyrinthitis:** An infection or inflammation of the inner ear that causes dizziness and loss of balance
- Parkinson's disease.
- Stroke/TBI.
- Cerebral palsy.
- Old age.
- **Vestibular neuronitis:** An inflammation of the vestibular nerve that can be caused by a virus, and primarily causes vertigo.
- **Perilymph fistula:** A leakage of inner ear fluid into the middle ear.
- **Cerebellar degeneration:** Cerebellar dysfunction causes balance problems and gait disorders along with difficulties in coordination resulting in ataxia, uncoordinated movements, imbalance, speech problems (dysarthria), visual problems (nystagmus) and vertigo.
- Proprioceptive dysfunction like tabes dorsalis.
- **Other causes such as:** Hypotension, hypoglycemia, orthostatic hypotension, etc.

### *Assessment of Balance*

The person's ability to prevent the displacement of COG (counterpoising reaction) in lying, sitting, standing, as well as the ability to control the displacement of COG, as occurs in reaching with hands, turning the body in sitting/standing should be tested. The strategies in standing discussed below such as ankle strategies, hip strategies, stepping strategies, that help to maintain balance should be tested. The functional balance grading scale is a simple method of grading balance into: Normal, Good, Fair, Poor, Nil, which can be applied by therapists in clinical settings. Besides the simple methods to test balance, special assessment tests discussed below can also be used to assess balance (the details of such tests are not under the scope of this book).

- **BERG balance scale**: It looks primarily at stationary balance such as ability to stand with and without eyes closed, standing tandem, etc.
- **Dynamic gait index:** It assesses a patient's balance during walking while performing various tasks such as altering speed or stepping around an object.
- **Tinetti balance assessment:** The Tinetti-balance assessment test, also called performance-oriented mobility assessment (POMA) assesses a person's perception of balance and stability during activities of daily living and the fear of falling.
- **Timed up and go test**: Determines the fall risk in elderly population and patients such as Parkinson's disease and measure the progress of balance, for activities such as sit to stand and walking.
- **Functional reach test**: It is a clinical outcome measure and assessment tool for ascertaining dynamic balance in one simple task.

### *Balance Strategies*

- **Ankle strategy:** The "ankle strategy" occurs with minimal perturbation of balance and involves shifting of COM at ankles **(Fig. 14.9)**. Control is distal to proximal. When perturbed from front to back, balance is retained by ankle dorsiflexion followed by knee extension. When perturbed from

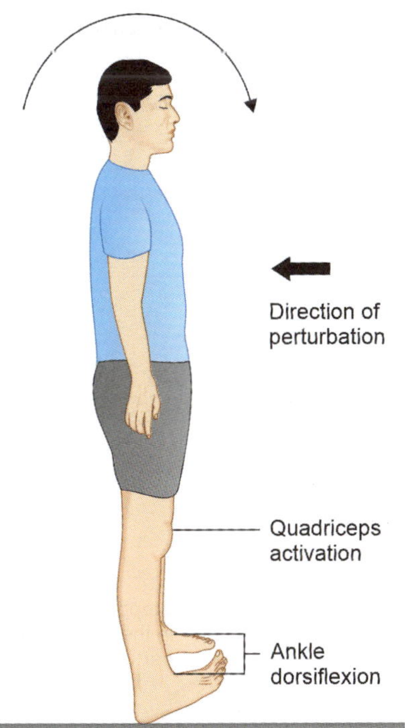


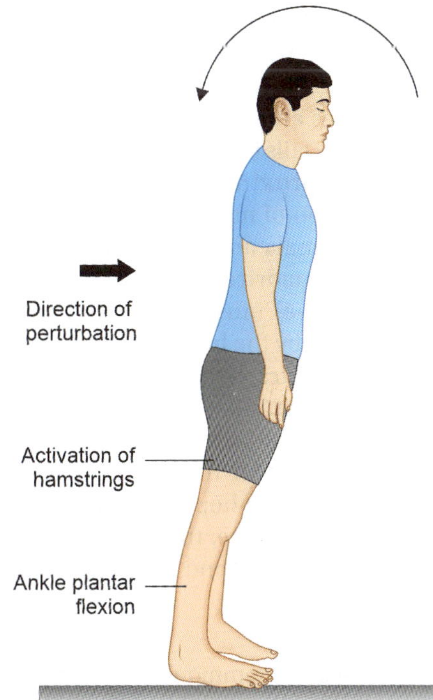


**Fig. 14.9:** The ankle strategies.

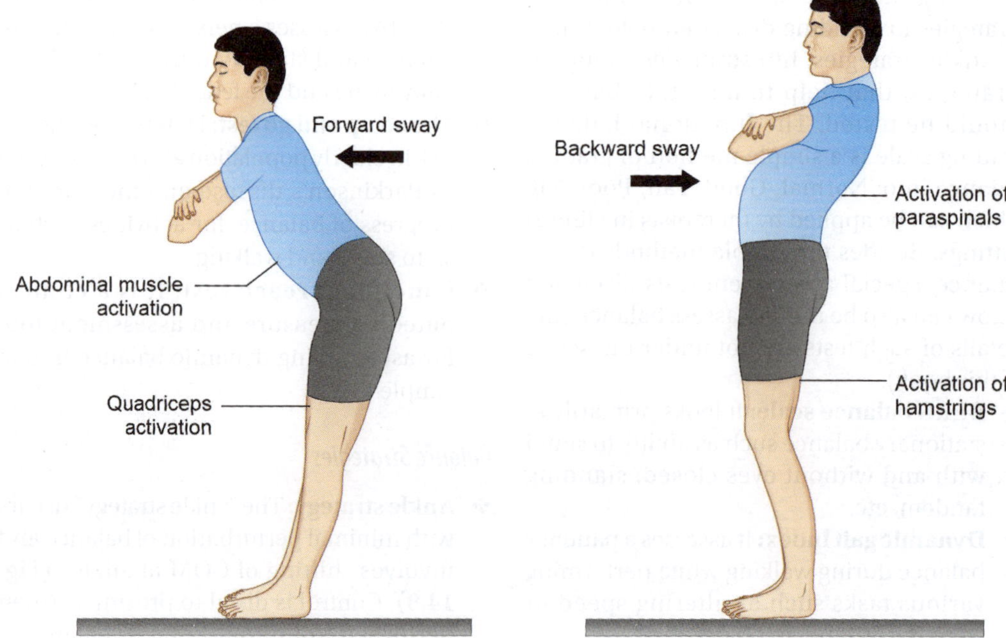


**Fig. 14.10:** The hip strategies.

back to front, balance is retained by ankle plantar flexion, followed by knee flexion.

- **The hip strategy (Fig. 14.10):** It involves shifting of COM by flexing or extending at the hips and is recruited when the ankle strategy fails (i.e., to larger perturbations). It has proximal to distal pattern of activation of muscles. With forward sway abdominals are activated first followed by the quadriceps. With backward sway, paraspinal muscles are activated first followed by the hamstrings.
- **Stepping strategy:** This strategy is recruited to larger perturbations, when ankle and hip strategies fail to retain balance. It realigns the BOS under the COM by rapid steps **(Fig. 14.11)** or hops in the direction of the displacing force, thereby increasing the base of support and retaining balance.

### *Balance Training*

Physiotherapy is commonly used to treat balance issues caused by neurological conditions. Interventions can include strengthening and endurance exercises, flexibility exercises, weight shifting and activities to improve

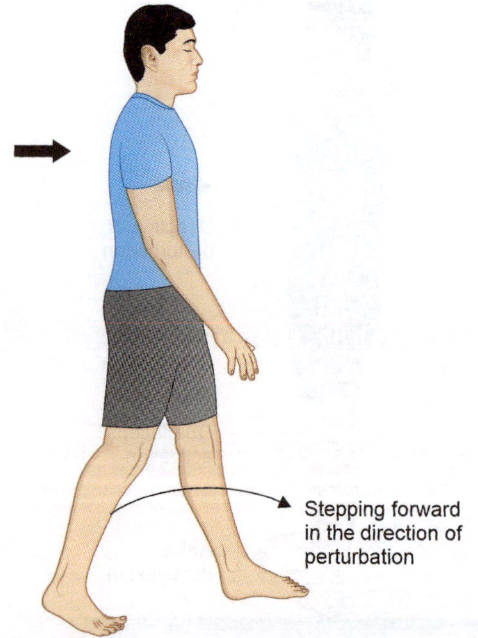


**Fig. 14.11:** The stepping strategy.

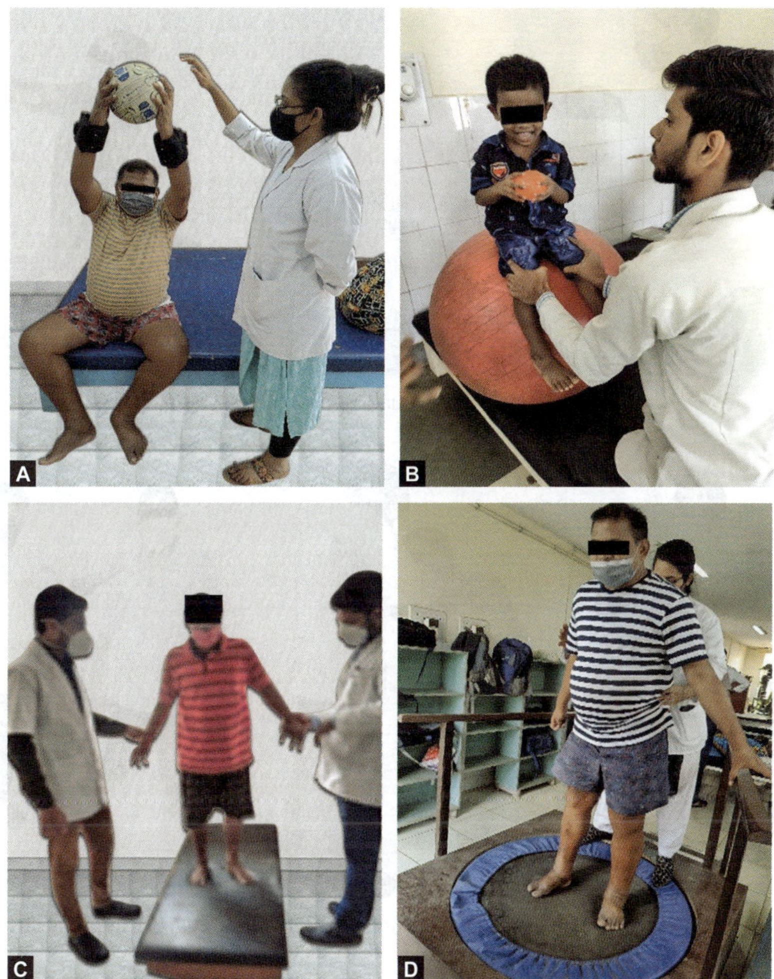

**Figs. 14.12A to D:** Shows balance training exercises; (A) Balancing exercise using ball and weight cuffs (to reduce tremor); (B) Exercises on Swiss ball; (C) Exercises on wobble board; (D) Exercises on trampoline.

proprioception, and instruction in the use of assistive devices (such as walkers or canes) to improve safety with walking. Balance exercises help to improve stability, mobility, endurance, ADL and IADL, etc. These exercises significantly reduces risk of fall and also improve athletic performance. Some balance training strategies used by therapist to develop balance are shown in **Figures 14.12 to 14.16**:

- Balancing exercises in sitting/standing **(Figs. 14.12A to D)**.
- Weight shifting in quadruped/kneeling **(Figs. 14.13A and B)**.
- Exercises to develop balance strategies in standing such as: Ankle/hip/stepping strategies **(Figs. 14.14A to C)**.
- Frenkle's exercises for patients with sensory ataxia.
- Virtual reality training **(Fig. 14.15)**.
- Postural mirror—biofeedback training **(Fig. 14.16)**.

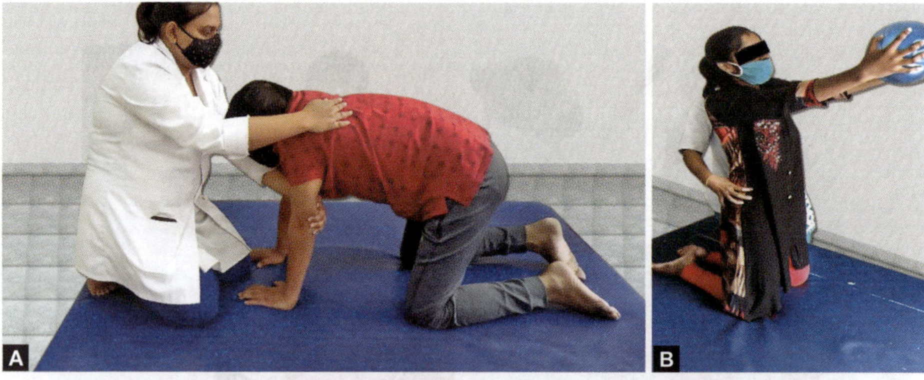

**Figs. 14.13A and B:** (A) Quadrped; (B) Kneel standing.

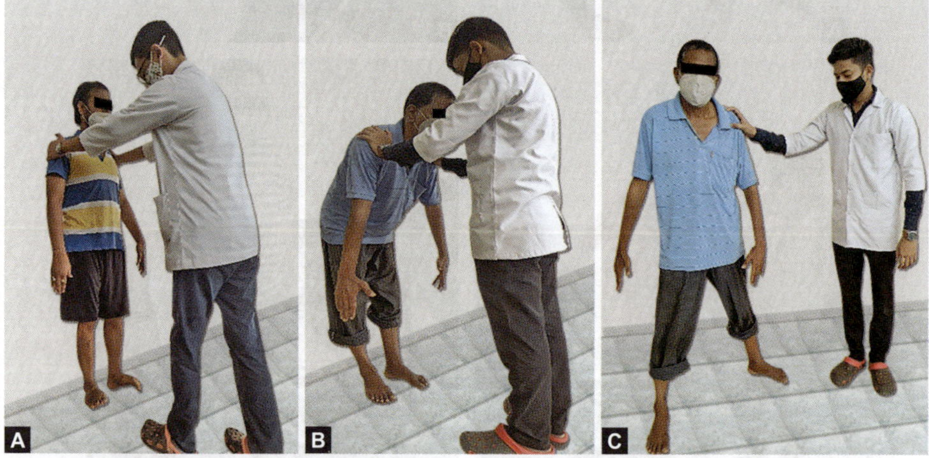

**Figs. 14.14A to C:** (A) Ankle strategy for balancing; (B) Hip strategy; (C) Stepping strategy.

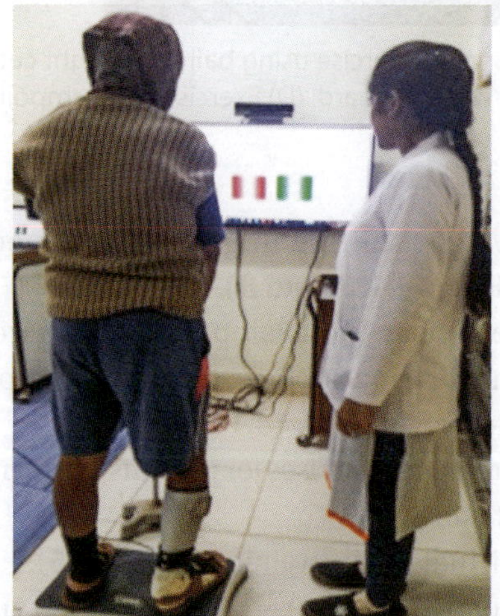

**Fig. 14.15:** Virtual reality training for balancing.

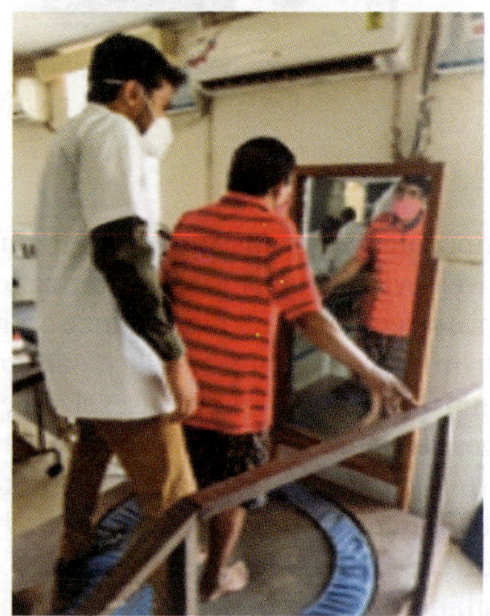

**Fig. 14.16:** Shows postural mirror biofeedback training on trampoline.

15

CHAPTER

# Suspension Therapy

## DEFINITION

**Suspension therapy is a special technique of therapeutic exercise in which a part or all of the body is suspended in the air in a special device called Gutheri-Smith suspension frame by ropes and slings attached to a fixed point above the body. The therapy is given to patients to increase range of motion (ROM), muscle power, and re-educate movement.**

## Principles of Suspension Therapy

It works under the principle of: (i) Friction, (ii) Pendulum, and (iii) Effect of gravity on movement.

### *Friction*

Friction occurs, during movement of one surface over other. If the friction between the surfaces is high, movement becomes difficult, and a weak muscle fails to overcome this frictional resistance to produce movement. In suspension therapy friction is less, causing smooth and easy movement.

### *Pendulum*

It works on the principles of pendulum, where application of force on pendulum, results in to and fro oscillatory movements. Very simple muscle contraction may initiate movement of joint, which behaves like a pendulum. The pendular to and fro motion in the human body is used to maintain joint ROM and muscle properties and strengthen muscles. It allows free/assisted/resisted movements.

### *Effect of Gravity on Movements*

It helps to eliminate gravity for free movements, as well as, utilizes gravity to either assist or resist movement as per the need. As per the muscle power, the impact of gravity can be used, either to assist, resist movements or to make movement free.

## Advantages

- It reduces the burden for the therapist.
- Easy to lift the limbs.
- Active movement can be performed easily with minimum friction.
- Many muscles can be strengthened in a session, using the device.
- It is a very good technique to exercise muscles with a grade of 1 or more, in recovering peripheral nerve injuries/neuropathies.

## Disadvantages

- Quite complex procedure.
- Requires many components/equipments.

## Suspension Instruments

- Suspension frame
- Supporting ropes
- Wooden cleat.
- Pulleys
- Slings
- S-hook and dog clips.

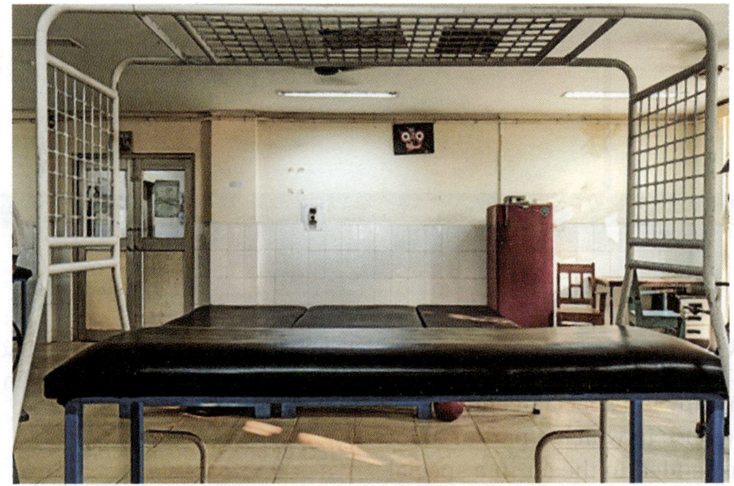

**Fig. 15.1:** Gutheri-Smith suspension frame.

## *Suspension Frame (Fig. 15.1)*

Invented by Late Mrs Guthrie Smith.

It is made up of stainless steel or plastic coated steel. In the top, head and foot end sides presents the 5-centimeter metal mesh, and the remaining sides are kept open. The measurement of the frame is 1 m or 2 m width × 2 m length × 2 m height. In the middle of the frame 2 m length × 1 m width × 1 m height couch is placed for the patient's accommodation.

## *Supporting Ropes*

It is 1.5 meters length and 3-ply hemp ropes are used for the suspension to avoid slipping. One end of the rope consists of a fixed ring and another end of the rope passes through the wooden cleat and is knotted in half-hitched manner **(Figs. 15.2A and B)**.

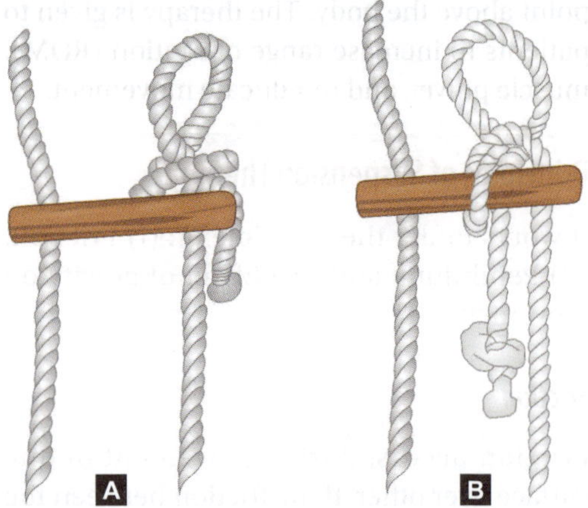


**Figs. 15.2A and B:** Half-hitched knotting: (A) Without tying the wooden cleat; (B) Knotting with the wooden cleat.

There are three types of supporting ropes: single rope, double rope, pulley rope.

1. **Single rope:** Has a ring fixed at one end by which it is hung up. The other end of the rope then passes through one end of the wooden cleat, through the ring of a dog clip and through the other end of the cleat and then knotted. The cleat is for altering the length of the rope and should be held horizontally for movement and pulled oblique when supporting. The rope is held on the cleat by frictional resistance. Length of rope required is 1.5 m **(Fig. 15.3)**.
2. **Double rope:** It consists of two pulleys at upper and lower attachments. This device gives a mechanical advantage of two as two pulleys are used. The rope is shortened by pushing the cleat down, allowing the lifter to move with gravity at the same

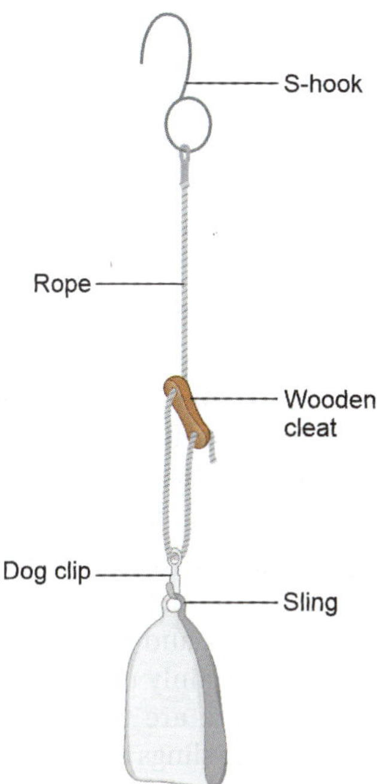


**Fig. 15.3:** The single rope system.

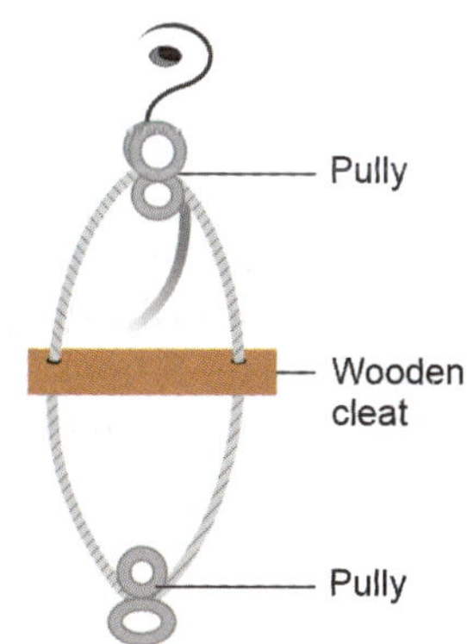


**Fig. 15.4:** The double rope system.

time as it offers a mechanical advantage of two. Such a rope is used to suspend the heavy parts of the body, such as the pelvis, thorax or heavy thighs when these are to be supported together **(Fig. 15.4)**.

3. **The pulley rope:** This has a dog clip attached at one end of the rope which then passes over the wheel of the pulley. The rope then passes through the cleat and a second dog clip. It is used for three dimensional movements of a limb **(Fig. 15.5)**.

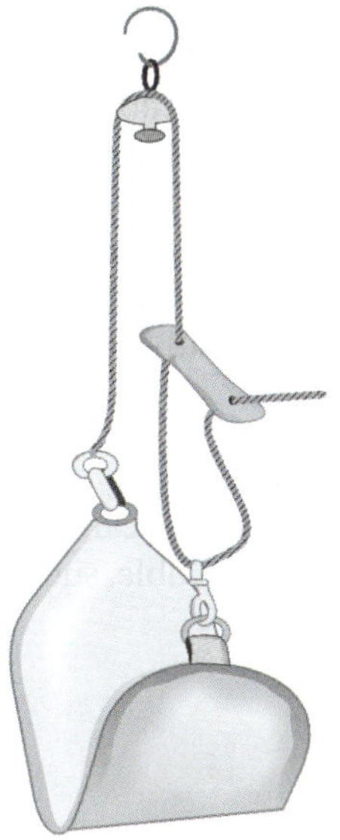

**Fig. 15.5:** The pulley rope system.

### *Wooden Cleat (Fig. 15.6)*

It is made up of wood and is used for altering the length of the rope. It has two or three holes for the rope passage. The rope itself holds the cleat by friction resistance. Sometime the wooden cleat is placed horizontally, for adjusting the length of the rope and the oblique alignment of the cleat is for friction resistance by the rope to avoid slippery.

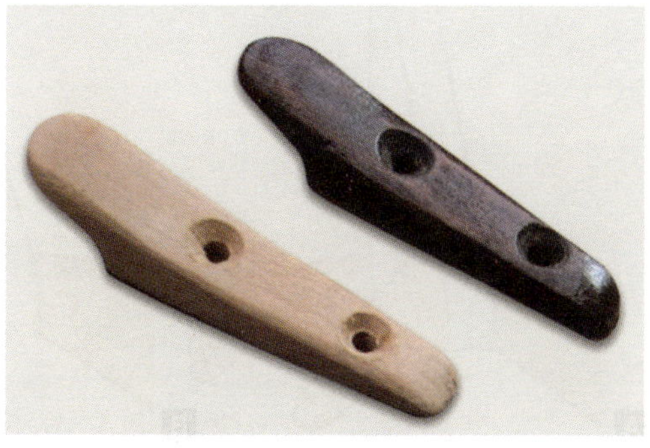

**Fig. 15.6:** Wooden cleats.

### *Pulleys*

It gives the mechanical advantage. Pulleys are used to reduce the burden of lifting whole body or body parts. Here sometimes single or double pulleys are used depending on the situation. If the body part is big, say for example, trunk, thorax, and thigh, double pulleys are used.

### *Slings*

The slings are made up of canvas. There are four varieties of slings available, such as **(Fig. 15.7)**:

1. Single sling
2. Double sling

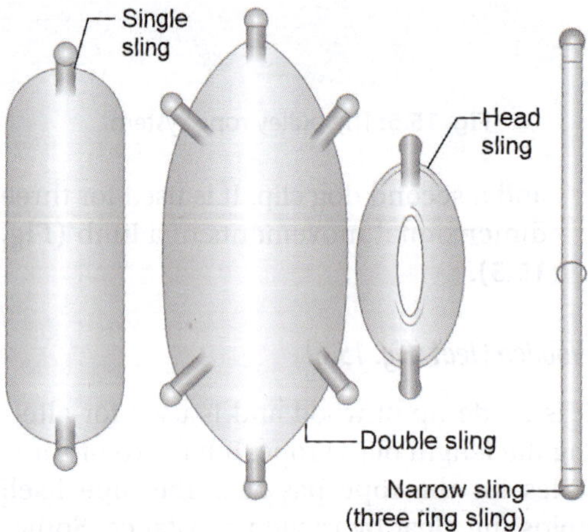


**Fig. 15.7:** Different slings used for suspension therapy.

3. Three-ring sling
4. Head sling.

**Single sling:** It is 68 cm length and 17 cm width, both the ends are having the D-rings for the attachment with the dog clip or S-hook. These types of slings are used for the elbow and knee region. It is sometime folded in 'figure of 8' manner to support the wrist and ankle.

**Double sling:** It is bigger than the single sling, it will have more than two sides with the D-rings. It is more useful for supporting the bigger parts like thorax, trunk, and thigh. It has 68 cm length and 28 cm width.

**Three-ring sling:** It is 75 cm length and 3–4 cm width and has three D-rings. Two at the both end of the sling and one in the middle kept moving. It is mainly used for wrist and ankle regions. There are three methods to support or apply the slings in wrist and ankle. It is shown in **Figures 15.8A to C**.

**Head sling:** It is used for head support. In the middle of the sling presents a slit for accommodation of occipital region while in supine or lower ear accommodation while inside lying.

**S-hook and dog clips:** The dog clip **(Fig. 15.9A)** attaches the rope to the slings supporting the body parts and the S-hook **(Fig. 15.9B)** connects the rope to the wire mesh.

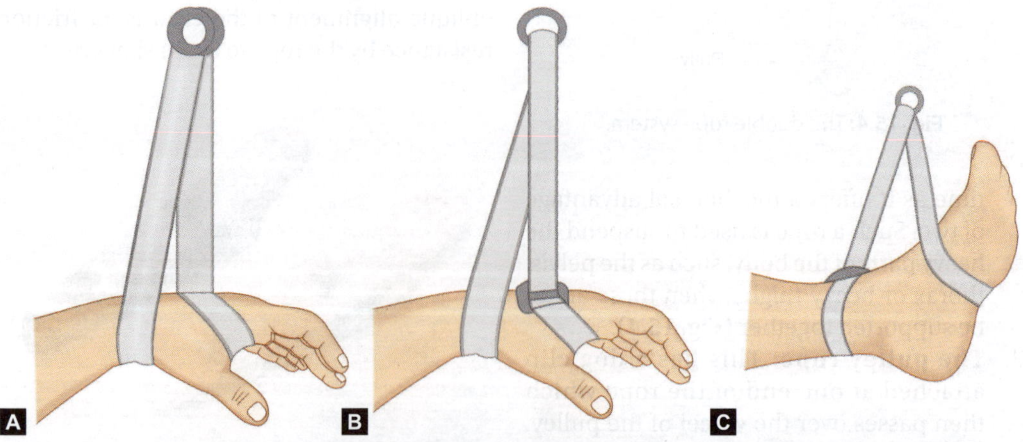


**Figs. 15.8A to C:** Mode of applying the three-ring sling: (A) Figure of 8 method in wrist; (B) Middle moving ring alone used for supporting as seen in picture; (C) Double loop support for ankle.

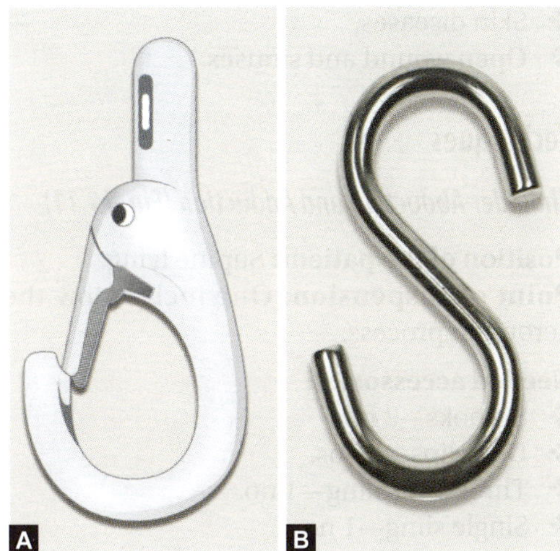


**Figs. 15.9A and B:** (A) Dog clip; (B) S-hook.

**Figures 15.10A to G** show the accessories for suspension therapy.

## Procedure of Use of Rope and Slings

One end of the supporting rope is attached by the S-hook with the mesh and another end passes through one hole of the wooden cleat, and taken out through another hole. The wooden cleat is used for adjusting the length of the rope, and another way of lengthening adjustment made by knotting the rope about the cleat. The other S-hook attaches the sling with the supporting rope in-between the two holes of the wooden cleat. The knotting should be half-hitched, so that it can be removed easily while altering the support or movement. Sometime padding is needed mainly for elbow and knee joint to avoid flexion movement.

## Types of Suspension

- Axial suspension
- Vertical suspension
- Pendular suspension.

### Axial Suspension

Joint axis is taken as the point of the suspension. The limb is supported by the slings above the axis of the joint. If the movement is initiated the limb moves both sides and the base of the swings shows the segment of the base of the cone shape. The part moves parallel to the floor.

**Uses:**
- Relaxation.
- Maintain muscular property.
- Increase the blood circulation.
- Increase the venous drainage.
- Increase the lymphatic drainage.

### Vertical Suspension

The center of gravity of the body part or the body is taken as the point of suspension. In general, the center of gravity of the segments of the limb is located at the junction of the

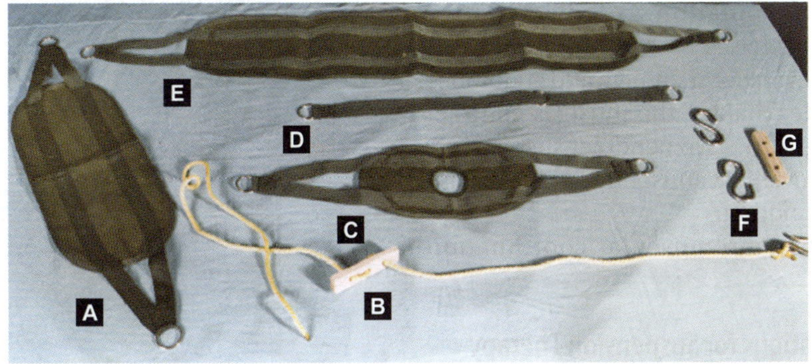


**Figs. 15.10A to G:** Suspension accessories: (A) Single sling; (B) Supporting rope; (C) Head sling; (D) Three ring sling; (E) Single sling for trunk or thorax; (F) S-hook; (G) Wooden cleat.

upper 1/3rd and lower 2/3rd of the segment. The body parts can be supported in these types of suspensions rather than strengthening or performing pendular movement of the limb.

**Uses:** It is used for support as it tends to limit the movement of the part to a small-range pendular movement on each side of the central resting point.

### *Pendular Suspension*

Here at first the axis of the joint is taken as the point of suspension, and then depending on the strengthening of the muscle group, the axis is changed towards medially or laterally, anteriorly or posteriorly. The muscles will be getting resistance if the axis is shifted opposite to that movement. For example, if the axis is shifted towards the abductor side the adductor muscles will be getting resistance during movement. However, to increase/maintain joint ROM, the axis is shifted towards the same side of the movement to be performed.

**Uses:**
- ❖ To strengthen the muscles.
- ❖ To increase and maintain ROM.
- ❖ To increase the endurance.

## Indications for Suspension Therapy

- ❖ For re-education and strengthening of weak muscles. Sometimes suspension therapy is combined with faradic type current stimulation to provide active assisted exercises.
- ❖ For improvement of strength and endurance of muscles making the muscles contract against gravity, as in pendular suspension.
- ❖ For improvement and maintenance of joint range of motion.
- ❖ For early neuromuscular coordination training.

## Contraindications for Suspension Therapy

- ❖ Acute soft tissue injuries and fractures.
- ❖ Hypermobile joints.
- ❖ Skin diseases.
- ❖ Open wound and sinuses.

## Techniques

### *Shoulder Abduction and Adduction (Fig. 15.11)*

**Position of the patient:** Supine lying.
**Point of suspension:** One inch below the acromion process.

**Needed accessories:**
- ❖ S-hooks—2 nos.
- ❖ Dog clips—2 nos.
- ❖ Three-ring sling—1 no.
- ❖ Single sling—1 no.
- ❖ Supporting-rope with wooden cleat—2 nos.

**Procedure:**
- ❖ One inch below the acromion process is taken as the suspension point by primary supporting rope, which is connected by the S-hook with the mesh.
- ❖ Secondary supporting rope attached in the same S-hook.
- ❖ Three-ring sling is used to support the wrist.
- ❖ Single sling is used to support the elbow.
- ❖ The primary supporting rope is attached with the wrist sling.

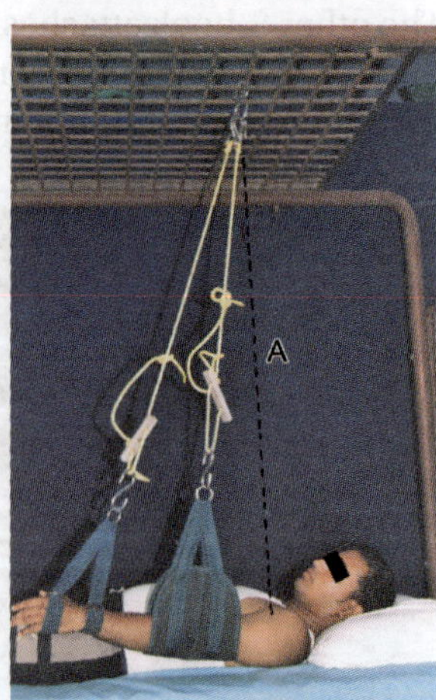


**Fig. 15.11:** Suspension for abduction and adduction of shoulder joint.

- ❖ Secondary supporting rope is attached with the elbow sling.
- ❖ Patient is instructed to perform the abduction-adduction movement of the shoulder.
- ❖ For strengthening the abductor muscles, medial shifting of the axis is carried out, vice versa for adductor muscles strengthening.

### *Shoulder Flexion and Extension (Fig. 15.12)*

**Position of the patient:** Side lying.
**Point of suspension:** Greater tuberosity.

**Needed accessories:**
- ❖ S-hooks—2 nos.
- ❖ Dog clips—2 nos.
- ❖ Three-ring sling—1 no.
- ❖ Single sling—1 no.
- ❖ Supporting-rope with wooden cleat—2 nos.

**Procedure:**
- ❖ Greater tuberosity is taken as the suspension point by primary supporting rope. Which is connected by the S-hook with the mesh.
- ❖ Secondary supporting rope attached in the same S-hook. Three-ring sling is used to support the wrist.

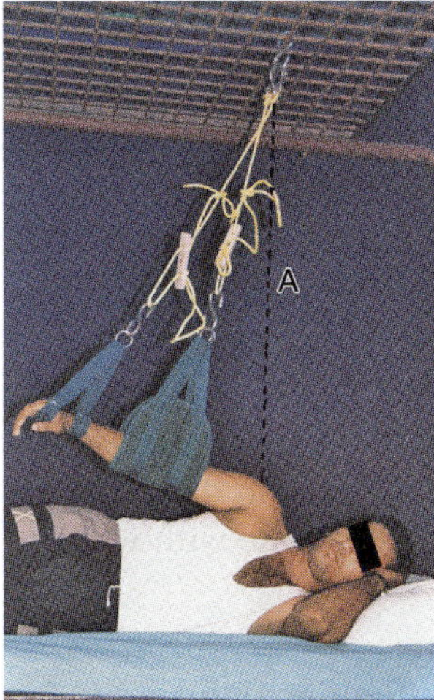


**Fig. 15.12:** Suspension for flexion and extension of shoulder joint.

- ❖ Single sling is used to support the elbow.
- ❖ The primary supporting rope is attached with the wrist sling.
- ❖ Secondary supporting rope is attached with the elbow sling.
- ❖ Patient is instructed to perform the flexion and extension movement of the shoulder.
- ❖ For strengthening the flexor muscles, posterior shifting of the axis is carried out and vice versa for extensor strengthening.

### *Shoulder Medial and Lateral Rotation (Fig. 15.13)*

**Position of the patient:** Supine lying.
**Point of suspension:** Olecranon process of ulna.

**Needed accessories:**
- ❖ S-hook—2 nos.
- ❖ Dog clips—2 nos.
- ❖ Three-ring sling—1 no.
- ❖ Single sling—1 no.
- ❖ Supporting-rope with wooden cleat—2 nos.

**Procedure:**
- ❖ Shoulder is flexed 90° with the elbow in 90° flexion. The olecranon process is taken as the suspension point by primary supporting rope which is connected by the S-hook with the mesh.
- ❖ Secondary supporting rope is attached with head side mesh by another S-hook in the vertical suspension.
- ❖ Three-ring sling is used to support the wrist.

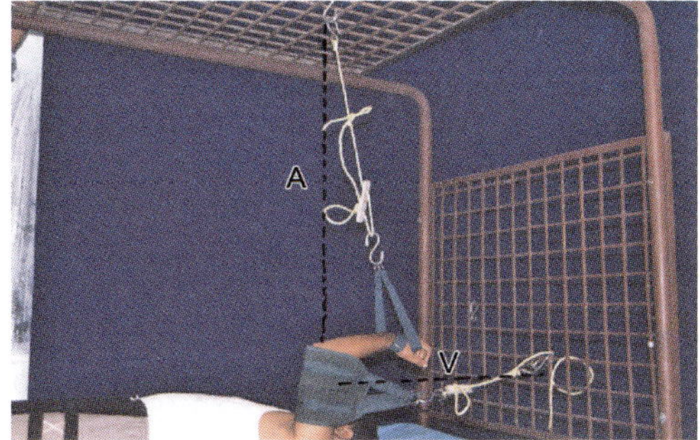


**Fig. 15.13:** Suspension for medial and lateral rotation of shoulder joint.

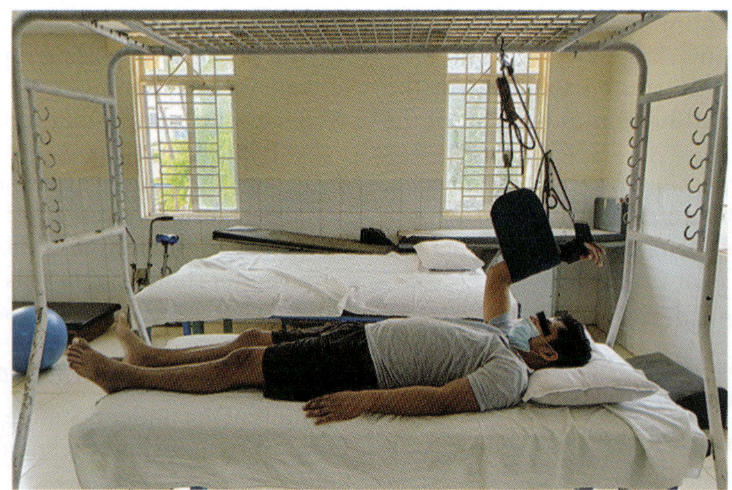

**Fig. 15.14:** Suspension therapy for shoulder rotation.

- Single sling is used to support the arm.
- The primary supporting rope is attached with the wrist sling.
- Secondary supporting rope is attached with the arm sling.
- Patient is instructed to perform the medial and lateral rotation movement of the shoulder.
- For strengthening the medial rotator, lateral shifting of the axis is carried out and vice versa for lateral rotator strengthening.

**Alternative arrangements for shoulder rotation:**

- Shoulder is flexed 90° with the elbow in 90° flexion. The olecranon process (that aligns with the shoulder) is taken as the suspension point.
- Single sling is attached to the forearm and the narrow sling/single sling is applied to the wrist and hand as shown in **Figure 15.14**.

### *Elbow Flexion and Extension (Fig. 15.15)*

**Position of the patient:** Sitting.
**Point of suspension:** Lateral epicondyle of the humerus.
**Needed accessories:**

- S-hooks—2 nos.

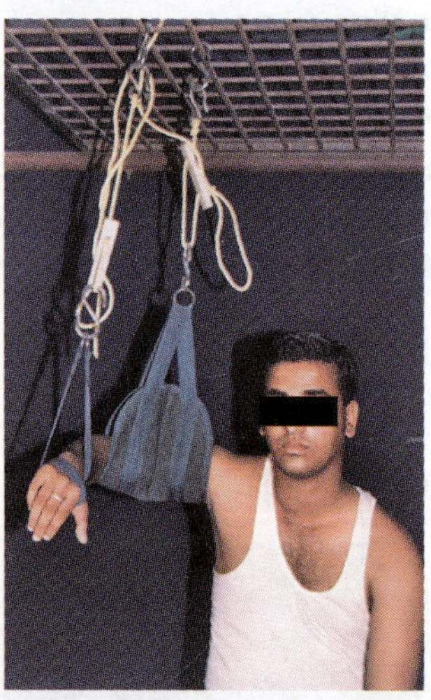

**Fig. 15.15:** Suspension for flexion and extension of elbow joint, one sling is used as vertical suspension and the another is as axial suspension.

- Dog clips—2 nos.
- Three-ring sling—1 no.
- Single sling—1 no.
- Supporting-rope with wooden cleat—2 nos.

**Procedure:**

- With shoulder abducted to 90° with the elbow in 90° flexion position the lateral epicondyle is taken as the suspension

point by primary supporting rope, which is connected by the S-hook with the mesh.
- ❖ Secondary supporting rope attached with the mesh by another S-hook in vertical suspension (from a point, above the junction of upper 1/3rd and lower 2/3rd of a line joining tip of acromion process and lateral epicondyle of humerus).
- ❖ Three-ring sling is used to support the wrist.
- ❖ Single sling is used to support the arm.
- ❖ The primary supporting rope is attached with the wrist sling.
- ❖ Secondary supporting rope is attached with the arm sling.
- ❖ Patient is instructed to perform the elbow flexion and extension movement.
- ❖ For strengthening the flexor lateral shifting of the axis is carried out and vice versa for extensor strengthening.

### *Hip Flexion and Extension (Fig. 15.16)*

**Position of the patient:** Side lying.
**Point of suspension:** Greater trochanter of femur.

**Needed accessories:**
- ❖ S-hooks—2 nos
- ❖ Dog clips—2 nos
- ❖ Three-ring sling—1 no.
- ❖ Single sling—1 no.
- ❖ Supporting-rope with wooden cleat—2 nos.

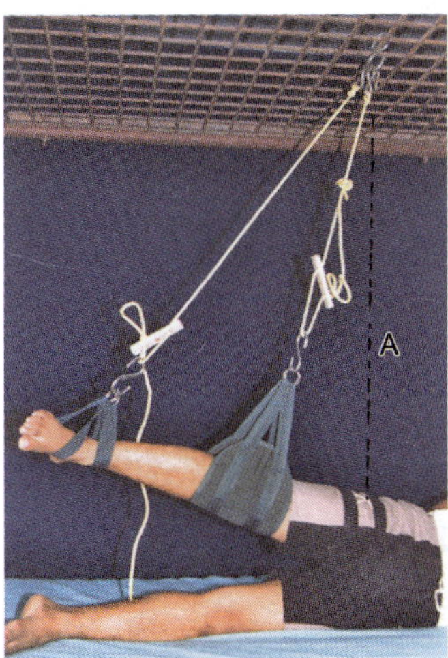


**Fig. 15.16:** Suspension for flexion and extension of hip joint.

**Procedure:**
- ❖ Greater trochanter is taken as the suspension point by primary supporting rope which is connected by the S-hook with the wire mesh.
- ❖ Secondary supporting rope attached with the same S-hook.
- ❖ Three-ring sling is used to support the ankle.
- ❖ Single sling is used to support the knee.
- ❖ The primary supporting rope is attached with the ankle sling.
- ❖ Secondary supporting rope is attached with the knee sling.
- ❖ Patient is instructed to perform the flexion and extension movement of the hip.
- ❖ For strengthening the flexor posterior shifting of the axis is carried out vice versa for extensor strengthening.

### *Hip Abduction and Adduction (Fig. 15.17)*

**Position of the patient:** Supine lying.
**Point of suspension:** From a point above the hip joint line (2 inches below the ASIS).

**Needed accessories:**
- ❖ S-hooks—2 nos.
- ❖ Dog clips—2 nos.

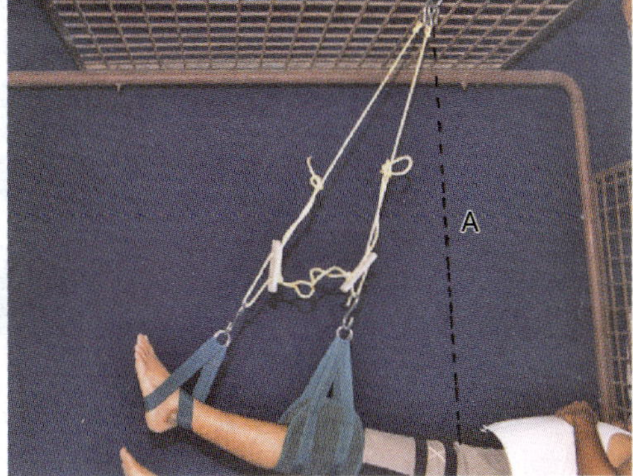


**Fig. 15.17:** Suspension for abduction and adduction of hip joint.

- Three-ring sling—1 no.
- Single sling—1 no.
- Supporting-rope with wooden cleat—2 nos.

**Procedure:**

- Point of suspension is from a point on the wire mesh, over the hip joint, which lies at the junction of lateral 2/3rd and medial 1/3rd of the line joining symphysis pubis and ASIS, or ½ inch below the mid inguinal point or 2 inches below the ASIS. The primary supporting rope, is connected by the S-hook with the mesh in line with hip joint.
- Secondary supporting rope attached with the same S-hook.
- Three-ring sling is used to support the ankle.
- Single sling is used to support the knee.
- The primary supporting rope is attached with the ankle sling.
- Secondary supporting rope is attached with the knee sling.
- Patient is instructed to perform the abduction and adduction movement of the hip.
- For strengthening the abductor medial shifting of the axis is carried out and vice versa for adductor strengthening.

### *Hip Medial and Lateral Rotation (Fig. 15.18)*

**Position of the patient:** Supine lying with hip and knee flexed at 90 degrees.

**Needed accessories:**

- S-hooks—2 nos.
- Dog clips—2 nos.
- Three-ring sling—1 no.
- Single sling—1 no.
- Supporting-rope with wooden cleat—2 nos.

**Fixation point:** Over the hip joint (apex of patella is taken as reference point, when hip and knee are flexed 90 degrees).

The three ring sling is applied to the ankle, and the single sling is attached to the leg.

For strengthening of the medial rotator medial shifting of the axis is carried out and vice versa for lateral rotator strengthening.

### *Knee Flexion and Extension (Fig. 15.19)*

**Position of the patient:** Side lying.
**Point of suspension***:* Lateral joint line of knee.

**Needed accessories:**

- S-hooks—4 nos
- Three-ring sling—1 no.
- Single sling—1 no.
- Supporting-rope with wooden cleat—2 nos.

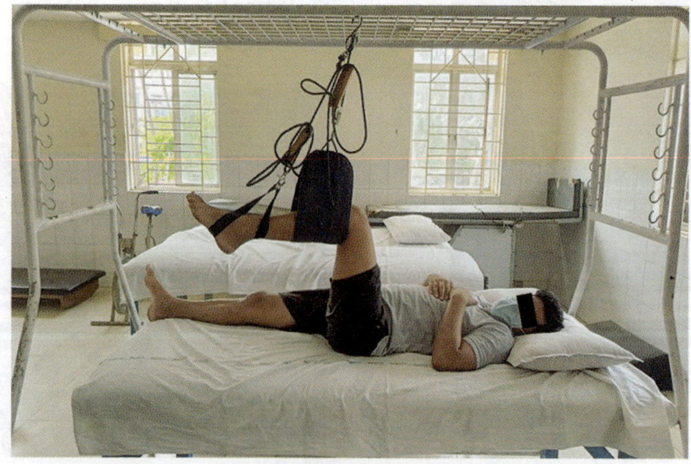

**Fig. 15.18:** Suspension for hip—medial and lateral rotation.

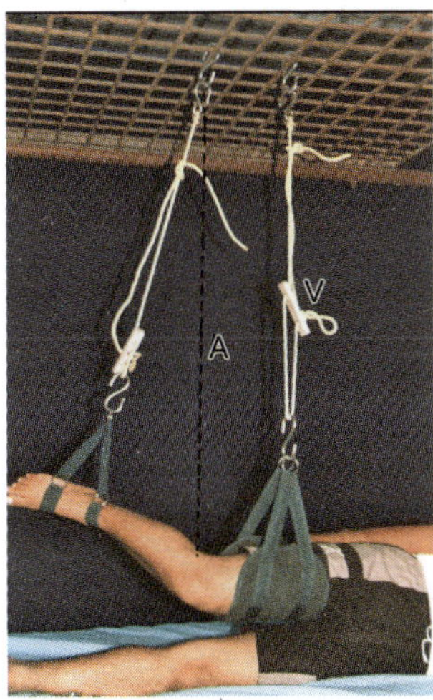


**Fig. 15.19:** Suspension for flexion and extension of knee joint, one sling is used as vertical suspension and the another is as axial suspension.

**Procedure:**

- Lateral joint line is taken as the suspension point by primary supporting rope. Which is connected by the S-hook with the mesh.
- COG of the thigh (proximal 1/3rd and distal 2/3rd of thigh) is taken as the suspension point by the secondary supporting rope, connected by S-hook with mesh.
- Single sling is used to support the thigh.
- The primary supporting rope is attached with the ankle sling.
- Secondary supporting rope is attached with the thigh sling.
- Patient is instructed to perform the flexion and extension movement of the knee.
- For strengthening the flexor anterior shifting of the axis is carried out and vice versa for extensor strengthening.

**Suspension Therapy for Trunk**

- **Upper trunk:**
  - **Side flexion (Fig. 15.20).**
    **Position of patient:** Supine lying.
    **Fixation point:** The ropes connecting the double sling supporting the thorax and head sling supporting the head should be connected to a point in the wire mesh just above the level of umbilicus. After the head and thorax are elevated the patient is asked to swing the body sideways.
  - **Flexion and extension:** The subject is placed in side lying. The head sling supporting the head and large sling supporting the thorax are connected by ropes to a point on the wire mesh in line with the umbilicus. The head and trunk are elevated and the patient is asked to swing the body forward and backward.
- **Lower trunk:**
  - **Flexion and extension (Fig. 15.21):**

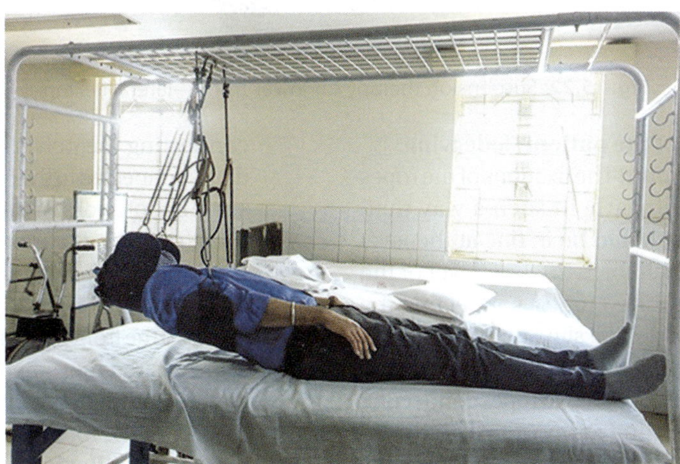

**Fig. 15.20:** Suspension therapy for upper trunk—side flexion.

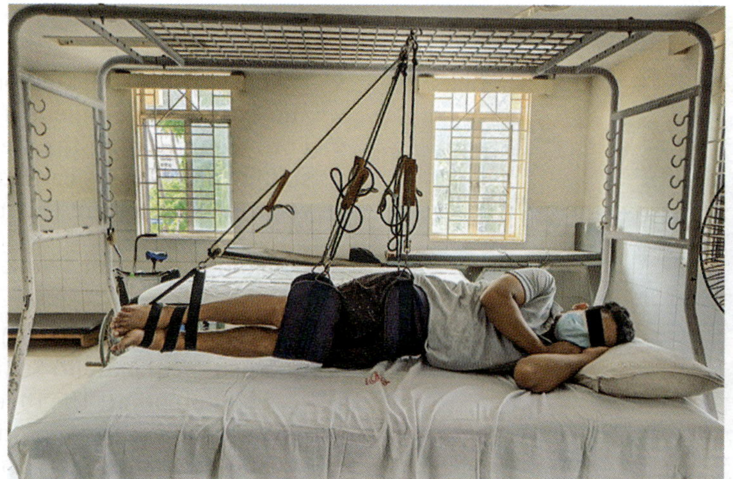

**Fig. 15.21:** Suspension therapy for lower trunk—flexion and extension.

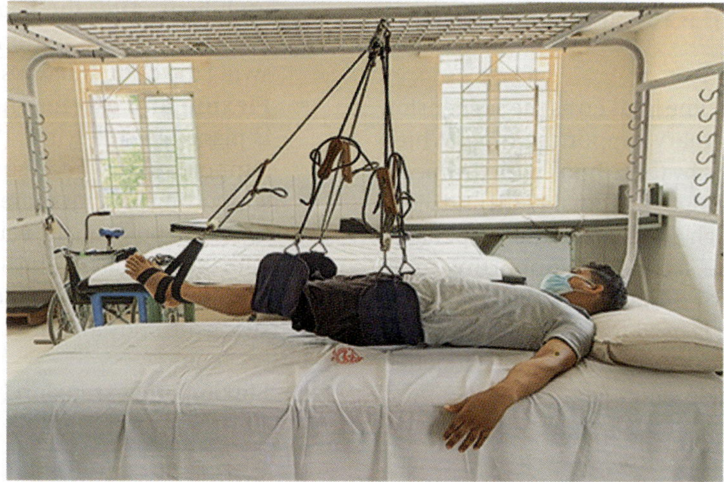

**Fig. 15.22:** Suspension therapy for lower trunk—lateral flexion.

**Position of the patient:** Side lying.

**Fixation point:** The fixations of the ropes are done linearly in such a way that, the hooks should be in line at the level of the 3rd lumbar vertebra (level of the umbilicus). Two ropes, connecting the large sling/double sling under the pelvis are fastened to the outer ends of the line of hooks. The other two ropes connecting the single sling supporting the thighs are connected to the mesh through two hooks that are placed between two hooks connecting the pelvis. One single rope that is connected to the central-most hook in the line of hooks is connected with each three ring slings connecting each foot. If flexion is the desired movement, the thigh and foot ropes are moved to be fixed lateral to the front pelvic rope. If extension is the desired movement, then the thigh and the foot ropes are moved to outside the rear pelvic rope.

- **Side/lateral flexion (Fig. 15.22):** The patient in supine position lying with pillows placed under head and upper trunk. The arrangements of slings and ropes are done in same manner as described for flexion extension, i.e., the hooks are placed in one line over the L3 vertebra, with the two hooks for the pelvis being most outermost, followed by two hooks supporting the thighs and a central hook that supports the feet through the three ring slings. After arrangements of the slings, the ropes are shortened in an order, i.e., knee, followed by feet and pelvis to keep the lower body off the bed.

# 16 CHAPTER Mobility/Walking Aids

## DEFINITION

Mobility aids are the assistive devices provided to individuals with sensory and motor deficits to facilitate stable posture and locomotion. These are useful to assist people who have difficulty in standing and walking or people who cannot walk independently.

These devices are mostly prescribed for the below mentioned cases:

- Painful joints.
- Muscle weakness/paralysis
- Problem in balancing
- Fractures (delayed union/nonunion)
- Joint diseases (arthritis).
- Traumatic conditions (soft tissue injuries).
- Lack of proprioception (Charcot's joint).

(In simple view: Mobility aids are useful for musculoskeletal and neuromuscular problems). These mobility aids reduce the weight-bearing on the lower limbs, increase stability and promotes mobility. There are six (6) major varieties of mobility aids **(Figs. 16.1A to J)**:

1. Crutches
2. Canes
3. Walkers
4. Wheelchairs
5. Braces and splints (orthosis)
6. Prothesis.

## CRUTCHES

Crutches are used mostly to relieve the weight-bearing in the one or both the lower extremities and provide additional support where the balance is impaired for the patients. At present three types of crutches are available:

- Axillary crutch
- Elbow crutch
- Gutter crutch.

### Axillary Crutch (Fig. 16.1A)

Axillary crutch provides the maximum stability and support to the patient than any other crutches. It gives >80% of stability, so that it can be recommended for the patient having marked instability in walking. It is made of aluminium, steel materials, and sometimes by the wood.

#### *Parts of Axillary Crutch*

**Axillary pad:** Axillary pad situated at the top portion of the crutch. It should be placed 5 cm below the axilla, if not the axillary pad compresses the axilla causing the neuropraxia of the axillary nerve and most commonly the radial nerve or brachial plexus. Normally, this axillary pad is made-up of metal and is covered by the cushion materials to avoid the damage to the lateral aspect of the chest wall. The axillary pad is placed in the lateral wall of the chest to provide the improved lateral stability.

**Handgrip:** It is made-up of plastic material, and sometimes covered by the cushion material. Handgrip normally comes in line with the greater trochanter area of the person using it. It has the adjustable clips or screws to adjust the height and push button handgrips are also available.

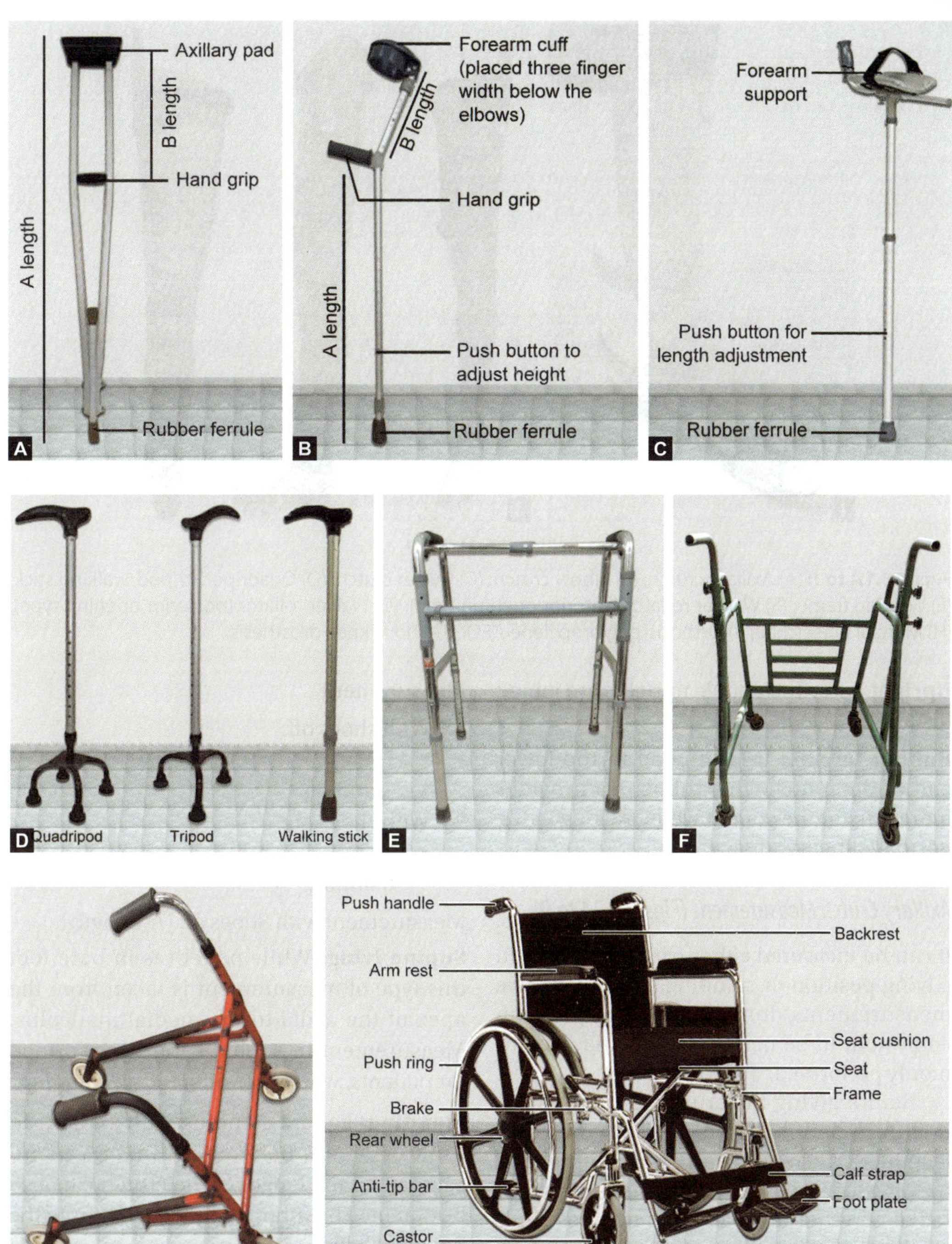


**Figs. 16.1A to H**

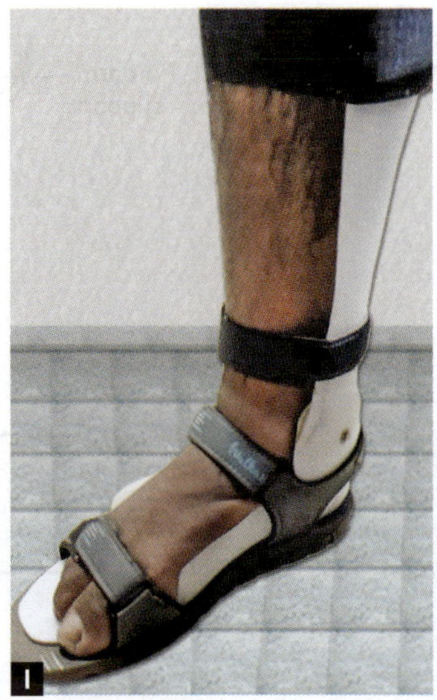

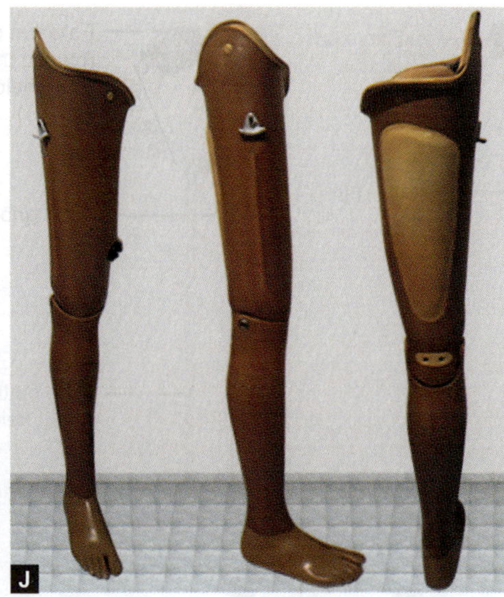

Figs. 16.1I and J

**Figs. 16.1A to J:** (A) Axillary crutch; (B) Elbow crutch; (C) Gutter crutch; (D) Quadripod/tripod/walking stick; (E) Walking frame; (F) Wallker rollator (anterior opening type); (G) Walker rollator (posterior opening type); (H) Manual wheelchair; (I) Orthosis-polypropylene AFO; (J) Above knee prosthesis.

**Upright bars:** The double uprights are joined distally by a single leg.

**Rubber ferrule:** It is situated in the lower end of the crutch. This rubber tip provides more grip for the patient while walking in the normal/slippery surface.

### *Axillary Crutch Measurement (Figs. 16.2A to D)*

It can be measured either with the patient in a lying position or standing, as follows. The measurements done in standing position comes out to be most accurate and is commonly performed.

Before giving the crutch to the patient, it should be measured perfectly because lengthier crutch may cause the compression over the axilla, which leads to neuropraxia of radial nerve (crutch palsy). Sometimes if it is small, the patient's gait pattern may change or it may cause some other complication like back-ache.

**Measurement**

1. With shoes off:
   - Lying
   - Standing
2. With shoes on:
   - Lying
   - Standing

Measurement with Shoes off (A-Length)

**Supine lying:** While patient is in bare foot this type of measurement is taken from the apex of the axilla to the medial malleolus. Measurement in supine lying is performed for patients, who poses difficulty in standing.

**Standing:** Patient standing with support in front of a wall. Before standing, a general estimate of the length of the crutch can also be obtained by subtracting 16 inches from the patient's height. Measurement is taken from 2 inches below the apex of axilla to 2 inches lateral and the 6 inches anterior to the foot.

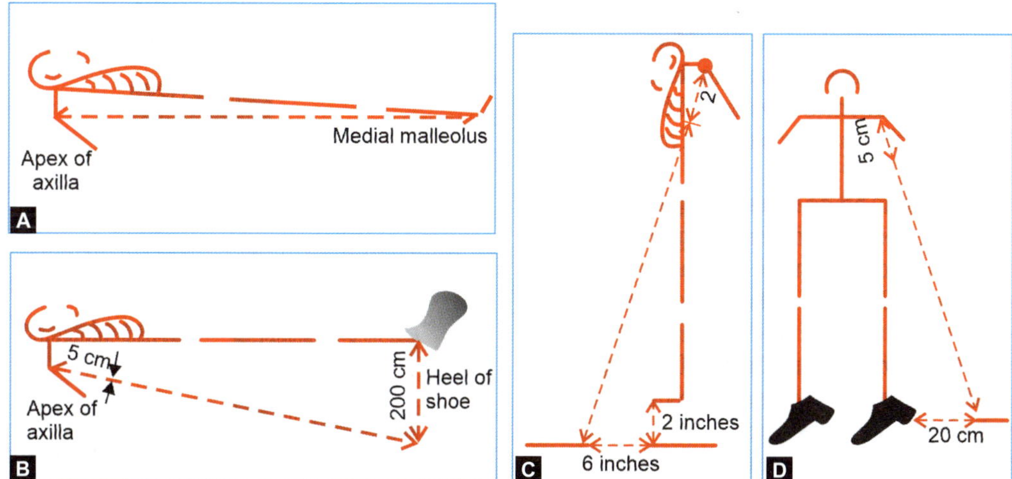


**Figs. 16.2A to D:** Axillary crutch measurement: (A) Lying shoes off; (B) Lying shoes on; (C) Standing shoes off; (D) Standing shoes on.

Measurement with Shoes

**Supine lying:** This type of measurement is taken with the patient wearing the shoes. The measurement is taken from 5 cm below the apex of axilla (from anterior axillary fold) to 20 cm lateral to the heel of the shoe. It is not accurate method of measuring the crutch length.

**Standing:** Patient standing with support in front of a wall. Measurement is taken from 2 inches below the apex of axilla to 20 cm lateral to the heel of the shoe.

Handgrip Measurement
(B-Length Measurement)

**In supine lying:** With the elbow flexed to 20-30°, measurement is taken from a point 5 cm below the apex of the axilla to the ulnar styloid process.

**In standing**: With the shoulder relaxed, the hand grip should be adjusted to provide 20-30 degrees of elbow flexion.

### Weight Transmission

Elbow is extended and the weight is transmitted to the handpiece. So that the pressure over the axilla is reduced.

## *Pre-crutch Training*

Before making the patient walk with the crutches, the therapist has to assess the patient whether the patient is capable of using the crutch by his own or not. The important thing that is needed to walk the crutches should be assessed and improved, which include:

- Psychological state of the patient
- Crutch muscle power.
- Balancing
- Gait pattern
- Ability to walk and gait pattern

### Psychological State

The mental acceptance is the very important factor to make the patient practice the crutch walking. First of all patient has to cooperate with the therapist to learn the gait pattern with the help of his mental stability and support. If the patient does not have the mental acceptance of the crutches, the therapist should explain about the problems and the needs of the crutch for the ambulation and independence. Mainly the therapist has to gain the confidence of the patient to make him practice the crutch walking. Normally, many of the patients do not accept to adopt the crutch due to their social and economical status. Making the mental acceptance of the patient plays the main role in the gait-training program.

### Crutch Muscles Power

To walk with the crutches the patient needs good strength or power in some group of muscles. So, the therapist should assess the crutch muscles to establish whether it has normal power or not. They are:

- **Shoulder girdle:** Depressors, extensors, adductors.
- **Elbow:** Extensors
- **Wrist:** Extensors
- **Finger:** Flexors
- **Hip:** Extensors, abductors
- **Knee:** Extensors
- **Ankle:** Plantar flexors
- **Toe:** Flexors.
- **Core muscles:** The core muscles, including the abdominal and back muscles, play a crucial role in maintaining balance and stability while using crutches. These muscles provide support to the spine and pelvis, allowing the user to transfer weight from one leg to the other smoothly.

If the muscle power is less, it should be strengthened. The strengthening program can be given with the crutches itself, along with strengthening with weights, springs and other resisted instruments.

*Examples*

- **Supine lying:** Shoulder abduction, adduction, elevation, depression can be done with the crutches.
- **Side lying:** Shoulder flexion and extension can be done with crutches.
- **Standing:** All the above-mentioned exercise can be done.
- **Sitting:** Doing push ups on bed/chair/wheelchair. It is helpful for the patient's bed activities as well as for strengthening the upper limb.

### Balancing (Figs. 16.3A and B)

Balancing is the important criteria to be assessed, because lack of balance leads to falling while walking which causes some other complication like injury or fracture. If the patient lacks balance in sitting or standing, it has to be treated first before going for crutch walking. The balancing training has to be given as mentioned in the chapter functional re-education training.

Besides, balancing exercises and activities, balancing with crutches, such as standing

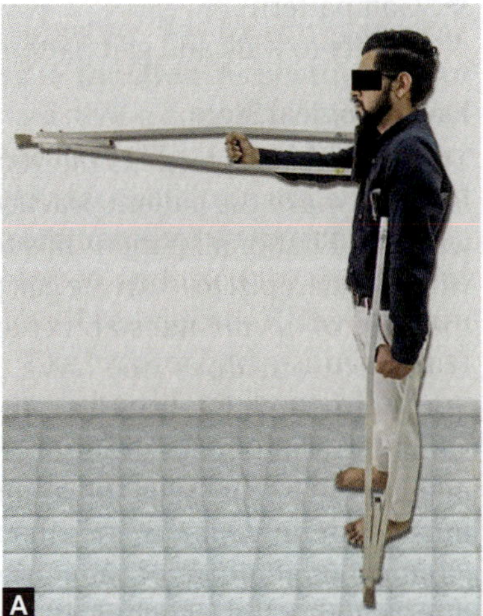

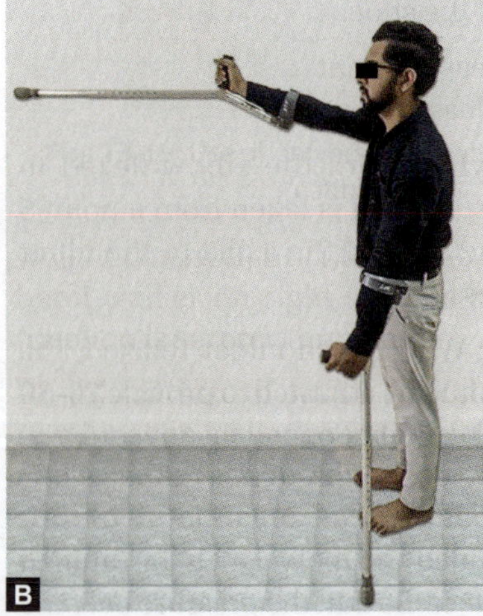

**Figs. 16.3A and B:** (A) Balancing with axillary crutches; (B) Balancing with elbow crutches.

with crutches, lifting crutches alternatively forwards, backwards and to the sides and placing on the ground, helps for balancing with crutches.

**Assessing the ability to walk and gait pattern:** The therapist or the assistance has to support the patient while walking first time to avoid the imbalance of the patient. The pattern of walking with support is observed and analyzed. Before making the patient walk with crutches, he/she should be made to walk in the parallel bar. Until he gets the stability and balance, the same need to be continued.

Preparation for Crutch Walking

- **Preparation of upper limbs:** Muscles of crutch walking such as scapula depressor, shoulder extensors and adductors and elbow extensors, wrist extensors, finger flexors must be assessed and strengthened before the patient starts walking. The hand grip must also be tested to see that the patient has sufficient power and mobility to grasp the hand piece. If the patient is found to have weaker grip, grip strength must be increased, before the patient is made to use the crutch.
- **Preparation of lower limbs:** The strength and mobility of both legs should be assessed and muscles, if weak should be strengthened. Main attention should be given to the hip abductors and extensor, the knee extensors, and the ankle plantar flexors.
- **Training transition from sitting to standing and vice versa:**
  - *Using axillary crutches:* for sitting to standing, the patient is asked to hold both the crutches on the affected side and sit at the edge of the chair with the affected leg placed forwards. The sound side hand is placed over the hand rest of chair. By pushing the crutches with affected side hand, and pushing the arm rest with the sound side hand, the patient raises the body and stands up **(Figs. 16.4A and B)**. The same procedure is followed for sitting on chair from standing.
  - *Using elbow crutches:* for standing from sitting using elbow crutches, the patient is made to sit at the edge of bed/chair, with the base of the crutches, slightly anterior to the sound limb and the affected limb placed anteriorly. The patient is asked to push with the crutches and sound limb and attain

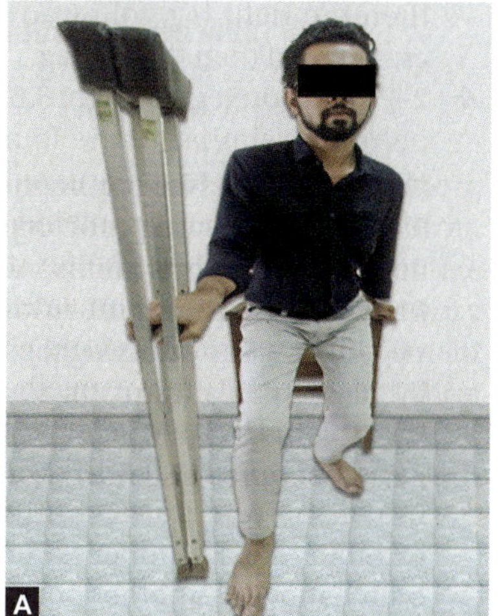


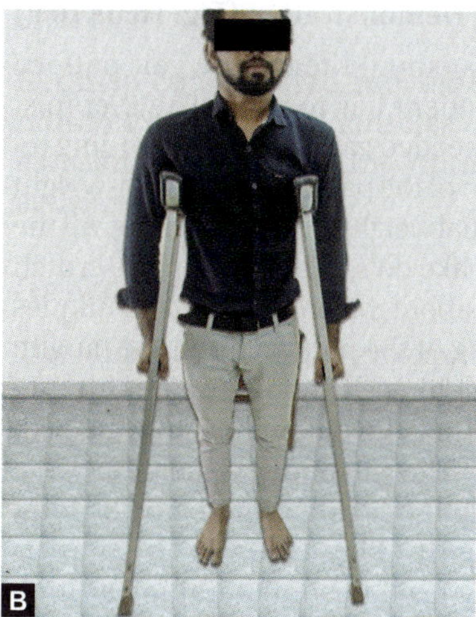


**Figs. 16.4A and B:** Sit to standing and vice versa using axillary crutches (the affected right lower limb is placed forward).

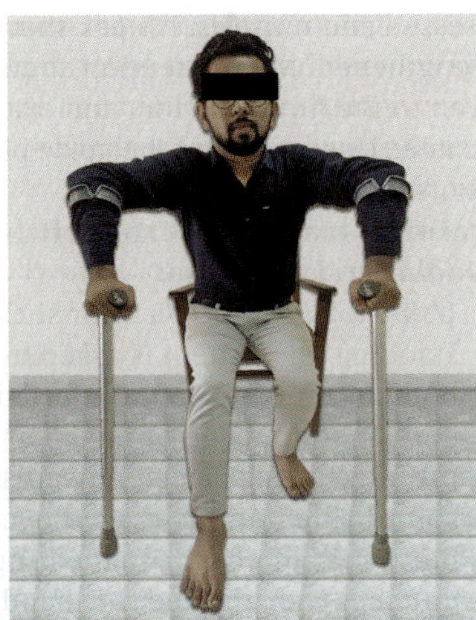

**Fig. 16.5:** Sit to standing and standing to sitting using elbow crutches (The affected right lower limb is placed forward).

standing. The same procedure is used for sitting from standing, holding on the elbow crutches **(Fig. 16.5)**.

- **Development of balance with crutches:** Patient's standing balance with the crutches must be assessed, and balance training with crutches should be given before he/she is made to walk with the crutches.

**Gait Pattern Demonstration (Fig. 16.6A to F)**

The therapist should teach the gait pattern which the patient has to walk. The therapist teaches the needed gait pattern depending on the condition of the patient, that is non-weight bearing/partial weight-bearing walking. All the instructions like do's and don'ts in the crutch walking and about the progression techniques and changing of the pattern has to be taught. The therapist himself should walk in front of the patient, how the patient has to walk with the crutches. The gait patterns include:

- **Non-weight bearing crutch gait/3-point crutch gait (Fig. 16.6A):** This gait is generally used for unilateral lower limb amputees, acute fractures in one lower limb, joint replacement in one knee or hip and patients after surgery for fractures in lower limb, where weight bearing is not permitted. The patient is made to stand with a triangular base, i.e., crutches either in front or behind the weight bearing leg. The crutches serve as two points and the normal limb that bears load acts as the third point. While walking, the patient should take both the crutches with affected leg without the affected leg touching the ground, followed by the normal/weight bearing leg.
- **Partial weight bearing crutch gait (Fig. 16.6B):** This is a modification of the three point pattern. During forward progression of the involved lower extremity, weight is borne partially on both crutches and on the affected leg. In this, both the crutches and the affected leg are taken forward and put down together. Weight is then taken through the crutches and the affected leg, while the unaffected leg is brought through.
- **4-Point crutch gait (Fig. 16.6C):** This gait pattern is used when there is a lack of coordination, poor balance, and muscle weakness in both lower extremities. In this gait pattern, one crutch is advanced and then the opposite leg is advanced. For example, the left crutch is moved forward, then the right leg, followed by the right crutch, and then the left leg.
- **2-Point crutch gait (Fig. 16.6D):** This gait pattern is similar to the four point gait. However, it is less stable as only two points of floor contact are maintained and the use of such gait requires better balance. This pattern more closely simulates normal gait, i.e., lower extremity along with opposite upper extremity move together along with the crutch. That means left lower extremity and right upper extremity with the crutch moves as one point, and right lower extremity and left upper extremity with the crutch move as another point, making the two-point gait pattern.
- **Swing to gait (Fig. 16.6E):** This gait is commonly used for patients of spinal

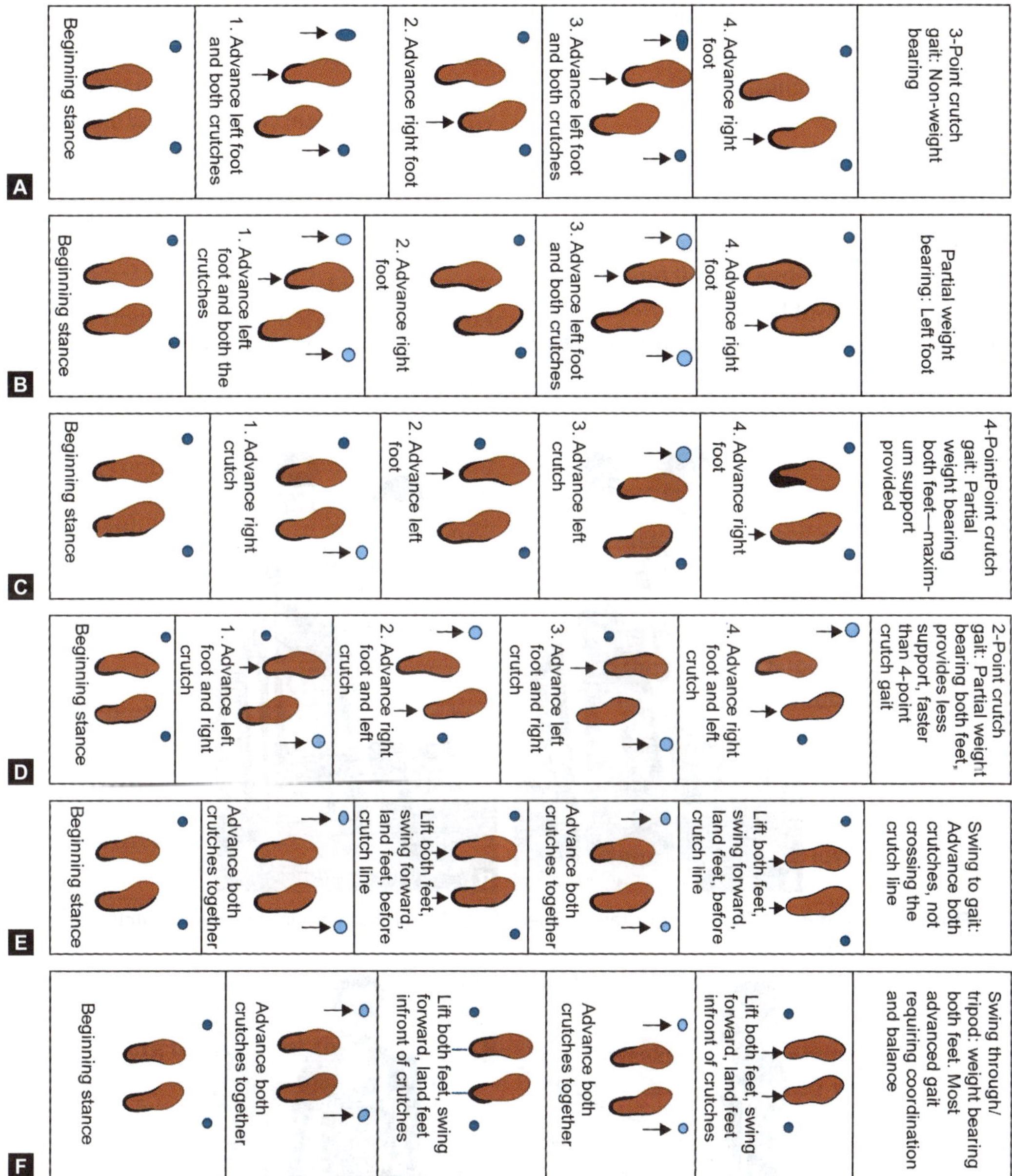


**Figs. 16.6A to F:** (A) Shows 3-point gait pattern; (B) Shows partial weight bearing gait pattern; (C) Shows 4-point gait pattern; (D) Shows 2-point gait pattern; (E) Shows swing to gait pattern; (F) Shows swing through gait pattern.

cord injury, who have bilateral lower extremity involvement. This gait involves forward movements of both crutches simultaneously, shifting weight to the hands and swinging the lower extremities to the crutches, not crossing the crutch line.

- **Swing through gait (Fig. 16.6F):** In this gait which is also used for patients with spinal cord injury, the crutches are moved forward together, weight is shifted onto the hands and the lower extremities are swung beyond the crutches.

### Stair Climbing

**Rules:**

- ❖ Leg placed first while climbing up, and Crutch placed first while coming down **(Figs. 16.7A and B)**.
- ❖ Good to heaven, bad to hell **(Figs. 16.8 and 16.9)**

**Climbing-up Stairs**

Non-weight-bearing

- ❖ **Three-point crutch gait:** Unaffected leg → affected side crutch → unaffected side crutch.
- ❖ **Two-point crutch gait:** Unaffected leg → affected side and unaffected side crutches.

Partial Weight-bearing

**Four-point crutch gait:** Unaffected leg → Affected leg → affected crutch → unaffected crutch.

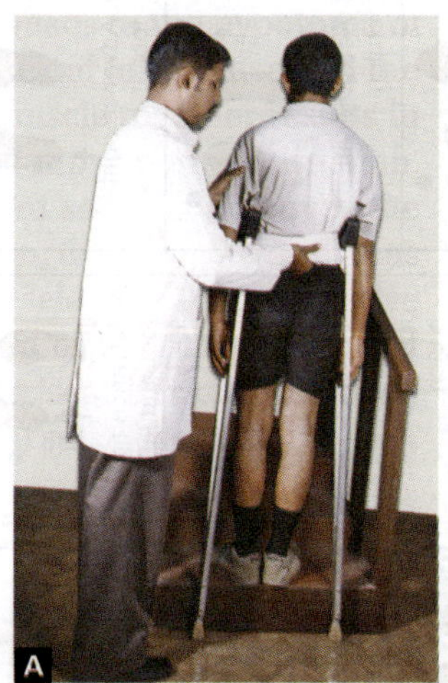

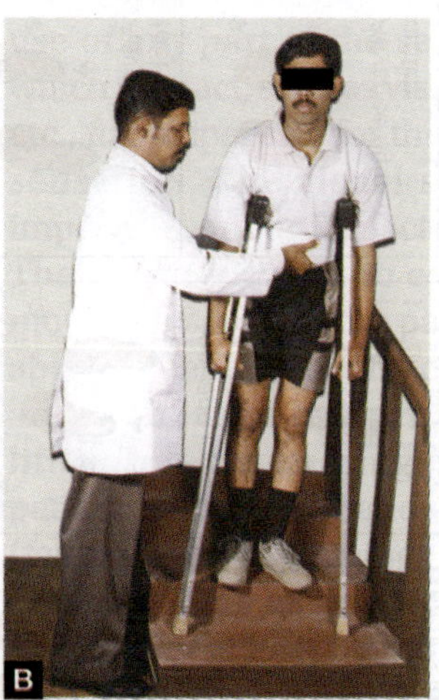

**Figs. 16.7A and B:** (A) Climbing up stair with legs first; (B) Climbing down stairs with crutches first.

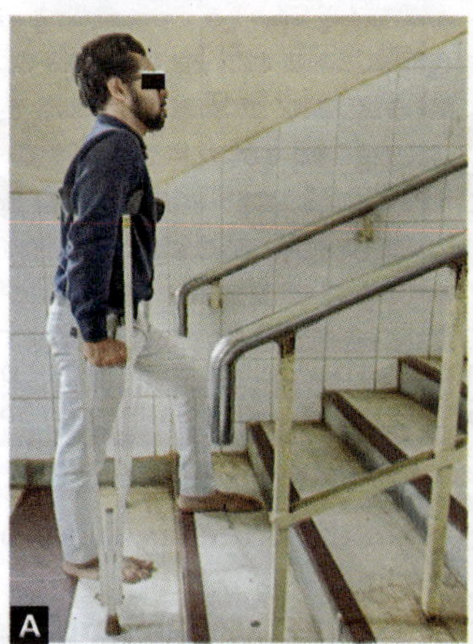

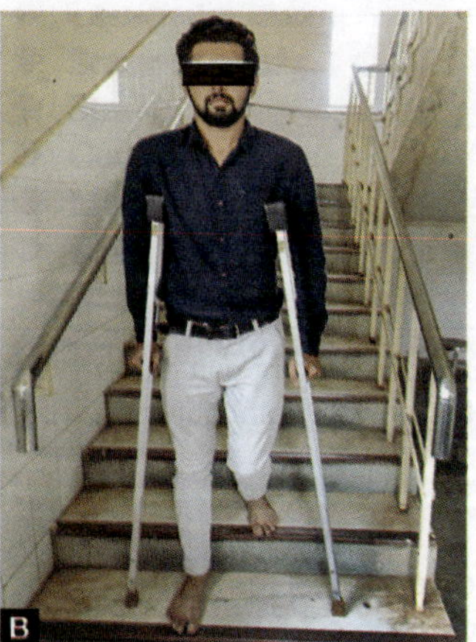

**Figs. 16.8A and B:** (A) Climbing up using axillary crutches with left (sound leg) leg first; (B) Climbing down using axillary crutches with right (affected leg) first.

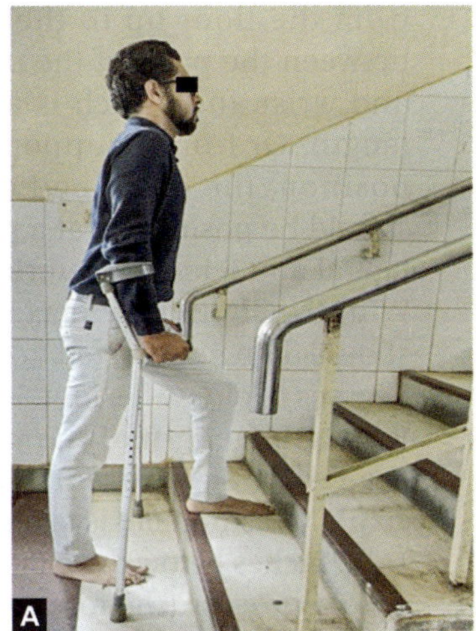

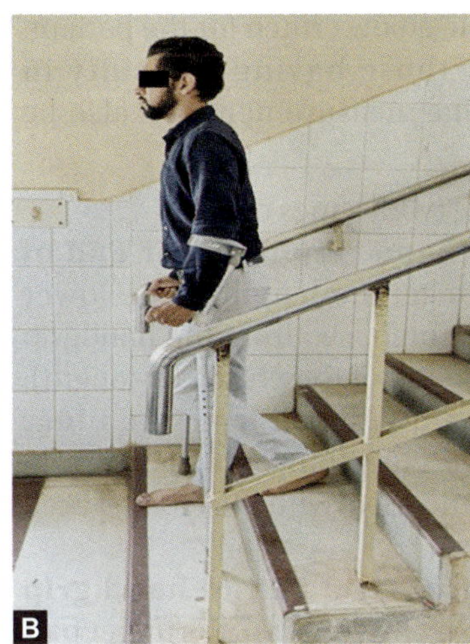


**Figs. 16.9A and B:** (A) Climbing up using elbow crutches with left (sound leg) leg first; (B) Climbing down using elbow crutches with right (affected leg) first.

- **Three-point crutch gait:** Unaffected leg → affected leg → affected and unaffected crutches.

### Climb Down Stairs

Non-weight-bearing

- **Three-point crutch gait:** Unaffected side crutch → affected side crutch → unaffected leg.
- **Two-point crutch gait:** Unaffected and affected crutches → unaffected leg.

Partial Weight-Bearing

- **Four-point crutch gait:** Affected crutch → unaffected crutch → affected leg → unaffected leg.
- **Three-point crutch gait:** Affected and unaffected crutches → affected leg-Unaffected leg.

## Elbow Crutch/Lofstrand Crutch (Fig. 16.1B)

It gives less stability than the axillary crutch. It renders 60% of stability to the patient using it. So, elbow crutches are recommended for the patient having the minimal instability in walking. It is made up of aluminium/plastic and sometime from stainless steel.

### *Parts of Elbow Crutch*

**Forearm cuff:** The forearm cuff is made of metal/plastic. It is placed just below the elbow joint.

**Single upright:** it has the proximal adjustable press clips and the distal adjustable press clips. The proximal press clips adjust the height of the forearm cuff and the distal press clip helps to adjust the height of the crutch.

**Handpiece:** Handpiece is placed junction between the proximal and digital adjustable press clips and the handpiece comes around the greater trochanter region of the person using it.

**Rubber ferrule:** It affords more grip even while walking in the slippery surface.

### *Weight Transmission*

Same like axillary crutches the weight is transmitted to the handpiece when the elbow is extended.

### *Elbow Crutch Measurement*

As per the measurement of axillary crutch, standing is also a method of choice to measure the length of the elbow crutch for the patient. However, for those having difficulty in standing, supine measurement can also be performed.

In Supine Lying (with shoes on)

- **A-length (hand grip to lower end of crutch):** To get the length of the lower part of the crutch, i.e., from the handgrip to the lower end of the crutch (A-length), measurement is taken from the ulnar styloid process to a point of 20 cm lateral to the heel of the shoe, with the elbow flexed to 20°–30°.
- **B-length (forearm cuff to hand grip length):** To get the length of the upper part of the crutch, i.e., forearm cuff to hand grip (B-length), measurement is taken from a point 1–1.5 inches below the elbow to the ulnar styloid process.

In Standing (Fig. 16.10)

- **A-length (hand grip to lower end of crutch):** Patient standing tall with the back against the wall, shoulders back with the elbows flexed at 20–30 degrees. Measurement is taken in an inch tape from the floor up to the deep crease between the palm of the patient's hand and wrist and 1 inch is added to this length. Or from a supported standing position, the distal end of the crutch should be positioned at a point 2 inches lateral and 6 inches anterior to the foot. With the shoulders relaxed, the height should then be adjusted to provide 20–30 degrees of elbow flexion.
- **B-length (length of the upper part of the crutch, i.e., forearm cuff to hand grip):** Measurement is taken from a point 1–1.5 inches below the elbow to the ulnar styloid process (the forearm cuff should be positioned over the proximal third of forearm, which is 1–1.5 inches below the elbow).

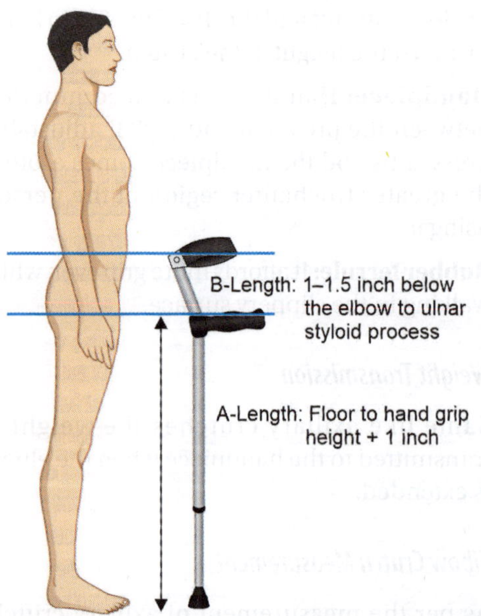


**Fig. 16.10:** Elbow crutch measurement in standing.

## Gutter Crutch (Fig. 16.1C)

This is also made up of metal and it contains the forearm pad with the supporting strap, adjustable handpiece and rubber ferrule. These types of crutches are mainly used for the rheumatoid hand and those who cannot weight bear through the wrist and hand. For example, fracture/dislocation of wrist. The length of the crutch and handpiece position can be adjustable.

### *Measurements of Gutter Crutch*

- **Measurement of forearm support:** Measured from 3 inches below the elbow, up to the wrist **(Fig. 16.11)**
- **Measurement of the vertical upright:** in supine lying, with shoes on—measurement is taken from the point of flexed elbow to 20 cm lateral to the heel of the shoe (with shoes on).

### *Walking Stick/Tripod/Quadripod (Fig. 16.1D)*

A walking stick, also known as a cane, is a long (sturdy), strongly built stick that is used to aid in walking. They come in a variety of shapes, sizes, and materials, such as wood,

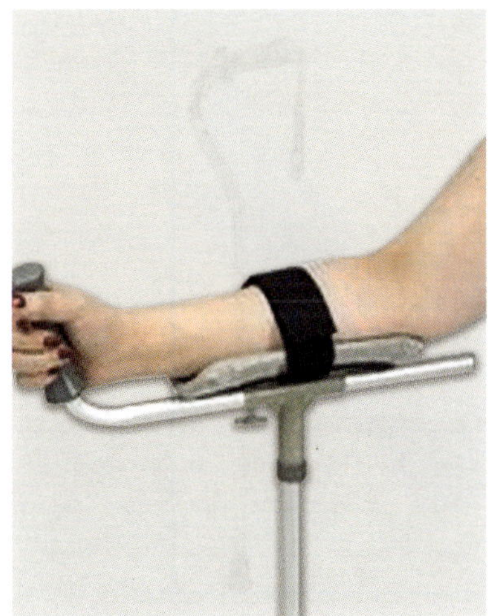

**Fig. 16.11:** The forearm support.

metal, or plastic. They can have a single point or multiple points of contact (tripod/quadripod) with the ground, depending on the design. Commonly all the sticks are having the handpiece and the rubber ferrule except the wooden made standard canes. The handpiece comes up to the greater trochanter level for the person using it.

The primary purpose of a walking stick is to provide support and stability to elderly with loss of balance as well as to promote protected/controlled weight bearing on the injured leg, minimizing impairment/disability. Walking sticks are a valuable tool for anyone who wants to improve their mobility and quality of life, after impairments from neuro-musculoskeletal diseases/disorders.

### Measurement of the Walking Stick

The length of the stick should be determined by the height of the individual. The stick should be long enough to support weight and provide balance while walking. Though the ideal height of the stick should be from the level of wrist to ground when the arm is hanging straight down by the side, the height of the stick/tripod/quadripod is measured from the level of greater trochanter of femur to a point on the floor (where the end of the stick/center of tripod/quadripod will be placed), approximately 6 inches from the lateral border of toes/shoes. While checking the length of the stick, the elbow should be flexed to about 20–30°, and the top of the hand grip should be at the level of the greater trochanter of femur.

### Types of Walking Sticks

There are different types of walking sticks available, each with its own unique features and benefits. The types include:

- **Cane:** A wooden, metal (aluminum), or carbon fiber made stick that provides support and balance.
- **Adjustable walking stick:** A lightweight and strong stick that can be adjusted to different heights.
- **Foldable walking stick:** A stick that can be folded and stored easily.
- **Walking stick with seat:** A stick that can fold out into a single-legged seat.
- **Walking stick with light:** A stick that has a built-in light for visibility and safety.
- **Smart Blind Stick:** The Smart Blind Stick scans the path in front of it with the help of ultrasonic sensor. Whenever the sensor detects any object in its path the buzzer starts to sound.

## CANES

There are various types of canes available, which the clinician recommends as per need of the patient.

### Standard Canes (Fig. 16.12)

- It is made-up of aluminum, wood or plastic.
- It has the curved or half-circled handpiece.
- It is not a height adjustable one. It has to be made depending on the height of the patient.
- It is inexpensive and can be carried anywhere.
- Normally, it is recommended for the elderly patients.

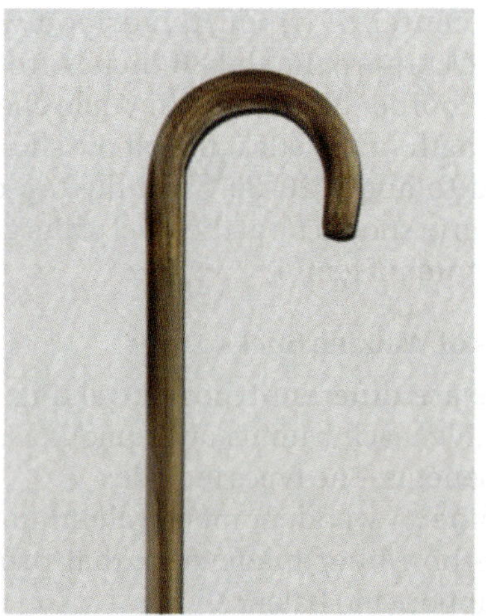

Fig. 16.12: The standard walking frame.

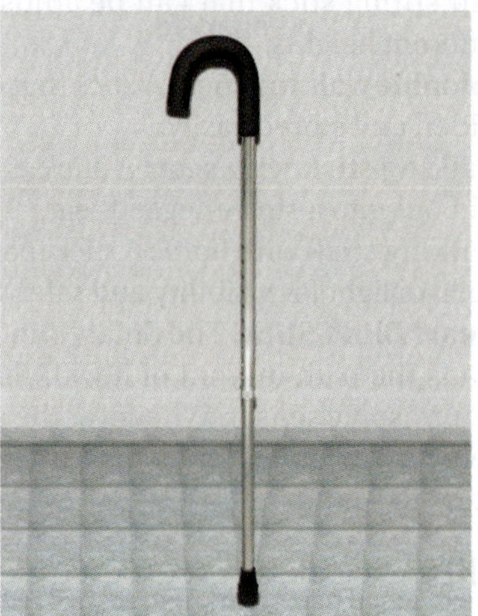

Fig. 16.13: Standard adjustable cane.

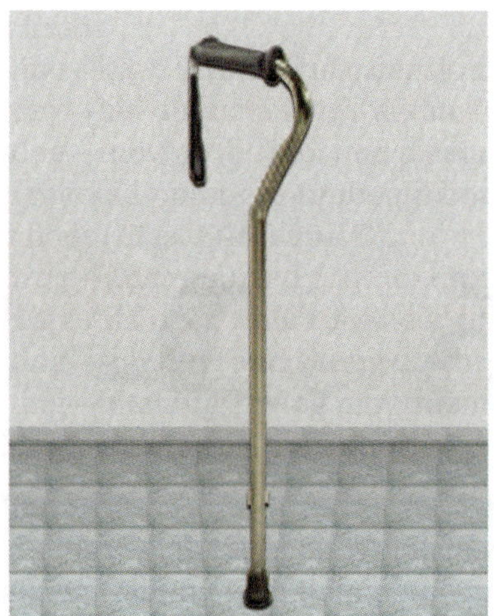

Fig. 16.14: Offset cane.

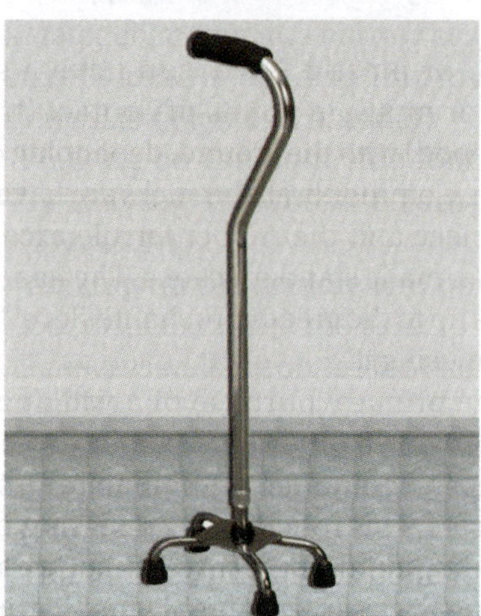

Fig. 16.15: Multileg cane (quadripod).

## Standard Adjustable Canes (Fig. 16.13)

- It is also made-up of aluminum and may be having the plastic covering.
- It has the curved or half-circled handpiece.
- It is having the height adjustable press clips.
- This is also easy to carry anywhere else.

## Offset Canes (Fig. 16.14)

An offset walking cane is a cane that features a specialized handle which makes it easier for it to bear weight and for the user to grip. The upper half of the cane is offset anteriorly so that the LOG falls on the cane and it gives more stability. It may be available in the standard and standard adjustable canes. It too has the adjustable screws or press clips.

## Multiple-legged Canes (Fig. 16.15)

### *Quadripod and Tripod Canes*

- It has the 4 or 3 legs with the rubber tip and it gives the broader base. The BOS in this varieties of canes are huge.

- ❖ Sometime the upper portion of the cane is offset anteriorly.
- ❖ It gives more stability than any other varieties.
- ❖ This is more useful for the neurological cases like very old hemiplegic patients and other elderly patients who have the injury of the lower limb.
- ❖ Height adjustable clips or screws are available.
- ❖ It is difficult to carry the cane in the staircase if the base is broader.

## Hemi-walkers (Fig. 16.16)

The folding hemi-walker is a side-style walker designed for use with one arm. It provides optimal comfort and support for users who do not require/can not use a traditional walker but need more stability than a cane. The height of the walker should be adjusted, so that the hand grip is at the level of the greater trochanter.

## Bariatric Canes (Fig. 16.17)

It is a walking aid for persons, weighing significantly more than the average weight for their body type. The device is fabricated from wood/metal/carbon fiber, which can hold a load of about 500 pounds. It can have a single shaft or four base points, with or without oxygen tank holder and wheels. It helps to improve stability by transferring weight from weak/painful side to opposite arm.

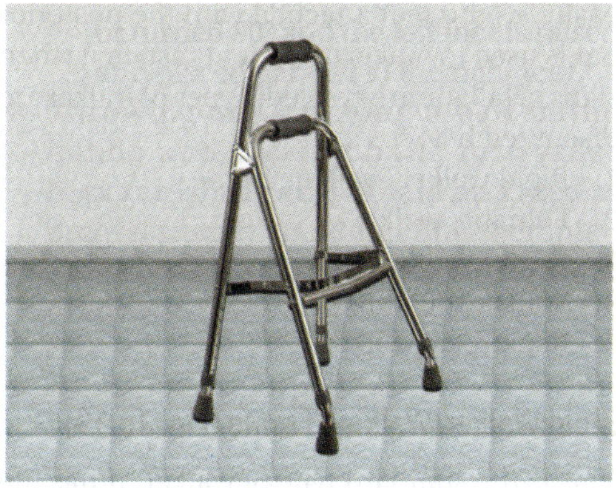

**Fig. 16.16:** The hemiwalker.

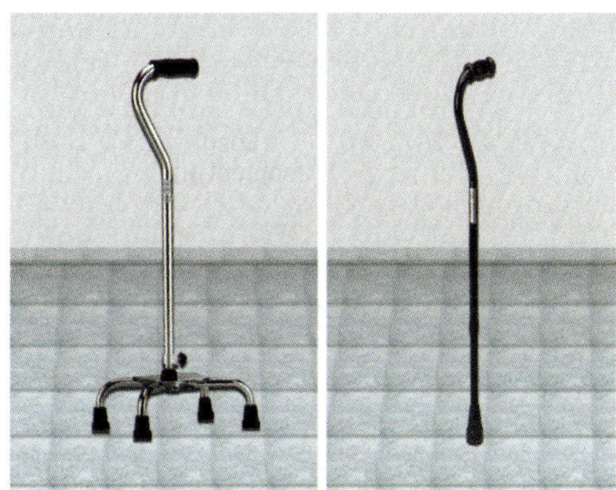

**Fig. 16.17:** The bariatric canes.

### *Procedure of Use*

To hold a walking stick, the handle of the stick should be held in the palm of the hand, wrapping the fingers around the handle, and placing the thumb on the top of the handle. The stick should be placed on the opposite side of the injured leg, to get maximum benefit while walking. For example, if the right leg is injured, the stick should be used on the left side **(Fig. 16.18)**. Use of a stick on the contralateral side decreases the joint reaction force on the affected side, due to the long moment arm. When going up and down stairs, the walking stick should be held on opposite hand and the handrail should be used for support. Stepping up should be with the stronger leg first, followed by the weaker leg up to the same step. When going down the stairs, weaker leg should be taken down first, followed by the stronger leg down to the same step.

## Gait Patterns with Canes

The patient's muscle power, stability, and the psychological state should be assessed as discussed under crutch training. If needed all the factors should be rectified before going for the gait training. Normally, while using the canes, the patient must have the maximum

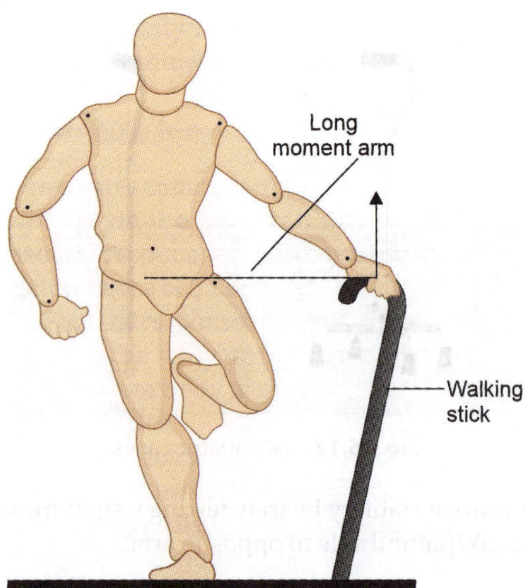


**Fig. 16.18:** Shows long moment arm, when stick used on opposite side.

weight-bearing capacity. The canes are used in the unaffected side and it is placed close to the body-line, otherwise the dynamic stability may be decreased. There are two types of gait patterns.

- **Three-point gait:** Cane → affected leg → unaffected leg.
- **Two-point gait:** Cane and affected side leg → unaffected side leg.

### *Stair Climbing Technique*

**Three-point Gait**

- Ascending steps:
  - Unaffected leg
  - Affected leg
  - Cane
- Descending steps:
  - Affected leg
  - Cane
  - Unaffected leg

**Two-point Gait**

- Ascending steps:
  - Unaffected leg
  - Affected leg and cane
- Descending steps:
  - Affected leg and cane
  - Unaffected leg.

## WALKING FRAMES/WALKER ROLLATOR (FIGS. 16.1E TO G)

They are light weight frames with four supporting bases, which can be adjustable in height. It may be useful for the non-weight-bearing, partial weight-bearing, gait pattern. It gives more stability as it has the broader base. Since the COG falls within the base of support, it gives anteroposterior as well as lateral stability.

In simple walking frames, patient lifts the frame forward then leans on it and takes steps. Frames with wheels such as rollator frames which can be pushed are used for individuals with better trunk stability. The reciprocal frame where each side moves independently are useful for ataxic patients. The weighted walker (walker with addition of weights to the frames) is considered for patients who have severe ataxia/involuntary movements. The walker/rollator frame may be either anterior opening type or posterior opening type (most commonly used). The anterior opening type is usually attached with a seat, over the posterior bar of the walker/rollator. The anterior opening type is selected for very weak patients with poor endurance, who fatigue very easily, as the seat attached with the posterior bar is used to make the patient rest on it when signs of fatigue are noticed. Types of walker are discussed below:

1. Rigid walker/walking frame.
2. Foldable walker
3. Gutter walker
4. Walker rollator.
5. Reciprocal walker.

### Rigid Walker/Walking Frame (Fig. 16.19)

This is the standard type of walker. It has the handgrip and rubber ferrule. The patient has

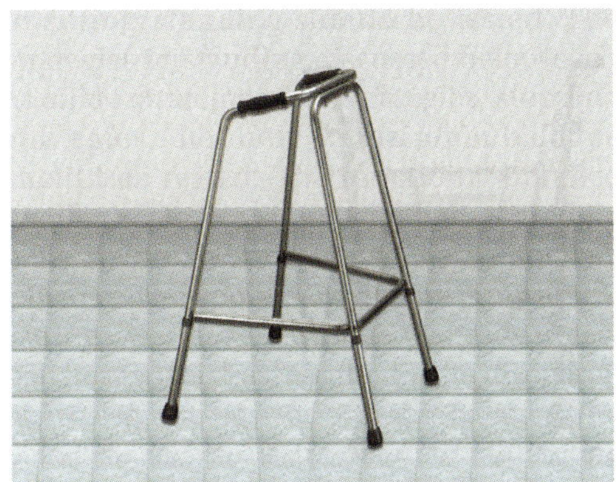

Fig. 16.19: The walking frame.

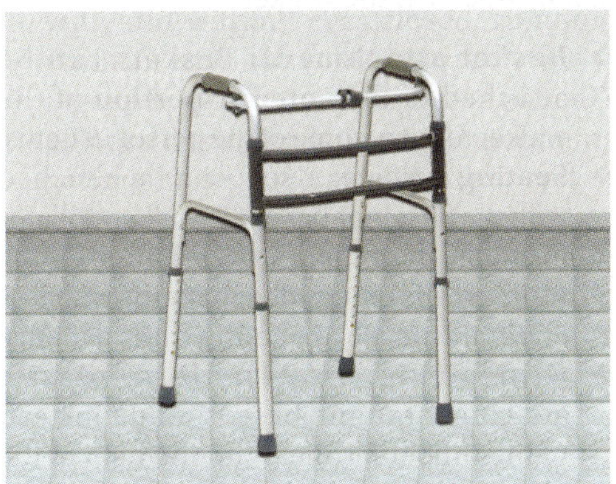

Fig. 16.20: Foldable walker.

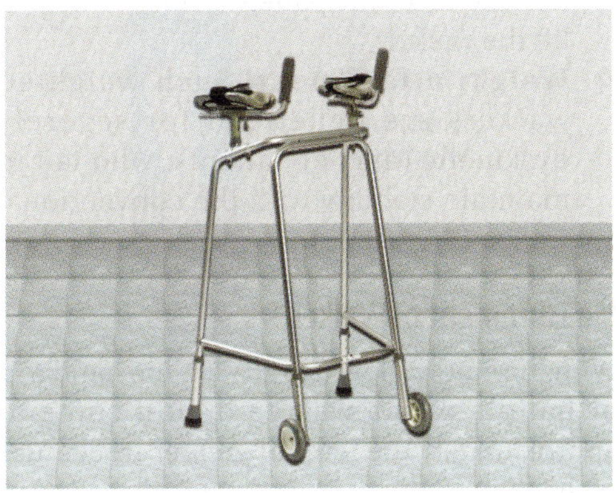

Fig. 16.21: The gutter walker.

to lift and place it front and walk. It is difficult to carry it in and out of the house.

## Foldable Walker (Fig. 16.20)

It has all the features of rigid walker except the folding nature. It is easily foldable and kept in a store place. It is also easy to carry while traveling.

## Gutter Walker (Fig. 16.21)

It is also having the entire feature like rigid walker and additionally it has the forearm platform instead of the handgrip. It is more helpful for the patient who has the problem over the wrist (RA, wrist bone fracture, wrist or hand injuries).

## Reciprocal Walker (Fig. 16.22)

This is designed to allow unilateral forward movement of one side of the walker. These types of walkers are useful for the patients who cannot lift and walk with the walker such as ataxic patients. There will be swivel joints present between the vertical and horizontal bars. While walking, one side of the walker moves forward with the opposite side leg followed by it and vice versa in a reciprocal manner, making each side of the walker moving forward alternatively.

## Walker Rollator (Figs. 16.23A and B)

The anterior vertical bars having the caster and lateral bar remains same as said in rigid

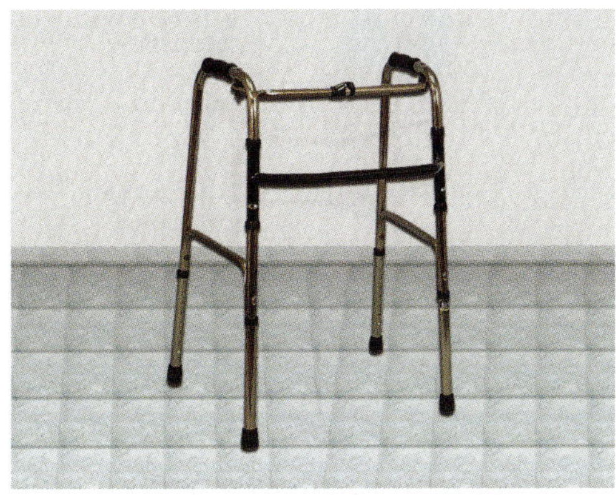

Fig. 16.22: The reciprocal walker.

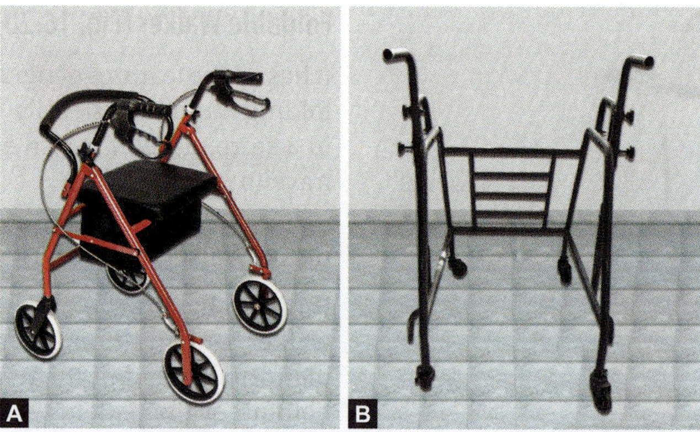
Figs. 16.23A and B: (A) Rollator (anterior opening type); (B) Rollator (posterior opening type).

walker. While walking the patient has to lift the rear bars off the ground and the wheels moved forward and ends with the rear bar placing on the ground. In patients who have better stability, rollators with 4 wheels may be used. The rollator could be of anterior opening type **(Fig. 16.23A)** or posterior opening type **(Fig. 16.23B)** (most commonly used). The anterior opening types have a seat over the posterior horizontal frame **(Fig. 16.23A)**, enabling the patient sit and take rest, while walking. Rollators are indicated for patients, who have good stability to move faster. It may not be recommended to the elderly patients because it may move fast if the patient loses his stability. Commonly, it is recommended for the children.

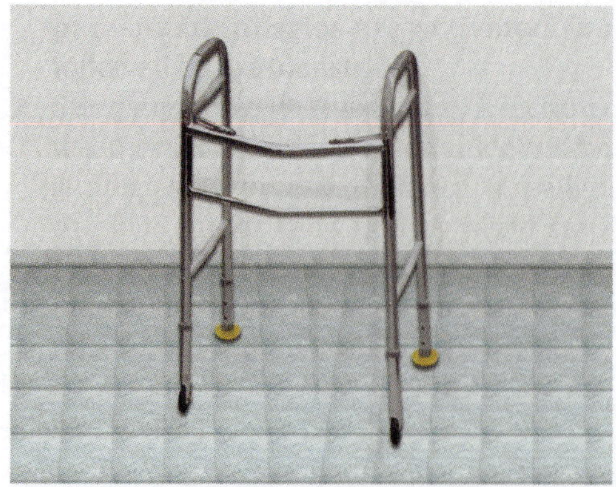
**Fig. 16.24:** Shows glides attached over the rear uprights.

## Modifications in the Walker

- **Basket attachment:** Baskets can be attached to the anterior portion of the walker to carry some of the personal items.
- **Seating surface:** A seat can be attached with the posterior bar of the walker/rollator to enable the patient sit (if required) while walking. It is required for patients with less endurance, such as quadriparesis patients.
- **Glides (Fig. 16.24):** Here, plastic attachment to the base is made instead of the rubber ferrule. With the help of the plastic attachment, the patient can drag or slide the walker forward in smooth surface. It is useful for the patient who is unable to lift the walker.
- **Weight attachment:** Such weighted walkers are beneficial for severely dyskinetic (ataxic) patients, who fail to maintain stability with the conventional walker **(Fig. 16.25)**.

## Measurement of Walker

With the elbows flexed to 20–30°, the handgrip or handle of the walker should come to approximately the level of greater trochanter of the femur.

# WHEELCHAIR

This is one of the variety of the mobility aids. The patient who has both lower limbs non-

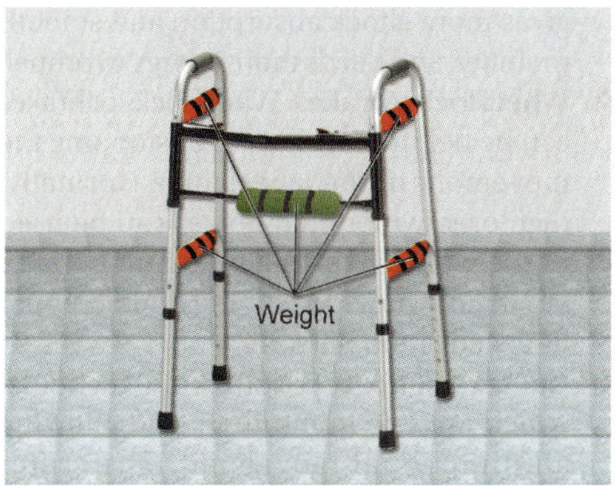


Fig. 16.25: Weighted walker.

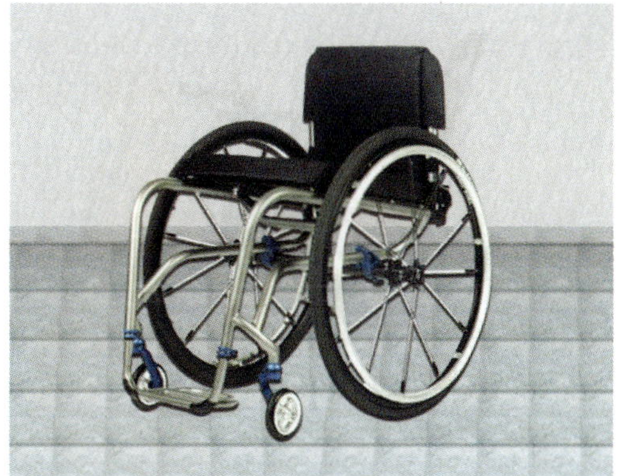

Fig. 16.26: The rigid wheelchair.

functioning or partially functioning has to be recommended for the wheelchair. It is the secondary house for the patient, because he has to spend most of the time with it. It may be modified depending on the condition of the patient. It gives 100% stability to the patient. Generally, wheelchairs are recommended for spinal cord injured/brain injured with paraplegia, quadriplegia and patients in the terminal stages of muscular dystrophy, etc. In the early stage of fractures involving lower limbs and spine, it is also used. The manual wheelchair with its parts has been shown in **Figure 16.1H**.

## Types of Wheelchairs

### *Rigid Wheelchairs (Fig. 16.26)*

The rigid wheelchairs are having the solid frame and also it is lighter. It is mainly used for the sports. It is difficult to carry while traveling. Such wheelchairs maximize energy transfer with each push, making them more efficient than folding wheelchairs. They are made from aluminum/titanium/carbon fiber.

### *Foldable Wheelchair (Fig. 16.27)*

Foldable wheelchair contains foldable frames and it is very much heavier. It occupies less space, so it is very much easy to carry while traveling also.

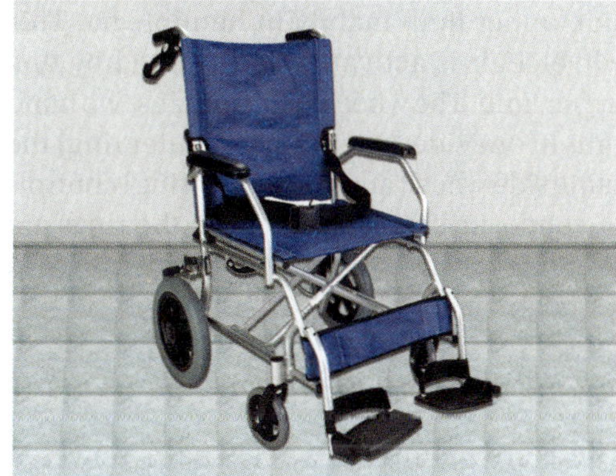

Fig. 16.27: The foldable wheel chair.

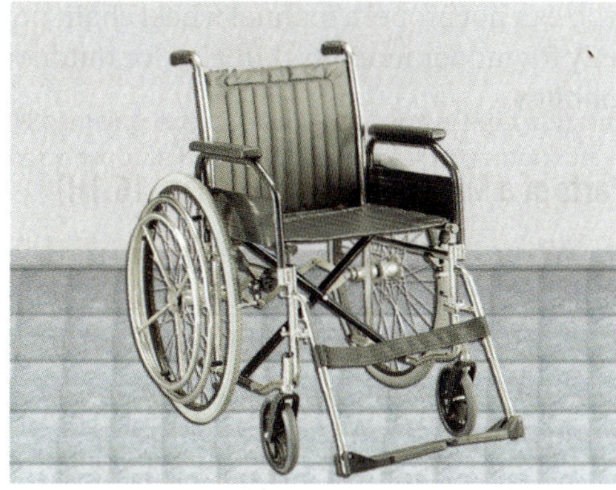

Fig. 16.28: The one arm driven wheelchair.

### *One Arm Driven Wheelchair (Fig. 16.28)*

One arm driven wheelchairs are used for the patient those who are not able to use their one

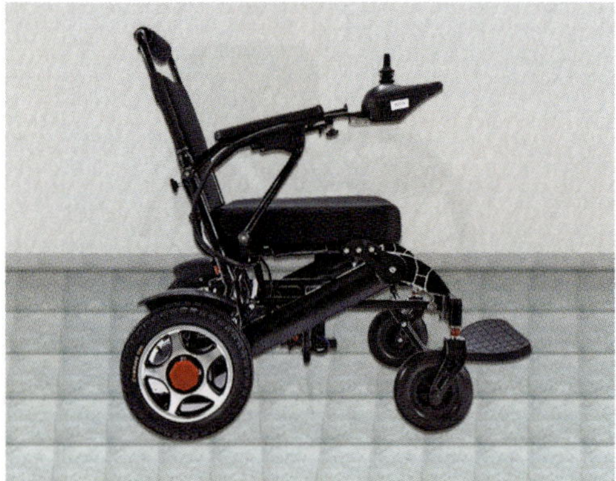

**Fig. 16.29:** The powered wheelchair.

side upper limb mainly in hemiplegia. This wheelchair is activated and steered by one upper limb. The wheelchair contains two hand rims in one side. One controls (outer ring) the same side wheel; another (inner ring) controls the opposite side wheel. If both the rings are simultaneously used the wheelchair moves in a straight line.

### *Powered Wheelchair (Fig.16.29)*

These are motorized wheel chairs powered by battery, rather than manually propelled. Though, costly, they are very useful for patients who can not propel a manual wheel chair, not only for indoor mobility, but also for outdoor mobility.

## Parts of a Manual Wheelchair (Fig. 16.1H)

- **Wheels:** The manually propelled wheelchair has 4 wheels. 2 small wheels (castors) in the front and 2 large wheels at the rear.
- **Tyres:** Hard polyurethane tyres or pneumatic tyres are used in wheelchairs. Hard polyurethane with smooth thread are designed for the indoor use or smooth surface maneuverability and does not provide the shock absorption. The pneumatic/air-filled tyres are generally used for the outdoor uneven surfaces. It gives more shock absorption and smooth mobility, and needs more energy to propel.
- **Wheel locks/brakes:** Wheel locks or brakes can be helpful for slowing or stopping the movement of the wheelchair. Normally, high or low mounted brakes can be used in the wheelchair. High mounted brakes are mainly provided for the limited upper limb activation person.
- **Casters:** These are the small wheels, which are two in numbers and allowing all directional movement. The caster wheel also may contain the polyurethane, pneumatic or semi-pneumatic tyres. Sometimes it also may have the wheel lock or brake.
- **Hand rim:** There are three types of hand rims, (1) standard metal rim, (2) friction rim, (3) projection rim. Standard rims can be used when the patient has no problem of grip. Friction rims are nothing but the standard rim with the surgical plaster tubing added for the additional grip. Projection rim can be used for the patient with the problem of gripping. It has the number of projection knobs; these knobs are perpendicular to the rim. If the knobs are more, more becomes the inconvenience. Only disadvantage is it increases the width of the wheelchair.
- **Footrest:** It may be fixed or movable. It keeps the foot in neutral position. The footrest with heel loop and leg strap added, helps maintaining the foot in neutral position.
- **Tilt bar:** It is the projection from the frame, which presents in the back portion of the wheelchair. It is used by the person who pushes the wheelchair. By pushing down the tilt bar with the leg, the wheelchair can be tilted backwards by lifting the caster up.
- **Seat and backrest:** The seat and the backrest normally are made-up of cushion. Sometimes metal or canvas seating may be made by depending on the economical state of the patient. The cushion is used

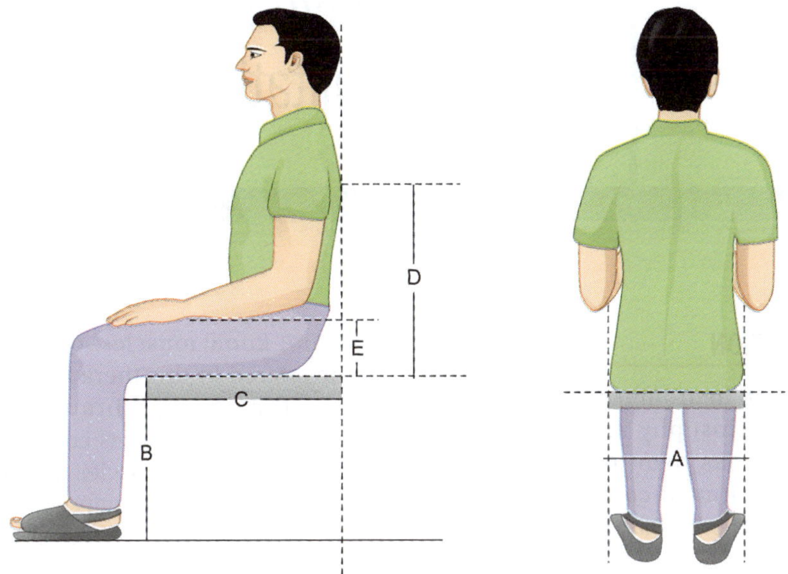


**Figs. 16.30A to E:** Measurement of wheelchair.

for the comfortability and to prevent the pressure sore and these cushions may be air filled or contour foamed. The height of the back-rest can be increased for the quadriplegic and high level spinal cord lesion patients.

## Measurement of Wheelchair (Figs. 16.30A to E)

**Seat width (Fig. 16.30A):** 1 or 2 inches added with the width of the widest part of the buttocks.

**Seat height (Fig. 16.30B):** Two inches added with the distance between the bottoms of the heel to the popliteal area.

**Seat depth (Fig. 16.30C):** Two inches added with the measurement taken from the popliteal area to the level of the buttocks.

**Backrest height (Fig. 16.30D):** Two inches less than the distance between the inferior angle of the scapula and the inferior part of the buttocks.

**Arm rest height (Fig. 16.30E):** Elbow kept in 90° flexion and the measurement taken from the buttocks level to the elbow level.

## Indications of Wheelchair

- Quadriplegia
- Paraplegia
- Hemiplegia
- Spinal cord injury
- Muscular dystrophy
- Amputation
- Lower limb fractures.

# 17 CHAPTER Proprioceptive Neuromuscular Facilitation Techniques

## INTRODUCTION

Proprioceptive neuromuscular facilitation (PNF) is a philosophy and a concept of treatment. It has been one of the most recognized treatment concepts in physiotherapy since the 1940s. Dr Herman Kabat and Margaret (Maggie) Knott started and continued to expand and develop the treatment techniques and procedures after their move to Vallejo, California in 1947. After Dorothy Voss joined the team in 1953, Maggie and Dorothy wrote the first PNF book that was published in 1956. The technique can be understood from the following definitions:

- **Proprioceptive:** Having to do with any of the sensory receptors that give information concerning movement and position of the body.
- **Neuromuscular:** Involving the nerves and muscles.
- **Facilitation:** Making easier

### Definition

Proprioceptive neuromuscular facilitation is a technique that involves stimulation of the proprioceptors for increasing the demand on the neuromuscular mechanism to obtain and facilitate its response for improving function.

The underlying philosophy of PNF signifies that all human beings, including those with disabilities, have untapped existing potential (Kabat 1950), which could be unveiled by appropriate stimulation of the proprioceptors. Beevor's Axiom, that discusses that the brain does not know muscles, only movements is considered in this therapeutic approach. As per the concept, brain registers the movements that muscles combine to make, not the individual muscles that are making the movements. The primary goal of treatment using the technique is to assist the patients so that they can achieve their highest level of function, and to reach this highest level of function, the therapist integrates principles of motor control and motor learning and uses the International Classification of Functioning (ICF) model in the treatment.

### Basic Principles of PNF

- PNF as an integrated approach, is directed at the total human being, not just at a specific problem or body segment.
- It states that all human beings have potentials that are not fully developed.
- As brain knows movements, not muscle actions (Beevor's axiom), movements resembling functional patterns, involving coordinated action of muscle groups should be emphasized.
- Based on the untapped existing potential of all patients, the therapist always focuses on mobilizing the patient's reserves.
- The treatment approach is always positive, reinforcing, and after using that the patient can actually perform, on a physical and psychological level.
- The technique recognizes that normal motor development proceeds in a cephalocaudal and proximodistal direction.

- It recognizes that early motor behavior is dominated by the reflex activity.
- The technique believes that, growth of motor behavior has some cyclic trends as evidenced by the shifts between flexor and extensor dominances.
- It identifies that goal-directed activity is made up of reversing movements.
- It states that normal movement and posture depend on "synergism" and a balanced interaction of antagonists.
- It states that developing motor behavior is expressed in an orderly sequence of total patterns of movement and posture.
- It states that normal motor development has an orderly sequence but lacks a step-by-step quality; overlapping occurs
- It states that improvement of the motor ability depends on motor learning.
- Frequency of stimulation and repetition of activity are used for the promotion and retention of motor learning and for the development of strength and endurance.
- Goal-directed activities, coupled with facilitation techniques, are used to hasten learning of total patterns of walking and of self-care activities.

### *Basic Neurophysiological Principles of PNF*

The work of Sir Charles Sherrington played a significant role in the development of the techniques of PNF. The neurophysiological principles abstracted from the work of Sherrington are:

- **After discharge:** The effect of stimulus continues after the stimulus stops. The feeling of increased power that comes after a static muscle contraction is a result of after discharge.
- **Temporal summation:** A succession of weak stimuli applied to the neuromuscular system combine to cause excitation of the said system.
- **Spatial summation:** Weak stimuli applied simultaneously to different areas of the body reinforce each other (summate) to cause excitation. This when combines with temporal summation produce increased activity of the neuromuscular system.
- **Irradiation:** This is the spreading and increased strength of a response that occur when either the number of stimuli or the strength of the stimuli is increased.
- **Successive induction:** An increased excitation of the agonist muscles follows the stimulation (contraction) of their antagonists. Techniques involving reversal of antagonists make use of this property.
- **Reciprocal innervations (reciprocal inhibition):** Contraction of the agonist muscles is accompanied by simultaneous inhibition of their antagonists. Relaxation techniques make use of this principle.

## Philosophy of PNF

- Positive approach with a strong start, achievable tasks are set up for success in a pain less environment.
- A functional approach (ICF), that include treatment on body structure and activity level.
- Mobilizes patient's potential by intensive training, active participation, motor learning and self training.
- The technique considers the person as a whole, with his/her environmental, personal, physical and emotional factors.
- The technique makes use of principles of motor control and motor learning, uses repetition in different contexts, respects stages of motor control and variability of practice.

## Basic Procedures of PNF

### *Body Position and Mechanics*

- The therapist's body should be in line with the desired motion or force **(Fig. 17.1)**. The resistance comes from the therapist's body, while the arms and hands remain relaxed.

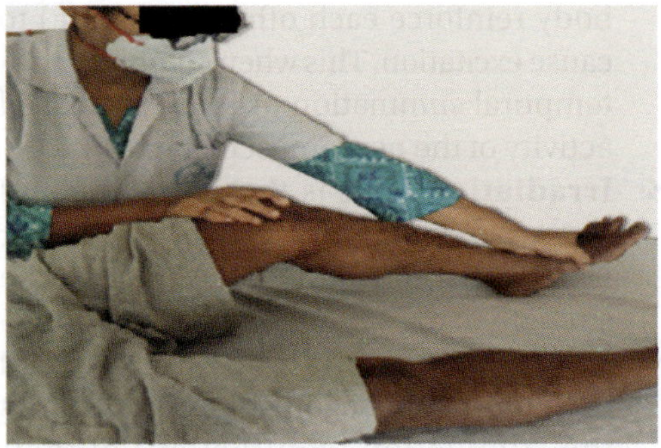

**Fig. 17.1:** Position of the therapist for applying PNF.

By using body weight, the therapist can give prolonged resistance without fatigue.

### *Manual Contact*

Pressure of the physiotherapist's manual contact on the patient provides a means of applying maximal resistance to movement in patterns. Touch contributes to facilitation by stimulating the exteroceptors. Manual contacts must be:

- **Purposeful:** Pressure must be firm, so that the patient must be aware of it.
- **Directional:** Pressure is applied only in the direction of the movement.
- **Comfortable:** Manual contacts which produce painful stimuli must be avoided.
- **Grip:** A lumbrical grip **(Figs. 17.2A and B)** is used by the therapist.

### *Command*

The therapist gives sensory cue by—touching, telling and visual demonstration. Verbal command tells the patient what to do, and when to do the movements.

### *Quick Stretch*

It facilitates muscle contraction and associated synergistic muscles. It is used as a stimulus to initiate voluntary motion, enhance quicker response in weak muscles, increase strength of muscles.

### *Traction and Approximation*

Traction (separation of joint surfaces) is used to stimulate flexion movements, whereas approximation (compression of joint surfaces) is used to facilitate extension movements, therefore promote stability and stimulate postural reflexes.

### *Maximal Resistance*

It is the greatest amount of resistance that can be applied to an active contraction allowing full ROM to occur or to an isometric contraction without defeating or breaking the patient's hold. This facilitates muscle contraction, increases motor control and learning, increases muscle strength and

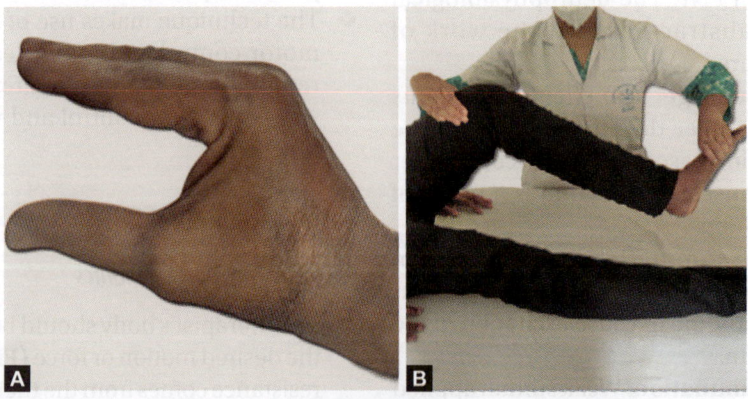

**Figs. 17.2A and B:** (A) Lumbrical grip; (B) Manual contact using lumbrical grip.

helps in the gain of awareness and direction of movements.

### Normal Timing

Timing is a sequencing of motion. It is the sequence of muscle contraction, which occurs in any motor activity, resulting in coordinated movement production. In normal developments, proximal control is evident before distal control, however, after coordinated purposeful movements have been acquired, timing and sequential contraction of muscles occur from distal to proximal. Hence, normal timing is from distal to proximal.

### Timing for Emphasis

Timing for emphasis involves changing the normal sequencing of motions to emphasize a particular muscle or desired activity. Kabat (1947) wrote that prevention of motion in a stronger synergist will redirect the energy of that contraction into a weaker muscle **(Fig. 17.3)**. The best results come when the strong muscles score at least "good" in strength.

### Irradiation and Reinforcement

Irradiation is spread of response from stronger muscles to weak muscles on stimulation. Reinforcement is to strengthen by fresh addition. Therapist reinforces weak muscles by the amount of resistance given to stronger muscles.

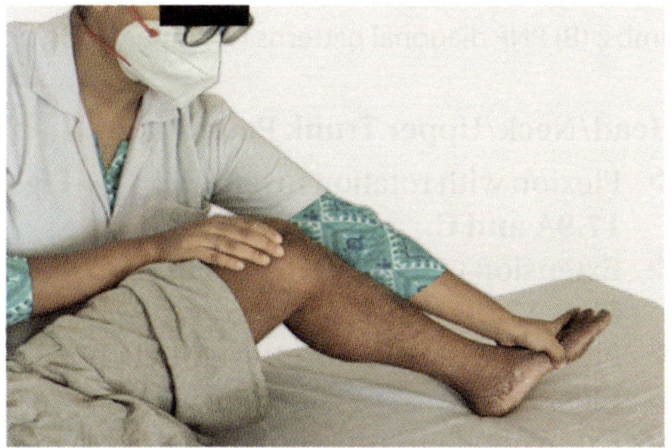

**Fig. 17.3:** Timing for emphasis: The strong motions of the hip and knee are blocked and the dorsiflexion-eversion of the ankle is promoted.

### Patterns of Facilitation

Mass movement patterns are used as the basis for all the techniques of PNF as these movements are similar to the normal functional movements. The pattern of movement is spiral or diagonal ($D_1/D_2$) **(Figs. 17.4A and B)** and they are observed in activities of everyday use, such as taking the hand to the mouth, reaching for food, walking, etc.

The upper extremity, lower extremity, head/neck/upper trunk and lower trunk patterns are described below:

**Upper Extremity Patterns**

- **$D_1$ flexion ($D_1$ fl):** Flexion-adduction-external rotation of shoulder, flexion/extension of elbow, forearm supination, wrist, fingers and thumb flexion **(Fig. 17.5A)**.
- **$D_1$ extension ($D_1$ ex):** Extension-abduction-internal rotation of shoulder, extension/flexion of elbow, forearm pronation, wrist, fingers and thumb extension **(Fig. 17.5B)**.
- **$D_2$ flexion ($D_2$fl):** Flexion-abduction-external rotation of shoulder, elbow flexion/extension, forearm supination, wrist, fingers and thumb extension **(Fig. 17.6A)**.
- **$D_2$ extension ($D_2$ ex):** Extension-adduction-internal rotation of shoulder, extension/flexion of elbow, forearm pronation, wrist, fingers and thumb extension **(Fig. 17.6B)**.

**Lower Extremity Patterns**

- **$D_1$ flexion ($D_1$ fl):** Flexion-adduction-external rotation of hip, knee flexion/extension, ankle dorsiflexion, foot inversion, toes extension **(Fig. 17.7A)**.
- **$D_1$ extension ($D_1$ ex):** Extension-abduction-internal rotation of hip, knee

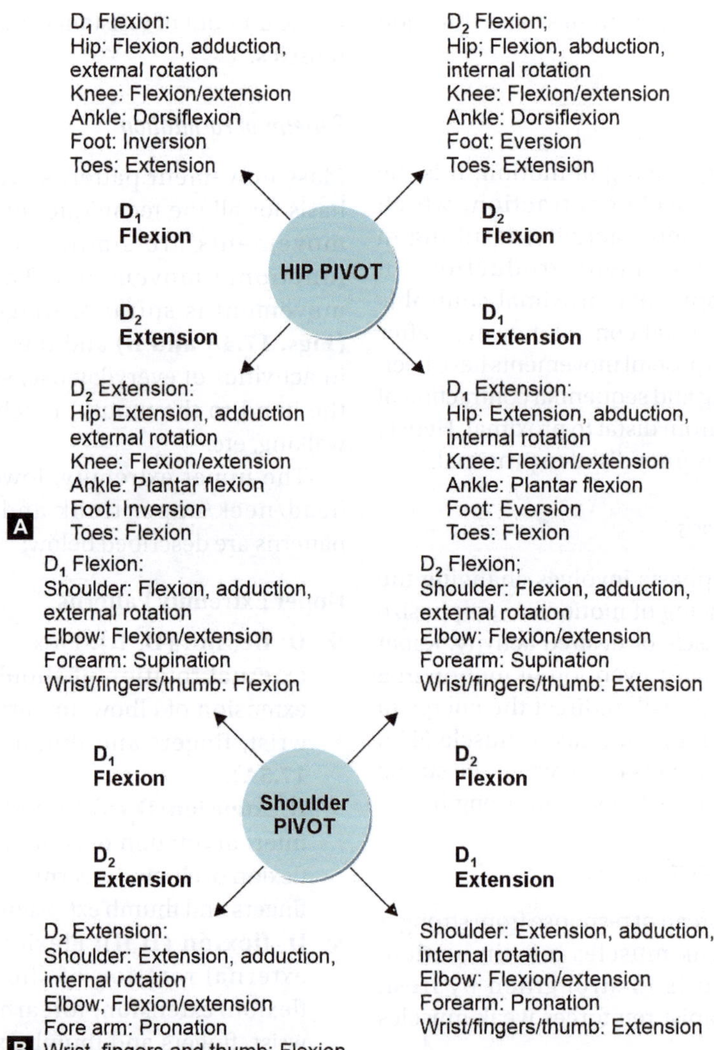


**Figs. 17.4A and B:** PNF diagonal patterns for lower limbs; (B) PNF diagonal patterns for upper limbs.

flexion/extension, ankle plantar flexion, foot eversion, toes flexion **(Fig. 17.7B)**.

- ❖ **$D_2$ flexion ($D_2$fl):** Flexion-abduction-internal rotation of hip, knee flexion/extension, ankle dorsiflexion, foot eversion, toes extension **(Fig. 17.8A)**.
- ❖ **$D_2$ extension ($D_2$ ex):** Extension-adduction-external rotation of hip, knee flexion/extension, ankle plantar flexion, foot inversion, toes flexion **(Fig. 17.8B)**.

**Head/Neck/Upper Trunk Patterns**

- ❖ Flexion with rotation to left (D fl. L)—**Figs. 17.9A and C**.
- ❖ Extension with rotation to right (D ex. R)—**Figs. 17.9B and D**.
- ❖ Flexion with rotation to right (D fl. R)—**Figs. 17.10A**.
- ❖ Extension with rotation to left (D ex. L)—**Figs. 17.10B**.
- ❖ Rotation to left (Ro. L)
- ❖ Rotation to right (Ro. R)

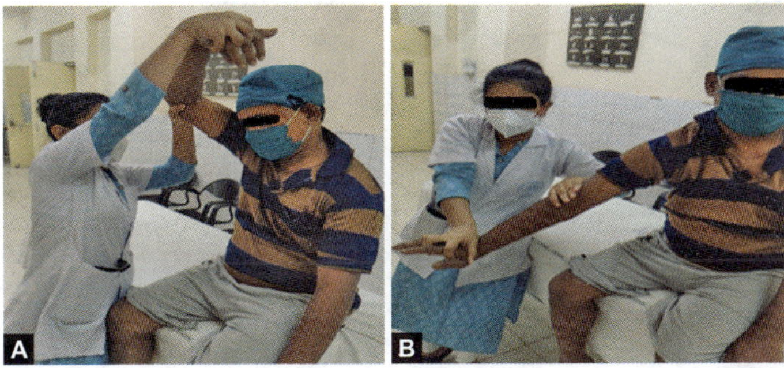

**Figs. 17.5A and B:** (A) $D_1$ flexion with elbow flexion; (B) $D_1$ extension with elbow extension.

(Note: The pattern can be with elbow flexion or elbow extension, such as $D_1$ flexion with elbow flexion/$D_1$ flexion with elbow extension, $D_1$ extension with elbow flexion/$D_1$ extension with elbow extension—the patterns are selected and trained as per need of the client, i.e., $D_1$ flexion with elbow flexion is selected for training the task of taking food to mouth, combing hair, etc., and $D_1$ extension with elbow flexion/extension can be selected for the task of reaching for objects).

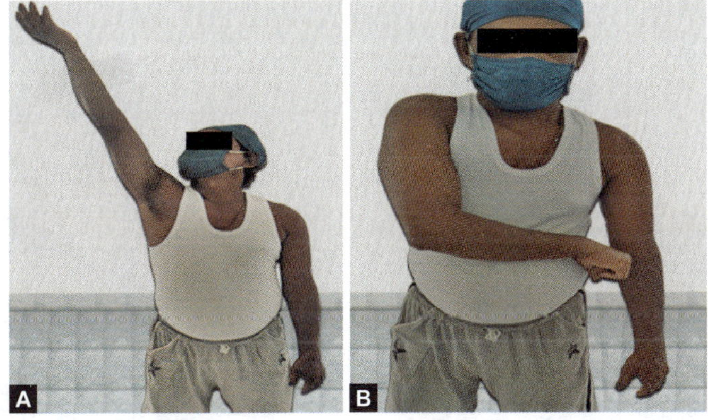

**Figs. 17.6A and B:** (A) $D_2$ flexion with elbow extension; (B) $D_2$ extension with elbow flexion.

(Note: Like $D_1$ pattern, $D_2$ pattern can be performed with both elbow flexion and extension as per need. A $D_2$ flexion pattern helps to reduce spasticity in the upper limb in stroke/head injury/cerebral palsy and used for activities like catching a ball/fruit falling from a superolateral location. A $D_2$ extension with elbow flexion pattern helps to pick up some object from the opposite side pocket of pant.).

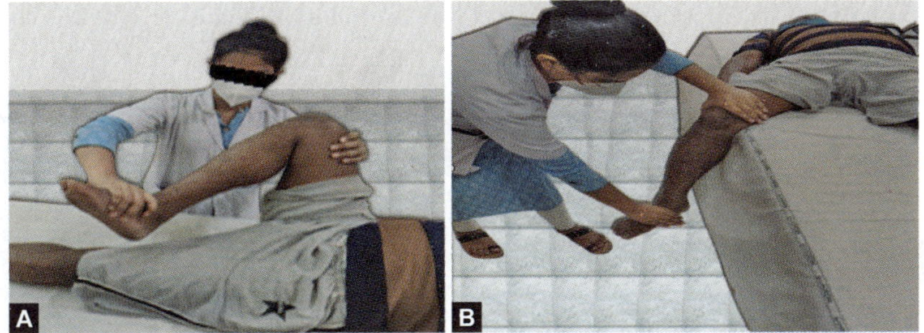

**Figs. 17.7A and B:** (A) $D_1$ flexion with knee flexion; (B) $D_1$ extension with knee flexion.

(Note: The pattern can be with knee flexion or knee extension, such as $D_1$ flexion with knee flexion/$D_1$ flexion with knee extension, $D_1$ extension with knee flexion/$D_1$extension with knee extension—the patterns are selected and trained as per need of the client, i.e., $D_1$ flexion with knee flexion is selected for training the task of clearing ground in the swing phase and $D_1$ flexion with knee extension can be selected for the task of heel striking on ground in stance phase).

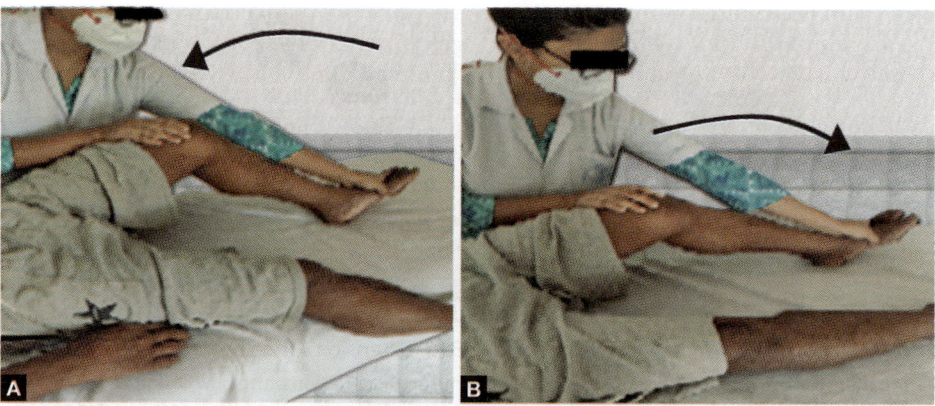

**Figs. 17.8A and B:** (A) $D_2$ flexion with knee flexion; (B) $D_2$ extension with knee extension.
(Note: Like $D_1$ pattern, $D_2$ pattern can be performed with both knee flexion and extension as per need).

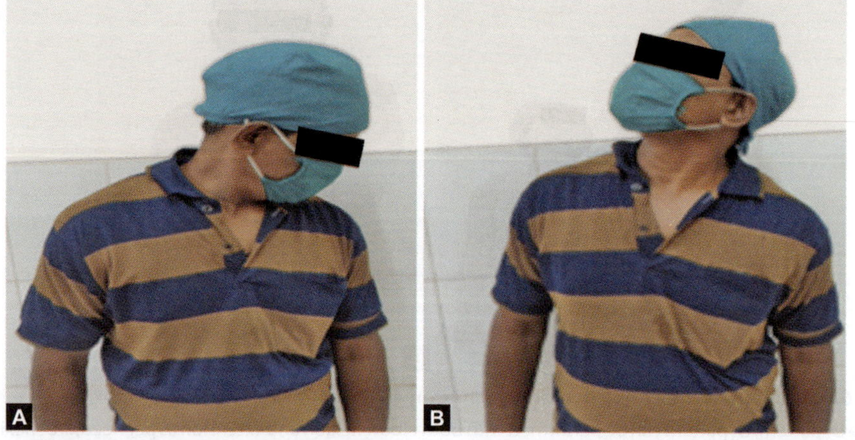

**Figs. 17.9A and B:** Neck pattern: (A) Flexion and rotation to left; (B) Extension and rotation to right.

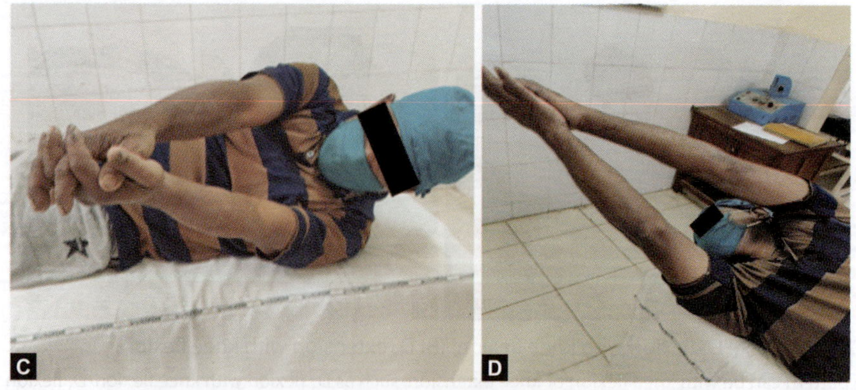

**Figs. 17.9C and D:** Head/neck/upper trunk pattern in lying:
(C) Flexion and rotation to left; (D) Extension and rotation to right.

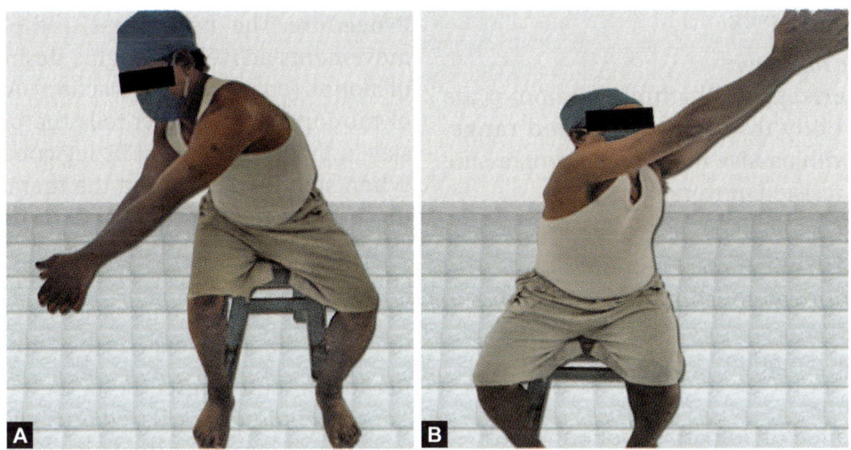

**Figs. 17.10A and B:** Head/neck/upper trunk pattern in sitting: (A) Flexion and rotation to right; (B) Extension and rotation to left.

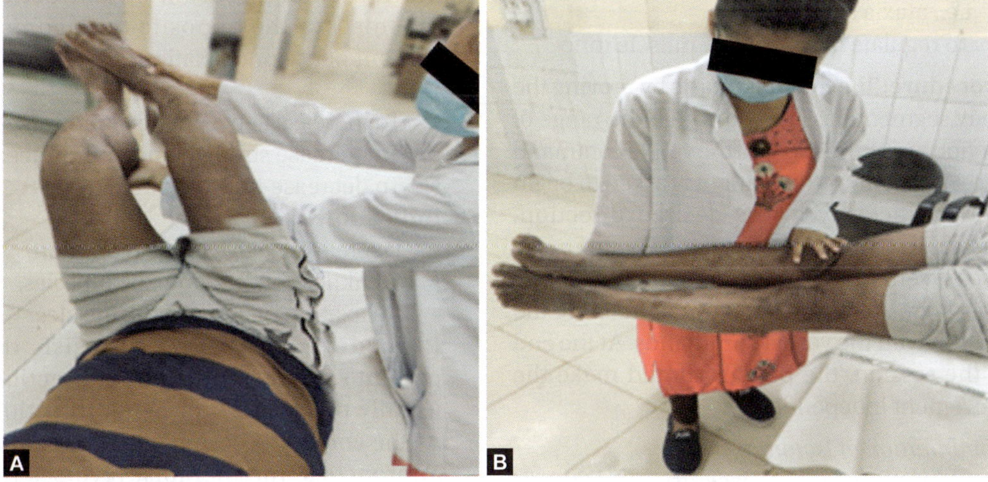

**Figs. 17.11A and B:** Lower trunk pattern: (A) Flexion and rotation to right; (B) Extension and rotation to left.

## Lower Trunk Patterns

- Flexion with rotation to right (D fl. R)—**Figs. 17.11A**
- Extension with rotation to left (D ex. L)—**Figs. 17.11B**
- Flexion with rotation to left (D fl. L)
- Extension with rotation to right (D ex. R)
- Rotation to left (Ro.L)—**Fig. 17.12**
- Rotation to right (Ro. R)

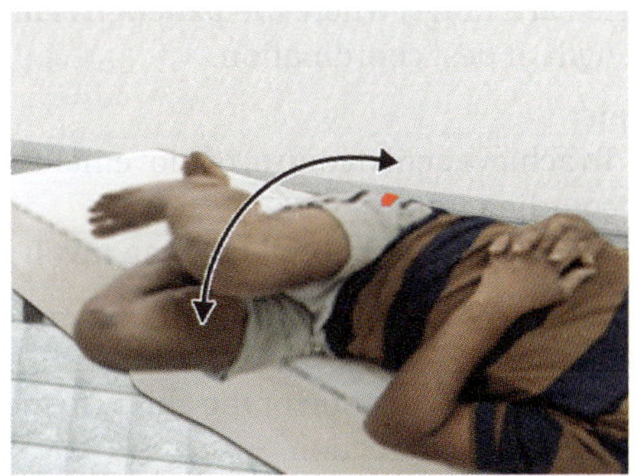

**Fig. 17.12:** Lower trunk rotation (left-right).

## Techniques of PNF

*Rhythmic Initiation*

**Characterization:** Rhythmic motion of the limb or body through the desired range, starting with passive motion and progressing to active resisted movement.

**Goals:**

- To aid in initiation of motion
- To improve coordination and sense of motion
- To teach motion

**Indications:**

- Difficulties in initiating motion
- Conditions like Parkinson's disease, where movement is too slow (Bradykinesias)
- Uncoordinated or dysrhythmic motion, i.e., ataxia and rigidity
- To regulate or normalize muscle tone

**Procedure:** The therapist starts by moving the body segment passively, through the range of motion, using the speed of the verbal command to set the rhythm. The patient is asked to begin working actively in the desired direction. The return motion is done by the therapist. As movement is produced, the therapist resists the active movement, maintaining the rhythm with the verbal commands. At the end of the session, the patient should make the movement independently.

*Combination of Isotonics*

Combined concentric, eccentric, and stabilizing contractions of one group of muscles (agonists) without relaxation. Treatment is started at a range, where the patient has most strength or best coordination.

**Goals:**

- To achieve active control of movement and coordination.
- To promote functional training involving eccentric control of movement

**Indications:**

- Lack of coordination or the ability to move in a desired direction
- Decreased eccentric control

**Procedure:** The therapist resists the patient's movements actively through a desired range of motion (concentric contraction). At the end of motion, the therapist tells the patient to stay in that position (stabilizing contraction). When stability is attained the therapist tells the patient to allow the part to be moved slowly back to the starting position (eccentric contraction). There is no relaxation between the different types of muscle activities and the therapist's hands remain on the same surface.

*Reversal of Antagonists*

These techniques are based on Sherrington's principle of successive induction (Sherrington 1961). They are of the following types:

- **Dynamic reversal/slow reversal:** Active motion changing from one direction (agonist) to the opposite (antagonist) without pause or relaxation.

  **Goal:**

  - To increase active range of motion.
  - To increase strength and endurance.
  - To decrease muscle tone.

  **Indications:**

  - Decreased active range of motion.
  - Weakness of the agonistic muscles.
  - Relaxation of hypertonic muscles.

  **Procedure:** The therapist resists the patient's movements in one direction, usually the stronger or better direction. As the end of the desired range of motion approaches, the therapist reverses the grip on the distal portion of the moving segment and gives a command to prepare for the change of direction. At the end of the desired movement, the therapist gives the action command to reverse direction, without relaxation, and gives resistance to the new motion starting with the distal part. When the patient begins moving in the opposite direction the therapist reverses the proximal grip so all resistance opposes the new direction **(Figs. 17.13A to C)**.
- **Stabilizing reversals:** Alternating isotonic contractions opposed by enough resistance to prevent motion. The command is a

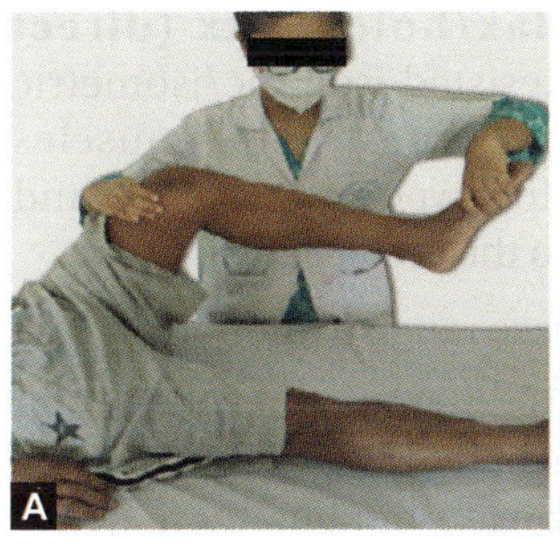

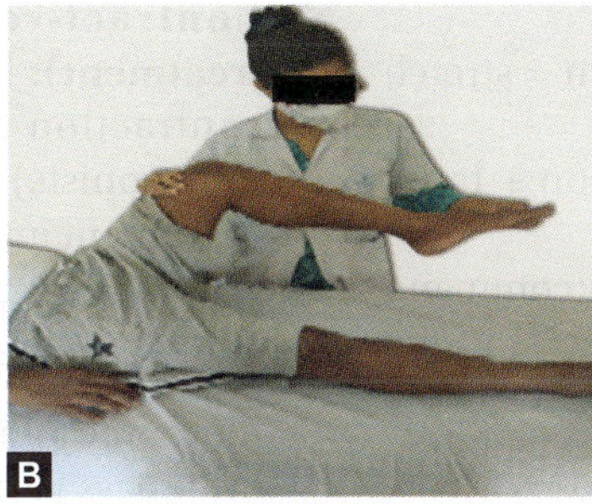

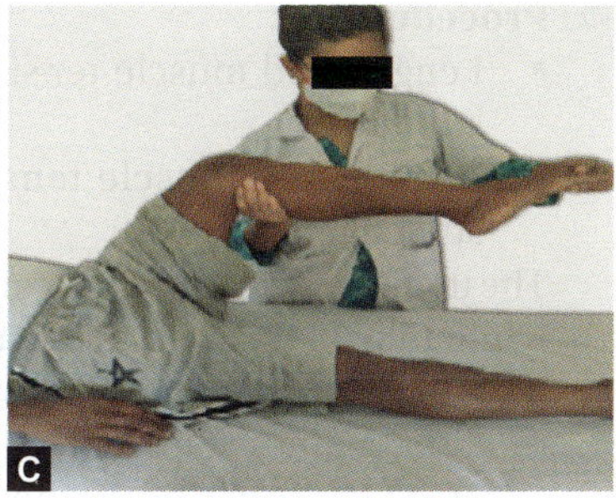


**Figs. 17.13A to C:** Dynamic Reversal/Slow reversal of the leg diagonal—flexion-adduction with knee flexion into extension-abduction with knee extension; (A) Resisting flexion adduction; (B) Distal grip changed and motion into extension-abduction started; (C) Resisting extension abduction.

dynamic command ("push against my hands", or "don't let me push you") and the therapist allows only a very small movement.

**Goal:** To increase stability and balance, increase muscle strength and coordination between agonist and antagonist.

**Procedure:** The therapist gives resistance to the patient, starting in the strongest direction, while asking the patient to oppose the force. Very little motion is allowed. Approximation or traction should be used to increase stability. When the patient is fully resisting the force the therapist moves one hand and begins to give resistance in another direction. After the patient responds to the new resistance, the therapist moves the other hand to resist the new direction.

**Goal:** To Increase stability and balance by increasing coordination between agonists and antagonists.

To increase muscle strength.

*Rhythmic Stabilization*

Alternating isometric contractions against resistance to agonists and antagonists. No motion is desired and only stability is intended.

**Goal:**

- ❖ Increase muscle strength and decrease pain. Increase stability and balance.
- ❖ To decrease muscle tone

**Procedure:** The therapist resists an isometric contraction of the agonistic muscle group.

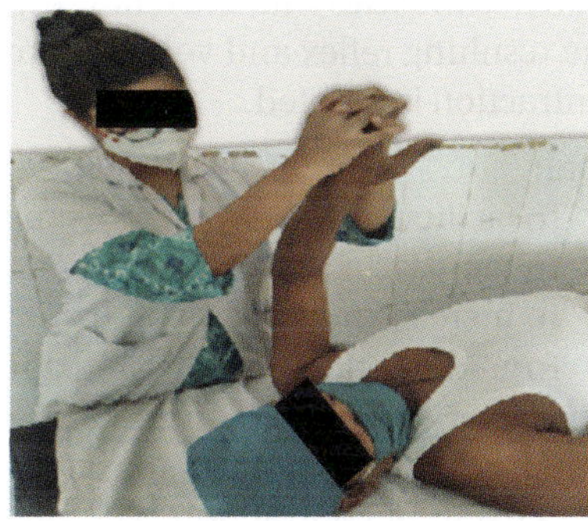

**Fig. 17.14:** Rhythmic stabilization of the shoulder in the diagonal of flexion-abduction/extension-adduction.

The patient maintains the position of the part without trying to move. The resistance is increased slowly as the patient builds a matching force. When the patient is responding fully, the therapist moves one hand to begin resisting the antagonistic motion at the distal part. Neither the therapist nor the patient relaxes as the resistance changes. Traction or approximation to the joints is applied as required. The reversals are repeated as often as needed. While applying the procedure. The therapist uses commands, such as " stay there", do not try to move **(Fig. 17.14)**.

*Repeated Stretch (Repeated Contraction):*

- ❖ **Repeated stretch from beginning of the range:** The stretch reflex elicited from muscles under the tension of elongation.

**Procedure:**

- Lengthened muscle tension = stretch stimulus
- Lengthened muscle tension + tap = stretch reflex

The therapist gives a preparatory command while fully elongating the muscles in the pattern. Particular attention is given to the rotation. A quick "tap" is given to lengthen (stretch) the muscles further and evoke the stretch reflex. At the same time as the stretch reflex, a command is given to link the patient's voluntary effort to contract the stretched muscles with the reflex response. The resulting reflex and voluntary muscle contraction is resisted.

**Goal:**

- To facilitate initiation of movement
- To Increase active range of motion
- To Increase muscle strength
- To guide motion in the desired direction

❖ **Repeated stretch through range:** The stretch reflex elicited from muscles under the tension of contraction. The therapist resists a pattern of motion so that all the muscles are contracting and tense. The movement can start with an initial stretch reflex. A preparatory command is subsequently given to coordinate the stretch reflex, with a new and increased effort by the patient. At the same time, the therapist slightly stretches the muscles by momentarily giving too much resistance. A new and stronger muscle contraction is asked for and is resisted. The stretch reflex is repeated to redirect the motion as the patient moves through the range. The patient must be allowed to move before the next stretch reflex is given and must not relax or reverse the direction of movement during the stretch.

**Goal:**

- To increase active range of motion
- To increase muscle strength
- To prevent or reduce fatigue
- To guide motion in the desired direction

❖ **Contract-relax/hold-relax (direct treatment):** Resisted isotonic/isometric contraction of the restricting muscles (antagonists) followed by relaxation and movement into the increased range.

**Goal:** To increase range of motion

**Procedure:** The therapist or the patient moves the joint or body segment to the end of the passive range of motion. The therapist asks the patient for a strong contraction (the contraction should be held at least for 5–8 seconds) of the restricting muscle or pattern. A maximal contraction in the most lengthened position of the muscle chain will provoke a structural change in the actin-myosin complex. After sufficient time, the therapist tells the patient to relax. The joint or body part is repositioned, either actively by the patient or passively by the therapist, to the new limit of the passive range. Active motion is performed by the patient at the new range and is resisted by the therapist. The technique is repeated until no more range is gained **(Fig. 17.15)**.

❖ **Contract-relax (indirect treatment):** The technique uses contraction of the agonistic muscles instead of the shortened muscles **(Fig. 17.16)**.

**Goal:** To increase range of motion.

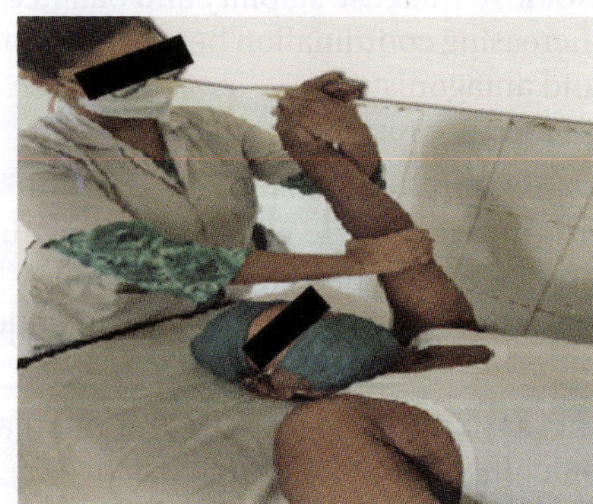

**Fig. 17.15:** Hold-relax or contract-relax: Direct treatment for shortened shoulder extensor and adductor muscles.

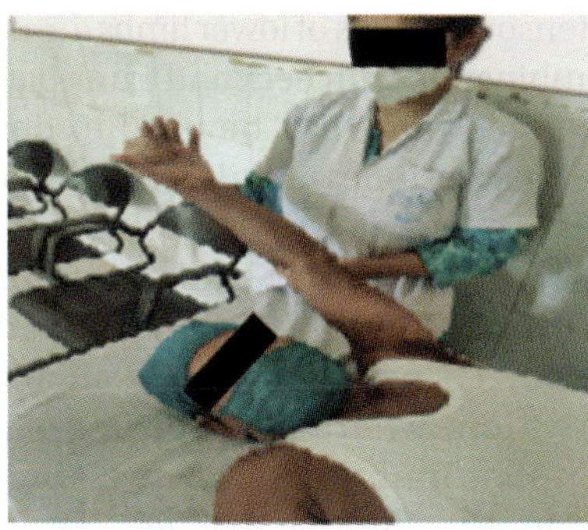

**Fig. 17.16:** Hold-relax or contract-relax (indirect treatment) for shortened shoulder extensor and adductor muscles.

**Indication:** The indirect method is performed, when the contraction of the range limiting muscle is too painful or too weak to produce effective contraction.

- **Replication:** A technique to facilitate motor learning of functional activities. Teaching the patient the outcome of a movement or activity is important for functional work (for example, sports) and self-care activities. The patient is placed in the "end" position of the activity where all the agonist muscles are shortened. The patient holds that position while the therapist resists all the components of movements. All the basic procedures are used to facilitate the patient's muscles. The patient is then asked to relax. The patient is then moved passively a short distance back in the opposite direction. Then he/she is asked to return to the end' position. For each replication of the movement the patient is moved to the starting position (beginning of the movement), and movements are challenged through a greater range of motion. At the end, the patient should perform the activity or motion alone, without facilitation or manual contact by the therapist.

**Goal:**

- Teach the patient the end position (outcome) of the movement
- Assess the patient's ability to sustain a contraction when the agonist muscles are shortened

**Clinical Application of PNF**

- **Stimulation of vital functions:** proprioceptive neuromuscular facilitation may be specifically applied to facilitate motions of the parts necessary or responsible for vital functions, such as:
  - **Respiration/breathing:** Techniques of proprioceptive neuromuscular facilitation can be applied to stimulate breathing and to strengthen the muscles responsible for breathing.
    The patterns helpful for inspiration are:
    - Neck extension
    - Upper and lower trunk extension
    - Flexor patterns of upper limbs

    The patterns responsible for expiration are:
    - Neck flexion
    - Upper and lower trunk flexion
    - Extensor patterns of the upper extremities

    The neck and trunk patterns combined with bilateral asymmetrical upper extremity patterns (chopping and lifting) and bilateral symmetrical upper extremity patterns promote breathing. Stimulation of muscles of respiration, such as diaphragm and intercostals can be facilitated using the technique. The accessory muscles that help in deep respiration can also be facilitated.
  - **Swallowing:** PNF is used to promote movement of tongue, lips, and to stimulate the gag reflex (stimulation of the gag reflex is helpful, because it demands response of the pharyngeal muscles with elevation of the soft

palate, which is automatically followed by a swallowing response.

- **To facilitate micturition and defecation:** The voluntary performance and control of micturition and defecation may be enhanced by performance of related patterns of facilitation against maximal resistance. The emptying of bowel and bladder can be promoted through flexor patterns of lower limbs and lower trunk. However stopping of the bladder and bowel emptying can be achieved through extensor patterns of lower extremities and lower trunk. The muscles of perineal region could be facilitated through performance of bilaterally symmetrical extension-adduction-external rotation patterns of the lower limbs.
- **To promote movement of eyeball:** The neck and upper trunk patterns promote the movement of the eyeball, as for example, neck extension and rotation pattern enhances upward and lateral movement of the eyeball. PNF can also be used for the treatment of nystagmus, where decrements in movement of the eyeballs are emphasized for stabilization and visual tracking.
- **To promote facial motion**
- **To reduce muscle tone:** PNF patterns like $D_2$ flexion with elbow extension in upper limb produces movements in an antispastic direction, hence reduces spasticity.
- **To develop posture and balance:** Rhythmic stabilization technique help to promote postural stability, where as the limb and trunk patterns help to restore balance.
- **To promote bed mobility:** To promote mobility on bed, such as rolling, creeping, crawling as well as mobility out of bed, such as walking, where the flexor and extensor patterns of lower limbs are used in combination with neck and trunk patterns. The technique can be used to develop motor milestones in children with cerebral palsy and developmental delay.
- **To improve upper limb function:** To improve functions, such as reaching for objects with the hand in an anterior direction, where $D_1$ extension pattern of upper limb is used. For taking food to mouth, combing hair, etc., $D_1$ flexion pattern with elbow flexion is used.

### Chopping Pattern

The chopping pattern which utilizes three dimensional movements referred to as spiral and diagonal patterns are used to improve activities, such as running, throwing, changing directions, etc. It challenges the individual's ability to maintain spine and hip position in all three planes of movement, while transferring force between upper and lower body. The chop exercise, commonly used in functional training, utilizes both $D_1$ and $D_2$ PNF patterns for the upper extremity **(Fig. 17.17)**.

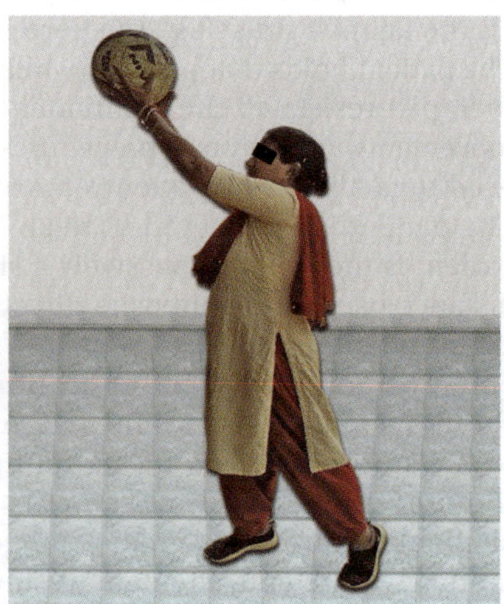

**Fig. 17.17:** PNF chopping pattern.

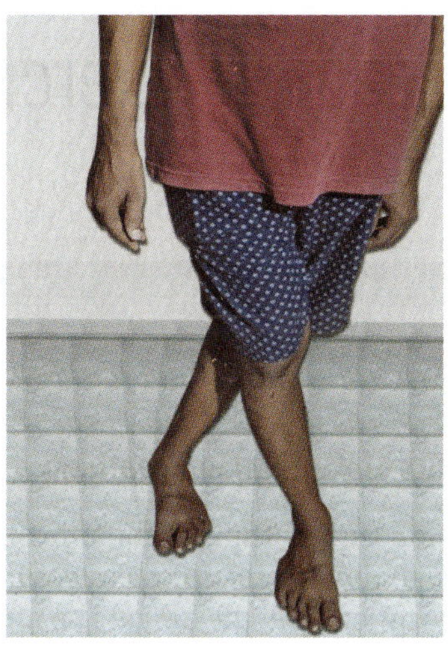

**Fig. 17.18:** PNF braiding pattern.

### Braiding Pattern/Technique

This traditional PNF pattern involving cross over stepping of the lower extremities is used in functional training for the lower extremity **(Fig. 17.18)**. This movement requires both $D_1$ and $D_2$ patterning from each hip when performing multiple steps. In order to increase difficulty in the PNF patterning, resistance bands can be used.

# 18 CHAPTER Breathing Exercise

## DEFINITION

Breathing exercises are a form of exercise that can be used for a variety of health-related reasons, to enhance the functioning of the respiratory system by improving ventilation; strengthening respiratory muscles; making breathing more efficient; and for stress reduction.

The exercises are intended to promote effective and healthy breathing and breath control that helps in improving respiratory function by maintaining lung volumes and capacities and controlling episodes of dyspnea, thereby improving the overall endurance and function. It is an effective tool in pulmonary rehabilitation.

Respiration is the sequence of events that result in the exchange of oxygen and carbon dioxide between the atmosphere and the body cells. In every 3–5 seconds, nerve impulses stimulate the breathing process, or ventilation, which moves air through a series of passages into and out of the lungs. After this, there is an exchange of gases between the lungs and the blood. This is called an external respiration. The blood transports the gases to and from the tissue cells. The exchange of gases between the blood and tissue cells is internal respiration. Finally, the cells utilize the oxygen for their specific activities—this is called cellular metabolism, or cellular respiration. Together, these activities constitute respiration.

### Mechanics of Ventilation/Breathing

Ventilation or breathing is the movement of air through the conducting passages between the atmosphere and the lungs. The air moves through the passages because of pressure gradients that are produced by contraction of the diaphragm and thoracic muscles. The process of air flowing into the lungs is called inspiration and air flowing out of the lungs is called expiration (described below). In normal breathing that occurs at a rate of 12–16 cycles per minute, the inspiration is an active process brought about by the contraction of diaphragm and external intercostal muscles and expiration is a passive process brought about by the recoil of elastic tissues. However, in forceful expiration, that usually occurs during airways clearance, the abdominals and internal intercostals muscles contract.

#### *Inspiration*

Inspiration (inhalation) is the process of taking air into the lungs. It is the active phase of ventilation that results from muscle contraction. During inspiration, the diaphragm, external intercostal muscles, and intercartilaginous portion of the internal intercostals muscles contract, and the thoracic cavity increases in volume. This decreases the intra-alveolar pressure, so that air flows into the lungs. During forceful inspiration/ labored breathing, the accessory muscles also undergo contraction along with diaphragm and external intercostal muscle.

### *Expiration*

Expiration (exhalation) is the process of letting air out of the lungs during the breathing cycle. During expiration, the relaxation of the diaphragm and elastic recoil of tissue decreases the thoracic volume and increases the intra-alveolar pressure. Expiration pushes air out of the lungs. However, during forceful expiration, the abdominals and interosseous portion of internal intercostals muscles contract.

## Respiratory Physiology

When we breathe in, air is inspired through the nose or mouth, through the conducting airways, and reaches the distal respiratory units, which contains the respiratory bronchiole, alveolar ducts, alveolar sacs, and alveoli. At full inspiration, the lungs contain maximum amount of air, called total lung capacity (TLC), which is the combination of so many volumes, such as tidal volume (TV), inspiratory reserve volume (IRV), expiratory reserve volume (ERV), and residual volume. The lung volumes and capacities and their normal values are discussed below **(Fig. 18.1)**.

### *Tidal Volume (TV)*

The amount of air inspired or expired, during normal resting ventilation is called tidal volume. Though normal TV is 500 mL, only 350 mL of air takes part in gas exchange and the remaining 150 mL of air remains in the conducting airways and does not take part in gas exchange.

### *Inspiratory Reserve Volume (IRV)*

After tidal inspiration, the amount of air that can be further inspired is called inspiratory reserve volume —2500 mL.

### *Expiratory Reserve Volume (ERV)*

The amount of air that can be expired forcefully after tidal expiration is called expiratory reserve volume—1,500 mL.

### *Residual Volume (RV)*

The amount of air remaining in the lungs after a forceful expiration—1,500 mL.

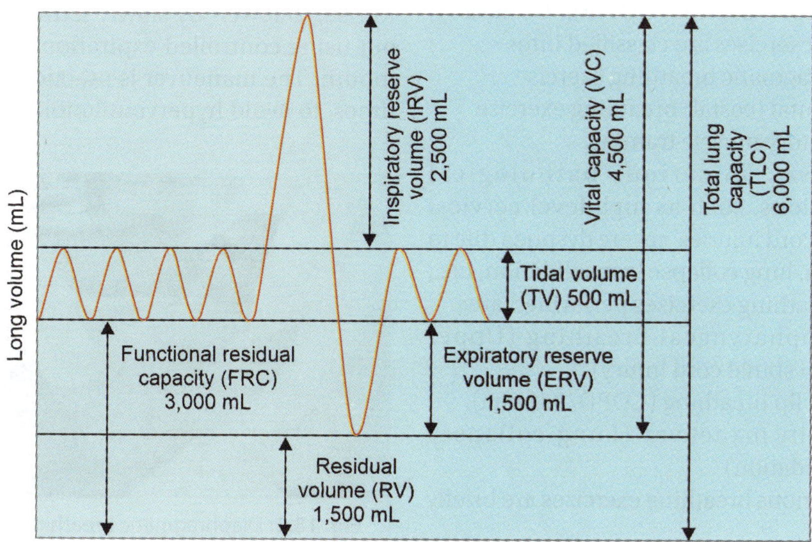


**Fig. 18.1:** Long volumes and capacities.

### *Inspiratory Capacity (IC)*

It is the amount of air that can be inspired after a tidal expiration. It is the sum of TV and IRV. Its value is 3,000 mL.

### *Functional Residual Capacity (FRC)*

It is the sum of ERV and RV. Its value is 3,000 mL.

### *Vital Capacity (VC)*

It is the maximum amount of air that can be inspired after a forceful expiration. It is the combination of three lung volumes, i.e., ERV, TV, and IRV. Its value in a healthy adult (male) is 4,500 mL.

### *Total Lung Capacity (TLC)*

It is the total air-holding capacity of lung, which is the sum of RV, ERV, TV, and IRV. Its value is 6,000 mL

**Types of breathing exercises:** Breathing exercises performed depend on the conditions for which they are applied. It may be deep breathing (for example in restrictive lung diseases), or controlled relaxed breathing (for example asthma/COPD). Generally, breathing exercises are classified into:

a. Diaphragmatic breathing exercise
b. Segmental (costal) breathing exercise
c. Ventilatory muscle training.
However, in serious pathological conditions, such as high level cervical spinal cord injuries, severe dyspnea due to asthma, lung collapse/consolidation, etc., the breathing exercises performed are:
d. Glossopharyngeal breathing (Upper cervical spinal cord injury)
e. Pursed lip breathing (COPD/Asthma).
f. Air shift maneuver (Lung collapse/consolidation)

The various breathing exercises are briefly discussed:

### *Diaphragmatic Breathing Exercise*

Diaphragm is the primary muscle for inspiration. Diaphragm controls breathing at an involuntary level. This contributes to about 60% of total work of breathing. A patient with primary pulmonary disease, such as COPD can be taught breathing control by optimal use of diaphragm and relaxation of the accessory muscles. This exercise also helps to mobilize secretions in the lungs in postural drainage. All breathing exercises start with diaphragmatic breathing, followed by segmental breathing and end with diaphragmatic breathing.

**Procedure**

The patient is placed in a relaxed position, where gravity will assist the descent of diaphragm, such as half-lying position with head and trunk elevated by 45° and hips and knees flexed with pillow support **(Fig. 18.2)**. Other positions, such as supine, sitting, standing may be used as the patient progress during treatment. The therapist places his/her hands over the rectus abdominis, just below the anterior costal margin. The patient is asked to breathe slowly and deeply via nose by keeping the shoulders relaxed and upper chest quiet, allowing the abdomen to rise, followed by slowly letting all the air out using controlled expiration through the mouth. The maneuver is practiced for 3 or 4 times, to avoid hyperventilation. The face of

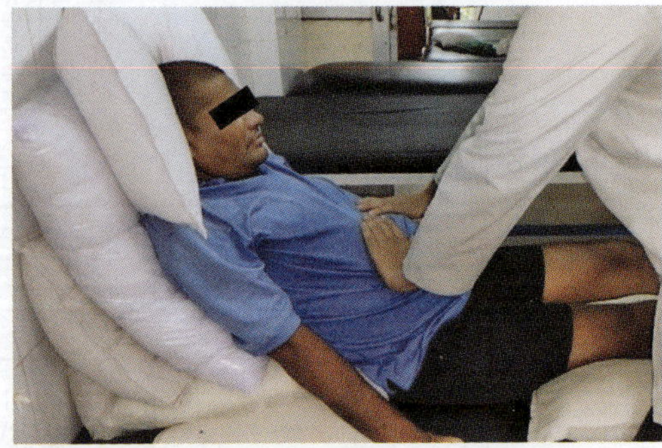

**Fig. 18.2:** Diaphragmatic breathing exercise.

the patient should be turned to sides, to avoid direct exposure to therapist/clinician.

### *Segmental Breathing*

It is performed on a segment of a lung, or a section of the chest wall that needs increased ventilation or movement. Hypoventilation that occurs in certain areas of the lungs, due to chest wall fibrosis, pain after surgery, atelectasis, trauma to chest wall, pneumonia, and post-mastectomy scar can be expanded by this procedure. This exercise when performed, prevents accumulation of pleural fluid and secretions, decreases paradoxical breathing, and panic episodes, and improves chest mobility. The segmental breathing exercises are briefly described below:

#### Lateral Costal Expansion/Lateral Basal Expansion Exercise

This exercise may be done unilaterally or bilaterally. The patient may be positioned in half-lying **(Fig. 18.3)**, sitting or supine/crook lying. The therapist places the hands along the lateral aspect of the lower ribs and asks the patient to breathe out through the mouth. As the patient breathes out, the therapist applies firm downward pressure into the ribs with the palms of the hands and guides the rib cage to move downward and inward during the phase of expiration. Then the patient is asked to deeply inhale air through the nose, while the therapist applies a quick downward and inward stretch to the chest, to facilitate contraction of external intercostals muscle, guiding the rib cage to move upward and outward. Light manual resistance can be applied to the lower ribs to increase sensory awareness, as the patient breaths in deeply and the chest expands. The procedure is repeated 3–4 times followed by performance of diaphragmatic breathing exercises as described above. The patient may be taught to perform the maneuver independently and to apply resistance with his own hand or towel/belt.

#### Posterior Basal Expansion Exercise

This form of segmental breathing is important for the postsurgical patients who are confined to bed for an extended period of time, as secretion often accumulates over the posterior segments of lower lobes. The patient is either made to remain in half-lying **(Fig. 18.4)**/sitting and leaning forward on pillows. The therapist places the hands over the posterior aspect of the lower ribs and follows

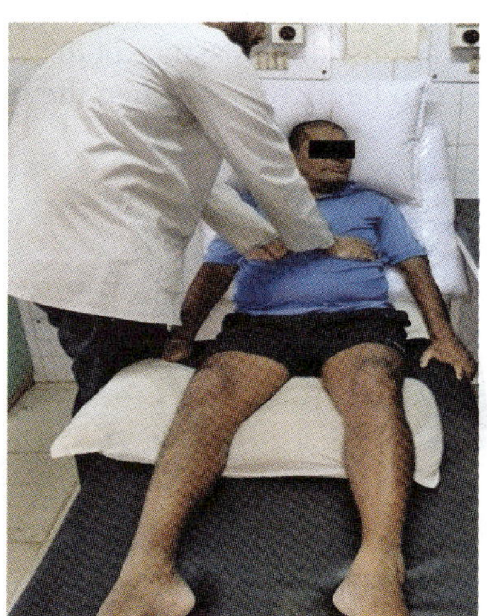

**Fig. 18.3:** Lateral costal expansion exercise.

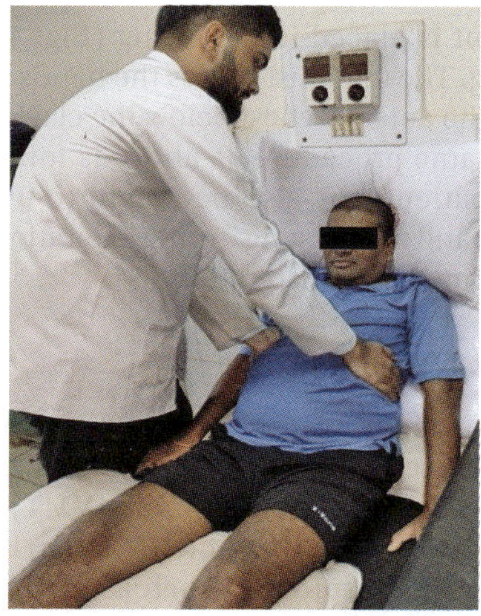

**Fig. 18.4:** Posterior basal expansion exercise.

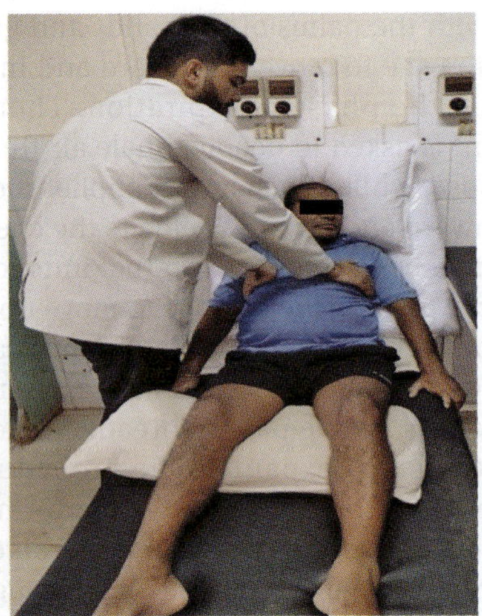
**Fig. 18.5:** Right middle/left (lingular) expansion exercises.

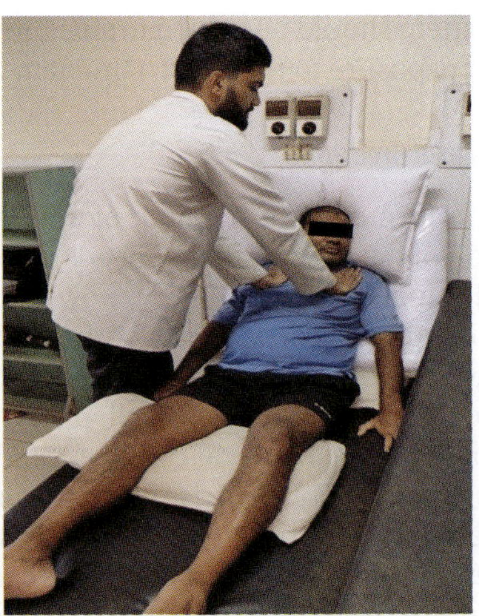
**Fig. 18.6:** Apical expansion exercise.

the same procedure as described for lateral basal expansion exercise described above.

### Right Middle-Lobe and Lingular Lobe (Left) Expansion Exercise

Patient is placed in sitting/half-lying. The therapist places the hands on either the right or left side of the patient's chest just below the axilla **(Fig. 18.5)**. The same procedure as above is followed.

### Apical Expansion Exercise

Patient is placed in half-lying **(Fig. 18.6)**/ sitting. The therapist places the hands/hand over the anterior chest below the clavicle(s). The same procedure as above is followed. The patient may also be taught to use his own hand for assisting during expiration and resisting during inspiration.

## *Ventilatory Muscle Training*

The process of improving strength and endurance of muscles of breathing is known as ventilatory muscle training (VMT). This technique usually focuses on primary muscles of inspiration such as diaphragm and intercostal muscles. The procedures involved are:

### Diaphragmatic Muscle Training Using Weights

The patient is placed in supine lying/crook lying **(Fig. 18.7)**. Place a small weight (1.30–2.20 kg) over the epigastric region of the abdomen. Tell the patient to breathe out through the mouth followed by deep inspiration through the nose, keeping the upper chest quiet. Gradually increase the time, that the patient breaths against the resistance of the weight. Weight can be increased, when the patient

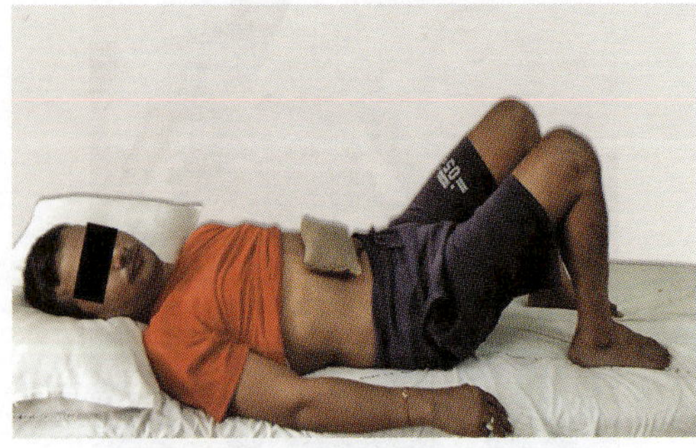
**Fig. 18.7:** Diaphragmatic muscle training using weight.

can sustain diaphragmatic breathing pattern, without the use of any accessory muscles of inspiration for 15 minutes.

### Inspiratory Resistance Training

The patient inhales through a hand-held resistive device that he or she places in the mouth. These devices are narrow tubes of varying diameters that provide resistance to airflow during inspiration and improve strength of inspiratory muscles. Gradually, the time is increased to 20–30 minutes.

### Incentive Spirometry

This is a form of low-level resistance training, where the patient inhales through a spirometer that provides visual or auditory feedback as he/she breaths deeply, with the mouthpiece placed in the mouth **(Fig. 18.8)**. The patient is placed in a comfortable position. Then, have the patient place mouthpiece of the device in the mouth and maximally inhale through the spirometer and hold the inspiration for few seconds and then exhale air through the mouth by removing the mouth piece.

### Glossopharyngeal Breathing

Glossopharyngeal breathing (GPB), also called "frog breathing", is a positive pressure breathing technique that uses muscles of the mouth and pharynx to propel small volumes of air ("gulps") into the lungs. It is a means of increasing the patient's inspiratory capacity, when there is severe weakness of muscles of inspiration. It is used primarily for ventilator dependent patients, due to abscence or incomplete innervations of the diaphragm because of high cervical cord injury or neuromuscular disorders. The patient takes several gulps of air (6–10 numbers). Then the mouth is closed and the tongue pushes the air back and traps it in the pharynx. The air is then forced into the lungs and the glottis is opened. This increases the depth of the inspiration and the patient's inspiratory and vital capacity.

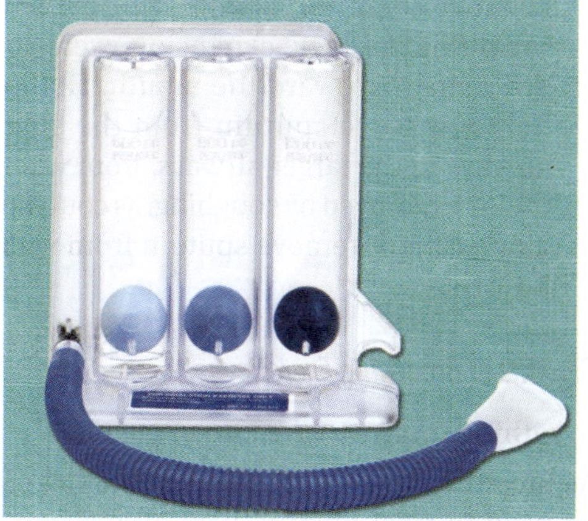

**Fig. 18.8:** The incentive spirometer.

### Pursed-lip Breathing Exercise

Pursed lip breathing is a technique that helps people living with asthma or COPD when they experience shortness of breath. Pursed lip breathing helps control shortness of breath, and provides a quick and easy way to slow patient's pace of breathing, making each breath more effective. This is a strategy that involves lightly pursing the lips together during controlled expiration. It helps to improve ventilation and releases trapped air in the lungs. Have the patient assume a comfortable position. Explain to the patient that expiration must be relaxed and passive and contraction of abdominals must be avoided. Instruct the patient to breathe slowly and deeply through the nose, and then breathe out gently through lightly pursed lips. By providing slight resistance, an increased positive pressure will generate within the airways, which helps to keep open small bronchioles that otherwise collapse. It can be applied as 3–5 minutes "rescue exercise" or an emergency procedure to counteract acute exacerbations or dyspnea in COPD and asthma.

### Air Shift Maneuver

Any individual with paradoxical breathing or a poorly expanding chest wall (due to intercostals weakness) during inspiration should learn to perform an air shift maneuver. When an individual has a dominant diaphragmatic breathing pattern that results in collapse of the anterior chest wall (as occurs in those with C4–T4 motor complete injuries), the volume of air moving into lungs does not act to expand the chest wall but instead moves in a caudal direction. An air shift is a maneuver in which a person inhales maximally, closes the glottis and relaxes the diaphragm to move the air upward toward the middle and upper lobes of the chest and creates expansion of these regions. This exercise is used to maintain chest mobility or expand the chest from ½ inch to as much as 2 inches. Position the patient in supine lying. Ask the patient to take deep breath, close the glottis and hold that breath. While holding the breath, therapist asks the patient to suck in the abdomen so that air will move from lower part to upper part of thorax. To learn this technique, the therapist places one hand on the patient's epigastric area, and the other hand on the upper part of the chest, and holds the hands in place. When the patient takes a deep breath, holds it, sucks in the stomach, and moves the air to the upper part of the chest, the therapist's top hand will rise. The patient is instructed to perform this exercise daily.

#### Heimlich Maneuver/Abdominal Thrust

This is an air shift maneuver performed to overcome inability to breathe caused by a blockage in the throat.

### *Active Cycle of Breathing Technique (ACBT)*

Active cycle of breathing technique combines different breathing techniques that help clear mucus from the lungs in three phases. It is an independent breathing exercise program consisting of breath control exercise, thoracic expansion exercise, and forced expiratory techniques. The components of ACBT are briefly discussed below:

- **Breath control exercise:** This is the first phase that relaxes the airways. It is the relaxed diaphragmatic breathing, where the patient is asked to breathe in through the nose and breathe out through the mouth with very little effort and relaxing the upper chest and shoulders. A good way to do this is to place one hand on the stomach as one breathes. He/she should breathe gently so that the airways are relaxed. By using the pursed lip technique when breathing out, a back pressure is created in the airways that stents the airway open longer. The breathing control is repeated for six breaths before moving to thoracic expansion exercises.
- **Thoracic expansion exercise:** This is the second phase that helps to get air behind the mucus and clear the mucus. The patient is asked to breathe in deeply (some people use a 3-second breath hold to get more air into smaller airways and behind the mucus) and then breathe out without forcing the air out. This may be done with chest clapping or vibration, followed by another cycle of breathing control.
- **Forced expiratory technique:** This is the third phase that helps to force the mucus out of the lungs. This is a maneuver used to move secretions, mobilized by deep breathing/thoracic expansion exercises, downstream toward the mouth. Huffing helps to move sputum from the small airways to the larger airways, from where they are removed by coughing, as coughing alone cannot remove sputum from small airways.

### *Benefits of Breathing Exercise*

#### Breathing Improves the Lung Function

As breathing increases lungs function, it can be used to treat obstructive and restrictive pulmonary conditions.

### Breathing Detoxifies and Releases Toxins

The body is designed to release 70% of its toxins through breathing. If the person is not breathing effectively, he is not properly ridding the body of its toxins ($CO_2$). When one exhales air from the body, he/she releases carbon dioxide that has been passed through from the bloodstream into the lungs.

### Breathing Releases Tension, Relaxes Mind/ Body and Brings Clarity

When a person is stressed, the muscles become tight and breathing becomes shallow. The body does not get adequate amount of oxygen as per need. Slow deep breathing exercises performed in such states of body induces relaxation, brings clarity by diverting attention and providing adequate oxygen to the brain to meet the needs of the body.

### Breathing Relieves Emotional Problems

Relaxed deep breathing exercises during negative emotional events and abnormal outbursts of emotion helps to overcome emotional problems.

### Breathing Relieves Pain

During episodes of pain, such as labor pain, individuals hold breath. It is found that breathing into the pain helps to ease it.

### Breathing Massages the Vital Organs

The movements of the diaphragm during the deep breathing exercise massage the stomach, small intestine, liver, and pancreas. The upward movement of the diaphragm also massages the heart. When air is inhaled, diaphragm descends, and abdomen expands. By this action, massage to vital organs improves circulation in them.

### Breathing Strengthens the Immune System

The oxygen that travels through the blood-stream by attaching to hemoglobin in the red blood cells enriches the body to metabolize nutrients and vitamins, strengthening the immune system.

### Breathing Improves Posture

Deep breathing techniques over a sustained period of time promotes good posture, thereby helps in correction of spinal deformities, such as kyphosis/scoliosis, when combined with spinal exercises and bracing.

### Breathing Improves Quality of the Blood

Regular deep breathing exercises remove all the carbon dioxide and increases oxygen in the blood and thus increases the quality of blood.

### Breathing Increases Digestion and Assimilation of Food

The digestive organs, such as the stomach receive more oxygen, and hence operate more efficiently helping in digestion and assimilation of food (into blood).

### Breathing Improves the Nervous System

The brain, spinal cord and nerves receive increased oxygenation and are more nourished. This helps to improve the function of the nervous system.

### Breathing Improves Tissue Healing

As breathing helps to provide the required amount of oxygen to the tissues, and helps in tissue metabolism, healing of injured tissues is facilitated more and more. Breathing improves cellular regeneration.

### Breathing Makes the Heart Stronger

Breathing exercises reduce the workload on the heart as it leads to more efficient lungs and increases oxygenation of blood. So, the heart does not have to work as hard to deliver oxygen to the tissues. Breathing exercises also produce a massaging effect on heart, increasing its efficiency.

### Proper Breathing Assists in Weight Control

In case of obesity, the extra oxygen burns up the excess fat more efficiently and reduces weight. In case of underweight, the extra oxygen feeds the starving tissues through increase of tissue metabolism.

**Breathing Boosts Energy Levels and Improves Stamina**

Due to this, breathing exercises are performed as a warm up exercise before resuming vigorous activities/sports. Breathing elevates moods—breathing increases pleasure by inducing neurochemicals in the brain to elevate mood and combat physical pain.

**Breathing Improves Endurance**

Breathing exercises improve both cardiorespiratory and muscular endurance.

# 19 CHAPTER Hydrotherapy

## INTRODUCTION

Hydrotherapy is a branch of alternative medicine and physiotherapy, that involves use of water for pain relief, joint mobilization, muscle strengthening and development of posture and balance.

The term hydrotherapy is coined from the Greek word—"Hydro" meaning "water" and "Therapeia" meaning "healing". It is a method of using the physical aspect of water for medical and relaxing treatments. The buoyancy effect of water minimizes the effects of gravity on weight bearing joints, assists and resists muscle work, the hydrostatic pressure exerts a circumferential force that helps to reduce edema and stabilizes unstable joints, and the warmth of water enhances blood flow and induces muscle relaxation.

Hydrotherapy refers to the use of multi-depth immersion pools or tanks that facilitate the application of various established therapeutic interventions including stretching, joint mobilizations, strengthening, etc. Water has an effect similar to a soothing massage on muscles by bringing more oxygen to the injured area. Movements that are extremely painful outside the water, can be conducted in water with minimum pain. Running, walking and floating in water have been found to be significantly effective.

### Principles of Hydrotherapy

Hydrotherapy for treatment of diseases and disorders are based upon the properties of water and heat. The properties of water that are used to assist or resist movement are:

#### *Buoyancy*

It is the upward force that works opposite to gravity when the body is placed in water. Buoyancy provides the patient with relative weightlessness and joint unloading allowing performance of active motion easily. It can be used to assist (when the body segment is made to move in a bottom to top direction) or resist movement (when the body segment is made to move in top to bottom direction).

#### *Hydrostatic Pressure*

It is the circumferential pressure exerted on the immersed objects inside water. This increased pressure reduces or limits effusion, assists venous return, centralizes peripheral blood flow.

#### *Viscosity*

It is friction occurring between molecules of liquid resulting in resistance to flow. It creates resistance to all active movements.

#### *Surface Tension*

The surface of the fluid acts a membrane under tension. Surface tension is measured as force per unit length. An extremity that moves through the surface will perform more work than if kept under water.

### Hydromechanics

Hydromechanics is the physical properties and characteristics of fluid in motion that affects movement. Its components include:

- **Laminar flow:** Movements where all molecules move parallel to each other resulting in typically slow movements.
- **Turbulent flow:** movements where molecules do not move parallel to each other, resulting in typically faster movements.

### Drag

The cumulative effects of turbulence and fluid viscosity acting on a object in motion, which may be used to resist movements.

### Warmth of Water

The properties of heat on body such as reduction of pain and spasm/spasticity, increase of metabolism and nerve conduction velocity are used to achieve desired therapeutic benefits in patients with diseases and disorders.

## Objectives of Hydrotherapy

- To relieve pain and edema.
- To promote relaxation.
- To Increase range of motion.
- To reduce muscle tone (spasticity).
- To strengthen muscles and enhance co-ordination and balance.
- To develop patient's confidence of holding a posture/moving.

## Clinical Applications of Hydrotherapy

The conditions treated by hydrotherapy include:

- Neck pain and back pain.
- Head and spinal injury sequel (except those having bladder and bowel incontinence)
- Cerebral palsy (children having no fear in water).

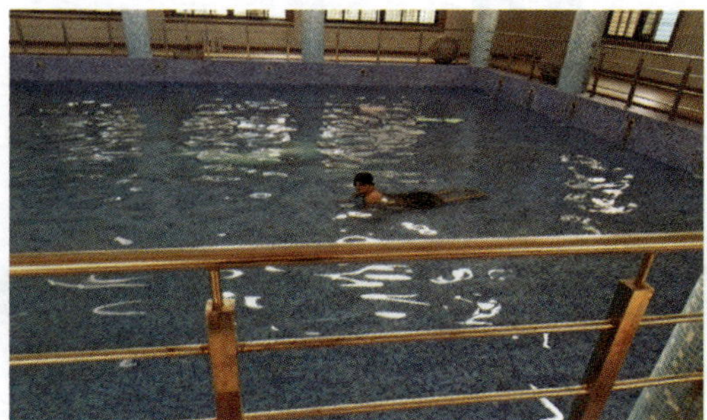

**Fig. 19.1:** The hydrotherapy pool.

- Arthritic conditions (rheumatoid arthritis, ankylosing spondylitis, etc).
- Sports injuries.
- Amputees.
- Orthopedic conditions.
- Stroke sequel causing hemiparesis/ quadriparesis.
- Women during prenatal and postnatal periods.

## Salient Features of Hydrotherapy Pool

The pool could be a stainless steel hydrotherapy pool, or a permanent concrete structure like a swimming pool **(Fig. 19.1)**. The swimming pool types has a floor with a slope which is shallow at one end and a deep at the other end. Hydrotherapy pools are often completely levelled with railings inside the pool to facilitate better physiotherapy.

The hydrotherapy pool room has a plant room, filtration system, and some kind of environmental control to provide air heating and dehumidification. The water temperature in the pool should be maintained at 28–30°C.

The water should be treated properly with disinfectants, filtration and heating. It should be tested in the laboratory to make sure that there is no infection.

## Advantages of Hydrotherapy

- In a hydrotherapy pool, the patient remains warm throughout the session.

- Hydrotherapy helps to handle the heaviest patients with great ease.
- Hydrotherapy can treat cases that are traditionally difficult.
- Hydrotherapy is applied to treat impairments like pain, decreased strength and stiffness.
- Hydrotherapy is used for treatment of disabilities to improve posture and mobility **(Fig. 19.2)**.
- Hydrotherapy improves cardiovascular and respiratory functions.
- Hydrotherapy positively influences overall as well as local metabolism.
- Hydrotherapy can easily be adapted to patient's specific needs and can simply be applied in a progressive way from a non-weight bearing to a full weight bearing program.

### *Procedure of Treatment*

The patient is advised to bring own costumes, swimming caps, etc., and should have a light tiffin before the hydrotherapy session. The contraindications for hydrotherapy such as fever, open wound, skin infections, epilepsy, etc., should be checked before each session. Patient should be asked to remove foot wear and take a shower before and after each hydrotherapy session. Patient should be advised to drink water before and after every hydrotherapy session. Individualized attention should be given to each patient in the pool. Use of floaters, and other exercise gadgets are made in the pool as required. The duration of each treatment session, is kept to about half an hour.

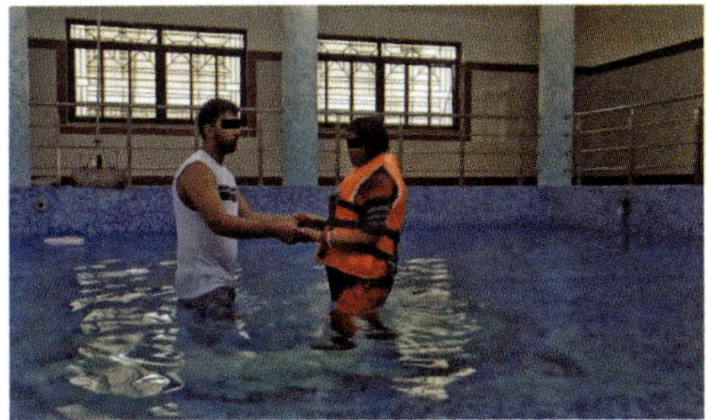

**Fig. 19.2:** Hydrotherapy to improve standing posture by stabilizing the knee through hydrostatic pressure.

### Therapeutic Effects and Uses of Hydrotherapy

a. **Strengthening of muscle:** Water provides a remarkable environment to produce very fine exercise progression. Muscles are strengthened by resistance offered by upward force (buoyancy), turbulence force, etc. Even manual resistance can be applied along with these forces inside water.
   **Uses:** Polyneuropathies.
b. **Endurance training:** Exercises in water improves both cardiorespiratory and muscular endurance, hence considered as an important treatment modality for patients with poor endurance.
   **Uses:** Ankylosing spondylitis.
c. **Joint mobility:** Relief of pain and muscle spasm by the warmth of the water and by the assistance of buoyancy, mobility of joints can be improved.
   **Uses:** Poly arthritis like rheumatoid arthritis.
d. **Coordination and balance:** The buoyancy of water relieves the patient from weight and makes the activities like walking and step climbing easy. The hydrostatic pressure exerted on unstable joints produces a strong proprioceptive stimulation and helps in restoring stability of joints and balance of body.
   **Uses:** Ataxic disorders like cerebellar ataxia.
e. **Pain relief:** The enhanced joint movement due to augmentation of muscular activities, combined with the warmth of water improves circulation and enable removal of waste metabolites and improves nutrition. This phenomenon combined with the effect of reduction of muscle spasm helps in reduction of pain.
   **Uses:** Low back pain.
f. **Swelling reduction:** The hydrostatic pressure, combined with enhanced blood

flow brought about by warmth of water and enhanced muscular contractions, help in reduction of swelling.

**Uses:** For stump edema.

## Contraindications and Precautions for Hydrotherapy

### *Contraindications*

- Infective wounds
- Hyperpyrexia
- Cardiac failure
- Deep vein thrombosis.
- Gastrointestinal disorder
- Hypo- or hypertension
- Epilepsy
- Low vital lung capacity
- Incontinence of bladder and bowel.

### *Precautions*

- Mentally retarded.
- Persons having fear for water.
- Persons wearing contact lens.
- Persons wearing hearing aids.
- Persons with cardiorespiratory anomalies such as angina pectoris.
- Small children.

# 20 CHAPTER

# Gait

## INRODUCTION

Gait is the style, manner, or a pattern of walking. The walking pattern or style may differ from individual to individual. It depends on the age, sex, mood, of an individual and may be affected by diseases and injuries. The body mass is propelled by the lower extremities, assisted by rotational movements of trunk and swinging of the upper extremities. It is the forward propulsion of the body by the lower extremities with the coordinated rotated movements of the body segment. The lower extremity support and carries the head, trunk and arm.

The head, neck, upper limb and trunk contributes to about 75% of body weight, among this head and upper limb contributes to about 25% of the total body weight, neck and trunk contributes to about 50% of the body weight, and lower extremities contribute to about 25% of the body weight. This activity requires more coordination, balance, kinesthetic sense and proper muscle strength.

### Definition

Normal human locomotion/normal gait, is the series of rhythmic alternating movements of the trunk and extremities, resulting in a forward progression of center of gravity. It is a cyclic motion of the body, called the gait cycle, which is measured from heel strike to heel strike of the same limb.

### Gait Cycle (Fig. 20.1)

The gait cycle consists of the phases such as: stance phase and swing phase as shown in **Figure 20.1.** There is also a period of double support, that occurs twice throughout one gait cycle. The relative contribution of different phases in the gait cycle are:

- **Stance phase—60% of the gait cycle:** The activities that occur, when the foot is in contact with the ground.
- **Swing phase—40% of the gait cycle:** The activities that occur, when the foot is not in contact with the ground.
- **Double support—20% of the gait cycle:** This is the time period, when both the feet are in contact with the ground.

In normal walking the stance phase contributes to 60% of the gait cycle and the swing phase to 40% of the cycle. When the one lower extremity begins its stance phase, the other lower extremity ends in the stance phase and moves to swing phase. **Tables 20.1 and 20.2** define activities, which occur during the stance phase and swing phase, as per the traditional method and Rancho Los Amigos (RLA) method [The Rancho Los Amigos Observational Gait Analysis system (Rancho OGA) is a standardized approach utilized to assess gait impairment for various diagnoses].

### Variables/Parameters in Gait Cycle

The temporal (time taken for the event) and spatial (distance covered in space)

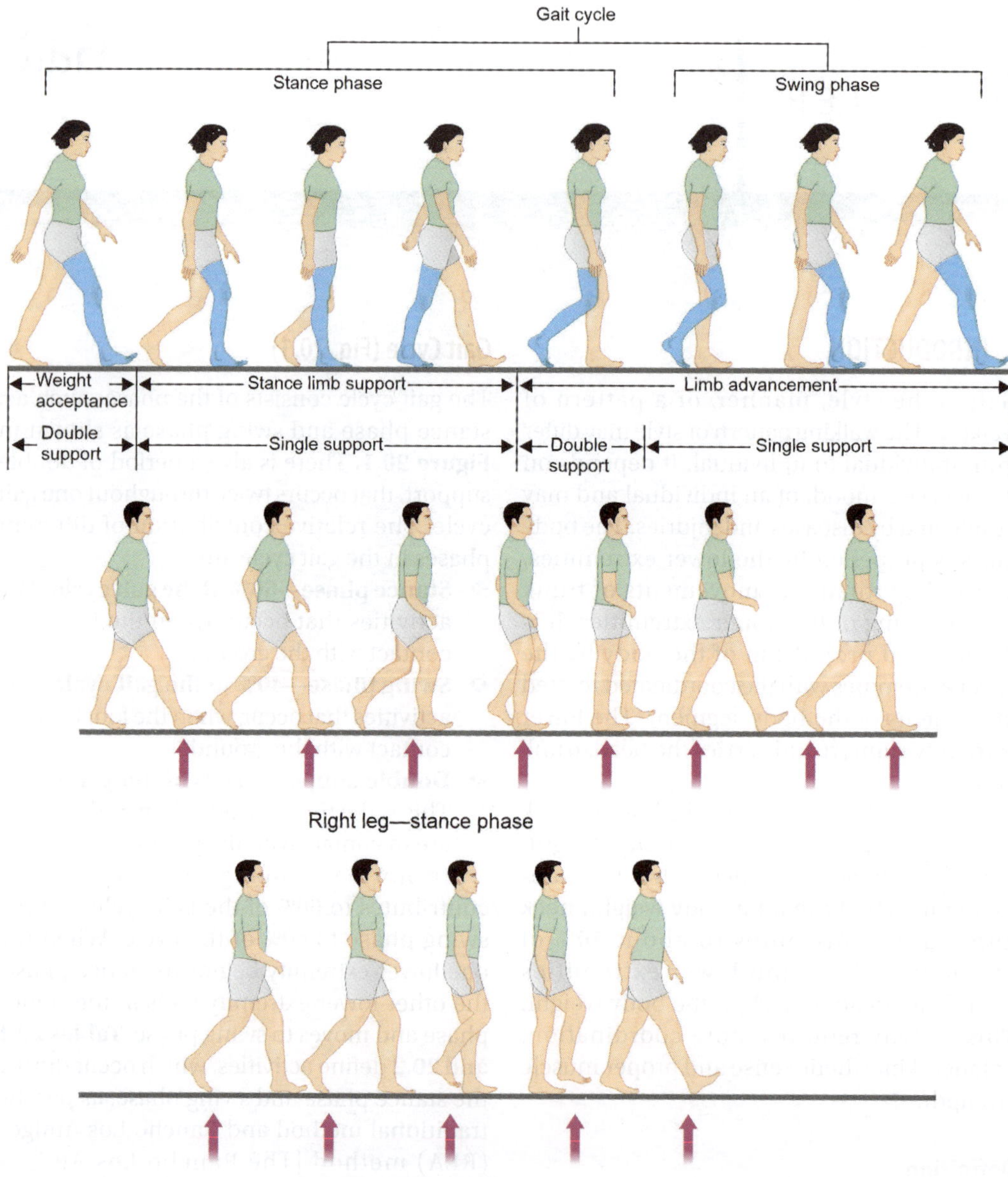


**Fig. 20.1:** Gait cycle and its phases.

parameters/variables of gait are important parameters, that that help the clinician identify normal and pathological gaits, and to provide gait training.

### *Temporal Parameters*

- **Stance time:** Time taken for the stance phase.
- **Swing time:** Time taken for the swing phase.

**Table 20.1:** Activities occurring during stance phase.

| *Traditional method* | *Rancho Los Amigo's (RLA) method* |
|---|---|
| 1. **Heel strike:** Heel of the loading extremity touches the ground. This is the beginning of the stance phase resulting in double support | 1. **Initial contact:** Heel of the leading extremity strike the ground |
| 2. **Foot flat:** The foot totally contacts the ground after the heel strike | 2. **Loading response:** Starts with the double support and it starts after the initial contact and continues till the contralateral extremity clears the ground |
| 3. **Mid-stance:** This is the stage where the weight is totally transmitted to the weight bearing lower extremity | 3. **Mid-stance:** Begins when the contralateral foot leaves the ground and continues until ipsilateral heel lifts off the ground. The body is supported by a single leg and remains in a straight line to the supporting limb |
| 4. **Heel-off:** This is the stage at which the heel of the stance phase lower extremity clears the ground after total weight-bearing | 4. **Terminal stance:** Begins from the end of mid-stance, when the heel leaves the floor and continues until the contralateral foot contacts the ground (initial contact of the contralateral limb) |
| 5. **Toe-off:** The stage at which the toe of the reference lower extremity clears the ground | 5. **Pre-swing:** This period begins, when the contralateral foot contacts the ground and continues until the ipsilateral foot leaves the ground |

**Table 20.2:** Activities occurring in swing phase.

| *Traditional method* | *Rancho Los Amigo's (RLA) method* |
|---|---|
| 1. **Acceleration:** It starts immediately from the toe-off of the reference lower extremity to the same extremity coming directly under the body | 1. **Initial swing:** It starts from the point of foot clearing the ground to the maximum knee flexion of the same extremity |
| 2. **Mid-swing:** When the swinging lower extremity swings directly beneath the body | 2. **Mid-swing:** It starts from the maximum knee flexion to the vertical position of the tibia |
| 3. **Deceleration:** It starts from the limb, which swings beneath the body to the knee extension and the preparation for the heel strike | 3. **Terminal swing:** It is the period from the tibia vertical position to the preparation of the initial contact of the heel |

- **Time for double support:** This is the time in one gait cycle, when both feet are supported on the ground.
- **Step time**: This is the time, that elapses from heel strike of one leg to the next heel strike of the opposite leg.
- **Stride time:** The time taken between two corresponding heel strikes in the same leg.
- **Cadence**: The number of steps taken in one minute. The normal value of cadence is: 80–130 steps per minute with an average value of 116 steps/min in adult female and 110 steps/min in adult males.

**Determination of Cadence**

- **Step length:** Larger the step length results in reduction in cadence, and the shorter the step length vice versa.
- **Gender:** Normally, in females the cadence is more due to their shorter step length and it is reverse in male. In normal walking the cadence in female is 116 and in male is 110.
- **Speed of walking:** The cadence depends on the speed of walking. In normal walking the cadence is between 80–130. If it goes more than 180 it is said to be running and if it falls below 70 is called slow walking. The

speed (velocity - meter/minute) of walking = Step length (m) × Cadence (steps/min). Average walking speed at a step length of 75 cm (0.75 m) and a cadence of 110 steps = 0.75 m × 110 = 82.5 meter/min.

### *Spatial Parameters (Fig. 20.2)*

#### Step Length

The distance from heel strike of one limb to corresponding next heel strike of the other limb. The normal step length in adult female is about 65 cm and in adult male is about 75 cm.

#### Stride Length

This is the distance between two consecutive heel strikes of the same leg. The average value of stride length for adult female is: 1.28 meter and for adult male is 1.46 meter.

#### Stride Width/Width of the Walking Base

This is the transverse distance between centers of right and left heels during normal walking. The normal value being: 5–10 cm.

#### Degree of Toe Out

This is the angle between the line of progression (line joining the centers of heels on the same side) and long axis of the foot. The normal value is about 5-7°, which may decrease in fast walking.

## Characteristics of Normal Gait

Normal walking has the following six characteristics such as:

- **Upward displacement of center of gravity:** The center of gravity of human body moves in a sinusoidal path in sagittal plane, with maximum upward displacement occurring during mid-stance and maximum downward displacement occurring during double support. The amount of displacement is about 5 cm.
- **Horizontal displacement of center of gravity:** The center of gravity which remains at the center of the body during double support, gets displaces from side to side (i.e., from one limb to other at mid-stance phases). The maximum displacement in the horizontal plane from right to left is about 5 cm.
- **Pelvic dip/rotation of pelvis in coronal plane:** During normal walking, the pelvis dips by about 5° on the swing phase side, which is counteracted by contraction of gluteus medius of the stance limbs with a reverse action, so that pelvis rotates about the same degrees over the femur of the stance limb, to assist effective ground clearance of the swing side limb.
- **Knee flexion during stance phase:** Shortly after heel strike, flexion of the knee begins and continues, during the early part of the stance phase, until approximately 20° of knee flexion is reached. This knee flexion, helps to smooth out the path of the center of gravity, by preventing its upward displacement.
- **Width of the walking base:** The distance between the mid points of successive heel contacts of each limb, called width of

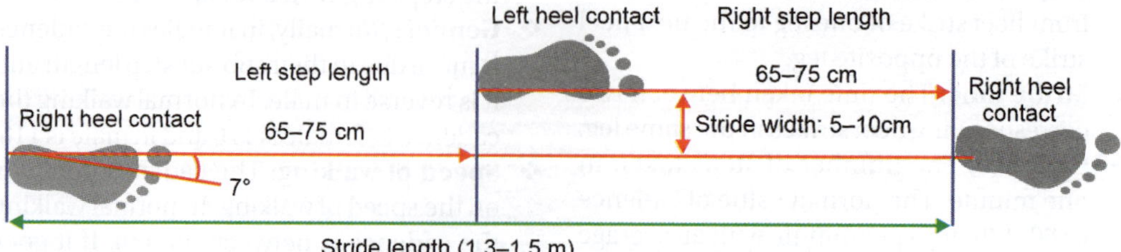


**Fig. 20.2:** The spatial parameters of normal gait.

the walking base normally has a value of 5–10 cm. Such narrow walking base helps to minimize the lateral displacement of center of gravity during normal walking.

- **Cadence:** The number of steps taken in a minute, which normally ranges from 80–130 steps/min. If the cadence increases, walking turns into running.

## Determinants of Gait

Though, description of the gait mainly focusses on the functioning of the lower extremities, however, apart from the lower extremities participation in gait, other events are happening to achieve the proper gait pattern. There is the coordinated movement of the trunk, upper limb, head to render the good gait pattern.

The determinants of gait are supposed to represent the adjustments made by pelvis, hip, knee and ankle/foot, that helps to minimize the movements of body's center of gravity, resulting in an energy efficient gait. These determinants help for the followings:

- Minimizes the vertical and lateral displacement of body's center of gravity.
- Decreases energy expenditure.
- Makes the gait more efficient.

The six determinants of gait are:

- **Rotation of pelvis in transverse plane:** The pelvis rotates in transverse plane up to an angle of 8° total, i.e., 4 degrees in a forward direction over the swing limb, and 4° in a backward direction over the stance limb.

  The forward rotation occurs during the relative extremity in swing phase. The forward rotation starts during the acceleration and ends in deceleration. During the midswing the pelvis comes to the neutral position, meanwhile opposite pelvis goes for backward rotation. After the midstance of the opposite extremity, there will be sudden dropping of the COG level. The forward and backward rotations help to prevent further reduction of the COG level. During deceleration the lower extremity lengthens and the same time the stance phase lower extremity (midstance) also relatively lengthened. The same time lengthening of both the lower extremities prevent the further reduction of the COG. The lengthening of the legs is possible due to the forward and backward rotation of the pelvis.

  **Result:** Forward and backward rotations help to minimize the hyper-reduction of the COG.

- **Lateral pelvic tilt (drop of pelvis in the frontal plane):** The pelvis that tilts laterally by an angle of 5° on the swing side, is controlled by contraction of gluteus medius on the supported side, thereby helping in the prevention of too much upward displacement of body's center of gravity.

  During the midstance period the COG reaches the peak level and the total body is supported by one lower extremity. To reduce the COG level, opposite side, i.e., swing phase pelvis tilts laterally, so that the COG comes little down, meanwhile the stance phase hip abductors helps to prevent the swing phase side pelvis drop.

  **Result:** Lateral pelvic tilt helps to reduce the COG level during the midstance period.

- **Knee flexion during stance phase:** It occurs to prevent excessive upward displacement of the body's center of gravity, as the body is carried forward over the stance limb. This determinant helps to reduce the COG level during the midstance period. If the swinging lower extremity knee remains in extended position, the COG still more increases in the midstance phase.

  **Result:** Knee flexion helps to reduce the COG level during the midstance period.

- **Knee, ankle and foot interactions:** The combined movements of knee, ankle and foot prevent the abrupt changes in the vertical displacement of the center of gravity from downward to upward direction.

The knee, ankle-foot interaction prevent the abrupt hike of the upward displacement of the COG when the foot passes from the heel strike to foot flat. Normally, after the heel strike huge upward displacement of COG occurs. To reduce that, there is some interaction between the knee, ankle, foot takes place (knee flexion, ankle plantar flexion, foot pronation) and also the same interaction takes place during the midstance to heel off. After the midstance there is sudden dropping of COG. To prevent the sudden drop of COG there is some changes happening in the knee, ankle and foot (ankle plantar flexion, knee extension, foot supination).

**Results:** Knee, ankle and foot interactions prevents abrupt changes in vertical displacement of COG.

- **Physiological valgus of knee:** This reduces the width of the walking base, due to which minimal lateral displacement of the pelvis is required, to shift the COG, from one lower extremity to another over the base of support.
- **Lateral displacement of the pelvis:** The pelvis that displaces laterally over the stance limbs can be kept to a minimum by a narrow walking base. By keeping the walking base narrow, little lateral movement of the pelvis is required to preserve balance.

These determinants are much more helpful to keep the COG in the minimal level to produce the efficient gait. First four determinants are helpful to maintain the vertical raising of the COG to a minimum. The fifth and the sixth determinant reduces the sideways movement of the COG. In normal walking pattern vertical displacement of the COG produces the sinusoidal curve. This is drawn by marking the COG level in each phase and the line connecting all the points gives a wavy curve called as sinusoidal curve **(Fig. 20.3)**. Disturbance in this curve results due to some pathology.

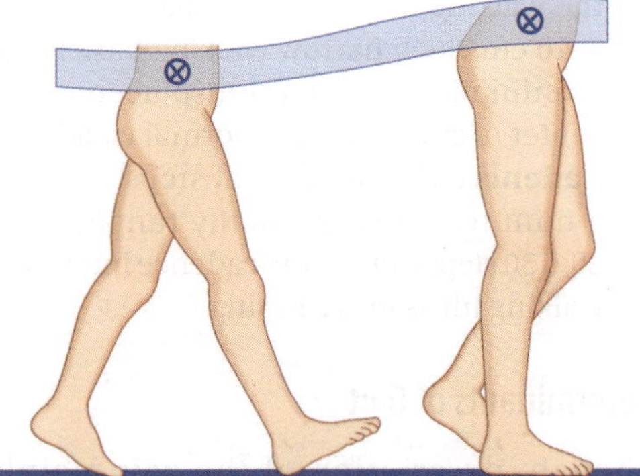

**Fig. 20.3:** Sinusoidal curve.

## Biomechanics of Normal Gait

Biomechanics of gait cycle refers to movements and forces of the lower extremities during walking.

This has two components such as:

### *Kinetics*

It is defined as the forces acting on the body, that are responsible for the movement. The forces are:

- Forces acting on the foot by the supporting surface (ground reaction force).
- Forces acting in the joints.
- Forces produced by the contracting muscles.
- Moments produced by the muscles crossing the joints.
- Mechanical power generated/absorbed by the muscles.
- Energy pattern of the body while walking.

### *Kinematics*

This is the term used to describe movements, without considering the internal or external forces that caused such movements. It includes:

- Positions of body segment.
- Velocity of body segments.
- Acceleration of body segments.

The kinematics and kinetic factors of normal gait in terms of joint motions and muscle actions are discussed below:

#### Initial Contact (Heel Strike)

| Joints | Kinematics/joint motion | Kinetic/muscles involved and nature of contraction |
|---|---|---|
| Hip | 20–30° flexion | Hip extensors contract eccentrically and hip flexors contract concentrically |
| Knee | 5° flexion | Eccentric contraction of quadriceps |
| Ankle | Neutral position | Concentric to eccentric contraction of dorsiflexors |

#### Loading Response (Foot Flat)

| Joints | Kinematics/joint motion | Kinetic/muscles involved and nature of contraction |
|---|---|---|
| Hip | Gradual extension | Concentric contraction of hip extensors |
| Knee | 10–15° of knee flexion | Eccentric contraction of quadriceps and concentric contraction of knee flexors |
| Ankle | Rapid plantar-flexion to 10° | Eccentric contraction of dorsiflexors |

#### Midstance

| Joints | Kinematics/joint motion | Kinetic/muscles involved and nature of contraction |
|---|---|---|
| Hip | Extended | Concentric contraction of hip extensors |
| Knee | 5° of knee flexion | Eccentric contraction of quadriceps |
| Ankle | Gradual dorsiflexion | Eccentric contraction of plantar flexors and concentric contraction of dorsiflexors |

#### Terminal Stance (Heel Off)

| Joints | Kinematics/joint motion | Kinetic/muscles involved and nature of contraction. |
|---|---|---|
| Hip | Extends until a maximum of 10° extension | Concentric contraction of hip extensors and eccentric contraction of hip flexors |
| Knee | Flexes from 5° of flexion | Eccentric contraction of quadriceps and concentric contraction of knee flexors |
| Ankle | Gradual dorsiflexion until a maximum of 10° dorsiflexion, before beginning to plantarflex | Eccentric followed by concentric contraction of plantar flexors |

#### Pre-swing (Toe Off)

| Joints | Kinematics/joint motion | Kinetic/muscles involved and nature of contraction |
|---|---|---|
| Hip | Begins to flex before foot leaves the ground | Concentric contraction of hip flexors |
| Knee | Begins to flex rapidly | Eccentric contraction of quadriceps |
| Ankle | Begins to plantarflex rapidly before foot leaves the ground | Concentric contraction of plantar flexors |

#### Early Swing (Acceleration)

| Joints | Kinematics/joint motion | Kinetic/muscles involved and nature of contraction |
|---|---|---|

| Hip | Gradually flexes | Concentric contraction of hip flexors |
|---|---|---|
| Knee | Rapid knee flexion until a maximum of about 60° | Eccentric contraction of quadriceps and concentric contraction of knee flexors |
| Ankle | Continues to plantarflex until a maximum of 20° before moving back towards a neutral position | Eccentric contraction of dorsiflexors, then concentric contraction of dorsiflexors and eccentric contraction of plantar flexors |

### Midswing

| Joints | Kinematics/joint motion | Kinetic/muscles involved and nature of contraction |
|---|---|---|
| Hip | Continues to flex until a maximum of just over 30° of hip flexion | Concentric contraction of hip flexors |
| Knee | Begins to extend | Eccentric contraction of flexors |
| Ankle | Maintains a neutral position | Concentric contraction of dorsiflexors |

### Late Swing/Deceleration

| Joints | Kinematics/joint motion | Kinetic/muscles involved and nature of contraction |
|---|---|---|
| Hip | Hip is flexed to around 30° | Concentric contraction of flexors and eccentric contraction of hip extensors |
| Knee | Extends until full extension, and flexes just slightly before initial contact | Eccentric, followed by concentric contraction of knee flexors |
| Ankle | Maintains a neutral position | Concentric contraction of dorsiflexors |

## Gait Deviation

A gait deviation is an abnormality in the gait cycle that can affect the trunk, hip, knee, or ankle joint. Gait deviations can stem from increased age and/or pathologies involving neuromuscular and musculoskeletal systems, causing pain, weakness and deformities in the lower limbs. The common gait deviations are briefly discussed below.

### *Gait Deviation Due to Musculoskeletal Pathology*

#### Trendelenburg Gait/Lurching Gait

Trendelenburg gait occurs when the gluteus medius is weak. The weakness of the involved side causes a contralateral pelvic drop during swing phase. This contralateral drop of pelvis might cause the quadratus lumborum, on the stance leg, to bring the pelvis back to neutral, by bending of the trunk towards the stance side. The patient walks with lateral trunk bending towards the weaker side, not only to prevent drop of pelvis on swing side, but also to reduce the weight arm over the stance hip, promoting efficiency of gluteus medius to prevent pelvic drop,

#### Posterior Lurch Gait

Posterior lurch gait is when the trunk leans posteriorly with a hyperextended hip, especially during the loading response due to a weak gluteus maximus. Such posterior bending brings the line of gravity to the posterior aspect of hip, producing extension moment of the hip.

#### Vaulting

In this type of gait, the patient walks with raising of heel on the affected side, to compensate for shortening of the affected lower limb.

#### Antalgic Gait

Antalgic gait is due to pain in the lower extremities that results in a limp that is associated with a shortened stance phase relative to the swing phase. This gait deviation, asymmetry, can be caused by issues that originate in the trunk, hip, knee, or ankle.

**Hand to Knee Gait**

This deviation of gait occurs due to weakness/ paralysis of the quadriceps on the affected side. The person uses his/her own hand to stabilize the knee during stance phase.

## *Gait Deviations Due to Nervous System Pathology*

**Hemiplegic/Circumductory Gait**

It is characterized by unilateral leg extension and circumduction, in which the paretic leg performs a lateral motion (circumduction) during the swing phase **(Fig. 20.4)**.

**Scissoring Gait**

When spasticity in the adductors is marked it results in a scissoring gait where the legs are crossed in the scissors-like pattern **(Fig. 20.5)**.

**Crouch Gait**

This gait is found in children of spastic cerebral palsy, where the child walks with hip and knees flexion and ankle dorsiflexion **(Fig. 20.6)**.

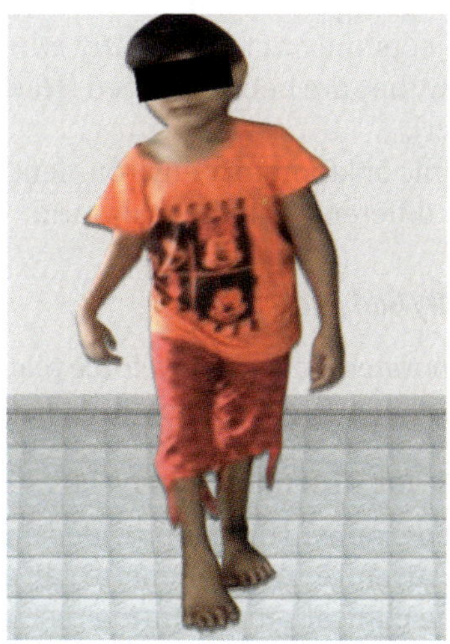

**Fig. 20.4:** Infantile hemiparetic child walking in circumductory gait.

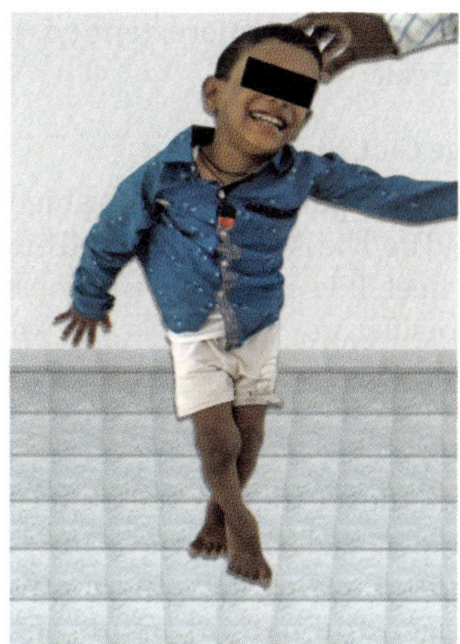

**Fig. 20.5:** Spastic CP child walking in scissoring gait.

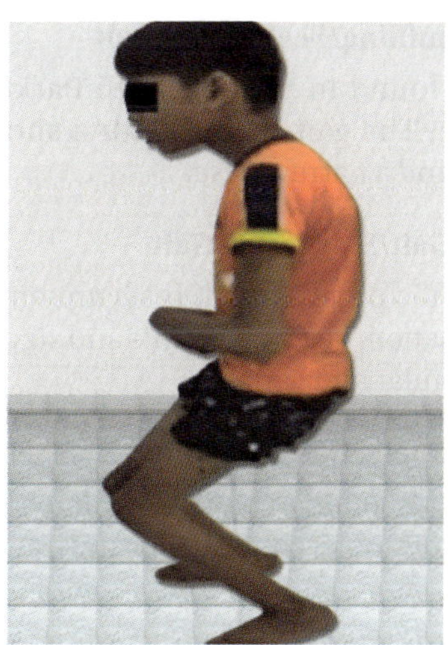

**Fig. 20.6:** Cerebral palsy child walking in crouch gait.

**Jump Knee Gait**

This gait is also found in children of spastic cerebral palsy, where the child walks with bilateral hips and knees flexion and ankle plantar flexion.

**Stiff Knee Gait**

This is found in children of spastic cerebral palsy, with ankle equinus, where the knee remains extended/hyperextended, causing stiff knee gait.

### Steppage Gait/Slapping Gait

In this gait, the patient lifts the leg higher than usual and he/she is unable to stand or walk on his/her heel. It is caused by weakness in the ankle dorsiflexors. This gait is also known as a slapping gait.

### Waddling Gait

This results due to weakness of gluteus medius muscles, that leads the pelvis on the swinging side to drop during gait. In an attempt to counteract, the patient bends the trunk towards the other side, resulting in the gait to appear waddling.

### Slow Shuffling/Festinating Gait

This is found in patients with Parkinson's disease. The gait is slow with a short step length and a narrow base.

### Ataxic Gait/Staggering Gait

The gait is broad based, insecure and lacks coordination. Leg movements and step length are irregular and variable.

### Hyperkinetic Gait

This gait is found in patients with dyskinesia, such as dystonia, chorea, ballismus, athetosis, etc.

### Athetoid Dance Gait

In this the child uses ATNR, a primitive reflex to promote activities in stance and swing phases, resulting in a dance pattern of walking.

## Gait Analysis

When, a person is not able to walk normally, or has difficulty in walking, either due to neuromuscular/musculoskeletal diseases/disorders, then in this case the walking pattern (gait) of the person should be analyzed and some appropriate exercises, walking aids and orthotic devices should be provided to make walking (gait) energy efficient. The methods of gait analysis are as follows:

### *Visual/Observational Gait Analysis*

This is the simplest form of gait analysis made by the unaided human eye. This, of course, neglects the remarkable abilities of the human brain to process the data received by the eye. Visual gait analysis is, in reality, the most complicated and versatile form of analysis available. Many clinicians include the observation of a subject's gait as part of their clinical examination. Visual gait analysis is entirely subjective and the quality of the analysis depends on the skill of the person performing it.

The limitations of this method are:

- ❖ It is transitory, giving no permanent record.
- ❖ The eye cannot observe high-speed events.
- ❖ It is only possible to observe movements, not forces.
- ❖ It depends entirely on the skill of the individual observer.
- ❖ It is subjective and it can be difficult to avoid assessor bias if the patient is undergoing treatment.
- ❖ Subjects may act differently when they know they are being watched (Hawthorne effect).
- ❖ A clinic or laboratory environment may be very different than the real world.

### *Laboratory Gait Analysis*

It incorporates videography, force plates, etc., to gather kinematic and kinetic data.

#### Methods for Kinematic Analysis

- ❖ **Videography:** This has provided one of the most useful enhancements to gait analysis in the clinical setting during recent years. Gait examination by video recording is not an objective method, since it does not provide quantitative data in the form of numbers. This helps to overcome two of the limitations of visual gait analysis such as—the lack of a permanent record and the difficulty of observing high-speed events. Two-dimensional (2D) and three-dimensional (3D) video-based motion analysis systems are available for gait analysis; however, their use is limited due to challenges with providing accurate data. It has the following advantages:

- It can be used as a record for future reference.
- The patient can be demonstrated about his/her gait pattern by showing the video of his walking.

- **Electrogoniometry:** Electrogoniometers provide an affordable means of measuring joint motion during walking. Early electro-goniometer designs included two rigid links connected by a potentiometer that converted movement into an electrical signal that was proportional to the degree of movement. Recently, designs use a flexible shaft and two small end blocks that are affixed to the proximal and distal segments of the joint.
- **Optical motion analysis systems:** These are computerized motion analysis systems, where markers are placed on body segments such as the trunk, hip, knee, and ankle that are tracked by automated systems **(Figs. 20.7A and B)**. Motion analysis systems primarily use either active [light emitting diodes (LED)] or passive markers (that requires an external source of illumination) for tracking motion.

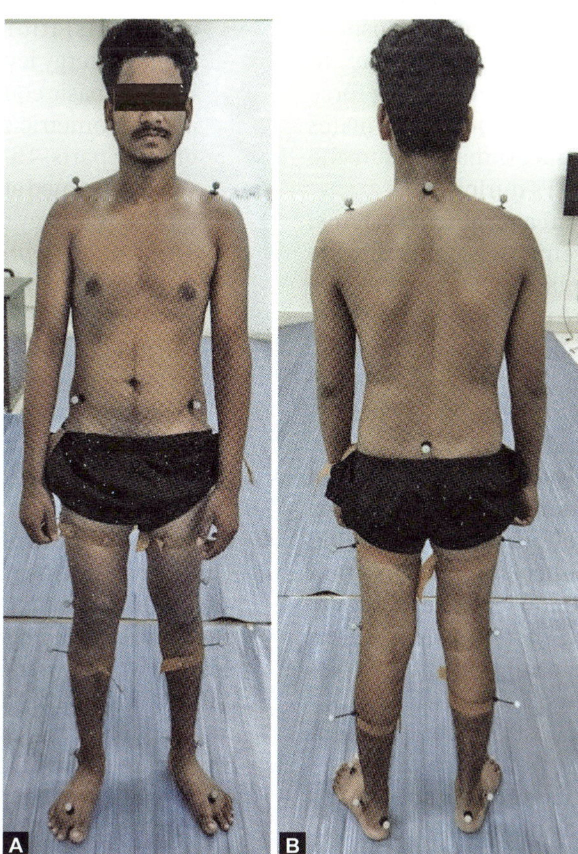


**Figs. 20.7A and B:** (A) Anterior view; (B) Posterior view.

- **Electromagnetic motion analysis systems:** The challenges with optical tracking systems is that T-motion analysis cameras need to be able to "see" the markers to track their position and subsequently calculate kinematic data. This alternative motion analysis technology employs electromagnetic tracking capabilities to determine the 3D coordinates of location and angulation of each sensor.

**Methods for Kinetic Analysis**

- **Force plate analysis:** This method focuses on analysis of the forces involved in gait, which include ground (floor) reaction forces (GRFs), joint torques, center of pressure (COP), center of mass (COM), mechanical energy, moments of force, power, work, joint reaction forces, and intrinsic foot pressure. The analysis usually starts with the forces being applied to the foot, which is determined by a force plates embedded in the floor. These plates contain load transducers that measure the COP, COM, and GRFs during gait.
- **Plantar pressure measurement systems:** Pressure measurement systems may be used with force plates. Plantar pressure measurements are used most commonly in gait analysis to determine the pressure distribution under the foot such as—foot-to-ground contact, foot-to-shoe contact, and shoe-to-ground contact.
- **Energy cost analysis (measurement of energy consumption) during gait:** Energy expenditure is an important consideration in gait analyses, particularly in neurological conditions, where muscular resources of energy may be low. There are three general approaches in determining energy costs which are as follows:
  - Physiological cost of energy expenditure.
  - Mechanical energy analysis.
  - Heart rate data analysis.
- **Physiological cost of energy expenditure:** It is the measurement of oxygen uptake/ maximum oxygen consumption volume ($VO_{2max}$), during walking, through open loop spirometry, in which exhaled air is sampled and analyzed for its oxygen content. Physiological cost analysis methods are most useful in comparing the energy cost of walking with normal values, which helps for determining the effects of energy costs of interventions such as use of orthoses, prosthesis, and walking aids.
- **Mechanical energy cost analysis:** There are two methods of measurement of mechanical energy costs such as:
  1. *Estimation of energy expenditure from the kinematic data:* The mass of the moving part and the COM are used to calculate the potential energy and translational and rotational kinetic energy levels of each body part through basic equations of motion and anthropometric constants for masses of body parts. The difference between values obtained at each time increment indicates energy cost.
  2. *The kinetic approach:* In this energy changes in body parts between subsequent instants in time are calculated from—the product of forces on each end of the joint and the velocity of the point of application, and from the muscle power, which are the product of each muscle moment and the angular velocity of the body part.
- **Energy expenditure from heart rate data:** This focuses on the measurement of heart rate during ambulation. The physiological cost index, which determines the relative costs of walking per unit distance walked, calculated as the difference between walking heart rate and the resting heart rate divided by average speed, is a method of calculation of energy expenditure from heart rate. The total heart beat index

provides an alternative approach for determining the relative energy efficiency of walking. It is calculated by dividing the total (cumulative) number of heartbeats during exercise by the total distance traveled in a given time period.

## Gait Training

The following procedures are be followed:

- After a thorough analysis, of the impairments of gait, the physiotherapist/clinician should make a problem list of kinematic impairments, such as decreased ROM in knee joint, that affects the ground clearance in swing phase, kinetic impairments, such as weak ankle dorsiflexors, that affects positioning of ankle during heel strike, etc.
- Assistive devices such as orthosis, walking aids/parallel bar/gait ladder **(Fig. 20.8A)**, etc., if required, should be selected as per the need of the patient.
- Gait training mats, postural mirror, gait ladder, etc., should be used to facilitate training.
- If training is to increase endurance of walking, heart rate, respiratory rate, and indices for energy consumption should be noted, before, during and after training and are documented.
- Support to the patient as required, should be provided by the therapist, either by manual contact or using belts/clothes, wrapped round the patient's pelvis **(Fig. 20.8B)**.

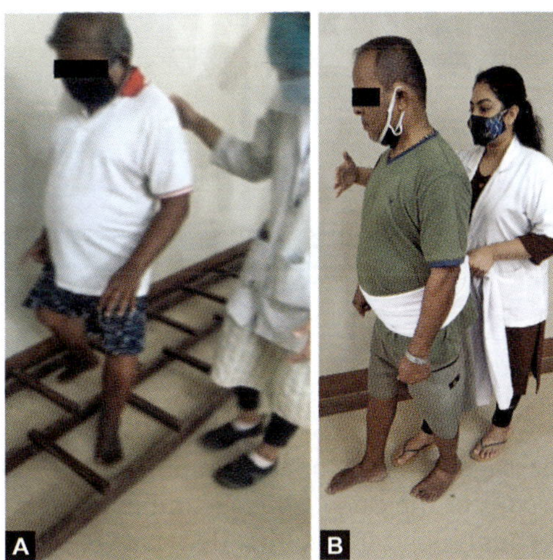


**Figs. 20.8A and B:** (A) Gait training on gait ladder; (B) Using bedsheet wraps for a patient of Parkinson disease.

# 21 CHAPTER Massage

## INTRODUCTION

Massage is the scientific manipulation of soft tissues of the body (muscle and connective tissues) to aid in healing, decrease tension, relieve stress, promote relaxation, reduce swelling and enhance function.

It is one of the ancient methods used for healing of soft tissues. Massage therapy has been used in many cultures around the world for a long time. Presently, the therapy has received wide acceptance among clinicians for recognized therapeutic effects.

### Classification of Massage

Massage is classified into various types on the basis of character of the technique, depth of the soft tissues manipulated as well as part of the body massaged.

**A. Classification on the basis of character of the technique**

- **Stroking massage:** The uninterrupted linear movement of hand along the whole length of segment is called stroking. It is further classified into:
  - *Superficial stroking:* It is the rhythmical movement of hand or parts thereof over the skin with the lightest amount of pressure in order to obtain sensory stimulation. It can be applied from proximal to the distal or vice versa **(Fig. 21.1)**.

    Uses: Used to induce relaxation of the segment/body.

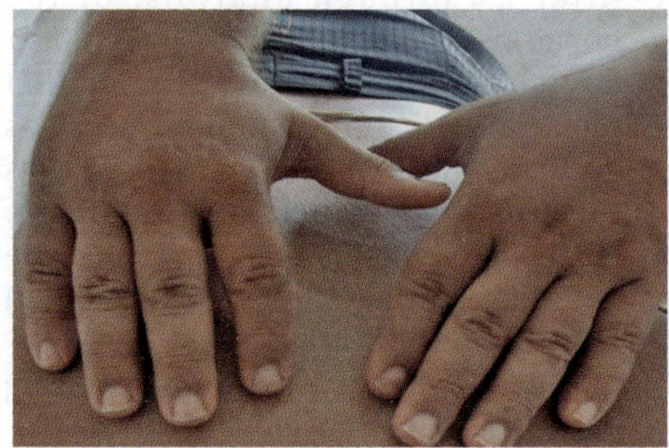

**Fig. 21.1:** Stroking massage.

  - *Efflurage (deep stroking):* Effleurage, a French word meaning "to skim" or "to touch lightly on", is a series of massage strokes used in Swedish massage to warm up the muscle before deep tissue work using petrissage. This is a soothing, stroking movement used at the beginning and the end of the facial and/or body massage. It is the movement of the palmar aspect of hand over the external surface of the body with constant moderate pressure, in the direction of the venous and lymphatic drainage **(Fig. 21.2)**.

    Uses: It aids relaxation, reduces stress, increases lymphatic and venous drainage.

- **Pressure manipulation/massage:**
  - *Kneading:* : In this group of techniques, the tissues are pressed down on to the underlying firm structure and intermittent pressure is applied in circular direction, parallel to the long axis of

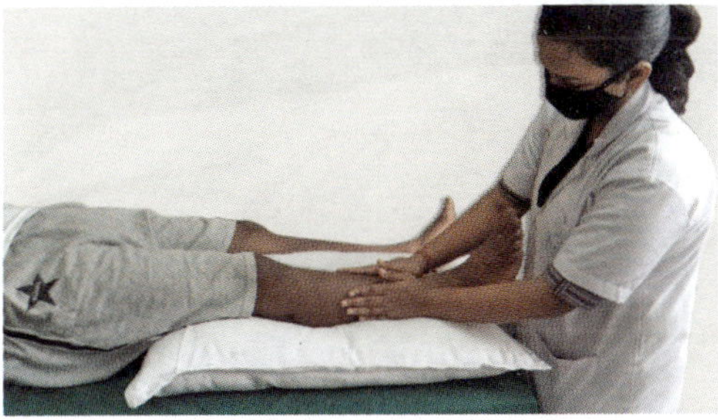

**Fig. 21.2:** Efflurage massage.

bone. It can produce many physiological effects, that include, increased capillarization, increased vasodilation, and increased tissue elasticity.

Uses: Used to increase flexibility of tight soft tissues, to decrease muscle spasm and pain and to reduce stress.

They are of the following types:

- Palmar kneading: Pressure is applied with the heel of palm **(Fig. 21.3)**.
- Elbow kneading: Pressure is applied with the olecranon process of elbow **(Fig. 21.4)**.
- Digital kneading: Pressure is applied with the fingers (finger kneading) or thumb (thumb kneading) **(Fig. 21.5)**.

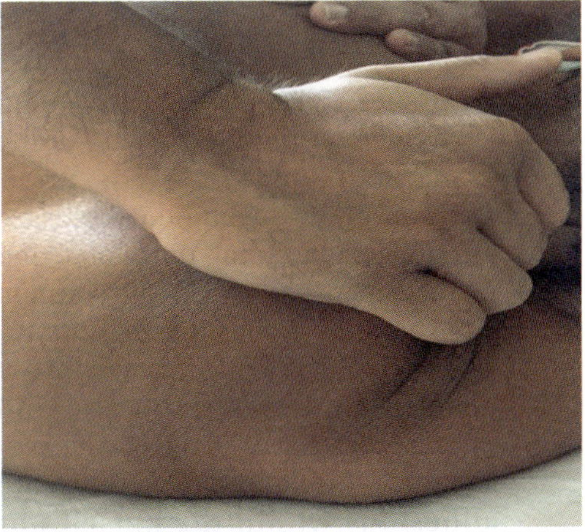

**Fig. 21.3:** Palmar kneading.

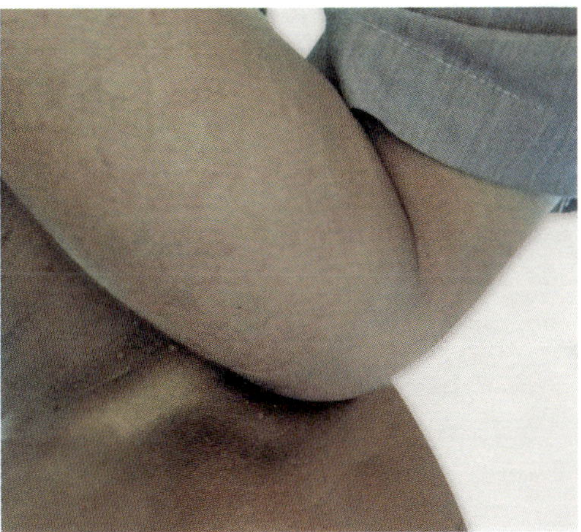

**Fig. 21.4:** Elbow kneading.

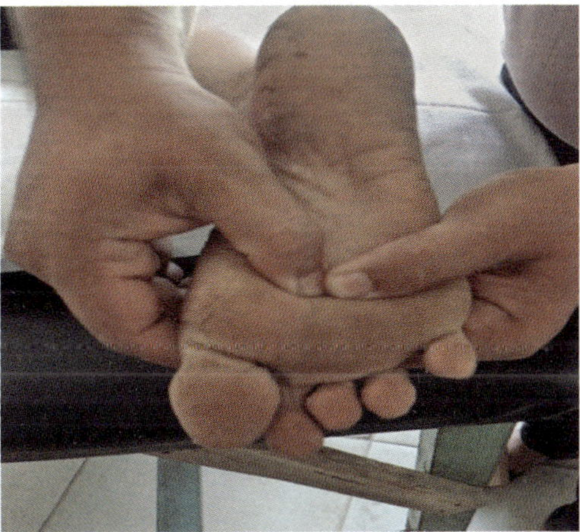

**Fig. 21.5:** Thumb kneading.

- Reinforced kneading: Both the hands, placed over one another, are used to apply pressure **(Fig. 21.6)**.

- *Petrissage:* In this technique, the tissues are grasped and lifted away from the underlying structures and intermittent pressure is applied to the tissues in the direction that is perpendicular to the long axis of the bone.

  Uses: It is used to improve blood circulation, loosen tight muscles and enhance the flexibility/joint range of motion.

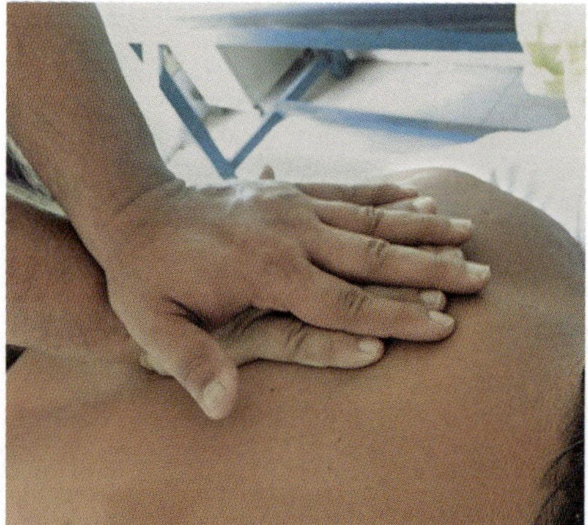
**Fig. 21.6:** Reinforced kneading.

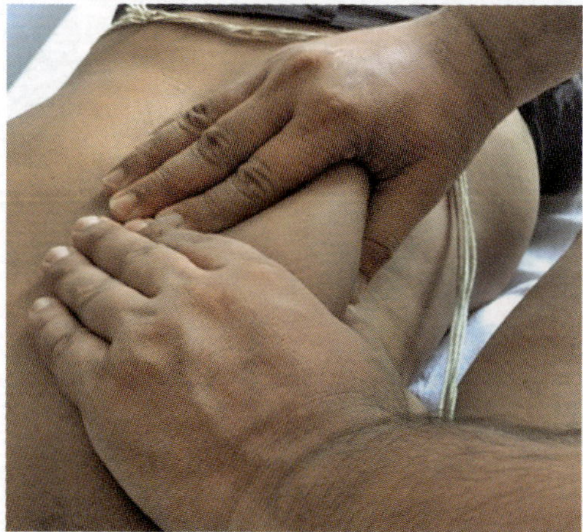
**Fig. 21.7:** Picking up massage.

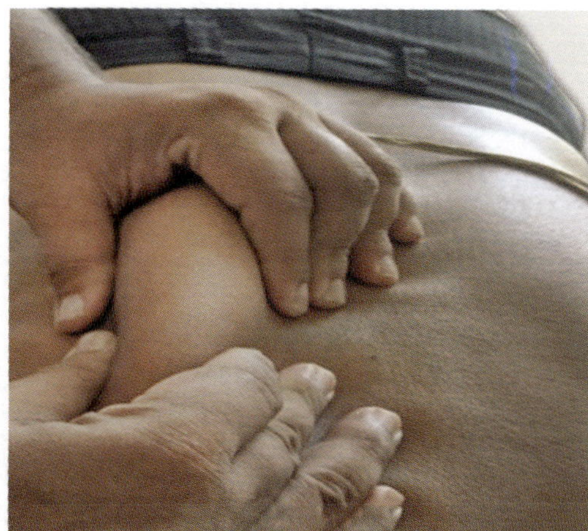
**Fig. 21.8:** Wringing massage.

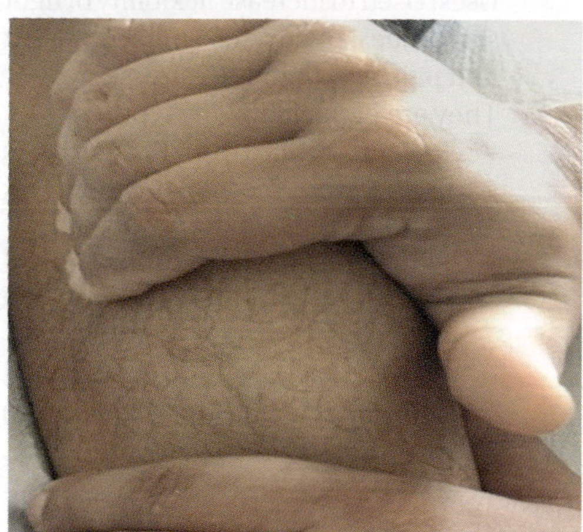
**Fig. 21.9:** Skin rolling.

They are of the following types:

- Picking up: In this technique, the tissues are lifted away from underlying structures, squeezed and then released using one or both the hands **(Fig. 21.7)**.
- Wringing: In this, the tissues are lifted away from the underlying structures, squeezed, twisted and then released, using both the hands **(Fig. 21.8)**.
- Skin rolling: The skin and fascia are lifted up with both the hands and moved over the subcutaneous tissues by keeping a roll of lifted tissue continuously ahead of the moving thumb **(Fig. 21.9)**.

- *Friction:* In this technique, the tissue are subjected to small range of to and fro movement performed with constant deep pressure of the finger or thumb.
  Uses: Friction is a massage technique used to increase circulation and release areas that are tight; particularly around joints and where there are adhesions within the muscles or tendons. It also prevents formation of adherent scars.

It is of the following types:
- Deep transverse friction: In this technique, to and fro movement is performed using the thumb or finger across the length of the structure **(Fig. 21.10)**.
- Circular friction: In this circular movements are given over the tissue using finger or thumb **(Fig. 21.11)**.

- *Myofascial release:* It is a technique that combines traction with varying amount of stretch to the muscles and underlying fascia, to produce a moderate sustained force in these tissues. The goal of this technique is to produce viscoelastic lengthening and plastic deformation of the fascia **(Figs. 21.12A and B)**.

  Uses: The technique is indicated for lengthening muscle and fascia, increase mobility between fascia layers, and to break adhesions. It also decreases pain and increases flexibility (ROM).

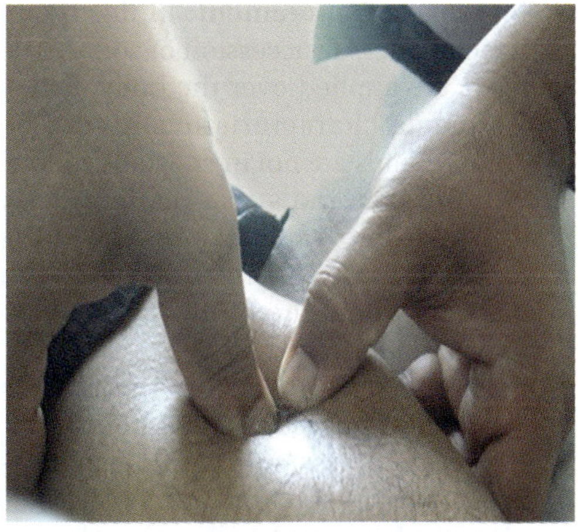

**Fig. 21.11:** Circular friction using thumb.

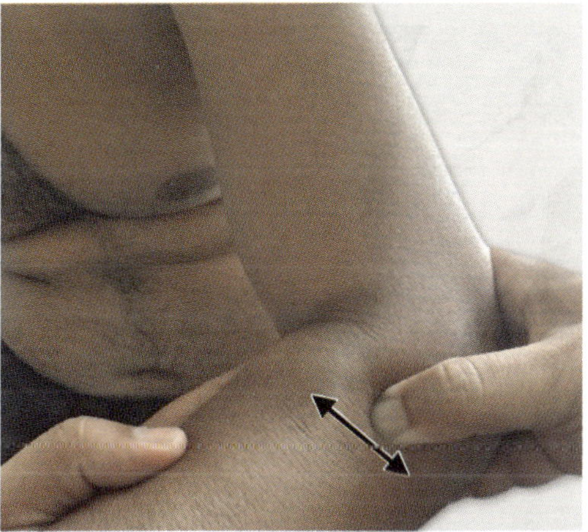

**Fig. 21.10:** DTFM, using thumb.

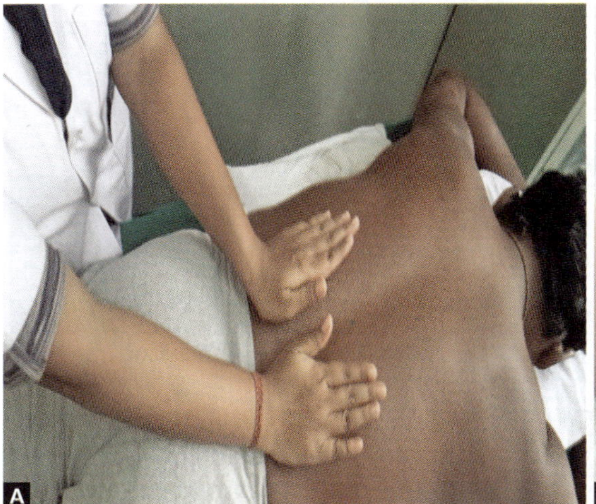


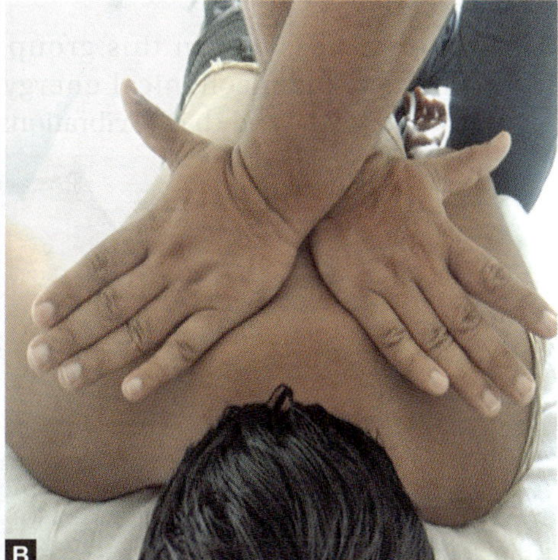


**Figs. 21.12A and B:** Myofascial release techniques.

- **Percussion/Tapotement:** In this group of techniques, a succession of soft, gentle blows are applied over the body, which produce a characteristic sound. The striking hands are not in constant contact with the skin and strike the body part at regular intervals. This results in the application of an intermittent touch and pressure to the body during these manipulations.
  *Uses:* It is used to loosen the muscle and fascia, increase ROM and flexibility, decrease soreness/stiffness. It also helps loosening secretion from the airways.
  It is of the following types:
  - *Clapping massage:* The technique is applied with the cupped hand **(Fig. 21.13)**.
  - *Hacking massage:* The technique is applied using ulnar border of the 5th, 4th and 3rd digits **(Fig. 21.14)**.
  - *Tapping massage:* The technique is applied using the pulp of the fingers **(Fig. 21.15)**.
  - *Beating:* The technique is applied using the anterior aspect of the clenched fist **(Fig. 21.16)**.
  - *Pounding:* The technique is applied using the medial aspect of the clenched fist **(Fig. 21.17)**.
- **Vibratory massage:** In this group of techniques, the mechanical energy is transmitted to the body by the vibrations of the distal part of upper limb, i.e., hand and/or fingers, which are in constant contact with the subjects skin, using the body weight and generalized co-contraction of the upper limb muscles.

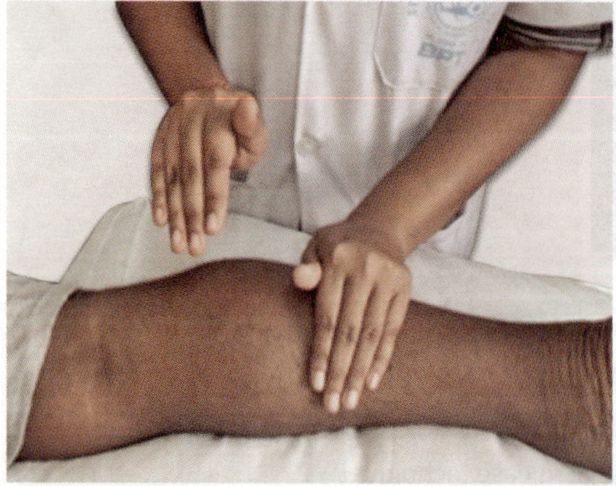

**Fig. 21.13:** Clapping massage.

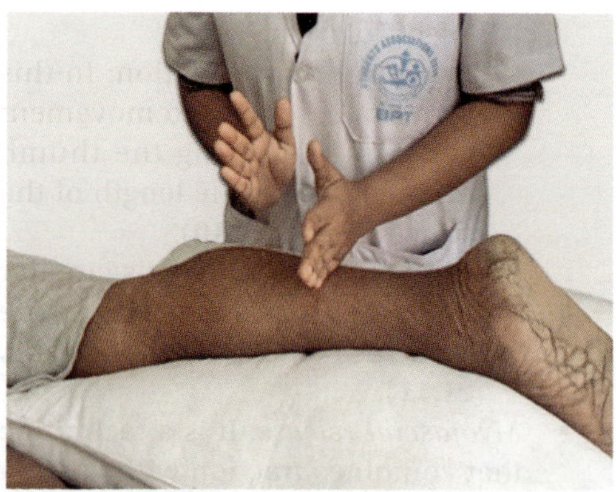

**Fig. 21.14:** Hacking massage.

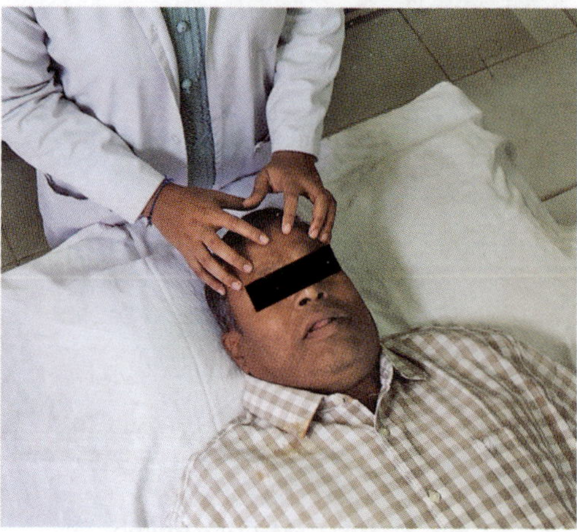

**Fig. 21.15:** Tapping massage.

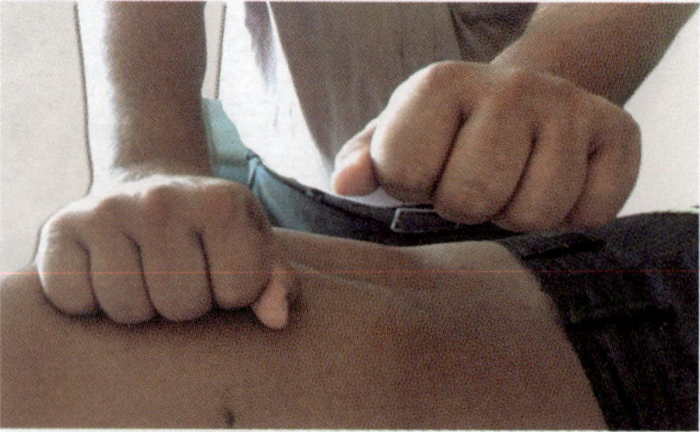

**Fig. 21.16:** Beating massage.

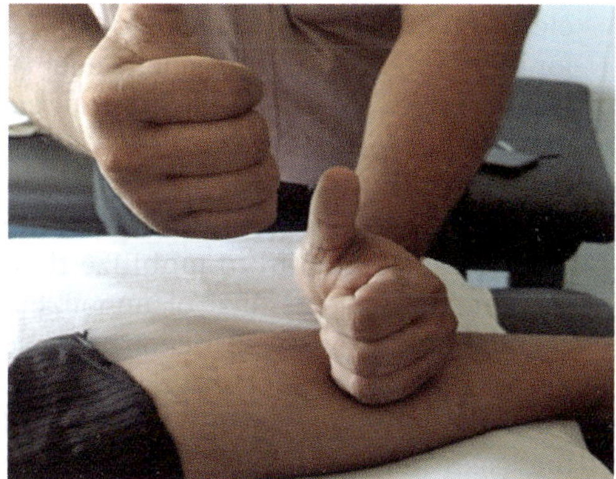

**Fig. 21.17:** Pounding massage.

This technique is mainly directed towards the lung and other hollow cavities.

*Uses:* Used to increase metabolism, increase ROM, improve vascularization, release trigger points, loosen secretions in the lungs.

They are of the following types:

- *Vibrations:* In this technique, the fine vibrations are produced, which tend to produce fine movement of hand in upwards and downward direction.
- *Shaking:* In this technique, coarse vibrations are produced, which tend to produce fine movement of hand in sideway direction.

**B. Classification on the basis of depth of tissue:**

- **Gentle/light massage:** The force applied during the maneuver are light, so that the effect of massage is confined to the superficial tissue only, e.g., stroking, tapping, etc.
- **Deep massage:** The forces applied during the massage are moderate to deep so that the effect of massage reaches to the deeper tissues like muscles, e.g., friction, kneading, etc.

**C. Classification on the basis of part of body massaged:**

- **Local massage:** When massage is administered in a particular area of the body segment, it is termed as local massage. For example, deep transverse friction massage for lateral epicondylitis.
- **General massage:** Massage applied to the entire body/large body segment, such as back or lower limb is usually termed as general massage.

**Swedish massage:** It is the use of five basic strokes put together in a sequence that will benefit the client. Pressure with a Swedish massage generally begins with light movements and increases gradually to medium to deeper pressure, and then returning to a lighter pressure to end body work in that specific area. The five basic strokes are—Effleurage, petrissage, friction, tapotement and vibration.

## Physiological Effects of Massage

### *Effect on Circulatory System*

The mechanical effect of massage help in pushing the venous blood and lymph towards the heart, resulting in prevention of pooling of blood and fluid in the distal body parts. The increased venous and lymphatic return also promotes increase of arterial blood flow, due to decrease of venous congestion, release of vasodilators, and activation of axon reflex.

### *Effect on Removal of Waste Metabolites*

As massage speeds up the lymphatic and venous flow, it promotes rapid disposal of the waste products of metabolism.

### *Effect on Nervous System*

Massage produces its effect on the sensory, motor as well as autonomic components of the nervous system, such as:

- **Sensory system:** Massage produces a strong sedative effect on the body when applied with slow rhythm. Deep stimulating massages, such as friction massage and kneading, etc., help in reducing pain due to the effects on the pain gate.

- **Motor system:** Massage has the effects of inhibition and facilitation on the motor function. Massage techniques that inhibit the motor system, causing a reduction of muscle tone include—petrissage and gentle effleurage. Massage techniques that increase the muscle tone, by stimulating the stretch reflex of the muscle spindle include—superficial stroking, tapping, hacking, etc.
- **Autonomic nervous system:** Massage has definite reflex effect and it can influence the functioning of visceral organ by modulating the autonomic nervous system through peripheral sensory stimulation.

### *Effect on Soft Tissues*

Massage has significant effect on certain properties of soft tissues, such as elasticity, plasticity and mobility. The adhesions present in the soft tissues are broken and mobility of soft tissues are promoted.

### *Effect on the Respiratory System*

Massage techniques, such as percussion, shaking, and vibration, assist in mobilization of secretions and drainage of the same towards the larger air ways, when combined with postural drainage. This results in efficient gaseous exchange in the lungs.

### *Effect on the Skin*

Massage techniques such as stroking (effleurage), petrissage help in improvement of nutrition to the skin through increase of blood flow. As a result, the skin becomes soft, supple and finer.

## Therapeutic Uses of Massage

Massage is used as a therapeutic modality to treat various conditions, such as:

- **Edema control:** Effleurage technique combined with elastic bandaging, elevation and active exercises is helpful for relief of both local and general edema. For example, lymphedema after radical mastectomy.
- **Scar mobilization:** Techniques, such as deep transverse friction, kneading massages are helpful to mobilize tight scar that restrict joint range of motion. For example, deep transverse friction massage to post-surgical scar after quadriceps plasty.
- **To increase circulation:** All types of massages and most particularly, petrissage and deep stroking and light digital kneading, etc., can be applied to increase circulation to tissues to promote repair. For example: Light finger kneading to margins of ulcers to increase blood flow to the ulcer, accelerating healing of the ulcer.
- **To reduce muscle spasm and pain:** Techniques, such as myofascial release, petrissage manipulation, etc., are found to be effective in reducing muscle spasm and pain. For example, spasm of paravertebral muscles in low back pain.
- **To induce general and local relaxation:** Techniques such as light stroking is helpful to induce general relaxation of the body and techniques, such as petrissage, myofascial release light percussion (tapping) are helpful to induce local relaxation of muscles. For example, light stroking is applied in the state of tension of body to induce relaxation, whereas light percussion (tapping) is applied to the forehead to induce local relaxation, in case of tension headache.
- **To mobilize secretions in lungs:** Certain percussion massage techniques such clapping, hacking and the vibratory techniques, such as vibration and shaking massages are applied to mobilize secretions in the lungs and drain them to the larger airways, when combined with postural drainage. For example, chest shaking in chronic bronchitis to drain secretions from the lungs.

## Contraindications of Massage

### *A. General Contraindications*

- High fever
- Hypersensitive skin
- Renal diseases
- Cardiac diseases
- Deep X-ray therapy
- Generalized osteoporosis
- Severe spasticity

### *B. Local Contraindications*

- Acute inflammation
- Skin diseases
- Recent fractures
- Open wound (Applicable to most of the techniques, except a few)
- Varicose veins
- Atherosclerosis
- Deep vein thrombosis.
- **Malignancy:** Where deep stroking, friction, kneading, etc., are not given to prevent metastasis.

## Massage Lubricants

Lubricants are used to decrease friction and control the amount of glide and drag, that occurs between the therapist's moving hands and the client's skin. The lubricants should be hypoallergenic and should be in the form of lotions, oils, creams and powders.

# 22 CHAPTER Traction

## DEFINITION

Traction is a form of medical treatment, in which weights and pulleys are used to gently pull or stretch an injured part of the body for a period of time.

It is a set of mechanisms for reducing fractured bones/correcting deformities due to musculoskeletal pathology or relieving pressure on the nerve roots in spine from a bulged disc, or stenosed intervertebral foramen.

The word traction is a derivative of the Latin word **"tractico"**, which means "a process of drawing or pulling". Various forms of spinal traction have been described, since the time of Hippocrates, for the relief of pain. James Cyriax popularized lumbar traction during the 1950s and 1960s as a treatment for disc protrusions, which is presently considered as a common modality for treating patients with cervical and lumbar disc bulge/spondylosis with arm/leg pain respectively.

### Types of Traction

Depending on the mode of application, traction are typed into the following types:

1. **Continuous traction:** Continuous or bed traction with very low load is applied for an extended period of time (may be several hours in a day and some times for 24 hours), to immobilize the injured part and provide rest to the patient. It helps in reduction of pain and muscle spasm, promoting reduction of dislocated joints and displaced fracture fragments.

In this type of traction, the traction force applied is not sufficient enough to overcome the coefficient of friction, [**The coefficient** of **friction (μ) is defined as the ratio of the frictional resistive force (F) to the applied perpendicular force (N) that pushes the objects together, i.e., μ = F/N. Lower the applied force, higher is the frictional resistance/coefficient of friction**], as the patient cannot tolerate such high force (sufficient to overcome the coefficient of friction) applied for hours/days. Though the traction force applied in this type of traction is insufficient to cause intervertebral separation, still it is used for patients with acute neck/back pain, for reduction of pain and spasm and promote recovery. This traction can be applied through two types of application.

i. *Skin traction:* Skin traction may be used as a definitive method of treatment as well as a first aid or temporary measure to immobilize joints, correct deformities, etc. The traction force is applied to the skin through adhesive straps/straps **(Figs. 22.1A and B)** for extremities, pelvic belts for lumbosacral spine and head halters for cervical spine, and the force is transmitted to bone and joints via the superficial fascia, deep fascia, and intermuscular septa. Though the maximum weight used for skin traction is about 10 lb (4.5–5 kg), the clinician should decide the weight, depending on the age and condition of the patient (particularly

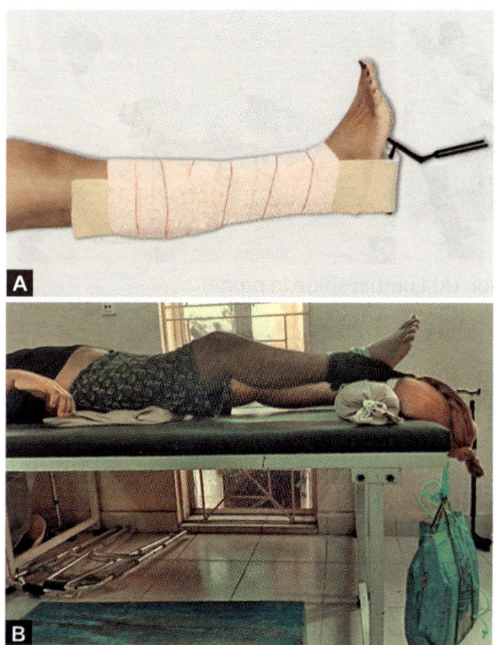

**Figs. 22.1A and B:** (A) Skin traction using adhesive straps; (B) Traction to deformed knee using ankle strap.

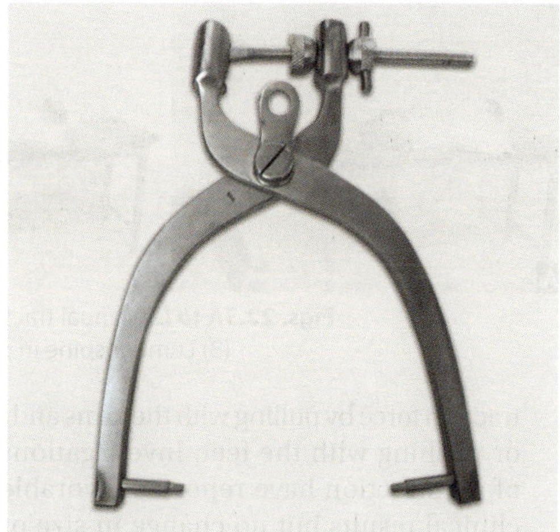

**Fig. 22.2:** Crutchfield tongs for skeletal traction.

for deformity correction, where continuous traction for few hours a day, with weight/traction force as tolerated, repeated for several sessions may be helpful).

ii. *Skeletal traction:* Skeletal traction is applied through direct fixation to bones through pins (Steinmann's pin for extremities), or crutch-field skull traction tongs **(Fig. 22.2)** to the skull (mostly applied for cervical injuries), to reduce displaced fractures/dislocations and to provide immobilization. The traction is applied through the use of pulleys, pins and weights, and a weight of 6–7 kg is attached to one end of the pulley in the traction mechanism. This procedure is performed by the Surgeon, using local anesthesia.

2. **Sustained traction/static traction:** This type of traction is used in physiotherapy clinics for treatment acute of cervical and lumbar pathologies. It involves application of load steadily for short periods of time, as per the conditions treated.
3. **Intermittent mechanical traction:** Intermittent traction is similar to sustained traction in its application, which utilizes a mechanical unit to alternately apply and release the traction force at preset intervals.
4. **Manual traction:** Manual traction is applied through the clinician's hands, that pulls on the patient's legs for lumbar traction in prone **(Fig. 22.3A)**/pulls on the pelvis for lumbar traction in supine **(Fig. 22.3B)**, and pulls on the mandible and occiput for cervical traction in supine **(Fig. 22.3C)**. It is usually applied for a few seconds duration to know whether, the symptoms are reducing with traction or not. If the symptoms reduce after applying manual traction in a particular position (say supine/prone for lumbar traction and neck neutral or slightly flexed for cervical traction), that position should be selected for application of traction.
4. **Autotraction:** Autotraction utilizes a especially designed table that is divided into two sections that can be individually tilted and rotated. The patient provides the

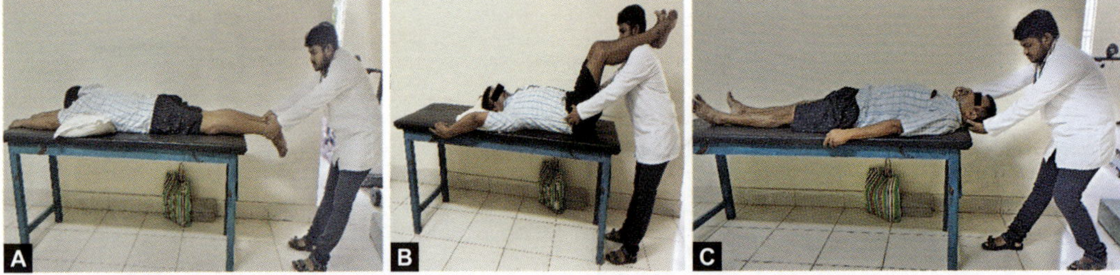

**Figs. 22.3A to C:** Manual traction for: (A) Lumbar spine in prone; (B) Lumbar spine in supine; (C) Cervical spine.

traction force by pulling with the arms and/or pushing with the feet. Investigations of autotraction have reported favorable clinical results but no change in size or location of lumbar disc herniation

6. **Positional traction:** This form of traction is applied to the thoracolumbar spine, by placing the patient in various positions using pillows, to apply a longitudinal pull on the spinal structures. It usually incorporates lateral bending with pillows placed on the opposite side (done for lumbar spondylosis with radicular pain in one leg) **(Fig. 22.4A)**, or forward bending, with pillows placed under the abdomen (lumbar spondylolisthesis without disc bulge) **(Fig. 22.4B)**.
7. **Gravity lumbar traction:** This involves using a chest harness to secure the patient as the treatment table is tilted to a vertical position, thereby using the weight of the lower half of the body to provide a traction force.
8. **Inversion table traction:** This is a difficult traction procedure, where the body is hung upside down, to apply a gravitational force on the spine. Though this traction is very effective, it carries risks, hence rarely performed today.

Though, various types of traction are used in clinical practice, the physiotherapists mostly apply spinal traction and skin traction using straps, such as traction to knee using ankle strap, to correct a knee flexion deformity, due to trauma/arthritis.

## Therapeutic Effects (Mechanism) of Traction

- Static traction, which is given in the acute spinal disorders stretches the spinal muscles, reducing paraspinal muscle

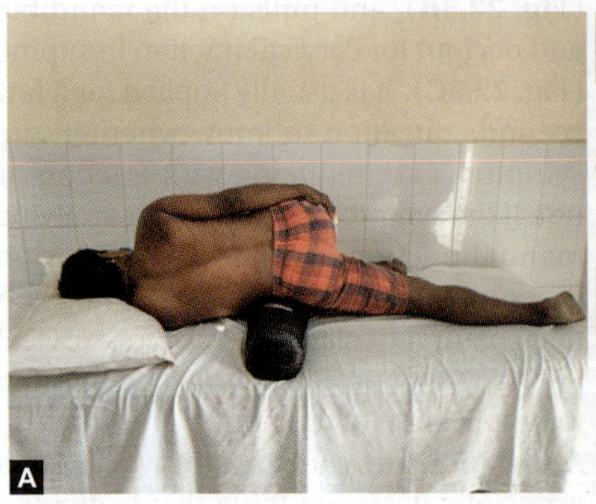

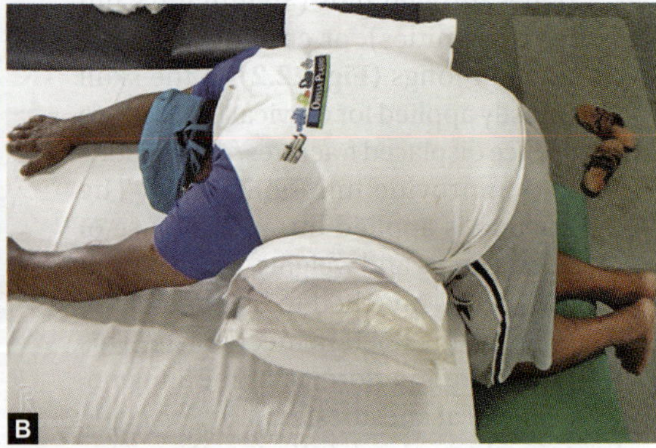

**Figs. 22.4A and B:** Positional traction: (A) Side lying over pillows with painful side upper most; (B) Trunk prone lying on pillows.

spasm and pain. Stretching of the adherent ligaments and tight capsules of the facet joints and releasing the adherent nerve roots help for pain reduction.

- Intermittent traction, that produces, repeated compression and relaxation, helps for mobilization of stiff intervertebral joints, releases adherent nerve roots at the intervertebral foramen, provides increased nutrition to the small facet joints, through the mechanism of increased fluid exchange, resulting in healing and reduction of inflammation. Improved circulation, reduction of adhesion and reduction of pain via pre-synaptic inhibition at the spinal cord level are the possible mechanisms of improvement with cervical traction.
- Traction in the sustained mode reduces the compression force over the intervertebral discs by widening the intervertebral space, that helps in reduction of the bulged disc through creation of a negative pressure and suctioning effect. This results in reduction of pressure on the nerve root, due to the bulged intervertebral disc. However, the duration of traction application in case of a bulged disc, should not exceed 10 to 11 minutes, or else, it may enhance the bulge due to fluid imbibition (though fluid imbibition is a natural process in healthy discs to absorb the required fluid for production of proteoglycans, necessary for supply of nutrients to the discs and promote recovery, excessive fluid absorption, may enhance the disc bulge).

## Parameters for Application of Traction

Before application of traction, the clinician/therapist is required to do a thorough clinical reasoning to decide the parameters of traction, that are to be selected, considering clinical needs of the individual patient. The parameters are briefly discussed below.

### *Selection of Traction Device*

Depending on the availability of the equipment, the mechanical traction units should be selected, which could be of the following types:

- **Simple mechanical traction:** In such mechanical traction devices, pulley and weights are used to apply the traction force are commonly used as home traction program **(Figs. 22.5A and B)**. While applying lumbar traction, the foot end of the bed is elevated as shown in the figure to achieve counter traction by the upper body, which remains inclined downwards. However, for cervical traction, the weight of the trunk applies counter traction, hence, there is no need to elevate the foot end of the bed.

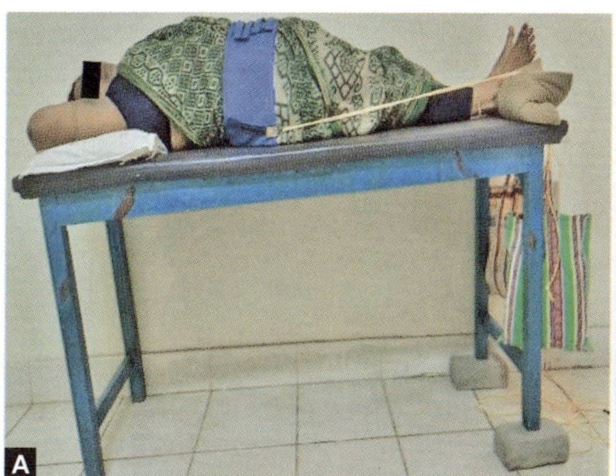
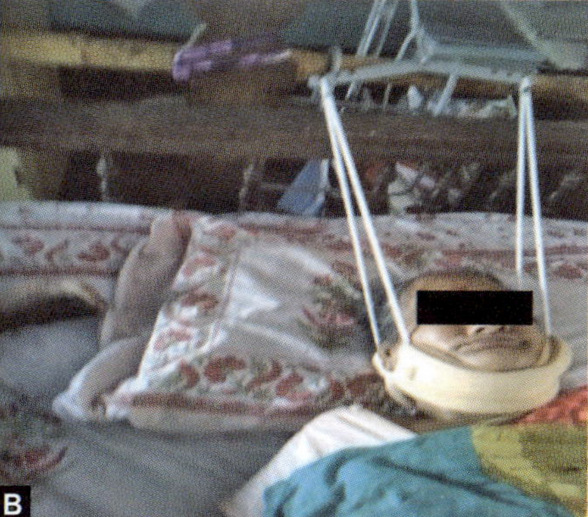

**Figs. 22.5A and B:** Mechanical traction: (A) Lumbar spine; (B) Cervical spine.

- **Motorized mechanical traction:** These devices use motors to produce the traction force. There is no need for elevating the foot end of the bed for lumbar traction, as besides the pelvic belt, a chest strap is used to fix the upper trunk for providing counter traction. The traction parameters are set manually in some machines, but currently machines are available, which are digitally controlled. The traction bed could be a simple flat bed or a split traction bed (which when used reduces friction and is preferred).
- **Pneumatic traction unit/pneumatic harness system and posture pump:** Pneumatic traction system is either a simple traction device, in which the device is kept on bed and after positioning of head on it, it is inflated by the patient **(Fig. 22.6A)**, or a very simple pneumatic harness, which is wrapped around the neck, and is inflated by the patient through a hand pump **(Fig. 22.6B)**. This can be used by the patient at home.

  Posture pump, is also a patient controlled pneumatic system, which is used to provide mechanical force to lumbosacral spine. However, such devices are not able to produce axial distraction.

### *Position*

- **Lumbar traction:** The clinician/therapist is required to take information from the patient, regarding the positional variations of symptoms, i.e., whether supine position is relieving the symptoms or the relief is produced in prone position. The position that produces relief is considered as the position for traction.
- **Supine position:** Supine is the position of flexion. If supine position is more comfortable and movement testing reveals pain in extension and relief in flexion (mostly occurs in lumbar spondylosis/spondylolisthesis) traction in supine is considered. However, to flatten the spine, some amount of hip flexion in supine is required. The most typical position for lumbar traction in supine, to cause vertebral separation, involves hips and knees flexion greater than 70° using a leg support platform/foot board (said as the Fowler's position) **(Fig. 22.7)**. However, if traction is desired for the lower lumbar spines, the hip flexion angles are reduced, and traction is applied by keeping a pillow under the knees. However, to localize the traction to the upper lumbar spines, the hip flexion angles are increased (Fowler's position is maintained)

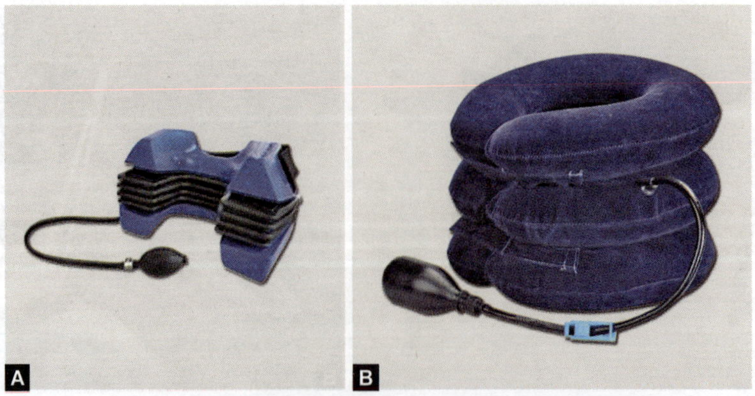


**Figs. 22.6A and B:** Pneumatic traction for cervical spine.

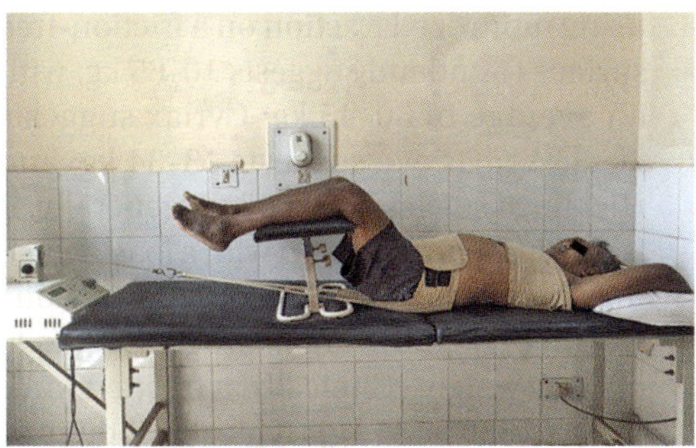

Fig. 22.7: Traction in supine with leg support platform/foot board, using Fowler's position.

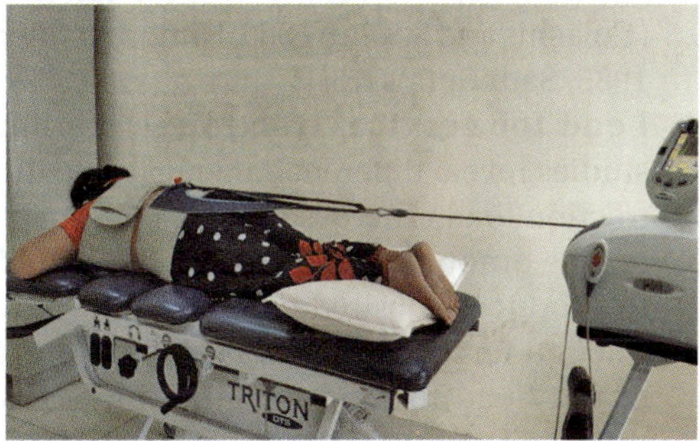


Fig. 22.8: Shows traction in prone.

- **Prone position:** As prone is the position of extension, patients who get pain in flexion (patients with PIVD), the prone position is selected for application of traction **(Fig. 22.8)**. One advantage of this position that, while traction is applied, other modalities, such as SWD/MWD/IR/Hot packs, etc., can be applied along with traction for better results. A pillow is placed under the legs to provide relaxion and support to the feet.

## Cervical Traction

Traction to cervical spine can be applied in supine/sitting **(Figs. 22.9A to C)**. The supine position has been shown to provide greater separation of intervertebral spaces from C4 to C7, than sitting, when the angle of pull and forces are controlled. For optimal results the neck should be flexed to about 20–30°, which stretches the muscles and soft tissues and opens up the intervertebral space. However, to localize traction to upper cervical spines, the neck flexion angles are reduced. The neck angle is kept at 0° for applying traction to C1-C2 segments.

### *Mode*

After the positioning, the clinician/therapist, should decide the mode, i.e., sustained/intermittent.

- **Sustained/static traction:** As already stated, sustained traction should be applied for acute conditions, where movements produce by intermittent mode is expected to produce more pain and discomfort. While treating acute disc disorders, it is always recommended to apply sustained traction for short periods of time to caused minimal fluid imbibition and suctioning in, of the bulged disc due to creation of negative pressure in the intervertebral space.
- **Intermittent traction:** While treating spinal disorders in the subacute and chronic stages, intermittent traction

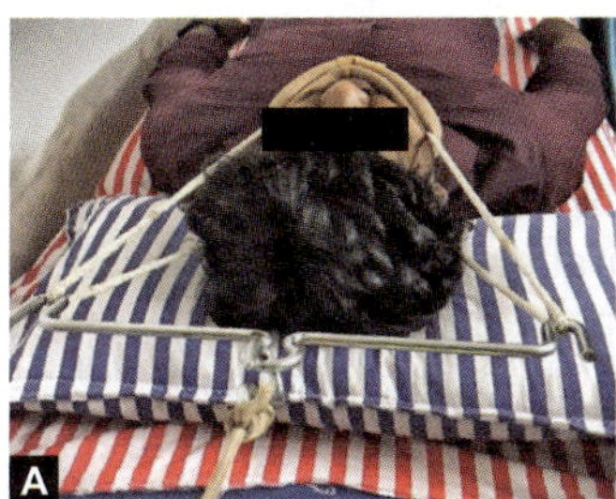


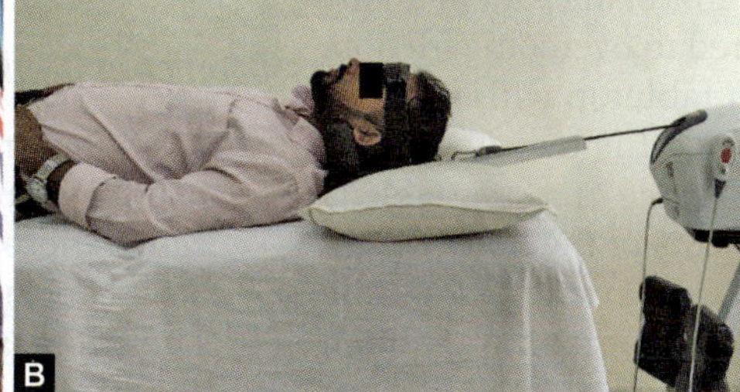


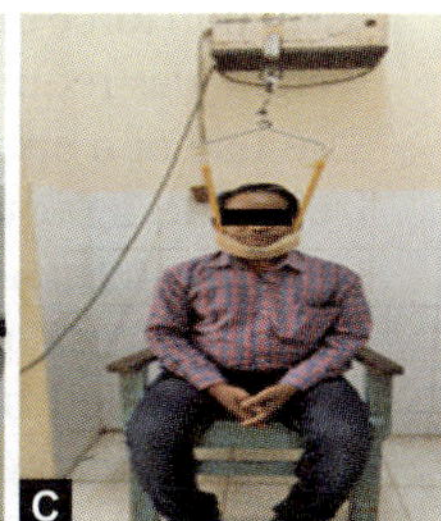


**Figs. 22.9A to C:** Cervical traction: (A) Supine using mandibular halter; (B) Supine using Saunder's halter; (C) Sitting using mandibular halter.

is the mode of choice. In this traction application, the hold to rest time ratio is kept high (may be 60 seconds hold time/10 seconds rest time) at the early days, when the conditions are less subacute, which are gradually decreased, by allowing more rest time as the conditions move towards chronicity. Though, there is no consensus on the choice or indications of the various forms of traction therapy, but it appears that intermittent motorized traction with the patient in the Fowler's position (i.e., supine with the hips and knees flexed, and the lower legs supported on a leg support platform/foot board) **(Fig. 22.7)**, is most effective for lumbosacral disorders, and hence ,frequently used (Maitland 1986).

For cervical spine, it has been found by researchers that, intermittent traction produces, twice the amount of vertebral separation as compared to sustained traction and presently is the mode of choice.

### *Load/Traction Force*

M Krause et al., 2000, found that, traction separates the vertebrae and it appears that large forces are not required. Vertebral separation could provide relief from radicular symptoms by removing direct pressure or contact forces from sensitized neural tissue.

- **Load for lumbar traction:** Generally for lumbar traction, the load selected should be sufficient enough to overcome the co-efficient of friction. Judovich showed that a traction force of 26% of the patient's body weight was required to overcome friction. The use of a split tabletop with friction-free rollers reduces this to a negligible amount. In the absence of a split table, a force in excess of 26% of the body weight must be used before any effect can be produced at the lumbar spine. Though different experts have given different views regarding selection of traction load using motorized traction on a friction-free surface (Maitland suggests 10–65 kg, with an average of 30–45 kg; Cyriax suggests 40–85 kg; Grieve suggests 13–34 kg; and Hicklings suggests 32–68 kg), generally, it is recommended to start with a load, which may be slightly higher than 1/3rd of body weight of the individual, progressing to ½ of body weight [Clinically, a traction force of up to 350N (35 kg) (typically about one half of body weight of a person weighing 70 kg) may be applied and the line of pull is generally kept at about 18° to the horizontal (Colachis and Strohm 1969, Hinterbuchner 1985, Saunders 1975)].
- **Load for cervical traction:** Different studies reveal different data regarding the traction load. There is no firm consensus on the amount of traction force needed to produce a desired clinical result. The traction force must be at least the weight of the head to produce any significant decompression of the cervical spine. It appears that at least 25–30 lbs (11–14 kg) of force are required to produce measurable separation of cervical vertebrae, which depends on the weight and clinical condition of the individual. However, the view of Hickling (1972), suggesting to select a traction load of 7–11 kg, applied for 15–25 minutes, seems clinically appropriate, which should be person specific. In general, a traction load of 1/8th of the individual's body weight may be selected initially, which may be enhanced to about 1/6th of body weight as per clinical need.

### *Duration of Traction*

- Sustained traction should not be applied for longer duration (>10–11 min), as it may cause increased fluid imbibition in the discs causing increase of symptoms.
- The meta-analysis done by Romeo et al. (2018), to find the efficacy of cervical traction reveals, longer traction times

resulted in better outcome in terms of pain and disability. Intermittent traction duration can be kept for 15–20 minutes, or slightly longer as per the response of the individual.

- **Hold to rest duration:** In intermittent traction application, a comfortable hold-rest time is set, as per the patient's condition. In subacute conditions, the rest time is kept shorter (say 50 seconds hold followed by 10 seconds rest in a cycle of 60 seconds), and as the condition improves (in chronic conditions), the rest time is gradually increased (say 40 seconds hold followed by 20 seconds rest) to cause frequent distraction and relaxation, causing increased mobility, fluid exchange, proprioceptive stimulation.

### Techniques of Application

Before traction is applied, the clinician/therapist, should check for contraindications listed below. After, the contraindications are checked, and patient is found suitable for traction, the therapist should perform manual testing, as shown in **Figures 22.3A to C** to decide, about the position, that will be most efficient and whether, traction is relieving the symptoms or not. If manual traction in a particular position produces relief, then patient should be taken for traction and the position as tested should be used. After setting the appropriate parameters, the therapist applies traction for the desired duration. The patient should be monitored for any discomfort/increase of pain/abnormal sensation, while traction is on, and in such case, traction should immediately be discontinued.

### Indications

- Continuous traction is used basically in the very acute stage for immobilization/provide rest to the affected body segments. It can also be used for deformity correction.
- Static traction for short duration should be considered by physiotherapist to treat acute PIVD/spondylosis, and to correct spinal deformities using the creep mechanism.
- Intermittent traction should be used in the subacute and chronic stages, to cause intervertebral separation, reduce radicular pain, and promote mobility.
- Traction to the limbs for correction of deformities and treat arthritic joints should be performed as indicated.

### Contraindications

Traction should not be applied in the following conditions:

- Acute traumatic conditions
- Infective disorders (Koch's spine)
- Rheumatoid arthritis affecting cervical spine
- Severe osteoporosis
- Malignant conditions
- Hemophilia
- Vascular pathologies, such as aortic aneurysm
- Severe hypermobility
- Pregnancy
- Myelopathies
- Vertebrobasilar insufficiency
- Midline herniated nucleus pulposus
- Untreated hypertension
- Prolonged steroid therapy.

# Multiple Choice Questions (MCQs)

1. **Which is true regarding a third order lever?**
   a. Effort is between fulcrum and weight
   b. Weight is between fulcrum and effort
   c. Fulcrum is between weight and effort
   d. None of the above
2. **Lever of power refers to:**
   a. 2nd order lever
   b. 3rd order lever
   c. 1st order lever
   d. None of the above
3. **Lever of speed refers to:**
   a. 1st order lever
   b. 2nd order lever
   c. 3rd order lever
   d. None of the above
4. **Which one of the followings is a white muscle fiber?**
   a. Type-IIa
   b. Type-I
   c. Type-IIb
   d. None of the above
5. **Gymnastic people have a greater proportion of:**
   a. Type-IIa fibers
   b. Type-I fibers
   c. Type-IIb fibers
   d. None of the above
6. **Which one of the followings is true regarding type-I muscle fibers?**
   a. These fibers contain more numbers of mitochondria and less amount of myoglobin
   b. These fibers contain more numbers of mitochondria and myoglobin
   c. These fibers do not contain significant amount of mitochondria and myoglobin
   d. None of the above
7. **Which one of the followings is true regarding type-IIa muscle fibers?**
   a. They produce ATP slowly through aerobic metabolism
   b. They produce ATP quickly through aerobic metabolism
   c. They produce ATP through anaerobic glycolysis
   d. None of the above
8. **Which one of the followings is true regarding carpometacarpal joints of thumb?**
   a. It is a hinged type synovial joint
   b. It is a plane type synovial joint
   c. It is a saddle type of synovial joint
   d. It is a condyloid type of synovial joint
9. **Outer range of muscle work refers to:**
   a. The muscle contracting from a position of full stretch, to a position half way through the full range of motion
   b. The muscle contracting to a position, halfway through the full range to a position, where a muscle is fully shortened
   c. The muscle contracting from a position of partial contraction to another position of partial contraction, not completing the full range
   d. None of the above

**10. Which one of the following is a fusiform muscle:**
a. Deltoid
b. Tibialis anterior
c. Biceps brachii
d. Rhomboids major

**11. Intervertebral joints (joints between vertebral bodies) come under:**
a. Primary cartilaginous joint
b. Secondary cartilaginous joint
c. Fibrous joint
d. Synovial joint

**12. What type of joint is facet joint?**
a. Fibrous joint
b. Plane type of synovial joint
c. Primary cartilaginous joint
d. Secondary cartilaginous joint

**13. What type of joint is wrist joint?**
a. Hinged type of synovial joint
b. Condyloid type of synovial joint
c. Pivot type of synovial joint
d. Primary cartilaginous joint

**14. What type of joint is knee joint?**
a. Condyloid type of synovial joint
b. Ball and socket type of synovial joint
c. Modified hinged type of synovial joint
d. Saddle type of synovial joint

**15. Shoulder joint is a:**
a. Hinged type of synovial joint
b. Ball and socket type of synovial joint
c. Condyloid type of synovial joint
d. Secondary cartilaginous joint

**16. ROM of foot eversion is:**
a. 30–40°
b. 5–10°
c. 40–50°
d. 15–20°

**17. Squatting is a type of:**
a. Open kinematic chain exercise
b. Closed kinematic chain exercise
c. Plyometric exercise
d. Isokinetic exercise

**18. Patients with wrist drop fail to make a grip, due to:**
a. Passive insufficiency of extensor digitorum communis
b. Active insufficiency of FDS and FDP
c. Both a and b
d. None of the above

**19. Which one of the following is true regarding eccentric exercise:**
a. The energy expenditure of this exercise is higher than concentric exercise
b. The energy expenditure of this exercise is lesser than concentric exercise
c. The energy expenditure is same as concentric exercise
d. None of the above

**20. Accommodating variable resistance exercise refers to:**
a. Isometric exercise
b. Isotonic exercise
c. Isokinetic exercise
d. None of the above

**21. Which one of the following is true regarding isometric exercise:**
a. The energy expenditure is lower than eccentric exercise
b. The energy expenditure is lower than concentric exercise
c. The energy expenditure is higher than concentric and eccentric exercises
d. None of the above

**22. For increase of muscle strength, using isokinetic system, which of the followings should be selected:**
a. High velocity exercises
b. Low velocity exercises
c. Both a and b
d. None of the above

**23. For increase of muscular endurance following injury, the velocity of isokinetic exercise should be:**
a. Low
b. High
c. Both a and b
d. None

**24. Which one of the following is true regarding energy expenditure of exercises?**

a. Eccentric < concentric < isometric
b. Isometric < eccentric < concentric
c. Concentric < isometric < eccentric
d. Concentric < eccentric < isometric

**25. Which one of the following true regarding exercises?**

a. Exercises stimulate the parasympathetic nervous system
b. Exercises stimulate the sympathetic nervous system
c. Both a and b
d. None of the above

**26. Which one of the followings is true regarding adaptations of exercise?**

a. Blood flow in the muscle increases to accommodate the increased metabolic activity
b. The nitric oxide released from the endothelial cells, produces increased blood flow
c. During vigorous exercise, blood flow from the renal and GI systems are shunted to the muscles
d. All of the above

**27. During exercise, respiratory rate increases due to:**

a. Increased production of $CO_2$ by working muscles
b. Reflex activity of respiratory centers
c. Hypersecretion of adrenaline
d. All of the above

**28. The difference in oxygen volume between an ideal, hypothetical oxygen uptake, and the actual uptake in real life is called as:**

a. Oxygen debt
b. Oxygen deficiency
c. Oxygen saturation
d. None of the above

**29. The extra volume of oxygen needed to restore all the energetic systems to their normal state after exercise is called as:**

a. Oxygen debt
b. Oxygen deficiency
c. Oxygen saturation
d. None of the above

**30. During vigorous exercise, urine flow decreases due to:**

a. Decreased blood flow to the kidneys
b. Increased fluid reabsorptions due to increased secretion of ADH
c. Both a and b
d. None of the above

**31. Which one of the followings are true regarding prolonged exercise:**

a. The urine flow decreases
b. Hemoconcentration in blood decreases
c. Body temperature increases
d. All of the above

**32. Which one of the following is true regarding strenuous exercise?**

a. There is release of growth hormone from pituitary gland, stimulating muscle and bone growth
b. The strenuous exercise decreases the gastric juice secretion and the stomach motility
c. Hemoconcentration occurs in blood, due to release of fluid from blood
d. All of the above

**33. Muscle power refers to:**

a. Ability of muscle to move weight with speed
b. Capacity of muscle to exert strong force against resistance in a single repetition
c. The submaximal force produced by the muscle groups for sustained period of time
d. None of the above

**34. Which of the followings is true regarding type-I muscle fibers?**
a. This has high oxidative and glycolytic capacity
b. This has low oxidative and high glycolytic capacity
c. This has high oxidative and low glycolytic capacity
d. None of the above

**35. Which of the followings take place in endurance activities?**
a. The slow twitch muscle fibers are recruited more and more
b. There is increase in the number of mitochondria
c. The gas exchange capacity of the myofibrils increases
d. All of the above

**36. Which of the following changes occur in strength training?**
a. It leads to hypertrophy of muscles and ligaments
b. It increases the bone mineral density
c. It increases blood pressure
d. All of the above

**37. The effect of exercise on blood pressure is:**
a. Strength training exercises increase blood pressure
b. Endurance training exercises decrease blood pressure
c. There is no change in blood pressure
d. None of the above

**38. Center of pressure (COP), refers to:**
a. The point, where the entire body mass is concentrated
b. The center of the distribution of the total force applied to the supporting surface
c. Both a and b
d. None of the above

**39. Which of the followings is true regarding base of support (BOS)?**
a. BOS $\alpha$ stability
b. BOS $\alpha$ 1/COG (center of gravity)
c. Both a and b
d. None of the above

**40. Lever of balance refers to:**
a. 2nd order lever
b. 1st order lever
c. 3rd order lever
d. None of the above

**41. Flexing the elbow with weight on hand is an example of:**
a. 2nd order lever
b. 3rd order lever
c. 1st order lever
d. None of the above

**42. Mechanical advantage is >1 in which type of lever:**
a. 1st order lever
b. 3rd order lever
c. 2nd order lever
d. None of the above

**43. Which of the following is true regarding movable pulley?**
a. Movable pulley acts like a 2nd order lever
b. Movable pulley reduces the restricting force into half
c. Both a and b
d. None of the above

**44. The tendency of a solid material, to undergo slow deformation, while subjected to persistent mechanical stress is called:**
a. Breaking stress
b. Fracture
c. Creep
d. None of the above

**45. While stretching a tight structure, the therapist should aim to:**
a. Cross the elastic limit and achieve creep
b. Cross the ultimate stress point, beyond which failure occurs
c. Move within elastic limit
d. None of the above

**46. Supination and pronation of forearm occurs in:**
a. Sagittal plane
b. Frontal plane
c. Transverse plane
d. None of the above

**47. The 3rd phase of problem oriented medical record (POMR) focuses on:**
a. Formation of effective data base
b. Identification of specific problem list from the data base
c. Identification of specific plan of care
d. Determination of effectiveness of plan of care

**48. Visual fields are tested by:**
a. Using Snellen chart
b. Testing blink reflex
c. Doing confrontation test
d. None of the above

**49. Impairment of lateral movement of eyeball could be due to:**
a. 3rd cranial nerve palsy
b. 4th cranial nerve palsy
c. 6th cranial nerve palsy
d. Both b and c

**50. Impairment of eyeball movement in lateral and downward direction could be due to:**
a. 2nd cranial nerve palsy
b. 3rd cranial nerve palsy
c. 4th cranial nerve palsy
d. 6th cranial nerve palsy

**51. Inability to move the eyeball in upward and medial direction, could be due to:**
a. 2nd cranial nerve palsy
b. 3rd cranial nerve palsy
c. 4th cranial nerve palsy
d. 6th cranial nerve palsy

**52. The part of the 8th nerve responsible for hearing is:**
a. Vestibular part
b. Cochlear part
c. Both a and b
d. None

**53. Taste sensation to posterior 1/3rd of the tongue is maintained by:**
a. 7th cranial nerve
b. 1st cranial nerve
c. 9th cranial nerve
d. None of the above

**54. Absence of gag reflex could be due to:**
a. 9th cranial nerve injury
b. 10th cranial nerve injury
c. Both 9th and 10th cranial nerve injury
d. None of the above

**55. If shrugging of shoulder is impaired, the cranial nerve implicated is:**
a. 9th cranial nerve
b. 10th cranial nerve
c. 11th cranial nerve
d. 12th cranial nerve

**56. In upper motor neuron injury to 12th cranial nerve, the deviation of tongue is:**
a. In the direction of side of lesion
b. In the opposite direction to the side of lesion
c. Absent
d. None of the above

**57. Which of the followings is true for an abnormal Rinne test?**
a. Air conduction is greater than bone conduction in the affected ear
b. Bone conduction is greater than air conduction in the affected ear
c. Bone conduction is same as air conduction in the affected ear
d. None of the above

**58. Epicritic sensation refers to:**
a. Sensations that provide discriminative analysis with regard to the environment
b. Sensations acting as a defensive agency against pathologic changes in the tissues
c. Both a and b
d. None of the above

**59. Dysesthesia refers to:**
- a. Abnormal sensations perceived without specific stimulation
- b. Painful sensations such as intense burning, elicited by a nonpainful cutaneous stimulus such as a light touch
- c. Both a and b
- d. None of the above

**60. Normal value of 2 point discrimination over the finger tips is:**
- a. 8–12 mm
- b. 30–40 mm
- c. 2–8 mm
- d. 20–30 mm

**61. The term pallesthesia refers to:**
- a. Ability to perceive joint position
- b. Ability to perceive vibration
- c. Ability to perceive joint motion
- d. Ability to perceive pain

**62. The term hyperpathia refers to:**
- a. A lowered threshold for painful sensation, resulting in exaggerated reaction to stimuli
- b. Painful sensation to nonpainful stimulus
- c. Abnormal sensations perceived without specific stimulation
- d. None of the above

**63. Hyperesthesia refers to:**
- a. Absence of touch appreciation
- b. Decrease of touch appreciation
- c. Exaggeration of touch sensation
- d. None of the above

**64. Extinction refers to:**
- a. Inability to identify objects from shape and size
- b. Inability to identify symbols drawn on skin
- c. Inability to perceive a sensory stimulus when corresponding areas on the opposite side of the body are stimulated simultaneously
- d. None of the above

**65. Topagnosia refers to:**
- a. Inability to localize stimuli to part of the body touched
- b. Inability to identify objects which are heavy/light
- c. Inability to identify joint position
- d. Inability to identify symbols drawn on skin

**66. The nipple region on front of trunk is innervated by:**
- a. T3 dermatome
- b. T4 dermatome
- c. T5 dermatome
- d. T6 dermatome

**67. The zone of skin between great toe and 2nd toe over the dorsum of foot is innervated by:**
- a. Sural nerve
- b. Superficial peroneal nerve
- c. Deep peroneal nerve
- d. Saphenous nerve

**68. Vibration sensation is tested using:**
- a. 512 Hz tunning fork
- b. 256 Hz tunning fork
- c. 128 Hz tunning fork
- d. None of the above

**69. The instrument used to test 2-point discrimination is called:**
- a. Goniometer
- b. Thermometer
- c. Aesthesiometer
- d. None of the above

**70. When there is considerable increase in muscle tone making passive movement difficult, the grade of spasticity as per Modified modified Ashworth scale:**
- a. Grade-I
- b. Grade-II
- c. Grade-III
- d. Grade-IV

**71. As per modified Tardieu scale dynamic component of spasticity is measured from:**
- a. R1 (resistance to quick stretch)
- b. R2 (resistance to slow stretch)

c. R1-R2
d. R2-R1

**72. The root value for cremasteric reflex is:**
a. S1, S2
b. L1, L2
c. T1, T2
d. L3, L4

**73. Absence of corneal reflex, indicates:**
a. 3rd cranial nerve injury
b. 4th cranial nerve injury
c. 5th cranial nerve injury
d. 2nd cranial nerve injury

**74. A very brisk tendon jerk with clonus indicates a grade of:**
a. 1+
b. 2+
c. 3+
d. 4+

**75. On examination, a patient was found to have, increased amplitude of tendon jerks with positive Babiniski sign. It indicates:**
a. UMN type of lesion
b. LMN type of lesion
c. Normal state of health
d. None of the above

**76. The maneuver to relax the patient while testing DTR is called:**
a. Phelp's maneuver
b. Jendrassik maneuver
c. Valsalva maneuver
d. None of the above

**77. The root value of knee jerk reflex is:**
a. L1, L2
b. L2, L3
c. L3, L4
d. L5-S1

**78. The root value of anal reflex is:**
a. S2–S4
b. S3–S4
c. S4–S5
d. L4–L5

**79. Maxillary reflex is tested to find integrity of:**
a. 7th cranial nerve
b. 9th cranial nerve
c. 5th cranial nerve
d. 4th cranial nerve

**80. Manual muscle testing using grades from: 0–10, comes under:**
a. Daniel's system of grading
b. MRC grading
c. Kendall system of grading
d. None of the above

**81. A positive sharpened Rhomberg test indicates:**
a. Cerebellar ataxia
b. Sensory ataxia
c. Vestibular ataxia
d. None of the above

**82. Apparent limb length discrepancy of lower limbs is measured from:**
a. Umbilicus to medial malleolus
b. Xiphisternum to medial malleolus
c. Umbilicus to lateral malleolus
d. Both a and b above

**83. Squaring of pelvis for an infrapelvic tilt is done by:**
a. Adducting the affected hip
b. Abducting the affected hip
c. Flexing the affected hip
d. Extending the affected hip

**84. Supratrochanteric shortening (if any) is found from:**
a. Femoral triangle
b. Bryant's triangle
c. Both a and b
d. None of the above

**85. Training heart rate is:**
a. RHR + (MHR + RHR) × % age of intensity of exercise
b. MHR + (MHR – RHR) × % age of intensity of exercise

c. RHR + (MHR – RHR) × % age of intensity of exercise
d. None of the above

**86. $VO_{2max}$ is determined from:**
a. Simple exercise test such as 6 minutes walk test
b. Cardiorespiratory exercise test such as treadmill test
c. Blood gas analysis
d. None of the above

**87. A gravity dependent goniometer is mostly used to:**
a. Measure range of motion of hips
b. Measure range of motion of shoulders
c. Measure pelvic tilt
d. None of the above

**88. In an electrogoniometer, the joint angle is measured from:**
a. Voltmeter
b. Ammeter
c. Potentiometer
d. None of the above

**89. During heel strike, the center of pressure is located at:**
a. Base of toes
b. Mid-foot
c. The heel
d. None of the above

**90. A coefficient of friction >1 suggests:**
a. Frictional more is more
b. Frictional force is less
c. Frictional force is negligible
d. None of the above

**91. During push off phase, the ground reaction force passes through:**
a. The heel
b. The mid-foot
c. The ball of toes
d. None of the above

**92. In normal standing the base of support is:**
a. 2–4 cm
b. 4–8 cm
c. 5–10 cm
d. 3–6 cm

**93. Sway back deformity is associated with:**
a. Anterior pelvic tilt
b. Posterior pelvic tilt
c. Lateral pelvic tilt
d. None of the above

**94. The pattern of muscle recruitment in ankle strategy is:**
a. Proximal to distal
b. Distal to proximal
c. Both a and b
d. None of the above

**95. The balance strategy recruited, on failure of fixed support strategies include:**
a. Stepping strategies
b. Counter poising reaction
c. Protective extension reaction
d. None of the above

**96. The pattern of muscle recruitment in hip strategy is:**
a. Distal to proximal
b. Proximal to distal
c. Both a and b
d. None of the above

**97. Box breathing is also known as:**
a. Diaphragmatic breathing
b. Costal breathing
c. Four square breathing
d. None of the above

**98. Progressive relaxation technique was described by:**
a. Mitchel
b. Jacobson
c. Bobaths
d. Vojta

**99. Physiological relaxation technique was described by:**
a. Mitchel
b. Jacobson
c. Bobaths
d. Vojta

**100. The technique of replacing unpleasant negative thoughts, visualizing pleasant and calming scenarios is called:**
a. Guided imagery
b. Body scan
c. Biofeedback
d. None of the above

**101. Anterior pelvic tilt is caused by:**
a. Tightness of hip flexors and lumbar extensor muscles
b. Weakness of abdominals and hip extensors
c. Both a and b above
d. None of the above

**102. Posterior pelvic tilt is caused by:**
a. Tightness of hip extensors, hamstrings and trunk flexor muscles
b. Weakness of lumbar extensors and hip flexors
c. Both a and b above
d. None of the above

**103. The muscles responsible for prevention of posterior pelvic tilt are:**
a. Lumbar extensors and hip flexors
b. Abdominal muscles and the hip extensors
c. Both a and b
d. None of the above

**104. The muscles responsible for prevention of anterior pelvic tilt are:**
a. Lumbar extensors and hip flexors
b. Abdominal muscles and the hip extensors
c. Both a and b
d. None of the above

**105. Normal lumbosacral angle is:**
a. 20° b. 40°
c. 60° d. 30°

**106. Which of the followings is true in anterior pelvic tilt?**
a. Lumbosacral angle is >30°
b. Lumbosacral angle is <30°
c. Lumbosacral angle remains unaltered
d. None of the above

**107. Lateral pelvic tilt occurs due to:**
a. Weakness of qudratus lumborum on ipsilateral side and shortening of gluteus medius on the contralateral side
b. Lengthening of quadratus lumborum on the ipsilateral side and weakness of gluteus medius on the contralateral side
c. Both a and b
d. None of the above

**108. Which of the followings are true regarding posterior pelvic tilt?**
a. It produces lordotic posture
b. It produces flat back posture
c. It produces sway back posture
d. Both b and c above

**109. Which of the followings are true regarding anterior pelvic tilt?**
a. Lumbar spine flexes and hip extends
b. Lumbar spine extends and hip flexes
c. Both a and b
d. None of the above

**110. Muscle setting exercises are used for:**
a. Maintenance of muscle power
b. Increasing muscle power
c. Both a and b above
d. None of the above

**111. Stabilization exercises involve:**
a. End range isometric contraction
b. Isometric contraction at the beginning of the range
c. Mid-range isometric contraction
d. None of the above

**112. In isometric strength training, the resistance applied should be:**
a. 40–50% of a muscle's force developing capacity
b. 50–60% of a muscle's force developing capacity
c. 60–80% of a muscle's force developing capacity
d. 80–90% of a muscle's force developing capacity

**113. In isometric strength training, muscle contraction should be sustained for:**
a. 4–5 seconds
b. 5–6 seconds

c. 6–10 seconds
d. 10–15 seconds

**114. During isometric strength training, increase of heart rate is due to:**
a. Decreased vagal tone
b. Increased discharge of cardiac sympathetic nerves
c. Both a and b above
d. None of the above

**115. Which of the followings are true regarding isotonic exercise?**
a. Tension/force produced by the muscles remain constant
b. Velocity of movement changes
c. Velocity of movement remains constant
d. Both a and b above

**116. Dynamic exercises are also called as:**
a. Isokinetic exercises
b. Auxotonic exercises
c. Isometric exercises
d. None of the above

**117. Which of the followings is true regarding eccentric exercise?**
a. It has lower metabolic demand
b. It produces high force, with less fatigue
c. It has low cardiovascular demand
d. All of the above

**118. DOMS is a complication of:**
a. Isometric resisted exercise
b. Concentric resisted exercise
c. Eccentric resisted exercise
d. Isokinetic exercise

**119. In eccentric resisted exercise, DOMS develops:**
a. 4–5 days after exercise
b. 1–2 days after exercise
c. 3–4 days after exercise
d. 7–8 days after exercise

**120. Which of the followings are true regarding open kinematic chain exercise?**
a. The distal part of the extremities are fixed to some surface
b. The distal part of the extremities move freely
c. Both a and b
d. None of the above

**121. Plyometric exercise involves:**
a. Explosive concentric followed by eccentric contractions
b. Explosive eccentric followed by concentric contractions
c. Repeated isometric contractions
d. None of the above

**122. Which of the followings is true regarding endurance exercise?**
a. Overload is applied through increase of load/intensity
b. Overload is applied through increase of volume of exercise
c. Both a and b
d. None of the above

**123. Cross training effect refers to:**
a. Gain in strength in upper limb, when strength training is given to lower limb
b. Gain in strength in one limb, when strength training is given to contralateral limb
c. Gain in strength in the limbs, when strength training is given to the trunk
d. None of the above

**124. Periodization protocol in strength training refers to:**
a. Systematic variation in exercise intensity at regular intervals over a specific periods of time
b. Systematic variation in exercise volume at regular intervals over a specific periods of time
c. Both a and b above
d. None of the above

**125. Which of the followings is true regarding aerobic exercise?**
a. High intensity exercise carried out over a short period of time
b. Lower intensity exercise carried out for a longer period of time

c. This exercise builds endurance
d. Both b and c

**126. Neural adaptations in strength training occurs due to:**

a. Decreased sensitivity of GTO
b. Increased firing at neuromuscular junction
c. Increased recruitment of motor units
d. All of the above

**127. Maximum hypertrophy of muscle occurs in:**

a. High volume moderate intensity exercise, performed eccentrically
b. Low volume moderate intensity exercise, performed eccentrically
c. High volume moderate intensity exercise, performed concentrically
d. Low volume moderate intensity exercise, performed concentrically

**128. Which of the following is true regarding 1 RM?**

a. It is the maximum weight (resistance), with which the muscle can contract through full/available ROM, for one time without fatigue
b. The muscle will be unable to perform the repetition for the second time
c. Both a and b
d. None of the above

**129. Which of the followings are uses of RM**

a. It documents a baseline measurement of dynamic strength of a muscle
b. It identifies an exercise load to be used during exercise
c. It finds out prognosis in reassessment and helps to alter the exercise regime accordingly
d. All of the above

**130. The training zone for sedentary people is:**

a. 30–40% of 1 RM
b. 50–60% of 1 RM
c. 60–70% of 1 RM
d. 80–95% of 1 RM

**131. Which of the following PRE method is based on 6 RM working weight?**

a. De Lorme and Watkins method
b. DAPRE method
c. Zinovieff method
d. MacQueen method

**132. Which one of the followings is true regarding circuit training?**

a. Each resistance exercise is performed at an exercise station for a specified number of sets and repetitions, without any rest between movements
b. It involves, alternating periods of high intensity exercise, with periods of rest or low intensity exercise
c. Each resistance exercise is performed at an exercise station for a specified number of sets and repetitions, with rest between movements
d. None of the above

**133. When the concave surface, moves over convex surface?**

a. Roll and glide occur in same direction
b. Roll and glide occur in opposite direction
c. Only roll occurs without any glide
d. None of the above

**134. When the convex surface, moves over concave surface?**

a. Roll and glide occur in same direction
b. Roll and glide occur in opposite direction
c. Only roll occurs without any glide
d. None of the above

**135. Codman's exercise is an example of:**

a. Static stretching
b. Static progressive stretching
c. Cyclic stretching
d. Ballistic stretching

**136. While performing stretching exercises, the duration of stretch is generally kept for?**

a. 60 seconds
b. 30 seconds
c. 40 seconds
d. 10 seconds

**137. Which of the followings regarding relaxed passive movements are true?**
a. 10-20 repetitions of movements, should be performed 4 times daily
b. 8-10 repetitions of movements, should be performed 2 times daily
c. The number of repetitions and sessions depends on patient's tolerance
d. None of the above

**138. Who, among the followings is regarded as father of orthopedic medicine?**
a. Geoffrey D Maitland
b. Robin McKenzie
c. Freddy Kaltenborn
d. James Henry Cyriax

**139. Superior radioulnar joint is:**
a. Plane type of synovial joint
b. Pivot type of synovial joint
c. Hinge type of synovial joint
d. None of the above

**140. Which of the followings is true regarding traction?**
a. The distal articulating surface moves perpendicularly over the proximal articulating surface
b. The distal articulating surface moves parallel to the proximal articulating surface
c. It involves the longitudinal pull on the long axis of the articulating bone to cause separation of joint surfaces
d. Both b and c above

**141. Which of the followings is true regarding loose packed position?**
a. The contact between the articulating surfaces are minimum
b. The capsule and ligaments are laxed in this position
c. The joint play is optimal in this position
d. All of the above

**142. Which of the followings are true regarding close packed position?**
a. Position with most amount of joint surface congruency
b. The capsule and supporting ligaments are maximally tight
c. The joint play is minimum in this position
d. All of the above

**143. Close packed position of shoulder is:**
a. Abduction of shoulder between 35 to 55°
b. Maximum abduction and lateral rotation of shoulder
c. Maximum abduction and medial rotation of shoulder
d. None of the above

**144. Capsular pattern of limitation of movements of shoulder are:**
a. Internal rotation limitation > Abduction limitation > Lateral rotation limitation
b. Lateral rotation limitation > Abduction limitation > Medial rotation limitation
c. Flexion limitation > Abduction limitation > Lateral rotation limitation
d. None of the above

**145. Capsular pattern of limitation of movements of hip are:**
a. Flexion limitation > Internal rotation limitation > Abduction limitation
b. Flexion limitation > External rotation limitation > Abduction limitation
c. Flexion limitation > Internal rotation limitation > Adduction limitation
d. None of the above

**146. Which of the followings is true regarding Ruffini corpuscles?**
a. These receptors are slow adaptive and have low threshold
b. These receptors are located around the hip, knee and shoulder
c. These receptors are located in the superficial joint capsule, periosteum, ligaments and tendons
d. All of the above

**147. Which of the followings are true regarding Pacinian corpuscles?**
a. These have low threshold and are rapidly adaptive
b. These are mainly found in lumbar spine, hand, foot and jaw
c. These are activated by change in joint position
d. All of the above

**148. Which of the followings are true regarding Golgi Mazzoni?**
a. These are stimulated during end range stretch
b. These are activated by joint mobilization techniques
c. These have inhibitive quality, hence regulate muscle tone
d. All of the above

**149. The end feel found in acute inflammation is:**
a. Soft end feel
b. Firm end feel
c. Hard end feel
d. Empty end feel

**150. The end feel found in capsular stretch is:**
a. Firm end feel
b. Hard end feel
c. Soft end feel
d. None of the above

**151. While mobilizing a stiff joint, the restriction of movement felt by the therapist is called:**
a. Pathological limit
b. First tissue stop
c. Anatomical limit
d. Both a and b above

**152. While mobilizing a stiff joint, a force more than that is required to cross the pathological limit will result in:**
a. Plastic deformation
b. Rupture if the anatomical limit is crossed
c. Both a and b
d. None of the above

**153. The joint mobilization technique should be performed within:**
a. Elastic limit
b. Pathological limit
c. Between pathological and anatomical limits
d. None of the above

**154. Which of the following Maitland grades of mobilization is used to reduce blocked facets?**
a. Grade I, II
b. Grade III
c. Grade IV
d. Grade V

**155. The oscillations of movements given in chronic stage is:**
a. Slow (30 oscillations in a minute)
b. Medium (60 oscillations in a minute)
c. Fast (120 oscillations in a minute)
d. None of the above

**156. Which of the following Maitland grades of mobilization is used to reduce pain?**
a. Grade I, II
b. Grade III
c. Grade IV
d. Grade V

**157. Which of the followings is true regarding Cyriax's grade B mobilization?**
a. Mobilization done within pain-free range
b. Sustained stretch given at the end range
c. High velocity, low amplitude manipulation, given at the end of range
d. None of the above

**158. Cord sign includes:**
a. Flaccidity and hyporeflexia
b. Spasticity, hyper-reflexia
c. Extensor plantar response and clonus
d. Both b and c above

**159. Reciprocal inhibition refers to:**

a. Relaxation of the contracting muscle
b. Relaxation of the antagonists to accommodate contraction of the agonists
c. Relaxation of the proximal groups of muscles
d. None of the above

**160. Autogenic inhibition involves:**

a. Stimulation of type Ia fibers of muscle spindle
b. Stimulation of type Ib fibers from GTO
c. Stimulation of type II fibers from muscle spindle
d. None of the above

**161. Which of the followings is true regarding hyperbolic stretching?**

a. It is an online program to increase flexibility and maintain fitness
b. It combines PNF stretching with static and dynamic stretches
c. Both a and b
d. None of the above

**162. Cryo-stretch involves:**

a. Ice immersion
b. Application of ice with active movements
c. Application of ice with stretching
d. None of the above

**163. The physical modalities help to facilitate stretching are:**

a. Heat
b. Cold
c. Massage
d. All of the above

**164. Which of the followings is true regarding development of engram?**

a. It is the abstract representation that stores the memory of rules of movements
b. A high repetitions of precise performance is required in order to develop an engram
c. Both a and b
d. None of the above

**165. Which of the followings are true regarding sensory ataxia?**

a. It affects patients with significant proprioceptive loss
b. The dorsal column of the spinal cord fails to carry proprioceptive information from the body to the brain
c. Patients have near normal co-ordination, when the eyes are opened
d. All of the above

**166. Which of the followings are true regarding cerebellar ataxia?**

a. This is caused by damage to cerebellum
b. There is loss of balance and co-ordination
c. There is dysmetria and dysdiadokokinesia
d. All of the above

**167. Which of the followings are true regarding finger to nose test?**

a. A patient with cerebellar ataxia, can perform the test with eyes closed
b. A patient with sensory ataxia, can not perform the test with eyes closed
c. A patient with sensory ataxia, can perform the test with eyes open
d. All of the above

**168. Frenkel's exercises are primarily designed to treat:**

a. Cerebellar ataxia
b. Vestibular ataxia
c. Sensory ataxia
d. None of the above

**169. While performing Frenkel's exercises:**

a. Progression should be from small range movement at low speed to large range movement at high speed
b. Progression should be from large range movement at high speed to small range movement at low speed

c. Both a and b
d. None of the above

**170. While using suspension therapy, the distal extremities are supported by:**
a. Single sling
b. Double sling
c. Three ring sling
d. None of the above

**171. Which of the followings is true regarding vertical suspension?**
a. The axis of the joint is taken as the point of suspension
b. The center of gravity of the body part is taken as the point of suspension
c. Both a and b
d. None of the above

**172. Using pendular suspension to assist hip abductors, the point of suspension should be from a point:**
a. Medial to hip axis
b. Lateral to hip axis
c. Anterior to hip axis
d. Posterior to hip axis

**173. The nerve most commonly affected in crutch palsy, using axillary crutch is:**
a. Axillary nerve
b. Radial nerve
c. Musculocutaneous nerve
d. None of the above

**174. In an axillary crutch, the axillary pad should be located:**
a. 4 cm below the apex of axilla
b. 3 cm below the apex of axilla
c. 5 cm below the apex of axilla
d. None of the above

**175. With shoes off, the length of the axillary crutch in supine lying is measured from:**
a. Apex of axilla to medial malleolus
b. Apex of axilla to lateral malleolus
c. 5 cm below the apex of axilla to 20 cm lateral to the heel
d. None of the above

**176. Length of hand grip of axillary crutch in supine lying is taken from:**
a. Apex of axilla to ulnar styloid process, with the elbow flexed to 20–30°
b. 5 cm below the apex of axilla to ulnar styloid process, with the elbow flexed to 20–30°
c. 5 cm below the apex of axilla to ulnar styloid process, with the elbow fully extended
d. None of the above

**177. For the unilateral lower limb amputee, the crutch gait used is:**
a. 3 point crutch gait
b. 2 point crutch gait
c. 4 point crutch gait
d. None of the above

**178. Partial weight bearing crutch gait is a progression from:**
a. 2-point crutch gait
b. 4-point crutch gait
c. 3-point crutch gait
d. None of the above

**179. Which of the followings is true regarding 2-point crutch gait**
a. This gait is more stable than 4-point crutch gait
b. This gait is less stable than 4-point crutch gait
c. This pattern closely resembles normal gait
d. Both b and c above

**180. The gait pattern, where the crutches are moved together and both lower limbs are swung beyond the crutches is called:**
a. 4-point crutch gait
b. Swing to crutch gait
c. Swing through crutch gait
d. None of the above

**181. The hand grip of the walking stick, should be up to the level of:**
a. ASIS
b. PSIS

c. Greater trochanter
d. None of the above

**182. Length of hand grip to floor of elbow crutch in supine lying with shoes on is measured from:**

a. Radial styloid to 20 cm lateral to heel of the shoe with elbow flexed by 20–30°
b. Ulnar styloid to 20 cm lateral to heel of the shoe with elbow flexed by 20–30°
c. Olecranon process to 20 cm lateral to heel of the shoe with elbow flexed by 20–30°
d. None of the above

**183. The rules for step climbing with crutches are:**

a. While climbing up, the crutches are placed on step followed by the feet, and vice versa for climbing down
b. While climbing up, the feet are placed first on step, followed by the crutches, and vice versa for climbing down
c. The normal leg proceeds first while climbing up, and the affected leg proceeds first while climbing down
d. Both b and c above

**184. Which of the following walking aids should be selected for very obese persons?**

a. Axillary crutches
b. Elbow crutches
c. Standard adjustable cane
d. Bariatric cane

**185. To minimize the stress on the affected lower limb, the walking stick is preferably used:**

a. On ipsilateral side
b. Contralateral side
c. On any side
d. None of the above

**186. The walkers of choice for ataxic patients are:**

a. Reciprocal walker
b. Weighted walker
c. Both a and b
d. None of the above

**187. Which of the followings are true, regarding sports wheel chair?**

a. It is rigid type
b. It is light weight and energy efficient
c. It can be folded, hence easy to transport
d. Both a and b

**188. Which of the followings is true regarding seat height of wheel chair?**

a. 1 inch added to distance between buttom of heel to popliteal fossa
b. 2 inches added to distance between buttom of heel to popliteal fossa
c. 3 inches added to distance between buttom of heel to popliteal fossa
d. 4 inches added to distance between buttom of heel to popliteal fossa

**189. Which of the followings is true regarding seat depth of wheel chair?**

a. 1 inch added to distance between popliteal area and level of buttock
b. 2 inches added to distance between popliteal area and level of buttock
c. 3 inches added to distance between popliteal area and level of buttock
d. 4 inches added to distance between popliteal area and level of buttock

**190. The back rest height of wheel chair is:**

a. Distance between the inferior angle of scapula and inferior part of buttock-1 inch
b. Distance between the inferior angle of scapula and inferior part of buttock-2 inches
c. Distance between the inferior angle of scapula and inferior part of buttock-3 inches
d. Distance between the inferior angle of scapula and inferior part of buttock-4 inches

**191. Which of the followings is true regarding Beevor's axiom?**

a. Brain knows individual muscle action
b. Brain knows movement patterns
c. Both a and b above
d. None of the above

**192. In PNF technique, an increased excitation of the agonist muscles, that follows the stimulation (contraction) of their antagonists is due to:**

a. Reciprocal innervation
b. Irradiation
c. Successive induction
d. None of the above

**193. Which of the followings are true regarding traction and compression in PNF?**

a. Traction facilitates extension, compression facilitates flexion
b. Traction facilitates flexion, compression facilitates extension
c. Both traction and compression facilitate flexion
d. Both traction and compression facilitate extension

**194. In PNF, the normal timing followed is:**

a. Proximal to distal
b. Distal to proximal
c. Both a and b
d. None of the above

**195. Timing for emphasis in PNF, uses the principle of:**

a. Irradiation
b. Reinforcement
c. Both a and b
d. None of the above

**196. D2 flexion pattern of upper limb is:**

a. Shoulder-flexion, adduction, external rotation, elbow-flexion/extension, forearm-supination, wrist and fingers-flexion
b. Shoulder-flexion, abduction, external rotation, elbow-flexion/extension, forearm-supination, wrist and fingers-extension
c. Shoulder-flexion, adduction, internal rotation, elbow-flexion/extension, forearm-pronation, wrist and fingers-flexion
d. Shoulder-flexion, abduction, internal rotation, elbow-flexion/extension, forearm-supination, wrist and fingers-flexion

**197. D1 flexion pattern of lower limb is:**

a. Hip-flexion, adduction, external rotation, knee-flexion/extension, ankle-dorsiflexion, foot-inversion, toes-extension
b. Hip-flexion, abduction, external rotation, knee-flexion/extension, ankle-dorsiflexion, foot-eversion, toes-extension
c. Hip-flexion, adduction, internal rotation, knee-flexion/extension, ankle-dorsiflexion, foot-eversion, toes-extension
d. Hip-flexion, abduction, internal rotation, knee-flexion/extension, ankle-dorsiflexion, foot-eversion, toes-extension

**198. Which of the following is true regarding PNF chopping pattern?**

a. It produces movements in all the 3-planes
b. It improves activities like running, throwing, changing directions
c. It combines D1 and D2 patterns of upper limb
d. All of the above

**199. The cross over stepping pattern of PNF is called as:**

a. Chopping pattern
b. Braiding pattern
c. Diagonal pattern
d. None of the above

**200. The nerve impulses stimulate breathing in every:**
a. 1–2 seconds
b. 2–3 seconds
c. 3–4 seconds
d. 3–5 seconds

**201. Normal breathing rate is:**
a. 10–12 breaths/minute
b. 12–16 breaths/minute
c. 20–24 breaths/minute
d. None of the above

**202. The muscles of inspiration are:**
a. The diaphragm, and abdominals
b. The diaphragm and external intercostal muscles
c. The diaphragm, external intercostal and intercartilaginous portion of internal intercostal
d. None of the above

**203. The muscles of forceful expiration are:**
a. Diaphragm and external intercostal muscles
b. Abdominals and external intercostal muscles
c. Abdominals and interosseous portion of internal intercostal muscles
d. None of the above

**204. Normal vital capacity in a healthy adult is:**
a. 3,000 mL  b. 4,000 mL
c. 4,500 mL  d. 5,000 mL

**205. Vital capacity can be calculated from:**
a. Combination of IRV, TV, ERV
b. TLC-RV
c. Both a and b
d. None of the above

**206. Which one of the followings is the primary muscles of inspiration?**
a. External intercostal
b. Internal intercostal
c. Diaphragm
d. None of the above

**207. Which one of the followings is true regarding, incentive spirometry?**
a. This is a form of low-level resistance training for muscles of ventilation
b. This provides visual feedback
c. This can be used as home exercise program
d. All of the above

**208. Active cycle of breathing technique is a combination of:**
a. Breath control exercise and thoracic expansion exercise
b. Breath control exercise and forced expiratory techniques
c. Breath control exercise, thoracic expansion exercise and forced expiratory techniques
d. None of the above

**209. Which of the followings are true regarding benefits of breathing exercise:**
a. The body is designed to release 70% of its toxins through breathing
b. It can be used to treat obstructive and restrictive pulmonary conditions
c. It relieves pain
d. All of the above

**210. Which of the followings are the principles of hydrotherapy used for treatment?**
a. Buoyancy
b. Hydrostatic pressure
c. Viscosity and surface tension
d. All of the above

**211. During hydrotherapy, stability of body is maintained by:**
a. Buoyancy
b. Viscosity
c. Hydrostatic pressure
d. None of the above

**212. Which of the followings are true regarding buoyancy?**
a. It resists movements, when the body segments move from bottom towards top in water

b. It assists movements, when the body segments move from bottom towards top in water
c. It resists movements, when the body segments move from top towards bottom in water
d. Both b and c

**213. The temperature of water in hydro-therapy pool, should be:**

a. 10–15° C
b. 20–25° C
c. 28–30° C
d. 35–40° C

**214. Double support constitutes:**

a. 10% of gait cycle
b. 20% of gait cycle
c. 30% of gait cycle
d. 40% of gait cycle

**215. Which of the followings are true regarding cadence?**

a. It is value is more in males and less in females
b. It is value is more in females and less in males
c. It is equal in males and females
d. None of the above

**216. Normal value of cadence is:**

a. 50–60 steps/min
b. 70–80 steps/min
c. 80–130 steps/min
d. None of the above

**217. The normal value of toe out is:**

a. 3–5°
b. 5–7°
c. 9–10°
d. None of the above

**218. Which of the followings is true regarding stride length?**

a. Stride length is more in females and less in males
b. Stride length is more in males and less in females
c. Stride length is equal in females and males
d. None of the above

**219. Normal step length in adult female is about:**

a. 75 cm
b. 85 cm
c. 65 cm
d. None of the above

**220. Normal stride length in adult male is about:**

a. 1.28 meter
b. 1.38 meter
c. 1.46 meter
d. None of the above

**221. Normal stride width in adult is:**

a. 2–4 cm
b. 5–6 cm
c. 5–10 cm
d. None of the above

**222. During normal walking, the drop of pelvis on swing side is about:**

a. 2°
b. 3°
c. 4°
d. 5°

**223. During normal walking, the maximum horizontal displacement of COG is about:**

a. 2 cm
b. 3 cm
c. 4 cm
d. 5 cm

**224. During normal walking, total rotation of pelvis in transverse plane is about:**

a. 5°
b. 6°
c. 7°
d. 8°

**225. Which of the followings are true regarding determinants of gait?**

a. It minimizes the vertical and lateral displacement of body's COG
b. It reduces energy expenditure
c. It makes the gait more efficient
d. All of the above

**226. During heel strike, the knee joint remains in:**

a. 0° flexion
b. 2° flexion
c. 4° flexion
d. 5° flexion

**227. During foot flat, the knee remains in:**

a. 5–10° flexion
b. 10–15° flexion
c. 15–20° flexion
d. None of the above

**228. The amount of knee flexion during early swing is:**

a. 30°
b. 40°
c. 50°
d. 60°

**229. Trendelenburg gait occurs due to weakness of:**

a. Quadriceps femoris
b. Gluteus maximus
c. Gluteus medius
d. None of the above

**230. Hand to knee gait is caused due to weakness of:**

a. Hamstrings muscle
b. Tibialis anterior muscle
c. Quadriceps femoris muscle
d. None of the above

**231. In jump knee gait, the individual walks with:**

a. Hip, knees flexion and ankle dorsiflexion
b. Hip, knee flexion and ankle plantar flexion
c. Hips flexion and adduction
d. None of the above

**232. A steppage gait results, due to:**

a. Weakness of hip extensors
b. Weakness of quadriceps
c. Weakness of tibialis anterior
d. None of the above

**233. Energy cost analysis during gait is done by:**

a. Estimating physiological cost of energy expenditure
b. Mechanical energy analysis
c. Heart rate data analysis
d. All of the above

**234. Which of the following massage is performed to reduce edema?**

a. Light stroking
b. Effleurage
c. Kneading
d. Friction

**235. To loosen secretions in the lungs, the massage performed is:**

a. Effleurage
b. Shaking and vibration
c. Clapping
d. Both b and c above

**236. The maximum weight used in skin traction is about:**

a. 2–3 kg
b. 3–4 kg
c. 4.5–5 kg
d. 10 kg

**237. The weight used in skeletal traction is about:**

a. 6–7 kg
b. 10–12 kg
c. 12–15 kg
d. None of the above

**238. The traction used in physiotherapy includes:**

a. Continuous traction
b. Static traction
c. Intermittent traction
d. Both b and c

**239. Which of the followings are true regarding static traction?**

a. It stretches the paraspinal muscles and reduces muscle spasm
b. It stretches the adherent ligaments and tight capsule of facet joints
c. It frees the adherent nerve roots
d. All of the above

**240. Which of the followings are true regarding intermittent traction?**

a. It mobilizes the stiff intervertebral joints

b. It releases the nerve roots off pressure in intervertebral foramina
c. It reduces pain via pre-synaptic inhibition in spinal cord
d. All of the above

**241. In acute PIVD, traction in sustained mode should not exceed:**

a. 15–20 minutes
b. 20–30 minutes
c. 10–11 minutes
d. None of the above

**242. The mechanism of reduction of disc bulge during static traction is:**

a. Fluid imbibition in disc
b. Creation of negative pressure in intervertebral space
c. Suctioning of disc material from outside to intervertebral space
d. All of the above

**243. Which of the followings hold true regarding fluid imbibition in discs?**

a. The discs absorb the necessary fluid to produce proteoglycans, necessary for supply of nutrients to disc, and promote recovery
b. Excessive fluid absorption by the disc increases the disc bulge
c. Both a and b
d. None of the above

**244. While applying mechanical traction at home, countertraction is produced by:**

a. Applying chest strap
b. Elevating the head end of bed
c. Elevating the foot end of bed
d. None of the above

**245. Which of the following holds true regarding supine position:**

a. It is the position of extension
b. It is position of flexion
c. This position is selected with necessary modifications, for patients who have pain in standing/extension
d. Both b and c

**246. For lumbar traction in supine, the hips and knees should be flexed:**

a. >30°  b. >40°
c. >60°  d. >70°

**247. For optimal results with cervical traction, the neck should be:**

a. Extended
b. Flexed to about 10–15°
c. Flexed to about 20–30°
d. None of the above

**248. Which of the followings are true regarding load applied for lumbar traction?**

a. A load >26% of body weight should be applied to overcome friction and cause vertebral separation, when split traction table is unavailable
b. Minimum load should be about 1/3rd of body weight
c. Maximum load should be about ½ of body weight
d. All of the above

**249. Which of the followings are true regarding load applied during cervical traction**

a. Generally, a load of 7–11 kg is applied, which is person specific
b. The minimum load should be 1/8th of body weight
c. The maximum load should be 1/6th of body weight
d. All of the above

**250. Which of the followings are true regarding cervical and lumbar traction?**

a. To apply traction to upper cervical spine, the neck should be slightly flexed/held in neutral
b. To apply traction to the upper lumbar spine, the Fowler's position is selected
c. To apply traction to the lower lumbar spine, hip flexion angles should be less than 70°
d. All of the above

## ANSWER KEY

| 1. a | 2. a | 3. c | 4. c | 5. c | 6. b | 7. b | 8. c | 9. a | 10. c |
|---|---|---|---|---|---|---|---|---|---|
| 11. b | 12. b | 13. b | 14. c | 15. b | 16. d | 17. b | 18. c | 19. b | 20. c |
| 21. c | 22. b | 23. b | 24. a | 25. b | 26. d | 27. d | 28. b | 29. a | 30. c |
| 31. d | 32. d | 33. a | 34. c | 35. d | 36. d | 37. b | 38. b | 39. c | 40. b |
| 41. b | 42. c | 43. c | 44. c | 45. a | 46. c | 47. c | 48. c | 49. d | 50. c |
| 51. b | 52. b | 53. c | 54. c | 55. c | 56. b | 57. b | 58. a | 59. b | 60. c |
| 61. b | 62. a | 63. c | 64. c | 65. a | 66. c | 67. c | 68. c | 69. c | 70. c |
| 71. d | 72. b | 73. c | 74. d | 75. a | 76. b | 77. c | 78. a | 79. c | 80. c |
| 81. c | 82. d | 83. b | 84. b | 85. c | 86. b | 87. c | 88. c | 89. c | 90. a |
| 91. c | 92. c | 93. b | 94. b | 95. a | 96. b | 97. c | 98. b | 99. a | 100. a |
| 101. c | 102. c | 103. a | 104. b | 105. d | 106. a | 107. b | 108. d | 109. b | 110. a |
| 111. c | 112. c | 113. c | 114. c | 115. d | 116. b | 117. d | 118. c | 119. b | 120. b |
| 121. b | 122. b | 123. b | 124. c | 125. d | 126. d | 127. a | 128. c | 129. d | 130. a |
| 131. b | 132. a | 133. a | 134. b | 135. d | 136. b | 137. b | 138. d | 139. b | 140. d |
| 141. d | 142. d | 143. b | 144. b | 145. a | 146. d | 147. d | 148. d | 149. d | 150. a |
| 151. d | 152. c | 153. c | 154. d | 155. c | 156. a | 157. b | 158. d | 159. b | 160. b |
| 161. c | 162. c | 163. d | 164. c | 165. d | 166. d | 167. d | 168. c | 169. b | 170. c |
| 171. b | 172. b | 173. b | 174. c | 175. a | 176. b | 177. a | 178. c | 179. d | 180. c |
| 181. c | 182. b | 183. d | 184. d | 185. b | 186. c | 187. d | 188. b | 189. b | 190. b |
| 191. b | 192. c | 193. b | 194. b | 195. c | 196. b | 197. a | 198. d | 199. b | 200. d |
| 201. b | 202. c | 203. c | 204. c | 205. c | 206. c | 207. d | 208. c | 209. d | 210. d |
| 211. c | 212. d | 213. c | 214. b | 215. b | 216. c | 217. b | 218. b | 219. c | 220. c |
| 221. c | 222. d | 223. d | 224. d | 225. d | 226. d | 227. b | 228. d | 229. c | 230. c |
| 231. b | 232. c | 233. d | 234. b | 235. d | 236. c | 237. a | 238. d | 239. d | 240. d |
| 241. c | 242. d | 243. c | 244. c | 245. d | 246. d | 247. c | 248. d | 249. d | 250. d |

# Index

Page numbers followed by *f* refer to figure and *t* refer to table.

## A



## B

## C

## D



## E

## F



## G

## H

## N

## O



## P

## Q



## R

## S

## T

## U

## V

## W